# Handbook of
# Colon and Rectal Surgery

**Marvin L. Corman, M.D.**
Vice-Chairman, Department of Surgery
North Shore–Long Island Jewish Hospital;
Associate Surgeon-in-Chief
Long Island Jewish Medical Center
Long Island, New York

**Stephen I. Allison, M.B.B.S., F.R.A.C.S.**
Senior Lecturer
Department of Surgery
University of Queensland;
Department of Surgery
Mater Misericordiae Hospital
Brisbane, Queensland
Australia

**Jonathan P. Kuehne, M.D.**
Voluntary Faculty
University of Southern California
Los Angeles County Medical Center
Los Angeles, California

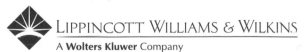
LIPPINCOTT WILLIAMS & WILKINS
A **Wolters Kluwer** Company
Philadelphia · Baltimore · New York · London
Buenos Aires · Hong Kong · Sydney · Tokyo

*Acquisitions Editor:* Lisa McAllister
*Developmental Editor:* Gina Gerace
*Production Editor:* Emmeline Parker
*Manufacturing Manager:* Benjamin Rivera
*Cover Designer:* Mark Lerner
*Compositor:* Lippincott Williams & Wilkins Desktop Division
*Printer:* Edwards Brothers

©2002 by **LIPPINCOTT WILLIAMS & WILKINS**
**530 Walnut Street**
**Philadelphia, PA 19106 USA**
**LWW.com**

Printed in the USA

**Library of Congress Cataloging-in-Publication Data**

Corman, Marvin L., 1939-
  Handbook of colon and rectal surgery / Marvin L. Corman, Stephen I. Allison, Jonathan P. Kuehne.
    p. ; cm.
  Includes index.
  ISBN 0-7817-2586-0
    1. Colon (Anatomy)—Surgery—Handbooks, manuals, etc. 2. Rectum—Surgery—Handbooks, manuals, etc. I. Allison,Stephen I. II. Kuehne, Jonathan P. III. Title.
    [DNLM: 1. Colon—surgery. 2. Recum—surgery. WI 520 C811h 2002]
  RD544.C673 2002
  617.5'547059—dc21

                                                    2001029919

10 9 8 7 6 5 4 3 2 1

# Contents

# Handbook of
# Colon and Rectal Surgery

# Contributing Authors

**Marvin L. Corman,** M.D., *Vice-Chairman, Department of Surgery, North Shore–Long Island Jewish Hospital; Associate Surgeon-in-Chief, Long Island Jewish Medical Center, Long Island, New York*

**Eric J. Daniels,** M.D., *UCLA School of Medicine, Los Angeles, California*

**Robert Gilliland,** M.D., *Research Fellow, Department of Colorectal Surgery, Cleveland Clinic Florida, Fort Lauderdale, Florida*

**Anthony A. Goodman,** M.D., *Professor of Medicine, Adjunct Professor of Medicine, Montana State University, Billings, Montana*

**Lester Gottesman,** M.D., *Assistant Professor, Columbia University College of Physicians and Surgeons, Division of Colon and Rectal Surgery, St. Luke's / Roosevelt Hospital Center, New York, New York*

**José Marcio N. Jorge,** M.D., *Instituto do Aparelho Digestivo, São Paulo, Brazil*

**Anthony M. Nyerges,** M.D., *Associate Clinical Professor, Co-Director, UCLA Pain Service, Department of Anesthesiology, UCLA School of Medicine, Los Angeles, California*

**Alberto Peña,** M.D., *Professor of Surgery, Albert Einstein College of Medicine, The Bronx; Chief, Pediatric Surgery, Long Island Jewish Medical Center, New Hyde Park, New York*

**John L. Petrini,** M.D., *Clinical Associate Professor of Medicine, University of Southern California, Los Angeles; Chief, Department of Gastroenterology, Sansum Medical Clinic, Santa Barbara, California*

**Daniel Rosenthal,** M.D, *Clinical Professor of Surgery, University of Texas Health Sciences Center, San Antonio, Texas*

**Ronald M. Stewart,** M.D., *Director of Trauma and Emergency Surgery, Assistant Professor of Surgery, University of Texas Health Sciences Center, Houston, Texas*

**Steven D. Wexner,** M.D., *Chairman, Department of Colorectal Surgery, Cleveland Clinic Florida, Fort Lauderdale, Florida*

# Note

This book is a synopsis of material published in *Colon and Rectal Surgery,* Fourth Edition, edited by Marvin L. Corman (Lippincott-Raven Publishers, 1998). Readers who seek more complete information regarding the topics covered in the present book, including references, should consult *Colon and Rectal Surgery, Fourth Edition.*

# Handbook of
# Colon and Rectal Surgery

# 1

# Anatomy and Embryology of the Anus, Rectum, and Colon

## EMBRYOLOGY

The primitive gut tube develops from the endodermal roof of the yolk sac. By the third week of development, it can be divided into three regions: the foregut in the head fold; the hindgut with its ventral allantoic outgrowth in the smaller tail fold; and, between these two portions, the midgut, which at this stage opens ventrally into the yolk sac. After the stages of (a) physiologic herniation, (b) return to the abdomen, and (c) fixation, the midgut progresses below the major pancreatic papilla to form the small intestine, the ascending colon, and the proximal two thirds of the transverse colon. The midgut (superior mesenteric) artery, with corresponding venous and lymphatic drainage, supplies this segment. The sympathetic innervation of the midgut and likewise the hindgut originates from T8 to L2, via splanchnic nerves and the autonomic abdominopelvic plexuses. The parasympathetic outflow to the midgut is derived from the 10th cranial nerve (vagus) with preganglionic cell bodies in the brainstem.

The distal colon (distal third of the transverse colon), the rectum, and the anal canal above the dentate line are all derived from the hindgut. Therefore, the hindgut (inferior mesenteric) artery, with corresponding venous and lymphatic drainage, supplies this segment. Its parasympathetic outflow comes from S2, S3, and S4 via splanchnic nerves.

The dentate line marks the fusion between endodermal and ectodermal tubes, where the terminal portion of the hindgut or cloaca fuses with the proctodeum, an ingrowth from the anal pit. Before the fifth week of development, the intestinal and urogenital tracts terminate in conjunction with the cloaca. At the sixth week, the urorectal septum migrates caudally and the two tracts are separated. The cloacal part of the anal canal, which has both endodermal and ectodermal elements, forms the anal transitional zone after breakdown of the anal membrane. During the 10th week, the anal tubercles, a pair of ectodermal swellings around the proctodeal pit, fuse dorsally to form a horseshoe-shaped structure and anteriorly to create the perineal body. The cloacal sphincter is separated by the

*1*

perineal body into urogenital and anal portions (external anal sphincter). The internal anal sphincter is formed later (6th to 12th week) from enlarging fibers of the circular layer of the rectum. The sphincters apparently migrate during their development; the external sphincter grows cephalad and the internal sphincter moves caudally. Concomitantly, the longitudinal muscle descends into the intersphincteric plane.

## ANATOMY OF THE COLON

In general, the colon surrounds the loops of small intestine as an arch. Its length is variable in the adult, averaging approximately 150 cm, about one quarter the length of the small intestine. Its diameter, which can be substantially augmented by distension, gradually decreases from 7.5 cm at the cecum to 2.5 cm at the sigmoid.

Three taeniae coli, anterior (taenia libera), posteromedial (taenia mesocolica), and posterolateral (taenia omentalis), represent bands of the outer longitudinal coat of muscle that traverse the colon from the base of the appendix to the rectosigmoid junction, where they merge. The muscular longitudinal layer is actually a complete coat around the colon, although it is considerably thicker at the taeniae. The haustra or haustral sacculations are outpouchings of bowel wall between the taeniae; they are caused by the relative shortness of the taeniae.

### Cecum

The cecum is the segment of the large bowel that projects downward as a blind pouch below the entrance of the ileum. It is a sacculated organ 6 to 8 cm in both length and breadth, usually situated in the right iliac fossa. The cecum is almost entirely invested with peritoneum. Its mobility is variable; however, in 10% to 22% of individuals it is abnormally mobile.

The ileum terminates in the posteromedial aspect of the cecum; the superior and inferior ileocecal ligaments maintain the angulation between these two structures. These ligaments, along with the mesentery of the appendix, form three pericecal recesses or fossae: superior ileocecal, inferior ileocecal, and retrocecal. The ileocecal sphincter, a circular sphincter, originates from a slight thickening of the muscular layer of the terminal ileum.

### Appendix

The vermiform appendix is an elongated diverticulum that arises from the posteromedial aspect of the cecum about 3 cm below the ileocecal junction. Its length varies from 2 to 20 cm (mean, 8 to 10 cm), and it is approximately 5 mm in diameter. The confluence of the three taeniae is a useful guide in locating the base of the appendix. Because of its great mobility, the appendix can occupy a variety of positions, possibly at different times in the same individual: retrocecal (65%), pelvic (31%), subcecal (2.3%), preileal (1.0%), and retroileal (0.4%). The mesoappendix, a triangular fold attached to the posterior leaf of the mesentery of the terminal ileum, usually contains the appendicular vessels close to its free edge.

## Ascending Colon

The ascending colon, extending from the level of the ileocecal junction to the right colic or hepatic flexure, is approximately 15 cm long. It ascends laterally to the psoas muscle and anteriorly to the iliacus, the quadratus lumborum, and the lower pole of the right kidney. The ascending colon is covered with peritoneum anteriorly and on both sides. As with the descending colon on its posterior surface, the ascending colon is devoid of peritoneum, which, instead, is replaced by an areolar tissue (fascia of Toldt) resulting from an embryologic process of fusion or coalescence of the mesentery to the posterior parietal peritoneum. In the lateral peritoneal reflection, this process is represented by the white line of Toldt, which is more evident at the descending–sigmoid junction. This line serves as a guide for the surgeon when the ascending, descending, or sigmoid colon is mobilized.

At the visceral surface of the right lobe of the liver and lateral to the gallbladder, the ascending colon turns sharply medially and slightly caudad and ventrally to form the right colic (hepatic) flexure. This flexure, which is supported by the nephrocolic ligament, lies immediately ventral to the lower part of the right kidney and over the descending duodenum.

### *Relationship to Ureters*

On both sides, the ureters rest on the psoas muscle in their inferomedial course; they are crossed obliquely by the spermatic vessels anteriorly and the genitofemoral nerve posteriorly. The right ureter lies laterally to the inferior vena cava and is crossed anteriorly by the right colic and ileocolic arteries, the root of the mesentery, and the terminal ileum. In its pelvic portion, the ureter crosses the pelvic brim in front of or a little lateral to the bifurcation of the common iliac artery, and descends abruptly between the peritoneum and the internal iliac artery. Before entering the bladder in the male, the vas deferens crosses lateromedially on its superior aspect. In the female, as the ureter traverses the posterior layer of the broad ligament and the parametrium close to the side of the uterus neck and upper part of the vagina, it is enveloped by the vesical and vaginal venous plexuses and is crossed above and lateromedially by the uterine artery.

## Transverse Colon

The transverse colon is the longest (45 cm) segment of the large bowel. It crosses the abdomen, and is relatively fixed at each flexure. In between, it is completely invested with peritoneum and suspended by a transverse mesocolon having an average width of 10 to 15 cm and providing variable mobility; the nadir of the transverse colon can reach the hypogastrium. The greater omentum is fused on the anterosuperior aspect of the transverse colon. The left colic (splenic) flexure is situated beneath the lower angle of the spleen and firmly attached to the diaphragm by the phrenocolic ligament.

## Descending Colon

A segment of the large intestine, the descending colon courses downward from the splenic flexure to the brim of the true pelvis, a distance of approximately 25 cm. As with the ascending colon, the descending colon is covered by peritoneum only on its anterior and lateral aspects. Posteriorly, it rests directly against the left kidney and the quadratus lumborum and transversus abdominis muscles. However, the descending colon is narrower and more dorsally situated than the ascending colon.

## Sigmoid Colon

The sigmoid colon, extending from the lower end of the descending colon at the pelvic brim to the proximal limit of the rectum, varies dramatically in length (15 to 50 cm; mean, 38 cm) and configuration. More commonly, the sigmoid colon is a mobile, omega-shaped loop completely invested by peritoneum. The mesosigmoid is attached to the pelvic walls in an inverted $V$ shape, resting in a recess known as the intersigmoid fossa. The left ureter, lying immediately underneath this fossa, is crossed on its anterior surface by the spermatic, left colic, and sigmoid vessels.

### *Rectosigmoid Junction*

Macroscopically, the rectosigmoid junction has been identified as the point where the taenia libera and the taenia omentalis fuse to form a single anterior taenia and where both haustra and mesocolon terminate.

## Rectum

The rectum is *felt* to be 12 to 15 cm in length, but both the proximal and distal limits are debatable. For example, the rectosigmoid junction is considered to be at the level of the third sacral vertebra by anatomists but at the sacral promontory by surgeons. Likewise, surgeons considered the distal limit to be the muscular anorectal ring and anatomists consider it the dentate line. The rectum occupies the sacral concavity and ends 2 to 3 cm anteroinferiorly from the tip of the coccyx.

The rectum has three lateral curves: the upper and lower are convex to the right and the middle is convex to the left. These curves correspond intraluminally to the folds or valves of Houston. The rectal valves do not contain all the muscle wall layers and do not have a specific function.

The rectum is characterized by the absence of taeniae, epiploic appendices, haustra, or a well-defined mesentery. An exception, however, is that a peritonealized mesorectum may be noted in patients with procidentia. The upper third of the rectum is anteriorly and laterally invested by peritoneum; the middle third is covered by peritoneum on its anterior aspect only. Finally, the lower third of the rectum is entirely extraperitoneal.

### Fascial Relationship of the Rectum

The walls and floor of the pelvis are lined by the parietal *endopelvic fascia*, which continues on the internal organs as a visceral pelvic fascia. Therefore, the fascia propria of the rectum is an extension of the pelvic fascia, enclosing the rectum, fat, nerves, and blood and lymphatic vessels. Distal condensations of this fascia form the lateral ligaments or lateral stalks of the rectum.

The *presacral fascia* is a thickened part of the parietal endopelvic fascia that covers the concavity of the sacrum and coccyx, nerves, middle sacral artery, and presacral veins.

The *rectosacral fascia* is an anteroinferiorly directed thick fascial reflection from the presacral fascia at the S4 level to the fascia propria of the rectum just above the anorectal ring. Anteriorly, the extraperitoneal rectum is separated from the prostate and seminal vesicles or vagina by a tough fascial investment, the visceral pelvic fascia of Denonvilliers. Both the rectosacral and the visceral pelvic fascia are important anatomic landmarks during rectal mobilization.

### Anal Canal

Two definitions found in the literature describe the anal canal. The "surgical" or "functional" anal canal extends for approximately 4 cm from the anal verge to the anorectal ring. The "anatomic" or "embryologic" anal canal is shorter (2 cm), extending from the anal verge to the dentate line, the level that corresponds to the proctodeal membrane.

The anus or anal orifice is an anteroposterior cutaneous slit that, along with the anal canal, remains virtually closed at rest. This is a result of tonic circumferential contraction of both the sphincters and the anal cushions. Posteriorly, the anal canal is related to the coccyx and anteriorly to the urethra in the male, and to the perineal body and the lowest part of the posterior vaginal wall in the female. Laterally, the ischiorectal fossa is situated on either side. The fossa contains fat and the inferior rectal vessels and nerves, which cross it to enter the wall of the anal canal.

## Epithelium

The lining of the anal canal consists of an upper mucosal and a lower cutaneous segment. The dentate (pectinate) line describes the "saw-toothed" junction of the ectoderm and the endoderm. It, therefore, represents an important landmark between two distinct origins of venous and lymphatic drainage: nerve supply and epithelial lining. Above the dentate line, the intestine is innervated by the sympathetic and parasympathetic systems, with venous, arterial, and lymphatic drainage to and from the hypogastric vessels. Distal to the dentate line, the anal canal is innervated by the somatic nervous system, with blood supply and drainage from the inferior hemorrhoidal system.

The pectinate or dentate line corresponds to a line of anal valves that represent remnants of the proctodeal membrane. Above each valve is found a little pocket known as an anal sinus or crypt. A variable number of glands are observed (4 to 12). Obstruction of these ducts, presumably by accumulation of foreign material in the crypts, can lead to abscesses and fistulas.

Cephalad to the dentate line, 8 to 14 longitudinal folds, known as the rectal columns (columns of Morgagni), have their bases connected in pairs to each valve at the dentate line. At the lower end of the columns are the anal papillae. This 0.5- to 1-cm strip of mucosa above the dentate line, known as the anal transition or cloacogenic zone, is the source of certain anal tumors (see Chapter 24). Cephalad to this area, the epithelium changes to a single layer of columnar cells and macroscopically acquires the characteristic pink color of the rectal mucosa.

The cutaneous part of the anal canal consists of modified squamous epithelium that is thin, smooth, pale, stretched, and devoid of hair and glands. The anal verge, which marks the lowermost edge of the anal canal, is sometimes the level of reference used for measurements taken during colonoscopy or surgery. Distal to the anal verge, the epithelium then acquires hair follicles; glands, including apocrine glands; and other features of normal skin.

## Internal Anal Sphincter

The internal anal sphincter (IAS) represents the distal (2.5 to 4 cm) condensation of the circular muscle layer of the rectum. As a smooth muscle in a state of continuous maximal contraction, the IAS is a natural barrier to the involuntary loss of stool and gas. The IAS is responsible for 50% to 85% of the resting tone, the external anal sphincter (EAS) accounting for 25% to 30%; the remaining 15% is attributed to expansion of the anal cushions.

### *Conjoined Longitudinal Muscle*

Whereas the inner circular layer of the rectum gives rise to the IAS, the outer longitudinal layer, at the level of the anorectal ring, mixes with fibers of the levator ani muscle to form the conjoined longitudinal muscle. This muscle descends between the IAS and the EAS, and ultimately some of its fibers (referred to as the corrugator cutis ani muscle) traverse the lowermost part of the EAS to insert into the perianal skin. Its role is rudimentary in humans.

### External Anal Sphincter

The EAS is the elliptic cylinder of striated muscle that envelops the entire length of the inner tube of smooth muscle, but it ends slightly more distal to the terminus of the IAS. The EAS encompasses three divisions: subcutaneous, superficial, and deep. The deepest part of the EAS is intimately related to the puborectalis muscle, which is actually considered a component of both the levator ani and the EAS muscle complexes. Others consider the EAS as being composed of a deep compartment (deep sphincter and puborectalis) and a superficial compartment (subcutaneous and superficial sphincter). Based on embryologic study, the EAS seems to be subdivided into two parts—superficial and deep—neither having any connection with the puborectalis.

### Levator Ani

The levator ani muscle, or pelvic diaphragm, is the major component of the pelvic floor. It consists of a pair of broad, symmetric sheets composed of three striated muscles: iliococcygeus, pubococcygeus, and puborectalis. A variable fourth component, the ischiococcygeus or coccygeus, is rudimentary in humans and is represented by only a few muscle fibers on the surface of the sacrospinous ligament. Ileococcygeus fibers arise from the ischial spine and posterior part of the obturator fascia and course inferiorly and medially to insert into the lateral aspects of S3 and S4, the coccyx, and the anococcygeal raphe. The pubococcygeus arises from the posterior aspect of the pubis and the anterior part of the obturator fascia. It runs dorsally alongside the anorectal junction to decussate with fibers of the opposite side at the anococcygeal raphe and insert into the anterior surface of the fourth sacral and first coccygeal segments.

The pelvic floor is "defective" in the midline. This defect, called the "levator hiatus," consists of an elliptic space situated between the two pubococcygeus muscles. The hiatal ligament, originating from the pelvic fascia, keeps the intrahiatal viscera together and prevents their constriction during contraction of the levator ani. A dilator function has been attributed to the anococcygeal raphe because of its crisscross arrangement.

The puborectalis, the most medial portion of the levator ani muscle, is situated immediately cephalad to the deep component of the EAS. It is a strong, *U*-shaped loop of striated muscle that slings the anorectal junction to the posterior aspect of the pubis. Between the two pubococcygeus muscles is a defect through which the lower rectum, urethra, and either the dorsal vein of the penis in men, or the vagina in women pass. The puborectalis, currently considered a part of both muscular groups—the EAS and the levator ani—has the same innervation.

The puborectalis contributes to the anorectal ring and the anorectal angle. The anorectal ring is a strong muscular ring that represents the upper end of the sphincter and the upper border of the IAS, around the anorectal junction. The anorectal angle is thought to be the result of the anatomic configuration of the U-shaped sling of puborectalis muscle around the anorectal junction. Whereas the anal sphincters are responsible for closure of the anal canal to retain gas and liquid stool, the puborectalis muscle and the anorectal angle are designed to maintain gross fecal continence by a continuous sphincteric, occlusion-like activity that is attributed to the puborectalis.

### Pera-anal and Pararectal Spaces

Potential spaces of clinical significance in the anorectal region include the following: ischiorectal, perianal, intersphincteric, submucous, superficial postanal, deep postanal, supralevator, and retrorectal spaces. A thin horizontal fascia subdivides the ischiorectal fossa into two spaces: the perianal and ischiorectal. The ischiorectal space comprises the upper two thirds of the ischiorectal fossa. It is pyramid-shaped, situated on both sides between the anal canal and the lower part of the rectum medially, and the side wall of the pelvis laterally. The apex is at the origin of the levator ani muscle from the obturator fascia; the base is the perianal space. Anteriorly, the fossa is bounded by the urogenital diaphragm and transversus perinei muscle. Posterior to the ischiorectal fossa is the sacrotuberous ligament and the inferior border of the gluteus maximus. On the superolateral wall, the pudendal nerve and the internal pudendal vessels run in the pudendal canal (Alcock's canal). The ischiorectal fossa contains fat and the inferior rectal vessels and nerves.

The perianal space surrounds the lower part of the anal canal. Continuous with the subcutaneous fat of the buttocks laterally, it extends into the intersphincteric space medially. The external hemorrhoidal plexus lies in the perianal space and communicates with the internal hemorrhoidal plexus at the dentate line. This space is the typical site of anal hematomas, perianal abscesses, and anal fistula tracts. The perianal space also encloses the subcutaneous part of the EAS, the lowest part of the IAS, and fibers of the longitudinal muscle.

The intersphincteric space is a potential space between the IAS and the EAS. The submucous space, situated between the IAS and the mucocutaneous lining of the anal canal, contains the internal hemorrhoidal plexus and the muscularis submucosa ani. Above, it is continuous with the submucous layer of the rectum, and, inferiorly, it ends at the level of the dentate line.

The superficial postanal space is interposed between the anococcygeal ligament and the skin. The deep postanal space is situated between the anococcygeal ligament and the anococcygeal raphe. Both postanal spaces communicate posteriorly with the ischiorectal fossa and are the sites of horseshoe abscesses.

The supralevator spaces are situated between the peritoneum superiorly and the levator ani inferiorly. Medially, these bilateral spaces are limited by the rectum, and laterally by the obturator fascia. The retrorectal space is located between the fascia propria of the rectum anteriorly and the presacral fascia posteriorly. Laterally are the lateral rectal ligaments; inferiorly is the rectosacral ligament; above, the space is continuous with the retroperitoneum.

## Arterial Supply

The superior and inferior mesenteric arteries nourish the entire large intestine. The limit between the two territories is the splenic flexure. Collateral circulation between these two arteries is formed by a "continuous" communicating arcade along the mesenteric border of the colon, the marginal artery, from which the vasa recta supply the bowel. In addition, the internal iliac arteries supply the anorectum.

## Superior Mesenteric Artery

The superior mesenteric artery (SMA), which originates from the aorta behind the superior border of the pancreas at L1, supplies the cecum, appendix, ascending colon, and the transverse colon. Additionally, the SMA supplies the entire small bowel, pancreas, and occasionally, the liver. After passing behind the neck of the pancreas and anteromedial to the uncinate process, the SMA crosses the third part of the duodenum and continues downward and to the right along the base of the mesentery. From its left side arises a series of 12 to 20 jejunal and ileal branches. From its right side arise the colic branches: middle, right, and ileocolic arteries. The ileocolic artery bifurcates into a superior or ascending branch, which communicates with the descending branch of the right colic artery, and an inferior or descending branch, which gives off the anterior cecal, posterior cecal, and appendicular divisions. Finally, it continues into the small-bowel mesentery as the ileal branch.

The right colic artery may also arise from the ileocolic or middle colic arteries and is absent in up to 20% of patients.

The middle colic artery is the highest of the three colic branches of the superior mesenteric artery, arising close to the inferior border of the pancreas. Its right branch supplies the right transverse colon and hepatic flexure, anastomosing with the ascending branch of the right colic artery. Its left branch supplies the distal half of the transverse colon. Anatomic variations of this artery include its absence in 4% to 20% of cases and the presence of an accessory middle colic artery in 10%.

## Inferior Mesenteric Artery

The inferior mesenteric artery (IMA) originates from the anterior surface of the aorta, 3 to 4 cm above its bifurcation at the level of L2-3, and runs downward and to the left to enter the pelvis. Within the abdomen, the IMA branches into the left colic artery and two to six sigmoidal arteries. After crossing the left common iliac artery, it acquires the name "superior hemorrhoidal artery" or "superior rectal artery."

The left colic artery, the highest branch of the IMA, bifurcates into an ascending branch, which runs upward to the splenic flexure to contribute to the arcade of Riolan, and a descending branch, which supplies most of the descending colon. The sigmoidal arteries form arcades within the sigmoid mesocolon, resembling the small-bowel vasculature, and anastomose with branches of the left colic artery proximally, and with the superior hemorrhoidal artery distally. The marginal artery terminates within the arcade of sigmoidal arteries. The superior hemorrhoidal artery descends in the sigmoid mesocolon to the level of S3 and then to the posterior aspect of the rectum. In 80% of cases, it bifurcates into right (usually wider) and left terminal branches; multiple branches are present in 17% of cases. These divisions, once within the submucosa of the rectum, run straight downward to supply the lower rectum and the anal canal. The branches that reach the level of the rectal columns condensate in capillary plexuses, mostly at the right posterior, right anterior, and left lateral positions, corresponding to the location of the major internal hemorrhoidal groups.

The major blood supply to the anorectum is through the superior and inferior hemorrhoidal arteries. The contribution of the middle hemorrhoidal artery varies with the size of the superior hemorrhoidal artery. The middle hemorrhoidal artery originates more commonly from the anterior division of the internal iliac or the pudendal arteries, and reaches the rectum and the lower third of the rectum anterolaterally, close to the level of the pelvic floor and deep to the levator fascia.

The paired inferior hemorrhoidal arteries are branches of the internal pudendal artery which, in turn, is a branch of the internal iliac artery. The inferior hemorrhoidal artery arises within the pudendal canal and is entirely extrapelvic throughout its course. It traverses the obturator fascia, the ischiorectal fossa, and the external anal sphincter to reach the submucosa of the anal canal, ultimately ascending in this plane.

## Venous Drainage

Venous drainage of the large intestine basically follows its arterial supply. Blood from the right colon, via the superior mesenteric vein, and from left colon and rectum, via the inferior mesenteric vein, reaches the intrahepatic capillary bed through the portal vein. The anorectum also drains, via middle and inferior hemorrhoidal veins, to the internal iliac vein and then to the inferior vena cava.

## Lymphatic Drainage

Lymphatic drainage from all parts of the colon follows its vascular supply. The submucous and subserous layers of the colon and rectum have a rich network of lymphatic plexuses, which drain into an extramural system of lymph channels and nodes. Colorectal lymph nodes are classically divided into four groups: epiploic, paracolic, intermediate, and principal. The epicolic group lies on the bowel wall under the peritoneum and in the appendices epiploicae. The paracolic nodes are situated along the marginal artery and on the arcades. The intermediate nodes are situated on the primary colic vessels, and the main or principal nodes on the superior and inferior mesenteric vessels. The lymph then drains to the cisterna chyli via the paraortic chain of nodes.

Lymph from the upper two thirds of the rectum drains exclusively upward to the inferior mesenteric nodes and then to the para-aortic nodes. Lymphatic drainage from the lower third of the rectum occurs both cephalad, along the superior hemorrhoidal and inferior mesentery arteries, and laterally, along the middle hemorrhoidal vessels to the internal iliac nodes. In the anal canal, the dentate line is the landmark for two different systems of lymphatic drainage: above, to the inferior mesenteric and internal iliac nodes, and below, along the inferior rectal lymphatics to the superficial inguinal nodes or, less frequently, along the inferior hemorrhoidal artery.

## Innervation

The sympathetic and parasympathetic components of the autonomic innervation of the large intestine closely follow the blood supply.

### Right Colon

Sympathetic innervation originates from the lower six thoracic segments. These thoracic splanchnic nerves reach the celiac, preaortic, and superior mesenteric ganglia, where they synapse. The postganglionic fibers then course along the superior mesenteric artery to the small bowel and right colon. The parasympathetic supply comes from the right (posterior) vagus nerve and celiac plexus. The fibers travel along the superior mesenteric artery, and finally synapse with cells in the autonomic plexuses within the bowel wall.

### Left Colon and Rectum

The sympathetic supply arises from L1, L2, and L3. Preganglionic fibers, via lumbar sympathetic nerves, synapse in the preaortic plexus, and the postganglionic fibers follow the branches of the IMA and superior rectal artery to the left colon and upper rectum. The presacral nerves, which are formed by fusion of the aortic plexus and lumbar splanchnic nerves innervate the lower rectum. Just below the sacral promontory, the presacral nerves form the hypogastric plexus (or superior hypogastric plexus). Two main hypogastric nerves, on either side of the rectum, carry sympathetic innervation from the hypogastric plexus to the pelvic plexus. The pelvic plexus lies on the lateral side of the pelvis at the level of the lower third of the rectum, adjacent to the lateral stalks.

The parasympathetic supply derives from S2, S3, and S4 splanchnic nerves. These fibers, which emerge through the sacral foramen, are called the "nervi erigentes." They pass laterally, forward and upward to join the sympathetic hypogastric nerves at the pelvic plexus. From the pelvic plexus, combined postganglionic parasympathetic and sympathetic fibers are distributed to the left colon and upper rectum via the inferior mesenteric plexus, and directly to the lower rectum and upper anal canal. The periprostatic plexus, a subdivision of the pelvic plexus situated on Denonvilliers' fascia, supplies the prostate, seminal vesicles, corpora cavernosa, vas deferens, urethra, ejaculatory ducts, and bulbourethral glands.

Division of both superior hypogastric plexuses or both hypogastric nerves resulting in sympathetic denervation, but with intact nervi erigentes, results in retrograde ejaculation from bladder sphincter dysfunction. An isolated injury of nervi erigentes will completely abolish erectile function. Finally, dissection near the seminal vesicles and prostate can damage the periprostatic plexus, leading to a mixed parasympathetic and sympathetic injury. This can result in erectile impotence as well as a flaccid, neurogenic bladder. In women, sexual complications also occur but are probably underdiagnosed. Most problems relate to discomfort with sexual intercourse.

### *Anal Canal*

#### *Motor Innervation*

The internal anal sphincter, supplied by sympathetic (L5) and parasympathetic nerves (S2, S3, and S4), follows the same route as the nerves to the rectum. The levator ani is supplied by sacral roots on its pelvic surface (S2, S3, and S4) and by the perineal branch of the pudendal nerve on its inferior surface. The puborectalis muscle receives additional innervation from the inferior rectal nerves. The EAS is innervated on each side by the inferior rectal branch of the pudendal nerve (S2 and S3) and by the perineal branch of S4. Despite the fact that the puborectalis and EAS have somewhat different innervations, these muscles seem to act as an indivisible unit. After unilateral transection of a pudendal nerve, EAS function is still preserved because of the crossover of the fibers at the spinal cord level.

#### *Sensory Innervation*

The upper anal canal contains a rich profusion of both free and organized sensory nerve endings, especially in the vicinity of the anal valves. Organized nerve endings include Meissner's corpuscles (touch), Krause's bulbs (cold), Golgi-Mazzoni bodies (pressure), and genital corpuscles (friction). Anal sensation, which is carried in the inferior rectal branch of the pudendal nerve, is thought to play a role in maintenance of anal continence.

## SUMMARY

Knowledge of colon and rectal anatomy, blood supply, lymphatic drainage, innervation, and muscle function and distribution are all extremely important to minimize complications of the surgical problems that are discussed in subsequent chapters.

# 2

# Physiology of the Colon

The primary physiologic purposes of the large bowel include the following: further breakdown of ingested materials by microfloral metabolism, absorption of water and electrolytes, secretion of electrolytes and mucus, storage of semisolid matter, and propulsion of feces toward the rectum and anus. These colonic functions act in concert to respond to the needs of the body while concomitantly producing fecal material suitable for evacuation. This chapter presents a current, general view of normal large-bowel physiology to facilitate the discussion of colonic pathophysiologic processes presented subsequently.

## FUNCTIONAL CLASSIFICATION

The large bowel, which is approximately 150 cm (5 feet) long, consists of the vermiform appendix, colon (cecum, ascending, transverse, descending, sigmoid), and rectum. This somewhat arbitrary segmentation of the large bowel is not strictly anatomic, as it is now widely appreciated that the large intestine is a heterogeneous organ with regional, biochemical, pharmacologic, and thus functional differences.

### Cecum and Ascending Colon (Right Colon)

Digested material enters the large intestine and remains in the right colon for an extended period, allowing aerobic and anaerobic metabolism of residual carbohydrate and protein by the intestinal flora, thereby producing multiple byproducts, most of which are then absorbed through the remaining colon. Also, the ascending colon (along with the transverse colon) is involved in regulating intraluminal fluid volume as well as sodium and water absorption.

### Transverse Colon

The transverse colon, generally believed to serve as a rapid conduit between the proximal (right) and distal (left) components of the large bowel, is also an important site for sodium and water absorption, a function that is critical to volume regulation.

## Left Colon

The left colon is the site for final modulation of intraluminal contents before evacuation. The distal large intestine also is thought to have a reservoir function or storage capacity, which some feel is important in maintaining anal continence.

With respect to the rectum, *in vitro* studies have demonstrated that little or no net absorption occurs there.

## DIGESTION

The healthy colon, despite its poorly recognized participation in the breakdown of foodstuffs to fulfill energy requirements, is capable of salvaging calories from poorly absorbed carbohydrates and proteins.

### Flora of the Large Intestine

The digestive processes of the colon are a consequence of the microorganisms that colonize the bowel and thereby participate in a symbiotic relationship with the host. More than 400 different species of gram-positive, gram-negative, and anaerobic types of bacteria have been identified. Studies have revealed up to $10^{12}$ bacteria per gram of wet feces. Given this amount, it is not surprising that bacteria make up 40% to 55% of fecal solids in individuals consuming a typical Western diet.

### Fermentation Substrates

#### *Nondigestible Starch*

Generally, it is accepted that approximately 10% of ingested starch will elude small-bowel digestion to reach the colon and be available for fermentation in individuals consuming a Western diet.

#### *Nonstarch Polysaccharides*

Nonstarch polysaccharides, the derivatives of plant material, include cellulose as well as noncellulose substrates. These and other physiologic variables, such as transit time, ultimately determine the extent of cellulose and noncellulose breakdown by the resident flora.

#### *Other Substrates*

Overall, the daily ileal effluent will make available 6 to 18 g of nitrogen-containing compounds for bacterial fermentation, compared with 8 to 40 g of carbohydrate.

### Products of Bacterial Metabolism

The principal products of microorganism fermentation of polysaccharides in the large bowel are short-chain fatty acids (SCFAs) or volatile fatty acids. These fatty acids contain from one to six carbons and are the predominant colonic anions. The three most abundant are acetate, propionate, and butyrate, with their production accounting for 85% to 95% of total SCFA generation.

### *SCFA Absorption*

More than 90% of SCFAs produced by bacterial fermentation is taken up by the colonic mucosal cells. However, the mechanism for uptake by the colonic epithelium remains unresolved.

### *Physiologic Actions of SCFA*

The SCFAs are produced as a result of bacterial fermentation. Once absorbed, they have been reported to contribute up to 7% of the basal metabolic requirements of humans. In fact, the colonic epithelium derives almost 75% of its energy needs from these fatty acids through metabolism to carbon dioxide, ketone bodies, and lipid precursors. Additionally, the absorption of SCFAs is tied closely to the transport of bicarbonate, sodium, and water, thus providing a mechanism to regulate intraluminal volume.

### *Other Products of Noncarbohydrate Fermentation*

The fermentation of peptides by microorganisms results in substances such as SCFAs, branched-chain fatty acids, isobutyrate, and methylbutyrate. In addition, the catabolism of amino acids results in the production of phenols, indoles, and amines, which have been implicated in disease states such as hepatic coma and colorectal cancer.

## COLONIC ABSORPTION AND SECRETION

The absorption and secretion of water, mucus, and electrolytes, particularly sodium, are complex and central processes of normal colonic activity.

### Sodium Absorption

Sodium movement across the colonic wall is an active process. Measurements of normal daily fecal water show 1 to 5 mEq of sodium, representing more than 90% absorption of the 200 mEq of sodium found in the ileal effluent.

## Transport Mechanisms

### Electrogenic Transport

In the distal colon, movement of sodium from the lumen into the mucosal cell occurs down an electrochemical gradient. The sodium ions, unable to permeate the phospholipid membrane, pass through protein channels characterized by their sensitivity to amiloride, a sodium transport blocker and aldosterone antagonist. This continues because of the $Na^+/K^+$-adenosine triphosphatase (ATPase) located on the basolateral aspect of the colonic epithelial cells that ensures an adequate difference between intracellular and intraluminal $Na^+$ concentrations.

### Electroneutral Absorption

An additional mechanism for the movement of sodium involves the concomitant absorption of the chloride ion. This electroneutral process occurs primarily through the coupling of apical sodium–hydrogen and chloride–bicarbonate ion exchanges.

### Effects of Aldosterone

As a steroid hormone, aldosterone crosses the cell membrane and binds to an intracellular receptor. This ligand–receptor interaction eventually leads both to acceleration of sodium absorption and $Na^+/K^+$-ATPase rates and to augmentation of sodium permeability in the distal colon.

### Chloride Ion Absorption

The mechanism of chloride ion transport across the human colonic apical membrane, which remains without clear definition, appears to result from several processes. Chloride absorption in the colon is generally accepted to occur by means of an energy-independent, passive mechanism. This process relies on the negative charge of the ion and the diffusion potential generated by electrogenic sodium absorption. Others have found that luminally directed bicarbonate gradients stimulated the uptake of chloride ions and concluded that an electroneutral chloride–bicarbonate transport contributes to the primary mechanism of sodium chloride absorption in the human proximal colon. Some authors have postulated that chloride–bicarbonate and chloride–hydroxyl ion channels possess unique functional features, with one involved in chloride transcellular transport and the other concerned with intracellular pH maintenance. Additional studies are needed to explore the detailed mechanism, regulation, and relative contributions of both active and passive chloride transport.

### Water Movement

One of the central functions of the large intestine is to control the level of fecal water. Average ileocecal flow for a healthy individual is approximately 1,500 to 2,000 mL/d. Of this amount, only 100 to 150 mL of water appears in the stool. The colon, which harbors a tremendous reserve transport capacity, is capable of absorbing as much as 5 to 6 L over a 24-hour period if challenged. The amount of water ultimately absorbed is regulated by any mediator of luminal flow, fluid composition, or net electrolyte transport.

### Bicarbonate Transport

The transport of bicarbonate ion across the apical membrane of colonic epithelium is generally considered a secretory process involving a chloride–bicarbonate ion antiport. Clearly, the most likely source of the intracellular bicarbonate ion is the conversion of carbon dioxide and water by carbonic anhydrase, whose levels have been found to be elevated in colonic mucosal cells.

### Potassium Transport

Currently, potassium absorption is believed to be predominantly a phenomenon of the distal colon that is electroneutral, sodium-independent, and mediated through an apical $K^+/H^+$-ATPase and a basolateral potassium ion channel.

Because the maintenance of potassium levels is critical to proper cell and body function, continuing interest in colonic regulation of this ion is of obvious importance.

## COLONIC MOTILITY

The phenomenon of gastrointestinal motility integrates a number of complex tissue functions, including smooth-muscle electrical activity, contractile activity, intraluminal pressure, and both extrinsic and intrinsic neural coordination. However, a clear understanding of the normal function, underlying motility, and regulatory patterns is often unappreciated.

A number of techniques have been used to improve knowledge in this area. Three methods of measurement have been employed—colonic manometry, radiographic observation (i.e., radio-opaque markers, fluoroscopy, defecography), and scintigraphy.

### Regulation

#### Myogenic

Electrical slow waves are the result of the rhythmic alterations in smooth-muscle membrane potentials as recorded on electromyogram studies. In the colon, these slow waves are of variable amplitude and frequency, but do not necessarily correlate with the contraction of muscle fibers. Muscle contraction occurs only with those slow waves that carry a strong initiating depolarization or spike. The cells responsible for production of slow waves, known as the pacemaker cells of the colon, are found in the circular muscle layer of the colonic wall.

### Neural

From a number of pharmacologic and histologic studies, four types of external nerves have been found to be active in colonic muscle. They are cholinergic and noncholinergic *excitatory* nerves and adrenergic and nonadrenergic *inhibitory* nerves.

The vagus and the sacral nerves provide cholinergic innervation of the large bowel. In addition, animal studies have shown that afferent fibers of the vagus nerve contain the following neuropeptides: substance P, somatostatin, gastrin, cholecystokinin, and vasoactive inhibitory peptide.

Vagal innervation of the myenteric plexus, which controls the intrinsic neural regulation of motility, is believed to contain two types of neurons. In addition to the well-characterized preganglionic cholinergic nerve, the vagus supply to the colon is believed to contain a preganglionic noncholinergic, nonadrenergic neuron. This type of neuron is thought to synapse with inhibitory neurons of the myenteric plexus and to use the vasoactive inhibitory peptide as a neurotransmitter.

Sympathetic innervation of the colon begins with cell bodies located in the dorsal horn of the lumbar spinal cord. The axons from these nerves course through several pathways to synapse with postganglionic adrenergic neurons found in the celiac, superior, and inferior mesenteric ganglia.

The sympathetic nervous system is well known to exhibit an inhibitory influence on the colon.s The neurotransmitters in the ganglion cells of the colonic wall are the same neuropeptides seen mediating parasympathetic function as well as numerous other activities unrelated to motility. Continued interest in and study of these neuropeptides will undoubtedly reveal important new information regarding the mechanisms of colonic function.

## CONCLUSION

The three central functions of the normal healthy colon are digestion, motility, and transport. All are important components of human physiology. They are being actively investigated and may, in time, lead to the introduction of new treatments for a host of conditions that affect the large bowel.

# 3

# Diet and Drugs in Colorectal Surgery

The role of diet in a healthy bowel has been a stimulating and controversial subject for two millennia. Data support a number of statements and recommendations, but controlled clinical trials defining the benefits of various foods and therapies are virtually nonexistent. In general, diets high in fiber and roughage help facilitate the normal passage of stool. In addition, they may be beneficial to the overall health of an individual by reducing cholesterol, maintaining blood sugar in the normal range, and decreasing the incidence of diverticulosis. Cruciferous plants also contain anticarcinogens that may reduce the incidence of colonic neoplasms. Furthermore, aspirin and other nonsteroidal antiinflammatory agents appear to reduce the incidence of colon cancer.

A number of conditions (e.g., irritable bowel syndrome, inflammatory bowel disease, diverticulitis, diarrhea, and constipation) can also often be ameliorated by dietary manipulation, even though the cause of the disorder may not be related to a specific food. This chapter focuses on some of the more common symptoms and conditions for which patients seek the attention of physicians trained in gastrointestinal disease and gastrointestinal surgery.

## BOWEL MANAGEMENT PROBLEMS

### Constipation

Constipation can be defined as either a decrease in the frequency of stools or an increase in difficulty in passing stools. Patients may also complain of hard bowel movements, small actions, inability to evacuate, or the sensation of incomplete evacuation. Those with fewer than three bowel movements per week are considered to have "constipation," but they may not be truly symptomatic or even seek medical attention. Those who do request help usually complain of either decreased frequency or difficulty in passing stool. Therapy, therefore, is directed at either increasing the water content (i.e., softening the stool) or increasing the frequency of bowel movements.

## History

A carefully obtained history is essential before recommending therapy. The history should include the duration of the complaints, dietary habits, the use of medications, and lifestyle. It is important to consider the more common endocrine conditions that can affect the bowels: hypothyroidism, diabetes mellitus, and hyperparathyroidism. Other diseases that predispose to constipation include uremia, porphyria, amyloidosis, and short-segment Hirschsprung's disease.

Because medications can frequently cause constipation, it is important to obtain the patient's history of medication use. Although the list is extensive, the more common ones to consider include opiates, analgesics, antipsychotics (particularly the monoamine oxidase inhibitors and tricyclic antidepressants), anticholinergics, iron and other heavy metals, antacids, anticonvulsants, calcium channel blockers, and diuretics.

## Evaluation

The perineum should be carefully inspected for obvious pathologic entities that may impede the passage of stool. Instrument examination, contrast studies, transit studies, gynecologic examination, ultrasonography, computed tomography, and physiologic studies may be required in selected patients. Certainly, gastrointestinal evaluation must be done at some point to rule out the presence of specific etiologic factors. Specific evaluations are discussed in the following chapters.

## Treatment

Standard treatment of nonspecific constipation begins with dietary manipulation, usually through increasing dietary fiber and fluid intake. Total daily fiber intake should be adjusted to approximately 30 g or more. In addition, several classes of medication are available to increase stool water or stool frequency. These include bulk laxatives, stool softeners, osmotic or saline laxatives, cathartics, and motility-enhancing drugs (prokinetics).

### Fiber Products

A fiber-containing bulk laxative may increase stool water-carrying capacity. The major disadvantage of bulking agents is the bloating and gas produced with the cellulose and lignin-based products. Lowering of serum cholesterol—the benefit of using bulk agents—is probably effected through the binding of bile salts and decreased reabsorption, so that the bile salt pool is lowered.

### Stool Softeners

Patients who are resistant to the bulking agents alone can increase the stool water content further with stool softeners or emollients. The principal agent is docusate, which inhibits the normal water-absorptive capacity of the colon while producing only a minimal decrease in the transit of fecal contents.

### Osmotic or Saline Laxatives

The preferred next step would be to use an osmotic or saline laxative. Magnesium, phosphate, sodium sulfate, and potassium tartrate are poorly absorbed chemicals. Ingestion increases the stool water content through an osmotic effect. They should be used with caution in individuals with renal, cardiac, or hepatic disease because they can cause a high serum phosphate level and impair cardiac contractility.

### Polysaccharides

Some carbohydrates are also poorly absorbed, which results in an osmotic effect that leads to enhanced water in the stool. These products include lactose, lactulose, and sorbitol. Side effects include gas, bloating, cramps, flatulence, and, of course, fluid loss at high doses.

### Lubricants

Mineral oil, a petroleum distillate, has been used to treat constipation. Its mechanism of action appears to be penetration of the stool by the oil, with resultant softening. However, because of the potential for complications, including decreased absorption of fat-soluble vitamins and essential fatty acids, chronic use should be avoided.

### Stimulant Laxatives

Cathartic laxatives are mucosally active agents that reduce net water and electrolyte absorption in addition to increasing bowel motility. Substances used most frequently include the diphenylmethane derivatives (phenolphthalein and bisacodyl) and the anthraquinone cathartics (senna, cascara sagrada, danthron). The primary side effect, in addition to diarrhea, is that of cramping. Furthermore, melanosis coli, a dark pigmentation of the colonic mucosa, may be a consequence of long-term use of senna and cascara.

### Motility Agents

Three agents are currently available that decrease transit time by accelerating the muscular activity of the bowel. Gastrointestinal motility can be enhanced through the use of metoclopramide, cisapride, or erythromycin. In pseudoobstruction, neostigmine has been reported to be useful in promoting normal motility.

## Summary

Long-term use of intestinal stimulants and cathartics can lead to fluid and electrolyte disturbances, including dehydration, hypokalemia, hyponatremia, hypoalbuminemia, steatorrhea, protein-losing enteropathy, and secondary hyperaldosteronism. Furthermore, because patients can become dependent on laxatives, what is known as a "cathartic colon" or a chronically flaccid colon can develop. A good general principle is that if laxatives are to be used, the lowest effective dose should be given; chronic use should be discouraged. Surgical intervention as a treatment for constipation should be offered only after an adequate trial of medical therapy and appropriate evaluation of the gastrointestinal tract (see Chapter 16).

## Diarrhea

Diarrhea is common; its causes include medications, infection, the consequences of radiation, hepatic or biliary disease, pancreatic insufficiency, intolerance to ingested food components, infiltration of the mucosa or submucosa with lymphocytes or eosinophils, neoplasm, inflammatory bowel disease, and irritable bowel syndrome. It is beyond the scope of this chapter to offer a comprehensive discussion of the causes and treatments of all possible conditions that can lead to the symptom of diarrhea.

The most common presentation is that of increased stool water. This leads to loose stools, watery stools, and increased stool volume, frequency, or both. By definition, diarrhea is classified as acute until symptoms have been present for more than 6 weeks. After this time, it is considered chronic.

### *Acute Diarrhea*

Acute diarrhea is often caused by medication or an infectious process, including bacterial enteritis, toxin ingestion, and infestation by the common intestinal parasites (e.g., *Giardia, Cryptosporidia, Isospora*). A discussion of the infectious and noninfectious colitides can be found in Chapter 33.

### *Principles of Management*

Treatment for acute diarrhea involves the identification of the offending agent and initiation of whatever specific measures are necessary to eliminate the source or eradicate the organism. Medications that decrease gastrointestinal motility in acute, febrile diarrheal illnesses should be avoided, as prolonged contact time can enhance the likelihood of transmucosal migration of the organism and lead to systemic infection. A better alternative is the use of pectin or bismuth compounds, such as kaopectin or bismuth subcitrate. These products bind shiga toxins and other cyclic guanosine monophosphate stimulatory toxins associated with bacterial infection, and decrease the net water and chloride secretion by the small bowel. If systemic signs and symptoms of infection are not present, the use of opiates to increase transit time and slow stool frequency offers symptomatic relief.

### Chronic Diarrhea

A wide variety of disorders that affect the hepatobiliary system, pancreas, and small or large bowel can cause chronic diarrheal illness. Individuals with chronic diarrhea present a challenge in differential diagnosis, which can inevitably lead to an extensive and expensive workup. Assuming that such an evaluation fails to establish a specific cause for the patient's symptoms, the most likely disorder is the so-called "irritable bowel syndrome." Treatment for this complaint is aimed at reducing the volume and frequency of bowel movements, so that the patient's lifestyle can be improved.

#### Treatment

The approach to the management of patients with chronic diarrhea without a definable cause begins with a carefully taken dietary history. Removing the offending agent usually reduces symptoms.

Medical therapy encompasses a wide variety of options. Those agents used specifically to treat diarrhea include the following:

The fiber-containing bulk agents, previously mentioned, decrease stool water when they are given with less than the recommended volume of liquid. Any of the bulk agents taken under these circumstances decreases the absorption of water through the gastrointestinal tract. Stool water can also be bound through the use of bile salt resins (e.g., cholestyramine).

Kaolin, a dehydrated aluminum silicate, and pectin, a carbohydrate (polygalacturonic acid), can also be used as adsorbents to treat diarrhea.

Opiates, the most effective form of therapy in the management of diarrheal illnesses, are usually given in the form of diphenoxylate or loperamide. They are also available in many other substances, including codeine phosphate and tincture of opium (paregoric). A patient whose diarrhea fails to resolve with any of these measures requires evaluation.

### Irritable Bowel Syndrome

Irritable bowel syndrome (IBS) is defined as abdominal pain with or without alterations in bowel habits and with no anatomic abnormality on diagnostic testing. Patients may present with a wide variety of complaints, but more than 90% will have two or more of the following: visible abdominal distension, increased frequency of bowel movements with the onset of pain, looser stools with the onset of pain, and relief of pain with defecation. Most patients typically complain of crampy, diffuse abdominal pain that is associated with alternating constipation and diarrhea.

### Cause and Pathogenesis

The cause of IBS is unknown. However, considerable evidence seems to implicate the roles of stress and psychiatric illness in its pathophysiology.

### Treatment

For most, IBS is a lifelong illness, with periods of health punctuated by episodes of symptoms.

The use of psychiatric therapy in this condition has been the subject of numerous studies. Hypnotherapy, stress reduction psychotherapy, dynamic psychotherapy, and relaxation techniques have all been used successfully.

No doubt, diet can play a role in IBS and lead to increased abdominal cramping or pain. Patients with diarrhea should be counseled with respect to foods that are likely to increase stool water and frequency. These include fiber, nonabsorbed carbohydrates, caffeine, and lactose. If constipation is the primary symptom, increased fiber and water intake may help reduce the difficulty in passing stools, but the consequences of bloating, cramps, and abdominal pain may make the use of this approach counterproductive.

For abdominal pain, the current first line of medications is the anticholinergic class of drugs. Anticholinergics can reduce the rate of spike activity, thereby decreasing tonic contractions in the colon. Antidepressants have also been shown to provide relief from the pain of IBS, often at doses far lower than those used to achieve an antidepressant effect.

Nonsteroidal antiinflammatory medications appear to have little role in the treatment of the pain of IBS, and absolutely no place exists for stronger pain medications such as opiates or narcotics.

Newer drugs, however, are becoming available to treat the diarrhea component of the disease.

### Short-Bowel Syndrome

Patients who have undergone resection of the small intestine, particularly the distal ileum, may present with symptoms of urgency and diarrhea (especially after meals), weight loss, or dehydration. When an extensive portion of the small intestine has been resected, sufficient surface area may not be available for absorption of nutrients. It has been estimated that the minimal length of small intestine necessary to sustain adequate enteral nutrition is approximately 1 m, although the presence of the colon may reduce that requirement. Individuals unable to achieve adequate enteral nutrition require parenteral hyperalimentation (see Chapter 30).

Recent studies have demonstrated that the colon can actually absorb a reasonable amount of calories, largely in the form of short-chain fatty acids. In addition to providing nutrient value to the cells of the colonic mucosa itself, 500 kcal/d may actually be absorbed into the systemic circulation.

The use of growth hormone and glutamine, with a diet of increased carbohydrates and decreased fat, has been demonstrated to increase the absorption of protein and to decrease stool output. In some individuals with small intestines too limited to provide adequate absorptive area, this regimen has decreased or completely eliminated the need for peripheral hyperalimentation.

Small bowel transplantation together with pancreatic transplantation has been used as a treatment option; however, to a degree, this is still experimental.

### Cholerheic Diarrhea

Individuals who have undergone resection of the distal ileum, particularly if the ileocecal valve has been removed, may exhibit symptoms of cramping, bloating, and diarrhea, often accompanying intake of food. The cause of these complaints is not clear, but it appears to be related to deconjugation of nonabsorbed bile salts by the colonic bacteria. Deconjugated bile salts are toxic to the lining of the colon; they initiate fluid and electrolyte secretion and lead to symptoms of cramping and diarrhea (cholerheic diarrhea). Treatment is a bile salt–binding medication, such as cholestyramine. Diarrhea can be further reduced by the use of loperamide or dephenoxylate in those individuals whose diarrhea persists despite bile salt–binding medications.

# 4

# Evaluation and Diagnostic Techniques

The evaluation of the symptoms frequently associated with diseases of the anus, rectum, and colon is covered in this chapter. In addition, the instrumentation and the studies available for the diagnosis of these conditions are presented. Although general principles of history taking and physical examination are discussed, the reader is advised to consult the appropriate chapter for evaluation of a particular entity.

## HISTORY

As in all fields of medicine, the patient history is the single most important piece of information that the physician can obtain. A carefully taken interview will probably either establish the diagnosis or at least suggest it. In pathology of the anus, rectum, and colon, a limited number of questions are pertinent.

### Bleeding

Blood may be pink, bright red, mahogany, black, or inapparent (i.e., occult). It may be noticed on the toilet paper, in the toilet bowl, or both. None of these rectal manifestations of blood is specifically diagnostic of the location or type of pathology. Blood that appears solely on the toilet paper is suggestive of a distal cause (e.g., hemorrhoids, fissure). Altered (e.g., dark) blood suggests a more proximal lesion (e.g., carcinoma of the cecum). Blood found in the toilet bowl may or may not indicate a greater blood loss.

Rectal bleeding may not be an isolated symptom. When associated with a painful lump and unrelated to defecation, it is usually the result of a thrombosed hemorrhoid. When related to defecation and associated with pain, it is often the result of an anal fissure, the most common cause of bleeding in the infant. When bleeding accompanies diarrhea, inflammatory bowel disease must be considered.

The physician must have a reasonable index of suspicion, as well as competent clinical judgment to determine whether additional studies are required to evaluate the cause of rectal bleeding.

## Pain

Anorectal pain is a frequent complaint. If continuous, it could be caused by a thrombosed hemorrhoid or abscess. If the pain is worse during and following defecation, examination will usually reveal the presence of an anal fissure. If the pain is deep-seated, intermittent, and unrelated to defecation, the patient is probably experiencing proctalgia fugax (i.e., levator spasm). If related to the coccyx and exacerbated by moving from a sitting to a standing position, coccygodynia is the probable cause. Anorectal pain is rarely associated with a tumor unless the lesion invades the internal sphincter to produce tenesmus—a painful, ineffective desire to defecate.

Abdominal pain that is colicky in nature can be caused by bowel obstruction, but most commonly it is caused by irritable bowel syndrome. Physical examination and plane abdominal films readily distinguish the two entities. When abdominal pain is continuous, it may be a consequence of peritoneal irritation from any of a number of causes. Here again, physical examination and determination of the presence or absence of peritoneal signs will lead the physician to pursue the appropriate course.

## Anal and Perianal Masses

The differential diagnosis of an anal or perianal lump involves the spectrum of benign and malignant neoplastic lesions as well as a host of dermatologic conditions. The most common cause is a thrombosed hemorrhoid. Others include prolapse of hemorrhoids, rectal prolapse, sebaceous cysts, lipomas, hypertrophied anal papillae, skin tags, and condylomata. With lesions of uncertain nature, biopsy is mandatory.

## Rectal Discharge

Mucous discharge and soiling of the underclothes are frequent complaints. The patient may have had prior anal surgery with deformity and scarring or may have sustained sphincter injury from surgical, accidental, or obstetric trauma or, if accompanied by a painful swelling, an anal or perianal abscess may be present.

Rectal discharge, however, is usually not related to the presence of a specific pathologic entity. Most individuals experience the difficulty because of dietary indiscretion or too vigorous attention to anal hygiene. Appropriate dietary and hygiene counseling may be all the treatment that is required (see Chapter 19). In patients with a lax anus, perineal strengthening exercises are advisable (see Chapter 13).

## Incontinence

Anorectal disease, fecal impaction, laxative abuse, or neurologic disease can cause fecal incontinence, but it can also be the result of trauma (see Chapter 13).

## Change in Bowel Habits

A change in bowel habit, one of the symptoms suggestive of colonic neoplasm, almost always requires endoscopy or radiologic investigation for adequate assessment.

A change in bowel habits may be as obvious as diarrhea when the patient has had a long history of constipation, or as subtle as the development of normal, easy bowel movements after many years of a difficult or irregular pattern. Bleeding occurring with a change in bowel habits increases the likelihood of the presence of a malignant neoplasm.

## PHYSICAL EXAMINATION

A general physical examination of the patient with a colorectal complaint is usually an unrewarding exercise.

The five basic approaches to colorectal evaluation include the following:

1. Inspection
2. Palpation
3. Anoscopy
4. Proctosigmoidoscopy or flexible sigmoidoscopy
5. Colonoscopy

For the purpose of simplicity, the term *proctosigmoidoscopy* is used interchangeably with the words *procto* and *sigmoidoscopy*. All three imply the use of the 25-cm rigid instrument.

### Positioning the Patient for Rigid Sigmoidoscopy

The prone jackknife position requires a special table that tilts the patient's head down (Fig. 4.1). The table is expensive, but it provides the examiner with the easiest access and the best view. It is the least comfortable position, however, for the patient.

The most comfortable position for the patient having this examination is the left lateral (i.e., Sims') position. The individual lies on the left side on the examining table or bed with the buttocks protruding over the edge, hips flexed, knees slightly extended, and right shoulder rotated anteriorly. The examiner can sit or stand, depending on the height of the table or bed.

The knee-chest position is probably somewhat more comfortable for the patient than the prone, but it is the most awkward for the physician. In our opinion, the knee-chest position should be abandoned.

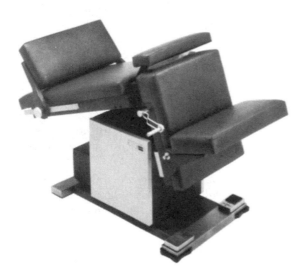

**FIG. 4.1.** The Ritter table, which is used for examination in the prone, jackknife position (Courtesy of Sybron Corp.)

No evidence suggests that this position either interferes with or facilitates insertion of the instrument to its full length.

To perform a satisfactory and reasonably comfortable examination and to obtain all necessary information, it is essential to inform the patient continually what is to be expected and what is happening.

### Inspection

Inspection of the anal area may reveal hemorrhoids, skin tags, a sentinel pile indicative of an underlying anal fissure, or dermatologic problems, including pruritic changes, abscess, fistula, scar, or deformity. Evaluation of the sacrococcygeal region may disclose a laminectomy scar, possibly suggesting a neurologic cause for incontinence. Pain on spreading the buttocks may indicate the presence of an anal fissure.

In addition to inspecting the perianal skin, it is important to evaluate the resting state of the anal opening. A patulous anal orifice may be seen with rectal prolapse, neurologic abnormality, sphincter injury, or in an anoreceptive person.

On straining, rectal prolapse, hypertrophied anal papilla, or, most commonly, hemorrhoids may protrude. In cases of suspected procidentia, the patient should optimally sit and strain on the toilet for the physician to identify this finding.

### Palpation

A water-soluble lubricant is applied to the gloved index finger. The patient is informed that a finger will be passed into the rectum and that this will make it feel as if the bowels will move, but they will not. Again, it is imperative to inform and reassure the patient continually.

The physician should examine the rectum and its surrounding structures in an organized approach. Assessment of sphincter tone and contractility is an important part of the rectal examination, and these should be noted routinely whenever a patient complains of problems with fecal control or discharge.

For the male patient, first feel the prostate anteriorly; assess it for hypertrophy, nodularity, and firmness.

For the female patient, palpate the cervix first, unless it is surgically absent. The uterine body may feel displaced posteriorly, and the presence of fibroid tumors may be noted. Bidigital examination (i.e., one finger in the rectum and the other in the vagina) will readily distinguish any anatomic or pathologic variations.

Then sweep the examining finger from anterior to posterior and back again, consciously thinking of a possible lesion that might be present. A submucosal rectal nodule may not be visible and would otherwise go undiagnosed if only direct visualization was used. It is often possible to feel a tumor or a diverticular mass in the sigmoid colon. Having the patient strain down (i.e., Valsalva's maneuver) sometimes reveals a lesion in the upper rectum or rectosigmoid that otherwise might not be palpable. Examination above the prostate in the male patient or in the cul-de-sac in the female patient may reveal a Blumer's shelf, which is a hard mass on the anterior rectal wall caused by metastatic tumor, usually of gastric or pancreatic origin. Attention to the presacral area may uncover an extrinsic mass (e.g., cyst, tumor, sacrococcygeal chordoma).

Finally, as the finger is withdrawn, the presence of anal pathology is noted (e.g., hypertrophied papilla, thrombosed hemorrhoid, stenosis, scarring). It is well recognized that digital examination of the anal canal is the most accurate means of diagnosing Crohn's disease in this area.

## Anoscopy

Anoscopy offers the best means to evaluate hemorrhoids, fissures, papillae, or other lesions of the anal canal. Together with proctosigmoidoscopy, it allows adequate anorectal evaluation. For any pathology noted or treated, the site should be recorded as follows: right anterior, left lateral, and so forth.

## Rigid Proctosigmoidoscopy

The sigmoidoscope is one of our most valuable diagnostic tools. It may reveal mucosal excrescences, polypoid lesions, cancer, inflammatory changes, stricture, vascular malformation, or anatomic distortion from extraluminal masses. It can also detect anal conditions, but should not replace the anoscope for this purpose.

### *Equipment*

A number of reusable or disposable rigid sigmoidoscopes are available, with proximal or distal lighting, and with or without fiberoptics. Reusable instruments require care and cleansing, whereas the disposable ones are obviously discarded.

Reusable instruments are available in a number of diameters, ranging from 1.1 to 2.7 cm. The medium (1.9-cm) instrument is an excellent compromise that offers the physician the ability both to screen the patient and to perform procedures.

In addition to the speculum tube, the instrumentation includes a light source, a proximal magnifying lens, and an attachment for air insufflation. It is also important to provide adequate suction. This can be accomplished by attachment to a vacuum pump or a water tap. Long swabs (i.e., chimney sweeps) are also helpful.

### Preparation

A small-volume enema (e.g., Fleet) is administered just before the procedure unless the patient has a history suggestive of inflammatory bowel disease. Vigorous catharsis and dietary restrictions the day before the examination are not necessary.

### Technique

Five principles should be adhered to in order to conduct a safe, competent sigmoidoscopic examination:

1. Be expeditious
2. Insufflate minimal air
3. Have a nurse or assistant always available
4. Keep talking to the patient: explain, reassure, distract
5. Do no harm

A digital rectal examination should always precede instrumentation. The well-lubricated sigmoidoscope is then inserted and passed to the maximal height as quickly as possible while causing minimal discomfort to the patient.

Air insufflation, which is of value in demonstrating the lumen of the bowel, provides even greater benefit in visualizing the mucosa when the instrument is withdrawn.

Successful insertion of the sigmoidoscope requires familiarity with the anatomy of the rectum and sigmoid colon. Knowing where the lumen is probably located without actually visualizing it permits the examiner considerable freedom in passing the instrument. When the sigmoidoscope is inserted, the low and midrectal areas are midline structures. As the upper rectum is reached, the bowel bends slightly to the left.

The physician should withdraw the instrument in a rotating fashion, carefully viewing the entire circumference of the bowel wall and ironing out mucosal folds to be certain that no small lesion is missed.

### Complications

### Perforation

Perforation from rigid sigmoidoscopy is extremely unusual. Perforation of the normal rectum or sigmoid colon should not occur from the instrument alone, but attempting to pass the rigid sigmoidoscope in a patient with inflammatory bowel disease, diverticulitis, radiation proctitis, or cancer can sometimes be a hazardous undertaking. Air insufflation can cause perforation of a diverticulum or of a walled-off abscess and, obviously, procedures such as biopsy and electrocoagulation can result in perforation.

### Bacteremia

Bacteremia can be associated with all endoscopic procedures of the lower gastrointestinal tract. Prophylactic antibiotic therapy is recommended for individuals considered at an increased risk, in accordance with the recommendations of the American Heart Association. This includes those who undergo proctosigmoidoscopy with biopsy, flexible sigmoidoscopy with biopsy, colonoscopy, or an anal procedure (e.g., rubber ring ligation of hemorrhoids). The following list illustrates the conditions for which prophylaxis is recommended.

### Cardiac Conditions Requiring Antibiotic Prophylaxis

Prosthetic cardiac valves, including bioprosthetic and homograft valves
Most congenital cardiac malformations
Surgically constructed systemic-pulmonary shunts
Rheumatic and other acquired valvular dysfunction, even after valvular surgery
Hypertrophic cardiomyopathy
Previous bacterial endocarditis, even in the absence of heart disease
Mitral valve prolapse with valvular regurgitation

However, postoperative coronary artery bypass graft surgery is not felt to require prophylactic antibiotic therapy, nor is such a regimen recommended for individuals who have cardiac pacemakers, implanted defibrillators, or physiologic, functional, or innocent heart murmurs.

Standard regimen of prophylactic antibiotic therapy is as follows:

Ampicillin, 2 g (50 mg/kg for children) intramuscularly or intravenously, plus
Gentamicin, 1.5 mg/kg (not to exceed 80 mg/kg) intramuscularly or intravenously (2 mg/kg for children)
Both administered 1/2 hour before the procedure.

For patients allergic to ampicillin, amoxicillin, or penicillin:

Vancomycin, 1 g (20 mg/kg up to 1 g for children) given intravenously slowly over 1 hour, plus gentamicin in the above dosages administered as described. Amoxicillin, 3 g orally 1 hour before procedure; then 1.5 g given 6 hours after initial dose.

### Procedures Performed Through the Sigmoidoscope

Three procedures commonly performed through the rigid proctosigmoidoscope are listed below:

1. Biopsy
2. Fulguration (i.e., electrocoagulation)
3. Snare excision

In recent years, fiberoptic and video-endoscopic procedures have virtually replaced rigid sigmoidoscopic procedures.

### Complications

If bleeding occurs from the pedicle, it may be secured by fulguration, by application of pressure with an epinephrine-soaked chimney sweep, or by the use of a long-armed (i.e., extended) rubber ring ligator (see Chapter 8).

In contrast to closed-system flexible endoscopy, electrocoagulation or snare excision with the open-ended sigmoidoscope does not require a full bowel preparation. Even when an explosive gas mixture may be present, venting should be adequate to prevent proximal bowel injury. However, bowel perforation under such circumstances is a potential hazard, albeit an uncommon one.

## BARIUM ENEMA

### Indications

A barium enema is useful in urgent or emergency circumstances to differentiate between small- and large-bowel obstruction, and acute appendicitis. It also has been successfully used in the therapeutic setting to reduce volvulus and intussusception.

### Preparation

The procedure is essentially a meaningless exercise without adequate preparation. A number of bowel preparations have been recommended, but basically they consist of some dietary restrictions the day before the procedure (e.g., a low-residue diet with a clear, liquid supper), a vigorous laxative, and a suppository or enema the day of the examination.

It is important to maintain adequate hydration when using a stimulant laxative preparation to avoid renal, cardiac, and electrolyte problems, particularly in the elderly.

## Alternatives to the Use of Barium

Water-soluble enemas or double-contrast barium enemas have primarily replaced single-contrast barium enema examinations. Water-soluble solutions of diatrizoate sodium (e.g., Hypaque, Gastrografin) provide reasonable radiopacity; they are nonirritating and relatively well tolerated if accidentally introduced into the peritoneal cavity. Therefore, they are safer in situations such toxic megacolon, peritonitis, and biopsy or snare excision of a polyp within 24 hours. The major limitation is that because of reduced opacification, visualization is sometimes less than adequate. In essence, there are no postevacuation residual results. Hypertonicity is a hazard in another respect; significant alteration in serum electrolytes can occur, especially in children and the elderly. Individuals with cardiac or renal disease are also at increased risk when these agents are used.

### *Double-Contrast or Air-Contrast Barium Enema*

The double-contrast (i.e., air-contrast) barium enema study has been advocated as an improved means of evaluating the colon, identifying small mucosal lesions, and diagnosing inflammatory bowel disease.

With the double-contrast examination, an attempt is made to coat the colon with a thin layer of contrast material and distend the bowel with air so that the entire mucosal circumference is visualized. However, an air-contrast enema has a number of disadvantages. First, the study inevitably results in considerably more radiation exposure; an adequate examination necessitates 10 or 12 overhead films plus several spot films. Second, it requires a cooperative patient who is able to roll around, support his or her own weight, and comprehend instructions. However, despite these concerns, with appropriate care, an air-contrast enema can be accomplished in virtually all individuals.

However, rather than elect the double-contrast approach for neoplasm screening, we almost exclusively use colonoscopy.

### *Complications of Barium Enema Examination*

Complications of barium enema examination, fortunately, are rare. However, when they occur, they can be of catastrophic consequence. A number of complications have been reported, as listed below.

Rectal perforation from enema tip or excessive balloon inflation
Rectal tear or hemorrhage
Colonic perforation
Barium peritonitis
Barium submucosal granuloma
Toxic megacolon
Septicemia
Venous barium embolism
Retrograde gastrointestinal filling with vomiting and aspiration in infants

Idiopathic colonic perforation has been reported to occur in 1 of 5,000 barium enema studies, with barium peritonitis historically associated with at least a 50% mortality rate, although the rate appears to have fallen considerably since the availability of more effective antibiotics and early surgical intervention. Although perforation at the tumor site, diverticulitis, ischemic colitis, and non-specific inflammatory bowel disease are the usual associated circumstances, perforation can occur in an otherwise normal bowel.

The timing of a barium enema examination following biopsy of the rectum or colon has been the subject of considerable debate. Our approach would be to carry on without delay if the biopsy indicates an exophytic lesion to avoid subsequent reexamination. Otherwise, the biopsy is performed after the x-ray study. The discussion, however, is moot, because we always use colonoscopy for proximal bowel evaluation in these circumstances.

### Management of Barium Enema Perforation

When free perforation is recognized, emergency surgical intervention is required. At laparotomy, it is necessary to remove as much of the contaminant as possible, with irrigation and mechanical wiping. Obviously, resection of the perforated segment and a diversionary procedure are mandatory.

Management of the patient with a rectal tear through which barium has extravasated poses a less clear-cut problem. Ultimately, a diversionary procedure may be required; but, depending on the extent of the injury, medical management should be considered, at least initially. Such management should consist of vigorous intravenous fluid replacement, antibiotics, and dietary restriction.

Perforation of the rectum or colon can also occur as a consequence of the double-contrast examination, with extravasation of air, but not necessarily of barium. As clinical signs of peritonitis may not be evident, it has been suggested that asymptomatic patients with radiographic findings of perirectal, mediastinal, or cervical emphysema be managed in the hospital with close observation rather than undergo immediate laparotomy. The success achieved with this approach may be attributable to the fact that the patients generally have undergone a complete bowel cleansing.

## DEFECOGRAPHY

Defecography is a radiologic technique whereby the lower bowel is examined with the patient in the sitting or squatting position in the act of eliminating the barium. The technique and clinical applications of defecography are discussed in Chapters 6, 16, and 17.

## RADIOLOGY OF THE SMALL INTESTINE

Although the small bowel represents 75% of the length and 90% of the mucosal surface of the alimentary tract, the incidence of small-bowel disease is low. Several indications exist for performing a small-bowel examination:

Unexplained gastrointestinal bleeding
Diarrhea or steatorrhea
Unexplained abdominal pain
Fever of unknown origin
The diagnosis of ulcerative colitis or Crohn's colitis

### Technique

Radiologic evaluation is done following an overnight fast. A large volume of barium is especially helpful in interpretation of diffuse lesions of the small bowel. Compression studies are used whenever necessary for better delineation of a lesion, and they are routinely used in demonstrating the terminal ileum. Initially, the patient is examined fluoroscopically, and if the barium meal has progressed sufficiently, a film is taken. Further filming, which depends on the rate of barium passage, is usually done once every 30 to 60 minutes until the material has reached the colon. Typically, in healthy persons, the barium column may take from 2 hours to as long as 6 hours. The terminal ileum must always be compressed. This segment of bowel tends to be hidden by overlapping loops in the pelvis, and because it is so often the site of disease, special study is required. This is obviously particularly true in cases of Crohn's disease.

### Enteroclysis

Enteroclysis involves the use of 250 mL of high-density barium. This is supplemented by methylcellulose, which acts to distend the small intestine. The material is inserted through a nasogastric tube with the tip of the small bowel ideally located at the ligament of Treitz. This permits a study equivalent to that of an air-contrast enema performed in the colon.

Enteroclysis is the most accurate available technique for contrast examination of the small intestine. It should be remembered that this technique is not the best method for evaluation of a problem related to the terminal ileal area.

## EXFOLIATIVE CYTOLOGY

Exfoliative cytology has never gained widespread acceptance, primarily because of the cumbersome methodology and the fact that colonoscopy is a far superior technique for the evaluation of the entire bowel. Unless it can be simplified and the results interpreted with accuracy, exfoliative cytology, in all probability, will become obsolete.

## OCCULT BLOOD DETERMINATION OF STOOL

Occult blood determination is probably the least expensive mass screening technique available for the detection of gastrointestinal pathology.

### Materials and Methods

For at least 48 hours before the collection of the first stool specimen, rare meat, turnips, melons, horseradish, salmon, and sardines must not be ingested. A high-fiber diet is usually advised, but concern has been expressed that the increased fecal weight significantly lowers fecal hemoglobin concentration, with the implication of a false–negative result. Medications such as aspirin and vitamin preparations, especially vitamin C (ascorbic acid) in excess of 250 mg/d, are excluded. Aspirin or other nonsteroidal antiinflammatory drugs should be avoided for 7 days before and during the test period.

The test is commenced on the third day, with the patient taking a sample from the stool and smearing it on the card. Samples from two or three consecutive bowel movements are recommended. In interpreting results, the American Cancer Society recommends that doubtful readings should be recorded as negative and trace readings as positive. A single positive slide is understood to mean that all determinations are positive. With such a conclusion, the physician is obligated to perform in sequential order a digital rectal examination, proctosigmoidoscopy or flexible sigmoidoscopy, and colonoscopy; if results of the colonoscopy are normal, upper gastrointestinal endoscopy and a small-bowel series should follow.

### Test Results

Numerous reports of the beneficial results and cost-effectiveness of mass screening for colorectal cancer have been published (see also Chapter 22).

Most authors believe that ample evidence suggests that occult blood determination of the stool should be an integral part of a complete physical examination, but how much screening reduces mortality is still an unanswered question. This view is being challenged in more recent publications. Increasingly, authors are suggesting that colonoscopy is the most appropriate screening tool and should replace all other modalities. This is being proposed to occur in patients aged between 50 and 60 years. If the colonoscopy is negative, then those patients probably tend not to form polyps and, therefore, probably do not require further bowel screening, as their risk of colorectal cancer is minimal. Whether this view becomes the norm and whether the community as a whole can afford the added cost of this screening is still unknown. The question, of course, remains: how much is a human life worth? We do not pretend to know the answer to that conundrum.

## FECES COLLECTION

Diarrhea and the frequency of infectious enteritis are symptoms requiring that the surgeon be familiar with at least the basic concepts of stool collection.

### Collecting Stool for Culture

The stool sample should arrive in the laboratory within ½ hour of having been taken, unless it is placed in a transport medium. Refrigeration is contraindicated. Swabs should not be used for collection.

Stool cultures are made by placing a sterile swab into the specimen and streaking a portion of several agar plates containing various inhibitory and noninhibitory agents to allow the recovery of both intestinal flora and pathogenic organisms (e.g., *Salmonella, Shigella, Campylobacter* [see Chapter 33]). The plates are examined at 24 hours, and suspect colonies are inoculated into identification media. If *Salmonella* or *Shigella* species are found, a subculture is sent for serologic typing or confirmation.

Certain organisms are somewhat unusual and difficult to identify in a stool specimen. A specific request is usually necessary for their culture because they require special techniques. These organisms include fungi (the test is generally limited to screening for *Candida*), *Mycobacterium*, pathogenic *Vibrio* (i.e., cholera), *Campylobacter*, and *Yersinia*. The discovery of certain organisms mandates reporting to the local public health authority.

### Collecting Stool for Examination for Ova and Parasites

The specimen must be less than 1 hour old when received by the laboratory. Three specimens are recommended for screening over a 5-day period. Collection can be done using a warm saline solution or Fleet enema.

Stool specimens for parasites are examined macroscopically for color and appearance (e.g., formed or liquid, with mucus or blood). They are also checked for adult worms or tapeworm proglottids (see Chapter 33).

A wet-mount preparation of stool on a glass slide with a drop each of saline solution and iodine is cover-slipped and examined microscopically for evidence of parasites (e.g., eggs, cysts, larvae) as well as for fecal leukocytes. A small portion of the specimen is also treated to concentrate the eggs and cysts, and later examined microscopically with wet mounts. Finally, a slide is streaked, trichrome-stained, and examined histologically with the oil immersion lens.

## INTRAVENOUS PYELOGRAPHY

With the frequent preoperative use of computed tomography, the status of the urinary tract is usually adequately appreciated without the need for the intravenous pyelography.

## PHYSIOLOGIC STUDIES

See Chapter 6.

# 5

# Flexible Sigmoidoscopy and Colonoscopy

The ability to visualize the colon, rectum, and anus has essentially paralleled the precision with which the surgeon has been able to diagnose and treat individuals with diseases of this area of the digestive tract. Flexible endoscopy of the colon began with the introduction of semirigid and then flexible upper gastrointestinal instruments (esophagogastroscopy). Subsequently, a major improvement in the quality of light transmission was made with the establishment of a glass-coated fiber, which permitted the transmission of illumination along nonlinear paths. When combined with a similar fiber bundle whose orientation was preserved, the illuminated image could be transmitted back to the observer. Initially, short, flexible fiberoptic instrument examinations of the rectum and distal colon were performed, but soon longer instruments were developed, usually gastroscopes that were applied to the bowel.

The latest advance in instrumentation is videoendoscopy, in which the image-transmitting fiberoptic bundle is replaced by a charged, coupled device (CCD) that provides an electronic image of the field of view. The endoscopist no longer needs to squint into the lens at the end of the instrument, but instead can work directly off of a high-resolution monitor. In addition, the digitized image can be handled like any electronic file: stored, printed, and annotated. This has proved to be a clearly superior method of record keeping and documentation.

## FLEXIBLE FIBEROPTIC SIGMOIDOSCOPY AND VIDEOENDOSCOPY

The term "endoscope" is derived from two Greek words: *endon*, meaning within, and *skopein*, to view. The diameters of the individual glass fibers in the image-conveying aligned bundles are similar, ranging from 9 to 12 μm. In the flexible fiberoptic instruments, the individual fibers are bound together at their ends, whereas the rest of the fibers remain loose and flexible. The fiberoptic endoscope can be made as long as necessary because light loss is negligible over several meters.

Flexible sigmoidoscopy (FS) is not a simple examination to master. The most difficult part of colonoscopy is negotiation of the sigmoid colon, and this problem pertains equally to FS; the only difference, perhaps, is that the physician does not usually have to use various straightening maneuvers, although this should be accomplished if necessary (see *Colonoscopy* section below). The examination requires skill and patience, and no substitute for experience exists.

Real and theoretic disadvantages to this examination include the following:

Cost
　Capital expense and repairs
　Personnel time for enema administration, cleansing
　Duration
Communicable disease
Complications
　Perforation
　Hemorrhage with concomitant procedure
　Explosion with electrocautery
　Compromise of adequate colon examination when colonoscopy is indicated

The use of flexible sigmoidoscopy is indicated in the following situations:

- As a substitute for rigid proctosigmoidoscopy in screening, evaluation of gastrointestinal complaints, and interim polyp and cancer surveillance between colonoscopic examinations
- To evaluate questionable radiologic findings in the sigmoid colon
- To confirm radiographic findings within range of the instrument
- For diagnostic and follow-up evaluation of a patient with inflammatory bowel disease, especially if the disease is confined to the left or distal colon
- To inspect colon anastomosis when it is within range of the instrument

Therapeutically, FS can be used (a) to reduce sigmoid volvulus and (b) in combination with the snare to remove a foreign body. Relative contraindications to this examination include fulminant colitis, toxic megacolon, peritonitis, acute diverticulitis, a poorly prepared bowel, and an uncooperative patient.

## Instrumentation

The specifications of the flexible sigmoidoscope vary somewhat among the manufacturers. Generally, the channel size ranges from 2.6 to 3.8 mm; diameter varies from 12.2 to 14.0 mm; and lengths range from 60 to 71 cm. Biopsy forceps, a cytology brush, or a snare and electrocautery can be passed through the working channel. The tip of the instrument is deflected by rotation of the larger dial in each direction. The smaller dial deflects the tip from side to side. When passing the instrument, it is advantageous to keep the dials in the neutral position as much as possible (see *Colonoscopy Technique*).

## Preparation

The use of FS requires only a limited bowel preparation. Two small enemas (e.g., Fleet) are given separately, the second approximately 10 minutes after the first has been eliminated. Dietary restrictions and oral laxatives are unnecessary.

## *Technique*

The patient is placed in the left lateral (Sims') position on a relatively high examining table. The patient's right leg is flexed more than the left, and the right shoulder is rotated anteriorly. It is usually easier for the physician to stand than to sit. Some physicians prefer a two-person team approach, one to handle the dials and the other to advance the instrument. This approach requires the use of a fiberoptic teaching attachment or videoendoscope. Conversely, many individuals believe that a single person can maneuver the dials with one hand and guide the instrument with the other, thereby permitting a more facile straightening maneuver, which may result in a more comfortable experience for the patient.

A well-lubricated finger is passed into the rectum, and then the instrument is inserted. Passing the blunt-ended FS through the anal canal without prior digital examination is difficult to accomplish and causes considerable apprehension and discomfort for the patient.

While insufflating air rather than redirecting the tip, the examiner passes the instrument to a depth of 10 or 12 cm, which usually permits visualization of the rectal ampulla. If a two-team approach is used, the person who advances the instrument has greater control of the course of the examination than the individual handling the dials.

The instrument is passed with the lumen, either under direct visualization or with the mucosa sliding past. The person on the distal end can judge how firmly to push while watching the mucosa rush by.

If further passage is impeded, the instrument is withdrawn slightly, the lumen is searched out by dial manipulation and rotation, and the instrument is advanced again. Various methods helpful in advancing the instrument have been described: torquing, dithering, and dither-torquing (i.e., accordionization—see later).

Negotiation of the sigmoid colon is the most difficult part of the procedure. If the physician is only able to stretch the colon through attempts at advancement, another maneuver must be tried. Counterclockwise rotation of the instrument produces the alpha loop. Clockwise rotation results in relative straightening of the sigmoid and the opportunity to advance the instrument into the descending colon. Another means of proceeding into the descending colon when the sigmoid loop has already been traversed is to withdraw the instrument while rotating it clockwise.

After the instrument has been passed to its full length or as far as possible, it is carefully and slowly withdrawn. Suction, irrigation, and air insufflation are used alternately, as indicated, to obtain clear visualization of the entire mucosa. It is important to remember that FS and colonoscopy are poor tools for evaluation of ampullary or distal rectal pathology. Particular care is required for examination of this area, and retroflexion is strongly recommended as the final maneuver.

Finally, the physician must not forget why the examination is being performed. If bleeding was the indication, it is not sufficient to reassure the patient that the FS was normal. Furthermore, FS is not the optimal tool for diagnosing pruritus ani, hemorrhoids, or fissure and, obviously, is not the appropriate instrument for evaluating the anal canal. Anoscopy and additional studies may be required.

## Complications

Complications (e.g., hemorrhage or perforation) should not occur with any greater frequency with a flexible than with a rigid instrument. Care obviously is required whenever the procedure is undertaken in the presence of bowel disease, especially active inflammatory disease, diverticulitis, and ischemia. Minimal air should be used under these circumstances. Explosions should not occur, because electrocautery should not be used for biopsy or snare excision with this instrument.

## COLONOSCOPY

In 1969, fiberoptic colonoscopy was introduced as a means of directly visualizing the colon and rectum, and, in many instances, even the terminal ileum. Within a few years, Wolff and Shinya demonstrated that by using a wire loop snare and electrocautery, polyps could be removed through the instrument, thus virtually rendering colotomy and polypectomy obsolete.

## Instrumentation

Instruments are made of varying working lengths, from approximately 115 cm to almost 180 cm. They are forward viewing and have a field of view up to 140°. As with flexible sigmoidoscopy, four-way angulation of the distal end is achieved from approximately 180° (up or down) and 160° (right and left) by manipulating the control knobs. Additional features include an air outlet, a forward water jet channel, and a suction or forceps channel. Air or carbon dioxide can be insufflated and liquid debris removed during the procedure. Accessories include a halogen light source and an electrosurgical unit, as well as photographic equipment. Requisite items for procedures include biopsy forceps, a diathermy snare, and grasping forceps, in addition to an instrument for brush cytology.

## Indications

It is generally agreed that colonoscopy supplements but does not replace the barium enema in the evaluation of colon disorders.

Indications for colonoscopy include the following:

Confirmation or refutation of suspected or equivocal radiologic abnormality (e.g., filling defects, narrowing [intrinsic versus extrinsic lesion], polyps)
Evaluation and follow-up of inflammatory bowel disease (e.g., dysplasia)
Differential diagnosis of diverticular disease or malignancy
Presence of a rectal polyp with or without barium enema abnormality (e.g., synchronous lesion)
Gastrointestinal symptoms (e.g., bleeding, abdominal pain, iron deficiency anemia) with or without radiologic investigation failing to reveal the source
Follow-up evaluation of patient with prior colon surgery
Acute lower gastrointestinal bleeding
Clinically significant diarrhea of unexplained origin
Endoscopic polypectomy
Reduction of sigmoid volvulus
Decompression of dilated colon (e.g., Ogilvie's syndrome)
Intraoperative colonoscopy; confirmation lesion location at time of laparotomy or during laparoscopic procedures

In many instances, the procedure is used either because the barium enema study has demonstrated a probable abnormality or because the barium enema has failed to indicate or identify the source when symptoms suggest colonic disease. Today, however, we feel that most colonoscopic procedures are carried out without the patient having undergone a previous barium enema study.

Diagnostic colonoscopy is generally not appropriate in some cases: (a) chronic, stable, irritable bowel complaints; (b) acute limited diarrhea, when bleeding is readily observed to come from an obvious source (e.g., fissure, hemorrhoids, peptic ulcer); (c) when patient management would be unaffected by the findings (e.g., metastatic carcinoma in the absence of bowel symptoms); and (d) routine screening for someone not at increased risk for malignancy.

Absolute contraindications to this examination are essentially limited to those patients with an acute cardiovascular problem (e.g., myocardial infarction), and those with an acute abdominal inflammation (e.g., peritonitis), acute diverticulitis, fulminant colitis, bowel perforation, and toxic megacolon. Relative contraindications include the last two trimesters of pregnancy, pregnancy at any stage if fluoroscopy is to be used, marked splenomegaly, or an abdominal aortic aneurysm. Patients who may be anemic because of a possible blood dyscrasia should undergo coagulation studies before colonoscopy, and those receiving the anticoagulant sodium warfarin (Coumadin) should have the medication changed to heparin.

## Patient Preparation

For safety and accuracy, a clean colon is required before proceeding with a colonoscopic examination. Formed stool presence can obscure the lumen and lead the endoscopist to apply forces in dangerous ways. Even a minor amount of stool can lead to confusion and misinterpretation.

A number of studies have been published that verify the safety and efficacy of polyethylene glycol (PEG) lavage in preparing a patient for colonoscopy and for barium enema examination, especially if bisacodyl (Dulcolax) is added to ensure evacuation of residual fluid. A volume of 4 L can be administered orally or by tube feedings, which is usually sufficient to produce adequate cleansing. The most frequent complaint about this method of cleansing the bowel, which is the primary drawback, is the discomfort and distaste associated with consumption of such a large quantity of fluid.

We prefer the patient taking Fleet Phospho-Soda (45 mL twice) the day before the examination, with the administration of a Fleet enema the evening before and the morning of the procedure. Fleet Phospho-Soda is not advisable for those individuals with the following conditions: renal failure, ascites, congestive heart failure, a history of myocardial infarction within 6 months, or for those taking a calcium channel blocker (e.g., Procardia, Calan [verapamil]). Hyperphosphatemia and hypocalcemic tetany have been reported in a patient with renal insufficiency.

## Results

A number of studies have been published that compare the various methods used to prepare the patient before colonoscopy: polythylene glycol (PEG), PEG with oral metoclopramide, and oral Fleet Phospho-Soda. Some investigators have found that all regimens were equally effective. However, the Phospho-Soda regimen was better tolerated and more likely to be completed than that of either of the other preparations.

## Sedation and Monitoring

Sedation with monitoring is usually advised whenever total colonoscopy is planned. The insufflation of air or carbon dioxide—the latter is more rapidly absorbed—and traction on the bowel from the instrument can cause considerable discomfort and anxiety. Complete anesthesia, however, is contraindicated. It is important for the examiner to be aware of any excessive discomfort that the patient is experiencing to avoid possible injury to the bowel wall, mesentery, or adjoining structures.

A number of combinations of medications have been advised to reduce discomfort, including sodium pentobarbital (Nembutal), meperidine hydrochloride (Demerol), hydroxyzine hydrochloride (Vistaril), diazepam (Valium), and midazolam (Versed). Care should be taken to avoid respiratory depression and hypotension because elderly patients and those with respiratory and pulmonary difficulties are at particular risk for the development of complications. Monitoring should include heart rate, blood pressure, and respiratory rate before, during, and immediately after the procedure. Pulse oximetry, a method that provides continuous noninvasive measurement of arterial hemoglobin and oxygen saturation, is required whenever conscious sedation is used.

## Antibiotic Prophylaxis

The risk of infective endocarditis or other infectious complications from colonoscopy is low. Still, a risk indeed exists. Recommendations for antibiotic prophylaxis, which are discussed in Chapter 4, are equally applicable to colonoscopy and FS.

## Examination Technique: General Principles

Colonoscopic examination is often viewed by the uninitiated as the process of pushing a tube up into the colon until the cecum is reached. On occasion, particularly in cases of a prior sigmoid resection, it may be almost that simple. However, most examinations require at least a modest amount of manipulation, and many are truly challenging. Furthermore, a clear understanding of colonic anatomy is essential. Each portion of the colon has its individual compliance; successful intubation largely depends on taking advantage of this compliance, as well as overcoming the varied obstacles to passage.

A number of properties of the colonoscope and maneuvers are used for successful intubation. These include tip deflection, shaft torquing, and shaft dithering. These physical movements of the instrument are combined with air insufflation, deflation, patient positioning, and abdominal pressure.

### *Tip Deflection*

The articulating deflection tip is the most critical element in the design of the colonoscope. Deflection permits the endoscopist to look around a bend or fold to see in just which direction the examination needs to proceed. This articulation is essential during therapeutic maneuvers in order to aim a snare or biopsy forceps in the proper direction. In selected instances, the deflection tip can be retroflexed to obtain a clearer view of an obscured area (e.g., the top of the anal canal or the cecal side of the ileocecal valve).

The articulating deflection tip, as essential as it is to facilitating intubation, can at the same time be the single greatest impediment to successful intubation, at least for the inexperienced colonoscopist. It also represents that part of the instrument most responsible for injury. Attempting to increase the deflection to more than 90° in an effort to see around a curve or angle of the bowel profoundly changes the distribution of forces against the colon wall. A greater proportion of the advancing force is distributed against the side wall of the bowel rather than in the forward direction of the lumen. Longitudinal advancement of the scope no longer follows the tip of the instrument. Instead, the deflection bend now becomes the leading edge of the instrument, with forward force transmitted directly to the wall of the colon. As a consequence, blunt or tearing trauma can easily occur.

In summary, use the least amount of deflection necessary to acquire the desired view. Limiting deflection to the use of the up-down dial only, while abjuring the simultaneous application of both controls, is helpful for minimizing inappropriate deflection.

### *Shaft Torquing*

Torquing is an essential maneuver for effective intubation as well as for optimal surface visualization during extubation. Shaft torquing can produce three major effects. When left-handed or counterclockwise torque is applied, there is a tendency to produce a loop in the redundant sigmoid colon. Second, if clockwise torque is applied, the sigmoid colon tends to straighten. The third effect is produced at the tip of the scope. When the shaft is torqued in either direction in the presence of modest tip deflection, strong leverage is transmitted toward the entrance to the more proximal bowel. Using torque with modest tip deflection is generally more effective in locating an elusive proximal segment than holding the shaft rigid while manipulating the deflection tip alone.

If the scope is relatively straight, the torque will transmit nearly 1 to 1 to the viewing lens of the instrument. However, if the scope shaft is within one or more loops, the results of torquing will have a much more profound effect on the bowel than on what is perceived through the viewing end of the instrument. If a so-called "alpha loop" is present in the sigmoid colon, the effect of clockwise torquing (especially when combined with shaft withdrawal) is to reduce that loop by "accordionizing" the bowel onto the scope. However, once reduced, the sigmoid loop will have a tendency to re-form, particularly if counterclockwise torque is applied during subsequent scope advancement. Therefore, to maintain reduction of a redundant sigmoid loop, the instrument must be advanced while the clockwise torque is maintained.

Occasionally, an extremely redundant sigmoid colon will develop two complete loops during intubation. Nearly always both are reducible. However, unlike the single loop configuration, remove the first loop by counterclockwise rotation and the second by clockwise rotation. Removing both loops is usually essential before proximal intubation into the descending colon can be accomplished.

Torque is also an important maneuver in manipulations in the area of the hepatic flexure. If the transverse colon is held in the upper abdomen, the scope takes a straight line to the hepatic flexure. At this point, clockwise torque is usually beneficial, as the gently deflected tip is directed down the ascending colon. Conversely, if the transverse colon is redundant, stretching down toward the pelvis, the hepatic flexure is then approached from below. When the ascending colon is viewed in this situation, a sharp deflection of the tip occurs. Once again, gentle scope withdrawal, along with clockwise torquing and intermittent desufflation, all combine to broaden the hepatic flexure and to drop the instrument into the ascending colon and cecum.

During extubation, as the instrument is withdrawn, the right hand is maintained on the shaft to apply torque. The left hand supports the scope head with the thumb free to move the up-down control. By combining back-and-forth torque with simultaneous small tip deflections, the colon surface can be continuously examined with minimal risk of overlooking lesions. This permits the colon that has been accordionized onto the scope to be dropped off, a bit at a time. If, rather than torquing, the instrument is simply withdrawn while using both hands of the dial controls, the view behind prominent folds is likely to be inadequate. Furthermore, if the colon is redundant, the bowel will likely fly off the scope at an uncontrollable rate.

### *Advancement or Withdrawal ("Dithering")*

When instrument progression is unimpeded by severe tip deflection, a redundant colon can be encouraged to accordionize along its length. This is most likely to occur if the scope is repeatedly advanced and withdrawn, a process referred to as "dithering." When combined with torquing in the sigmoid or descending colon, short dithering strokes can often reduce sigmoid redundancy as the scope is advanced, thereby avoiding the creation of a full loop. In less-tethered segments (e.g., with a redundant transverse colon), it is often advantageous to perform long (30 to 50 cm) dithering strokes to accordionize the excess bowel onto a limited segment of instrument.

### *Gas Insufflation*

Insufflation of gas is essential for effective visualization during colonoscopy. However, excess gas can lead to abdominal distention that results in severe discomfort and a possible vasovagal reaction. This works against the process of intubation, particularly at a flexure or when a redundant loop is being negotiated. Gas distention pushes the proximal end of the loop or flexure away from the end of the scope. As a consequence, the angle becomes more acute and, therefore, more difficult to pass. Conversely, when air is aspirated, the bowel is shortened. Concomitant torquing facilitates this maneuver.

### *Patient Position and Abdominal Pressure*

Although no single ideal position exists, the construction of most endoscopes and the right-handedness of most physicians tend to favor the patient assuming the left lateral position. Those with a colostomy or ileostomy may be more comfortable in either the lateral or supine position. In patients with poor abdominal wall muscle tone (e.g., paraplegia, large hernia, prior dehiscence), examination in the prone position may be helpful.

If forward progress stalls during the examination, it is often beneficial to change positions. This maneuver not only alters the relationship of the instrument to the colon, but it also redistributes organ pressures within the abdominal cavity. External pressure can be beneficial. In particular, pressure from just to the right of the umbilicus and directed toward the left iliac fossa will discourage sigmoid looping. Similarly, central abdominal pressure will help keep the redundant transverse colon from dropping deeply into the pelvis.

## General Approach

Before actually starting the procedure, it is important to check that the instrument is in proper working order. This includes such basic maneuvers as switching on the suction and ensuring that the line is attached. Air insufflation and lens washing are tested. The deflection tip should be maximally flexed and examined for both the degree of deflection and integrity of the covering surface. Ensure that the dial controls are maintained in the unlocked position.

Some endoscopists prefer to use a two-person approach to colonoscopy: one handles the dial-control housing while an assistant advances and torques the shaft. Others use a single operator technique. The expert colonoscopist should be able to perform an expeditious and thorough examination by avoiding the formation of bowel loops that interfere with advancement. The colonoscopist can detect the subtle clues that indicate that a loop is starting to form: the loss of the one-to-one correspondence of instrument insertion to image movement; a gradual increase in resistance to forward motion; and signs of patient discomfort. As mentioned, instrument withdrawal often facilitates subsequent passage. Advancement of the scope should nearly always be under direct vision. The "slide-by" technique, whereby the viewing tip is partially buried in the colon wall, should be avoided. Although it is often necessary to accept less than a totally clear view, insertion when blind to lumen orientation is strongly discouraged. Be aware of the possibility of causing injury if the colonic mucosa blanches or if the patient experiences pain.

### *Fluoroscopy*

Although not required for most examinations, fluoroscopy can be invaluable for difficult cases. When previous examinations have been inadequate or confusion exists to the anatomy and lesion locations, consider fluoroscopic guidance.

### *Electronic Imaging*

Real time electromagnetic imaging has been applied as an aid to colonoscopy. By this means, three sets of generator coils are placed beneath the endoscopy table, producing pulsed, low-strength electromagnetic fields outside of the patient. These fields are detected by a series of sensor coils positioned at 12-cm intervals along the length of a catheter that is inserted down the biopsy channel of the colonoscope. From the electrical signal produced in the sensor coil, the exact position and orientation of each coil can be calculated. This modality is not in general use at present.

## Sedation

Without sedation, colonoscopy of the entire colon can be an intolerably painful experience, thereby precluding a comprehensive evaluation. We prefer to initiate the examination after administering a small intravenous dose of demerol and midazolam (Versed), which can be supplemented, if necessary, depending on the patient's sensory and physiologic reactions. Do not strive to avoid medication but rather to provide a safe and reasonably comfortable examination for the patient (see previous discussion).

## Performing the Examination

### Rectal Examination

A digital rectal examination is a requisite initial step for every patient. As discussed in Chapter 4, it is not unusual to find important pathology (e.g., large hemorrhoids, an anal fissure, or a prostatic nodule or anorectal mass). Furthermore, extrarectal lesions cannot be identified by the instrument alone. Digital examination also permits the examiner to gauge anal sphincter tone. Finally, the examiner's finger prepares the patient for the subsequent instrument insertion.

### Anorectal Intubation

Because the anus has been prelubricated with jelly during the digital examination, only a light coating need be placed along the shaft. Care should be taken to avoid the application of lubricant to the lens, because it is not easily removed by the cleansing water jet. The tip should be gently guided through the anal canal at an angle by using the index finger to support the flexible end. Once the tip of the scope has been inserted approximately 10 cm above the anal verge, tip deflection will respond properly, and the middle and upper rectum can be readily visualized with adequate insufflation.

### Sigmoid Intubation

Once the rectosigmoid has been reached, the stage is set for sigmoid intubation. With the instrument tip positioned in the rectosigmoid, take the control section with the left hand while positioning the right hand on the shaft. Tip deflection is managed virtually exclusively by rotation of the larger up-down control, using the thumb from beneath the control housing. This keeps the index or middle finger free to operate the suction or air insufflation.

### Sigmoid-Descending Colon Intubation

While holding the control housing with the left hand, use the right hand to firmly grasp the shaft no more than 10 to 15 cm from the anus. A conscious effort is made to avoid bringing the right hand up to the dial controls, as this prevents the examiner from using the effective maneuver of simultaneous deflection and torquing. By keeping the hand on the shaft close to the anus, the instrument can be better controlled and less tendency exists to simply push excess scope into the colon.

The three methods of traversing the sigmoid colon are intubation by elongation, looping (alpha maneuver), and accordionization ("dither-torquing"). By using these principles, the operator can more deliberately and effectively control the process of intubation.

### Intubation by Elongation

Intubation by elongation merely refers to the process by which the instrument is inserted until either no apparent place is found to go or no more scope is left. Indeed, this is probably the most commonly used approach when one performs flexible sigmoidoscopy. If the sigmoid is minimally redundant, the examiner may have a reasonably straight shot through the sigmoid and descending colon to the level of the splenic flexure. However, if a redundant sigmoid colon is present, another maneuver is usually required.

### Intubation by Looping (Alpha Maneuver)

The relatively mobile sigmoid colon is fixed proximally at the descending colon junction and distally at the rectum. In contrast to simple advancement, counterclockwise torque with gentle tip deflection stretches the mid-sigmoid first in a ventral direction and then toward the right lower quadrant of the abdomen. As the scope is advanced using continuous counterclockwise torque, it courses back across the upper pelvis to the sigmoid–descending colon junction. This intentionally created broad curve flattens the angle at the sigmoid–descending colon junction into a gentle curve. Once the tip of the scope has passed to the level of the mid-descending colon, reduction can be undertaken, to remove the loop, while clockwise torque is applied. Then, the scope can be readily advanced to the splenic flexure by maintaining clockwise torque during advancement of the shaft. This is an efficient technique for negotiating a moderately redundant sigmoid colon if multiple tightly adherent loops are absent.

### Intubation by Accordionization ("Dither-Torquing")

When the colon segment to be intubated is not a "straight shot" or if unable to create a large, gentle loop, it is often best to use a "dither-torquing" approach. This method attempts to straighten a tightly nested colon as the scope is advanced. In this approach, try to accordionize as much colon as possible onto a limited length of instrument.

The technique, as mentioned above, uses simultaneous application of both "dithering" and "torquing."

### *Splenic Flexure and Transverse Colon Intubation*

If the sigmoid colon has been "accordionized" onto the scope and is straightened into a gentle, smooth curve, it is usually not difficult to negotiate the splenic flexure. The deflection tip is rotated into the distal transverse colon, but be aware of the hazard of creating an excessive deflection bend. Once the instrument has been passed to the level of the mid-transverse colon, this splenic flexure loop can generally be removed with a counterclockwise rotation.

Advancing the colonoscope through the transverse colon is usually uneventful. This part of the colon is distinguished by its well-defined triangular appearance. If the transverse colon is without redundancy, the intubation will proceed directly across the upper abdomen to the hepatic flexure. Redundancy of the transverse colon can result in a loop that has the configuration of the Greek letter gamma when viewed by fluoroscopy. This loop is optimally removed by clockwise rotation of the shaft before attempting to proceed into the ascending colon. Once this has been accomplished, it will usually stay derotated. If the transverse colon is redundant, the "dither-torquing" technique can also be used when progress is impeded.

## Hepatic Flexure and Ascending Colon

The hepatic flexure is often recognized by a bluish discoloration of the wall where the liver is in close proximity.

If the transverse colon has been negotiated straight across, or straight down from a high splenic flexure, then intubation into the ascending colon is usually accomplished by clockwise torque, flattening of the deflection tip, and simultaneous gas aspiration. These three mechanisms combine to drop the scope into the cecum. If the transverse colon is excessively redundant, it may not be able to be maintained in the upper abdomen, even if abdominal pressure is applied. The instrument, therefore, approaches the hepatic flexure from below rather than from across. Inevitably, the deflection tip will require a 180° bend to negotiate this area. Repeated efforts of clockwise torque and gas aspiration are usually required to progressively gather more colon onto the instrument, and finally drop the scope into the ascending colon and cecum.

Finally, if negotiation of the hepatic flexure continues to be a problem, changing the position is often beneficial. Initially, the patient should be rotated to the prone position. If this is not helpful, the right lateral decubitus position should be attempted.

## Cecum and Distal Ileum Intubation

The most reliable landmarks for visual confirmation of reaching the cecum are as follows:

- Appendiceal orifice
- Triangulation of the tinea

- Ileocecal valve
- Intubation of the distal ileum

Palpation of the right lower quadrant with concomitant movement of the colon endoscopically, as well as transillumination of the abdominal wall in the right iliac fossa, are less dependable signs. Fluoroscopy is helpful, but keep in mind that the cecum is not always in the right iliac fossa. Clearly, the least reliable indicator that the cecum has been reached is the "impression" that no colon remains. If the usual landmarks of an ileocecal location are not present and there seems to be no remaining colon, the endoscopist has probably stretched a more proximal segment into a blind recess (e.g., the proximal transverse colon).

Sometimes it is important to intubate the distal ileum, especially in the evaluation of an individual with inflammatory bowel disease. The success rate for accomplishing this maneuver increases with experience and is generally reported to be in the range of 80%.

When intubation of the distal ileum is indicated, recognize that the entrance is at an angle that is less than 90° to the axis of the ascending colon. This angle is made even more acute because of the caudad displacement of the cecum produced by air insufflation when complete colon intubation has been accomplished. The tip of the instrument must be positioned on the cecal side of the valve. The deflection tip is then angled toward the valve, prying the orifice open as the shaft is slightly withdrawn. A combination of torquing and suction usually directs the scope into the terminal ileum. The mucosal surface is recognized by its roughened, ground-glass appearance. This is in contrast to the smooth texture of the distended, adjacent cecum.

## Withdrawal and Examination

Inspection of the colon should be a smooth and continuous process. If the instrument is simply withdrawn, the accordionized colon will fly off the end of the scope in an uncontrolled fashion at various points along the way. Hidden areas behind folds will go unexamined. Expeditious withdrawal, therefore, usually results in a poor evaluation of the colon.

Sometimes, muscular spasm or irritability of the colon interferes with optimal visualization during withdrawal. This problem can sometimes be ameliorated by administering glucagon (1 mg) intravenously. However, this is not effective when the underlying impediment is caused by a fibrotic stricture or bowel wall thickening associated with diverticulitis.

Examination of the colon during extubation is most efficiently performed by keeping the right hand on the shaft while controlling tip deflection with the left hand. The view of the lumen can be continuously readjusted while the shaft is being withdrawn. The inner aspects of the proximal side of both the hepatic and splenic flexures are areas that must be carefully dropped from the scope to avoid missing what can be large lesions.

## Cleansing the Instrument

In the United States, government regulation through the Centers for Disease Control and Prevention has produced a number of recommendations for instrument cleansing. Vigorous mechanical cleansing using an enzymatic detergent immediately after the procedure, followed by a disinfectant and thorough rinsing, is considered the most effective method. Likewise, the channels should be cleansed and air dried. Ultrasonic sterilizers, scope washers, and automatic computer programmed disinfectors have been developed to reduce the possibility of toxic effects to the patient and to the personnel who handle the chemicals. Companies, products, and concepts continue to evolve in this area.

It is important to note that following disinfection the instruments should be thoroughly washed with plain water. A type of chemical colitis—a complication believed to be caused by contamination of the air–water channel with potentially toxic cleansing chemicals—has been observed in a number of individuals.

## Therapeutic Colonoscopy

### *Indications*

Probably the primary indication for the use of colonoscopy as a therapeutic tool is for polypectomy or biopsy. Therapeutic colonoscopy is also indicated for treatment of bleeding lesions (e.g., vascular anomalies, ulcerations, tumors, and bleeding at the polypectomy site). Additional applications include decompression of cecal and sigmoid volvulus, colonic decompression in Ogilvie's syndrome, foreign body removal, balloon dilatation of stricture, and palliative treatment of stenosing or bleeding malignant lesions.

### *Equipment*

Performance of polypectomy requires an electrical generating power source that, for endoscopic use, is transmitted by means of a wire loop snare or coagulating electrode. Polypectomy is undertaken through the accessory channel of the instrument.

Gas insufflation during polypectomy is a matter of particular concern because of the potential hazard of an explosive mixture being present. Consequently, adequate bowel preparation is essential. Frühmorgen reported no instance of gas explosion using standard methods of bowel preparation in more than 2,700 colonoscopy–polypectomy procedures.

Many cold and hot biopsy forceps, snares, baskets, and hooks for retrieval are commercially available to perform polypectomy. Shapes include oval, eccentric, and hexagonal.

The laser, an acronym for light amplification by stimulated emission of radiation, produces an intense monochromatic light that can destroy tissue to varying depths of penetration. The argon laser is considered most useful for treating mucosal lesions, because energy from this source penetrates only 1 mm of tissue; the Nd-YAG laser is better for deep and exophytic lesions, because it penetrates 3 to 4 mm of tissue. Optical fibers have been produced to fit through the open channel of most endoscopic instruments. Lasers have been used most effectively in the treatment of angiodysplastic lesions, but have also been applied to benign and malignant tumors, as well as to a variety of anatomic abnormalities.

### *Technique*

Maintaining adequate visualization and holding instrument position is essential to the performance of a polypectomy. By maneuvering the tip of the colonoscope and sometimes the patient, the wire loop can be advanced and the head of the polyp encircled. Small lesions can be removed simply with the biopsy instrument. The loop is drawn down to the pedicle until the latter is secured. The endoscope is then maneuvered to hold the polyp away from the bowel wall to avoid injury and possible perforation. The current is then applied and the polyp excised. It can then be removed using forceps, a hook or basket, or suction. When other polyps are present, they can be removed individually or collected by straining the stool over the ensuing hours. Pathologic confirmation is required.

Large polyps (i.e., those >2.5 cm) can be removed by the above-described technique if adequate visualization of the pedicle is possible and the head can be ensnared. Failing this, however, it can be removed piecemeal, and the specimens collected as described. Sometimes it is helpful to elevate a sessile polyp above the plane of the colon wall by injecting saline into the submucosa. This provides greater separation between the muscularis propria and the polyp base. In addition, the improved tissue hydration facilitates electrocoagulation. Even with the increased possibility of perforation, a properly informed patient may be well served by colonoscopy–polypectomy even if operative intervention occasionally is required for a complication (see *Complications*). The bowel is well prepared, and morbidity and mortality should be low. Colotomy, polypectomy, or more usually, resection, are reserved for lesions too large to be removed via the endoscope.

The proper application of electrocautery is essential for safe and effective polypectomy. No single combination of cutting and coagulation current or wattage must be used or is preferred. The general approach favored by many uses short bursts of monopolar, blended, cutting current while squeezing the snare. By using intermittent bursts, deep tissue cooling is permitted, thereby minimizing the likelihood of a full-thickness burn.

Malignant polyps, even if technically removable at colonoscopy, may require a subsequent resection (see Chapter 22). Such lesions are unlikely to be palpable at the time of operation. Accurate localization is important, particularly if intraluminal landmarks are absent and fluoroscopic control is unavailable. Some have advised the performance of a localizing preoperative barium enema. An alternative is to place a clip on the lesion using a plane abdominal radiograph for localization. An injection of particulate India ink or charcoal suspension, applied submucosally with a sclerotherapy needle, will persist indefinitely and allow identification of the dye on the serosal aspect at the time of laparotomy.

### *Results*

Shinya and Wolff report no mortality in their experience in endoscopically removing 7,000 polyps. Most series report approximately two thirds of the lesions as adenomatous polyps (i.e., tubular adenomas), a few as villous adenomas, and the remainder as malignant tumors, other benign neoplasms, and nonneoplastic conditions. The significance of polyps, their distribution, and the follow-up of patients are discussed in Chapter 21.

### Complications

The sheer volume of examinations that have been performed since the introduction of colonoscopy has resulted in a broad spectrum of complications from both diagnostic as well as therapeutic endeavors. The following table lists the complications of colonoscopy and colonoscopy–polypectomy:

- Hemorrhage caused by intraluminal or mesenteric injury, seromuscular tear, splenic trauma
- Perforation
- Retroperitoneal abscess
- Retroperitoneal and mediastinal emphysema
- Pneumoscrotum
- Pneumothorax
- Explosion
- Postcolonoscopy distention
- Postpolypectomy coagulation syndrome
- Colonic obstruction
- Loss of polyp
- Volvulus
- Bacteremia
- Infections
- Medical problems (e.g., pulmonary, cardiovascular, renal)
- Mechanical failure

### *Hemorrhage*

Bleeding is the most common complication following polypectomy. Hemorrhage can also be caused by biopsy, laceration of the mucosa by the instrument, or tearing of the mesentery or the splenic capsule. At particularly high risk are those who take salicylates regularly, are on therapeutic warfarin (coumadin), or have other bleeding disorders. Familiarity with the electrical equipment, the use of coagulating current, and the clinical experience of the endoscopist reduce the risk of hemorrhage. The endoscopist should be especially cautious when attempting removal of a polyp with a thick pedicle. In such circumstances, many experienced endoscopists suggest using blended current (i.e., coagulation with cutting). Intermittent application offers the best control and most likely helps avoid precipitous transection. By alternately loosening and tightening the snare during the course of current application, a controlled division of the pedicle can be achieved more effectively.

Deciding how to manage the problem of bleeding depends on the magnitude of the hemorrhage. If bleeding is recognized at the time of polypectomy, the area should be resnared (if the pedicle is still apparent) and strangulated for at least 5 minutes. Electrocautery should not be used, particularly if no pedicle is present. If the area is within reach of the rigid proctosigmoidoscope, it can be controlled by one of the means suggested in Chapter 4. In-hospital observation is mandatory if control has not been established with certainty, and operative intervention may be necessary if the bleeding persists. Symptoms include the usual signs of hemorrhage (e.g., weakness, syncope, pallor, hypotension, and tachycardia), but abdominal pain and distention as well as left shoulder pain may also be observed. A falling hematocrit is obviously ominous. The greatest aid to an early diagnosis is the knowledge that this complication can indeed occur.

To manage these patients, some authors recommend that technetium-tagged red blood cell scintigraphy may be used to identify those individuals who have ongoing bleeding and in whom additional invasive and possibly therapeutic procedures (e.g., arteriography or repeat endoscopy) are warranted in an attempt to avoid surgical intervention. However, most surgeons believe resection of the identified portion of bowel is a better therapeutic option than performing further investigations that do not alter the management.

### Perforation

Perforation of the colon with pneumoperitoneum usually becomes manifest almost immediately or within a few hours following the procedure. The incidence of perforation has been reported to range from 0.03% to 0.65% for diagnostic colonoscopies and from 0.073% to 2.1% for therapeutic endoscopies. Perforation is usually caused by polypectomy, disease in the colon (e.g., diverticulitis), or vigorous manipulation, rotation, or angulation of the instrument. Overdistension with air or gas can also precipitate a perforation.

The classic presentations of transmural burn are fever, localized abdominal pain, tenderness, focal peritoneal signs, distention, and leukocytosis. Again, inpatient treatment is required. Occasionally, the patient's symptoms may be minimal relative to the amount of gas that is apparent on abdominal roentgenogram. Nonsurgical management may be considered reasonable under the following circumstances:

• Stable condition
• Late diagnosis

- Good bowel preparation
- Pneumoperitoneum not expanding
- No evidence of peritonitis
- No distal obstruction
- Improvement with supportive care
- Absence of underlying pathology that would demand ultimate resection

Frequent follow-up evaluation is required. The patient should be kept from oral intake; intravenous fluid replacement and broad-spectrum antibiotics are advisable. A limited Gastrografin enema may also be considered in the equivocal situation (see Chapter 4).

Laparotomy should be undertaken if the patient exhibits signs and symptoms of peritonitis. Furthermore, surgery is most definitely indicated in the presence of a large perforation demonstrated either colonoscopically or radiographically and in the setting of generalized peritonitis or ongoing sepsis. Any concomitant pathology present at the time of the perforation (e.g., a large sessile polyp that may be malignant, intractable colitis, or a perforation proximal to a colonic lesion) that inevitably will require surgery may force the physician to recommend immediate operation. Fever and leukocytosis alone or in combination are not necessarily absolute indications for surgical intervention, but the burden of responsibility falls on the surgeon for unwarranted delay. A perforation that has sealed or even a negative laparotomy should not evoke criticism.

When a perforation is recognized shortly following the endoscopy, the hole or tear usually can be closed primarily without the need for a diversionary procedure if the bowel has been well prepared. If a resection is considered advisable, it can be safely undertaken without the need for proximal colostomy or ileostomy unless sepsis or gross contamination is observed.

It has generally been observed that perforations from therapeutic colonoscopy occur by a different mechanism than from diagnostic colonoscopy and may be selectively managed without an operation. Usually, perforations from diagnostic colonoscopy result in larger defects, and these are much more likely to require operative management.

The risk of perforation is greatly reduced if intermittent bursts of current are applied, which reduces the risk of more extensive tissue injury, a consequence of transfer of heat into the deeper tissues or of contact of the polyp head with the bowel wall. When possible, an attempt should be made to suspend the polyp within the intestinal lumen during electrosurgical removal.

Subcutaneous, retroperitoneal, and mediastinal emphysema, as well as pneumoscrotum and pneumothorax, have been reported after colonoscopy. These presentations do not necessarily constitute indications for surgical exploration (i.e., free perforation of the colon is not implied). With retroperitoneal gas, nonsurgical treatment should be the initial approach. In fact, as suggested earlier, close observation with antibiotic administration may be reasonably considered even with a pneumoperitoneum.

### Explosion

Explosion should not occur in a well-prepared colon. The use of an inert gas (e.g., carbon dioxide) has been advocated by some, but is probably an unnecessary caution. The examiner should be wary of using electric current if dissatisfied with the adequacy of the bowel preparation.

### Postcolonoscopy Distention

A postcolonoscopy syndrome has been described, manifested by abdominal distention, discomfort, and dilated loops of bowel on the roentgenogram. Patients do not exhibit signs of peritonitis. Treatment consists of observation and medical management.

### Postpolypectomy Coagulation Syndrome

The patient with postpolypectomy coagulation syndrome may develop localized signs of peritonitis, pain, fever, and leukocytosis without evidence of perforation being seen on radiologic examination. The condition is believed to be caused by transmural thermal injury of the bowel at the site of the polypectomy. Treatment may require inpatient observation, intravenous fluid therapy, and broad-spectrum antibiotics.

### Obstruction and Hernia Incarceration

Colonic obstruction can be precipitated by colonoscopy, usually at the site of underlying sigmoid disease. Volvulus has also been reported, possibly secondary to the alpha maneuver or to overinsufflation of air. Incarceration of the colonoscope in an inguinal hernia that would not permit reduction of the hernia or removal of the instrument has been reported, along with the technique for extraction.

### Loss of Polyp

All removed polyps should be submitted for histologic examination. Those less than 8 mm in diameter may be suctioned through the accessory channel of the colonoscope with the aid of a mucus trap. If the polyp cannot be removed by the standard methods of suctioning onto the tip of the instrument or snare recapture, an enema must be administered. The polyp is then evacuated with the fluid into a bedpan. Unfortunately, despite all reasonable efforts, the polyp is sometimes not recovered.

### Bacteremia

Bacteremia has been reported to be associated with colonoscopy, but other studies have failed to confirm this observation. Routine antibiotic prophylaxis is indicated for the patient at high risk (e.g., valvular heart disease, valve prosthesis; see Chapter 4).

### Medical Problems

Hypotension, bradycardia, tachycardia, and myocardial infarction have all been observed during and after colonoscopy.

### Mechanical Failure

Numerous problems can develop from malfunction of the instruments and accessories (e.g., breakage of the colonoscope with entrapment of the instrument). Defective electrical equipment and inexperience with its use are two of the most common reasons for polypectomy hemorrhage and bowel wall necrosis. The snare wire can break or become fused with the polyp. Incomplete division of the pedicle can occur with the snare completely closed.

### Summary

Despite the long list of complications, colonoscopy and colonoscopy–polypectomy can be undertaken with low morbidity and rare mortality–certainly lower mortality than may be anticipated after operative intervention.

## Special Situations

### Foreign-Body Removal

The problems of removal of foreign bodies inserted into the rectum or ingested are addressed in Chapter 15. The colonoscope has been successfully employed for such extractions.

### Volvulus

Colonoscopy has been successfully applied to the treatment of sigmoid volvulus. Although rigid proctosigmoidoscopy is more readily available and easier to use, an occasional situation arises when an attempt at reduction with a colonoscope may be indicated. The diagnosis and therapy of volvulus is discussed in Chapter 28.

### Intraoperative Colonoscopy

Intraoperative colonoscopy may be considered in several situations:

- When prior conventional colonoscopy has been unsuccessful
- To evaluate the remainder of the colon when a partial resection is contemplated

- To avoid contamination when an unsuspected polyp is found during a "clean" operation
- To localize the site of a lesion or prior excision site, particularly if contemplating laparoscopic resection
- To complement arteriography in the diagnosis of the source of gastrointestinal hemorrhage

Ideally, the patient is placed in the perineolithotomy position as if for combined abdominoperineal resection of the rectum. The abdominal surgeon guides the instrument through the bowel, thus expediting the procedure.

### *Pediatric Colonoscopy*

Pediatric colonoscopy can be performed with a narrow caliber endoscope or with the standard instrument, depending on the age of the patient. A general anesthetic is usually recommended for infants and young children. Preparation in infants usually consists of a clear liquid diet for 24 hours, but a laxative is usually advised for older children. The most common indications for use of the procedure in children is to evaluate rectal bleeding, and in cases of suspected polyps, inflammatory bowel disease, and congenital anomalies. Colonoscopy is not useful in the evaluation of children with constipation and isolated recurrent abdominal pain.

As a standard part of pediatric colonoscopy, emphasis is placed on intubating the terminal ileum because of its importance in the evaluation of Crohn's disease.

### BARIUM ENEMA VERSUS COLONOSCOPY

Generally speaking, most agree that colonoscopy is more successful in detecting small excrescences than is a barium enema examination, even with optimal preparation and double-contrast technique. Furthermore, colonoscopy is recommended as the primary colonic evaluation for individuals with occult or obvious blood in the stool. Some investigators even recommend it as part of a complete physical examination for asymptomatic, Hemoccult-negative men aged more than 50 years.

Most physicians who discover and remove a polyp at the time of proctosigmoidoscopy move directly to total colonoscopy rather than to barium enema or air-contrast enema. The need for a "road map" of the colon is no longer felt to be a requisite.

Protocols have been developed for follow-up evaluation of patients with rectal polyps (see Chapter 21), all involving the use of colonoscopy. In fact, we use barium enema exclusively for evaluation of patients in whom a neoplasm is not suspected (e.g., extrinsic lesion or compression, diverticular disease, as part of physiologic assessment, concomitant with defecography), although a computed tomography scan should certainly be considered if an extramural or mass lesion is suspected.

# 6

# Setting Up a Colorectal Physiology Laboratory

Assessing and testing the function of the colon and anorectum have become an increasingly popular exercise during the last decade. This has not simply advanced our understanding of the complex physiology but has also provided diagnostic information necessary for the optimal management of many conditions. Outlined in this chapter are the choices of equipment available to examine the colon and anorectum, with discussions of the advantages and disadvantages of each, to enable clinicians to make informed decisions regarding which equipment to purchase when setting up a laboratory.

No single test can adequately define the status of the anorectum in either health or disease. Accurate diagnosis depends on the integration of an adequate history and clinical examination as well as physiologic investigations.

## MANOMETRY

Anorectal manometry is an objective method used to assess anal muscular tone, rectal compliance, and anorectal sensation, and to verify the integrity of the rectoanal inhibitory reflex. Although several methods are available for obtaining and analyzing this information, no single method is universally accepted. Regardless of the method chosen, it is imperative to perform manometry in a precise and reproducible manner and to clearly define the parameters to be measured.

### Indications

Manometry has been widely used in patients with fecal incontinence to (a) identify the presence of sensory or muscular defects; (b) document sphincter function before procedures that can affect continence or require optimal continence (e.g., colonic or ileal pouch-anal anastomosis); and, possibly, (c) help in the evaluation of chronic constipation.

## Patient Preparation

The following factors are common to the performance of all static manometric examinations. The use of enemas to clear the rectum prior to the study is somewhat controversial. The purpose and nature of the procedure should be explained to the patient to allay any anxiety. It should be emphasized that anorectal manometry is painless. Examinations should be performed in the left lateral decubitus position with the patient's hips flexed to as near 90° as is comfortable. During the acquisition of the data, patients should be discouraged from excessive talking or motion, which can introduce artifact into the recording.

## Anorectal Manometry Systems

Three basic types of systems are used to perform manometric examinations: air- or water-filled balloon systems, water perfusion systems, and solid-state microtransducer systems.

### *Air- or Water-Filled Balloons*

In air- or water-filled balloon systems, fluid- or air-filled balloons are placed within the anus and rectum and then connected to transducers via small catheters.

This system is relatively simple and, therefore, can be performed by one operator. The presence of the rectoanal inhibitory reflex and information on rectal sensitivity and compliance can be reasonably obtained. Only determinations of the global resting and squeeze pressures of the anal canal can be obtained, however.

### *Water-Perfused Systems*

Water-perfused systems function by creating an artificial cavity between the anus and the catheter. As perfusion continues, full capacity is reached. Thereafter, fluid leaks into the rectal ampulla or out of the anus. The pressure required to overcome initial resistance after the space is filled is termed the *yield pressure*. As the pressure in the anal canal increases, the mucosa is brought into contact with the catheter ports, thereby impeding the flow of water. The yield pressure then becomes the pressure required to overcome this obstruction. This information is then transmitted via nondistensible capillary tubing to transducers that convert this pressure to electrical signals.

Water perfusion systems provide much reproducible data about the status of the anal sphincters and rectum. The one limitation is that they require the patient to be in the lateral decubitus position, which precludes ambulatory study.

### *Equipment*

#### *Catheters*

Catheters vary according to rigidity, diameter, and number and location of the ports. The external diameter should be 4 to 8 mm in order to minimize distortion of the anal canal. The number of lumens and ports ranges from 2 to 8 and they can be arranged either radially or longitudinally in a spiral fashion at 5- to 8-mm intervals. Additional ports for assessment of pressures inside rectal balloons can also be included.

### Withdrawal Motor

Unlike balloon catheters, withdrawal motors are designed to measure pressures along the whole length of the anal canal. Some investigators prefer a manual pull-through technique that can be performed by a skilled technician. However, the retraction rate is standarized more easily by using a withdrawal motor that can be controlled by computer software.

### Perfusion Apparatus

Hydraulic capillary infusion systems use nitrogen gas or compressed air to force water from a reservoir through small capillary tubes, thereby allowing perfusion of each transducer and catheter channel separately

### Transducers

The number of transducers required depends on the number of channels within the catheter.

### Recording Apparatus

Programs are available that automatically calculate many manometric parameters. Three-dimensional reconstruction of the pressure profile of the anal sphincter can demonstrate sphincter asymmetry and the presence of defects.

## Solid-State Noninfusion Catheters

Noninfusion transducer catheters usually contain three or more pressure channels. Although not as versatile as infusion catheters, they eliminate concerns about positioning so that recordings can be made with patients sitting    the preferred physiologic condition. Furthermore, these catheters can be used for ambulatory recordings.

## Technique of Manometric Evaluation

With the patient in the left lateral decubitus position, the catheter is inserted to 6 cm, and 20 to 30 seconds is allowed for the sphincter to recover from this insult and for the pressures to equilibrate.

Following this period of equilibration, various wave patterns may emerge, which demonstrate the presence of intrinsic cyclical activity attributed primarily to the internal sphincter. Three basic patterns are observed.

*Slow waves* are the most frequently encountered; these vary in frequency from 10 to 20 cycles/min with an amplitude from just above physiological baseline noise to 15 mmHg. The clinical significance of these waves is unknown.

*Ultraslow waves* are the second most common wave forms recorded. They have a frequency of 0.5 to 1.5 cycles/min and are of large amplitude (up to 100 mmHg). They are found more frequently in patients with high resting anal pressures, such as in those individuals with anal fissures, hemorrhoids, or primary anal sphincter hypertonia. They are seen most commonly in the region of maximal average resting pressure.

The *intermediate wave* is the least frequently observed type of oscillation (frequency, 4 to 8 cycles/min). They are most often noted in patients with neurogenic fecal incontinence or following ileal pouch-anal anastomosis. When present, they make interpretation of resting and squeeze pressures more difficult. *Resting pressure* should be assumed to be the mean of the peak and trough pressures at rest.

Following equilibration of the pressures, the patient is asked to perform a single maximal squeeze effort, followed by a period of rest, and then a maximal push effort. Thus, the high pressure zone, defined as that length of the anal canal through which pressures are greater than 50% of the average maximal pressure, can be calculated.

The catheter is then reinserted to a distance of 2 cm from the anal verge, and the latex balloon is insufflated with 40 mL of air over 2 to 3 seconds and kept inflated for 20 seconds to elicit the rectoanal inhibitory reflex. In response to distention of the lower rectum and upper anal canal, external sphincter contraction is followed by internal sphincter relaxation. If the reflex is not present, some feel it is important to repeat the test with increasing volumes of insufflation and at higher levels in the anal canal. Some patients, especially those with neurogenic fecal incontinence, decreased anal sensation, or megarectum, may respond only at a higher volume.

The catheter is then inserted to a distance of 6 cm from the anal verge, positioning the balloon in the rectal ampulla. The balloon is then slowly filled with core temperature water at a rate of approximately 1 mL/sec. The first sensation perceived by the patient is noted as the minimal sensory volume, and the mean intraballoon pressure is noted. Thereafter, balloon filling is continued until the maximal tolerable volume is reached and, again, the intraballoon pressure is noted. Using these values, rectal compliance can be calculated from the formula $\Delta V/\Delta P$.

The measurement of *compliance* is not a diagnostic test but supplements other investigations for evaluating the pathophysiology of anorectal disease. It is of particular value in patients with proctitis and incontinence through ascertaining whether the incontinence is caused by a lack of rectal reservoir function or diminished anal sphincter tone. Similarly, in some constipated patients, compliance may be abnormally high. This can reflect over accommodation and, therefore, a sensory contribution to the outlet obstruction.

## MANOVOLUMETRY

Limitations of manometry in assessing rectal compliance include the dependency on the subject's perception of the rectal balloon, and the use of deformable balloons that can lead to inaccuracy. Manovolumetry avoids these pitfalls and, therefore, may provide a more objective measurement of compliance.

## Procedure

Following emptying of the rectum with one or two Fleet's enemas, the patient is placed in the left lateral decubitus position. After the catheter is inserted, a series of distentions are commenced, beginning at a pressure of 5 cm of water and increasing stepwise by increments of 5 cm of water, emptying the balloon between each distention. Each distention lasts for at least 1 minute.

A graph of volume (mL) versus distention pressure (cm water) can be plotted and compared with the graph of normal controls. The compliance of the rectum can be determined at defined distention or pressure intervals, yielding reliable intrapatient comparisons.

## DEFECOGRAPHY (EVACUATION PROCTOGRAPHY)

Defecography is the fluoroscopic examination of the act of rectal expulsion. Almost all investigators perform this procedure with the patient in the seated position.

### Indications

Evacuation proctography is often used in the investigation of evacuatory complaints, particularly those of constipation and outlet obstruction. In addition, patients with colonic inertia often undergo defecography before colectomy to exclude pelvic floor dysfunction. The procedure may also be indicated to investigate the condition of individuals with solitary rectal ulcer syndrome or rectal pain. Its role in the evaluation of patients with fecal incontinence is less clear because the importance of the anorectal angle in maintaining bowel control is a subject of controversy.

### Equipment

#### *Imaging*

Defecography can be done in a standard fluoroscopic suite, with a table capable of supine and erect positioning. A video cassette recorder can be connected to the video output of the fluoroscopic system to record the procedure.

#### *Contrast Media*

A varying amount of liquid barium of the type used for double contrast enemas (58% wt/wt barium sulphate suspension) can be administered using a standard enema-tipped catheter to outline the rectum. In addition, most investigators use a high-density, high-viscosity barium paste to simulate stool. Finally, as the gun is removed, a small quantity of paste is inserted into the anus to outline the anal canal. With completion of the study, three lines of reference are drawn, so that the anorectal angle, puborectalis length, and extent of perineal descent can be assessed on the proctograms.

### *Anorectal Angle*

The anorectal angle is the angle formed by the axis of the posterior rectal wall and the axis formed by the anal canal; it is usually 70° to 140° at rest. This angle becomes more acute during the squeeze phase (75° to 90°) and more obtuse during evacuation (100° to 180° at maximal strain). The wide variation in observed normal values probably results from differences in interpretation. Therefore, the change in angle seen during the squeeze and push phases is more important than the actual measurement.

### *Puborectalis Length and Perineal Descent*

The *puborectalis length* is measured as the minimal distance between the antero-superior aspect of the symphysis pubis and the puborectalis notch. It ranges between 14 and 16 cm in the rest position, shortens to between 12 and 15 cm during the squeezing phase, and becomes elongated to 15 to 18 cm during the push phase. As with the anorectal angle determination, the change in these parameters is more important than their definitive value.

*Perineal descent* is assessed as the length of a perpendicular dropped from the pubococcygeal line to the anorectal junction. Perineal descent of either more than 3 cm in the rest phase or a further increase of 3 cm in the push phase is considered abnormal.

### *Interpretation*

A normal defecogram should demonstrate relaxation of the puborectalis as indicated by (a) an increase in the anorectal angle; (b) lengthening of the puborectalis, and (c) a blunting of the puborectalis notch. These changes should be accompanied by symmetric opening of the anal canal to form a cone that is wider cephalad than it is caudad. This process takes approximately 4 to 5 seconds. Contrast material in the upper rectum should subsequently be passed into the lower rectum and out the anus by rectal contraction, a process that can be facilitated by Valsalva's maneuver, squeezing the rectum onto the levator plate. Complete evacuation takes about 10 to 12 seconds when thickened contrast medium is used but is more rapid (8 to 9 seconds) when the mixture is more fluid.

In up to 50% of healthy patients, some infolding of the mucosa on the posterior wall of the rectum is a common finding during evacuation (~3 to 7 cm proximal to the anal canal). If these folds become circumferential and form a ring pocket, then an intussusception is truly present. Obviously, if this intussusception is extruded outside the anal canal, then it is termed a "rectal prolapse" or "procidentia."

Bulging of the anterior or posterior wall of the rectum is a relatively common finding on defecography, particularly in women. In women, an anterior *rectocele* of 2 cm, which empties on evacuation, is considered within normal limits. A nonemptying rectocele may be considered pathologic, but this finding should be interpreted in light of the patient's symptoms. The presence of a *sigmoidocele* is assessed during the maximal straining phase. The presence of a first-degree *sigmoidocele* (a sigmoid loop which is present within the true pelvis but does not reach or cross the pubococcygeal line) is considered a normal finding. A second-degree sigmoidocele, one that extends to or below the pubococcygeal line, is an abnormal finding. However, it may not be clinically significant. A sigmoid loop that extends below a line drawn between the coccyx and the ischial tuberosities, an uncommon finding, is termed a "third-degree sigmoidocele."

## Obstructed Defecation

In constipated patients, failure to evacuate or delayed evacuation of the rectal contents is a common finding. Most frequently, this inability to defecate is caused by inappropriate puborectalis or external sphincter contraction. This observation is known by a number of terms, including anismus, obstructed defecation, spastic pelvic floor syndrome, nonrelaxing puborectalis, and paradoxical puborectalis syndrome.

## EMPTYING STUDIES

The ability to evacuate normally and with equanimity in the presence of an audience is not one that all patients possess. Consequently, unsuccessful elimination can lead to a false–positive finding of outlet obstruction.

## Scintigraphy

Several authors have used radioactive isotopes and scintigraphy to perform a quantitative assessment of evacuation. This technique involves the rectal introduction of a semisolid material of a similar consistency to stool (e.g., oat porridge or scrambled eggs prelabeled with technetium-99 [$^{99m}$Tc]). A standard gamma camera is used to obtain images before and after the patient has evacuated in private. The percentage emptying can then be calculated. Although this test provides good quantitative information about the percentage of rectal contents evacuated per unit time, it has the disadvantages of requiring the patient to perform in public and provides no information about intussusception or other anatomic abnormalities.

## Fecoflowmetry

Fecoflowmetry assesses both the completeness of evacuation and the rate at which the evacuation occurs. After emptying the rectum, the patient assumes the left lateral decubitus position. A known quantity of water or barium paste is then instilled. Then, the patient is asked to walk until the desire to defecate is felt. The individual is then seated on the commode of a fecoflowmeter and permitted to defecate in private. This device consists of a weight transducer connected to an amplifier and an oscilloscope. The rate and extent to which the rectal contents are evacuated are calculated from the changing weight within the fecoflowmeter. Plotting weight against time results in a defecation flow curve. This technique, however, has yet to gain general acceptance.

## PERINEOMETRY

An alternative and simpler method of assessing perineal descent to the previously mentioned examinations is to use a device known as a St. Mark's perineometer. Although a simple test, perineometry adds little over defecography and is of minimal value in patient assessment.

## ENDOLUMINAL ULTRASOUND

### Indications

Endoanal ultrasonography provides an accurate two-dimensional image of the sphincter mechanism. The technique is applicable for patients with fecal incontinence, suspected occult perianal sepsis, complex or recurrent fistulas, undiagnosed anorectal pain, the preoperative staging and surveillance of anal carcinoma; for evaluating patients with congenital malformations of the sphincter mechanism; and for the preoperative staging and surveillance of rectal tumors.

### Equipment

Transducers of differing frequencies have been used. However, some controversy exists to whether a 10-MHz transducer (focal length 1 to 4 cm) gives a higher resolution of the anal sphincters than does the 7-MHz transducer (focal length 2 to 5 cm). Modern transducers are of the 360° rotating type.

A hard sonolucent cone covers the transducer head. It is carefully filled with water to ensure that all air bubbles are excluded because they will produce artifacts.

A condom containing ultrasound gel is placed over the probe, and a water-soluble lubricant is applied. The video output from the scanner can be connected to a video printer so that still pictures can be printed. The signal can be relayed through the printer to a standard VHS video recorder because real-time images are more informative than still pictures, especially when attempting to identify fistula tracks or abscess cavities.

### Interpretation

Examination takes place with the patient in the left lateral decubitus position, with the probe orientated so that the water spigot is in the upright position. The anal canal is divided into three regions: The upper anal canal begins at the pubo-rectalis muscle which appears as a *U*- or *V*-shaped band of mixed echogenicity passing behind the lumen of the anus. As the scanner is slowly withdrawn, the hypoechoic layer, which represents the internal sphincter, gradually increases in thickness, and the layer of mixed echogenicity meets anteriorly to form a con-tinuous band of muscle. The point of maximal thickness of the internal anal sphincter marks the mid-anal canal. As scanning continues distally, the internal sphincter gradually disappears to an almost imperceptibly thin strip. At this point, the hyperechoic superficial portion of the external anal sphincter at the level of the lower anal canal can be visualized.

## Conclusions and Recommendations

Ultrasound has a number of advantages when compared with other physio-logic and anatomic investigations. It is usually painless and is less expensive than is other imaging modalities such as computed tomography or magnetic res-onance imaging (MRI). It is also quicker to perform than these two techniques, and the patient is not exposed to radiation. Finally, because of its portability, the equipment can be taken to the operating room or used in the clinician's exami-nation room.

## MAGNETIC RESONANCE IMAGING

The advent of magnetic resonance imaging provided a new modality for the investigation of anorectal function. A number of the disadvantages and limita-tions associated with endoanal ultrasonography can be overcome using MRI in association with a surface or endoanal coil.

Magnetic resonance imaging has the advantage of not being operator depen-dent. Additionally, images can be obtained in either the sagittal or coronal planes. Although defecography remains the imaging modality of choice for the dynamic analysis of the anorectum, fast MRI has recently been introduced as an alternative. However, functional abnormalities occurring during defecation (e.g., intussusception, prolapse, and rectocele) cannot be detected.

## COLONIC TRANSIT STUDY

Although often caused by dietary insufficiency or evacuatory difficulties, colonic inertia is a common cause of constipation. It is also particularly resistant to standard medical treatment with dietary manipulation and cathartics. It is, therefore, important to be able to identify those who are suffering primarily from a disturbance in colonic motility (see Chapter 16). Currently, assessment of colonic transit is most commonly done through the use of either radiopaque markers or colonic scintigraphy.

## Radiopaque Markers

Initially, with ingestion of a single capsule of 20 radiopaque rings followed by daily abdominal roentgenographs, a normal finding is one in which 16 or more of the markers have passed by the fifth postingestion day, and all have been evacuated by the seventh day. Others have modified the test by suggesting the use of three boluses of 20 markers each, ingested at 24-hour intervals, and then taking two plain abdominal radiographs at 24 and 96 hours following the ingestion of the third bolus. Using modifications of these methods, transit through the right colon has been estimated to be from 6.9 to 13 hours; transit through the left colon from 9.1 to 15 hours; and transit through the rectosigmoid from 11 to 18.4 hours. Because the radiopaque marker study is simple, inexpensive, and reproducible, it is the most widely performed colonic transit evaluation.

## Colonic Scintigraphy

Colonic scintigraphy is a procedure that entails the tracking of a radionuclide-labeled bolus through the colon by using a gamma camera. Polystyrene pellets or resin particles labeled with $^{99m}$Tc or indium ($^{111}$In) can be incorporated into a gelatin capsule coated with a methacrylate polymer and ingested. This capsule will remain intact through the acid pH of the stomach and duodenum, but will dissolve in the distal small bowel where the pH is typically between 7.2 and 7.4. Multiple images can be obtained over 3 consecutive days without increasing radiation exposure. However, this type of intensive study makes considerable time demands on gamma camera use and is inconvenient for the patient. These difficulties can be ameliorated by limiting data acquisition to three times: at 28 hours, 52 hours, and 60 hours following ingestion. Image resolution, however, remains a problem leading to difficulty in interpreting the anatomic layout of the colon, loops of which can be superimposed or confused with small bowel.

## Recommendation

The patient is given a single capsule containing 24 radiopaque rings, and instructed to refrain from the use of laxatives or fiber products from the day before capsule ingestion until after completion of the study. Abdominal x-ray studies, which include the diaphragms and the pubis, are taken on days 3 and 5 following ingestion, and the total number of markers is counted on each film. No attempt is made to obtain values for segmental transit because no evidence suggests that segmental colonic resection is an appropriate option in the treatment of colonic inertia. However, if most markers are delayed in the rectosigmoid area, outlet obstruction is probable. The results of tests are deemed to be normal if 80% of the markers have been evacuated by the fifth day.

## SMALL BOWEL TRANSIT

It has generally been believed that prolonged oroanal transit times reflect mainly colonic transit abnormality. However, many patients with delayed colonic transit times may have a generalized motility disturbance of the gastrointestinal tract. Thus, before subjecting a patient to total colectomy, it may be advisable to obtain some measure of small bowel transit. Of course, an indication of small bowel transit time may be of benefit in the investigation of individuals with diarrhea, malabsorption, or increased stool frequency following coloanal or ileal pouch-anal anastomosis.

### Breath Hydrogen Analysis

The most widely used test of small bowel transit time involves breath hydrogen analysis. Strictly speaking, however, it is a measure of orocecal transit. Following an overnight fast, the patient ingests a nonabsorbable carbohydrate such as lactulose (1,4-β-galactofructose), which gives a value for liquid transit, or baked beans, which gives a figure for solid transit. On entering the cecum, these substrates are metabolized by colonic bacteria to hydrogen and short chain fatty acids. Hydrogen, which is highly diffusible and relatively insoluble in water, is rapidly absorbed into the blood, transported to the lungs, and exhaled.

Although it is a relatively simple test, a number of caveats apply to the interpretation of breath hydrogen analysis. First, 5% to 20% of the population are nonfermenters and do not produce hydrogen. In addition, oral bacteria can cause some breakdown of the substrate, but this can be easily overcome by the use of a mouthwash before the administration of the test meal. Similarly, small intestinal bacterial overgrowth will result in early metabolism of the substrate. Antibiotics consumed within 10 days before the test can deplete the colonic flora and result in a falsely prolonged result. Smoking and vigorous exercise should be avoided before the test because these factors can influence breath hydrogen. Also, some difficulty in interpreting the first peak of breath hydrogen can result in unreliable findings. Indeed, normal values from center to center often vary because of the different criteria used to identify the time of entry of the meal into the cecum.

### Small Intestinal Scintigraphy

Gastric emptying and small bowel transit time can be assessed by the ingestion of polystyrene pellets labeled with either $^{99m}$Tc or $^{111}$In or by labeling a meal of mashed potato with $^{99m}$Tc sulfur colloid or diethylenetriamine-penta-acetic acid. Methods using polystyrene pellets measure the small bowel transit of nondigestible solids, whereas the mashed potato meal is probably a measurement of liquid transit. Small bowel transit time is calculated as the time taken for a fixed quantity of the isotope (e.g., 10% or 50%) to empty from the stomach and enter the colon. Interpretation can be made difficult by small bowel loops overlying the cecum. This can be clarified by allowing the test to continue so that accurate images of cecal filling can be obtained.

## Recommendations

In our laboratory, small bowel transit study is used primarily as an adjunct to colonic transit studies in order to identify individuals with generalized intestinal hypomotility. We have found that measurements of orocecal transit using breath hydrogen is reliable, reproducible, and well tolerated.

We accept a rise of 3 ppm, which has been demonstrated to produce the lowest coefficient of variation between subjects and, therefore, is the value used to determine that the meal has reached the cecum. Patients who fail to produce an appreciable rise (>2 ppm) or sustained rise (more than three consecutive measurements) in breath hydrogen within 3 hours of ingestion are assumed to be nonfermenters.

## SMALL BOWEL, COLONIC, AND RECTAL MOTILITY

### Nonambulatory Studies

The relationship between the motor activity of the small bowel and the colon and rectum is not completely understood. Most studies have been performed on healthy volunteers and, therefore, the implications of abnormal activity in disease states is uncertain. No clear clinical implication is currently seen for using these investigations in the management of patients.

### Ambulatory Studies

Anally inserted manometric catheters usually require an empty colon. The laxative or enemas, themselves, are known to alter colonic motility. Two methods, radiotelemetry and tube-mounted transducers, have been developed which permit ambulatory monitoring without a bowel preparation. Both currently have little implication in clinical practice.

## ELECTROMYOGRAPHY

Anal electromyography (EMG) is a recording of the electrical activity from the muscle fibers of the external sphincter and puborectalis complex at rest, during maximal squeeze, during simulated defecation, and in response to various reflexes. It has been largely replaced by pudendal terminal motor latency (PTML) to assess nerve function.

## PUDENDAL NERVE TERMINAL MOTOR LATENCY

Because the pudendal nerve innervates the external anal sphincter, quantitative assessment of impulse transmission speed along this pathway can provide useful information in patients with incontinence, rectal prolapse, and constipation. Stimulation of the pudendal nerve and the time taken for the impulse to be transmitted is known as the "pudendal nerve terminal motor latency" (PNTML). In addition to bowel management concerns, the PNTML can be used to indirectly assess perineal nerve function in patients with urinary incontinence. A linear relationship is found between the terminal motor latencies of the perineal and pudendal nerves, the perineal nerve latencies being slightly longer.

### Equipment

#### *Electrode*

The Dantec (Dantec Medical Inc., Skovlunde, Denmak and Allentown, NJ.) St. Marks pudendal nerve stimulating device is used at most centers. This device consists of a thin strip of adhesive paper that is placed on the gloved finger with two stimulating electrodes, a larger anode and a smaller cathode, 1 cm apart at the tip, and two recording electrodes at the base, 4 cm distal to the anode.

#### *Electromyographic Equipment*

Electromyographic equipment involves a unit that can deliver a 50-V square-wave stimulus of 0.1 msec and can record the resultant motor unit potential.

### Recommendations

A single Fleet's enema is used to empty the rectum before the examination. The patient is placed in the left lateral decubitus position. An electrode is secured on the volar aspect of the examiner's gloved index finger. Following the application of electrode gel to the electrodes, the examiner's index finger is inserted into the rectum until the coccyx is palpated posteriorly. The finger is then moved laterally to the left and the left ischial spine palpated. This point is recognized by a strong contraction of the external sphincter around the examiner's finger and a coincident maximal amplitude motor unit potential of the recording apparatus. The terminal motor latency is the time interval between the onset of the stimulus and the onset of the motor unit potential. The motor unit potential image will be inverted on this side. The normal values for PNTML in most laboratories is 2.0 ± 0.2 ms.

## ANORECTAL SENSATION

Normal continence, in part, is maintained by anorectal sensation. Distal to the anal transition zone, the anal epithelium is sensitive to pain, temperature, and touch. Although proximally no pain fibers exist, numerous Golgi-Mazzoni bodies and pacinian corpuscles are sensitive to pressure changes.

The rectum is not sensitive to pain but is sensitive to distention of its lumen, giving rise to a feeling of fullness. It has been hypothesized that this sensation is not perceived at the mucosal level because of few nerve fibers, but it arises from stimulation of the pelvic floor muscles and receptors in surrounding structures.

The precise role of sensation in the maintenance of continence is unclear. The sampling reflex, which is important in enabling individuals to discriminate between flatus, liquid, and solid stool, is usually ablated following ileoanal or coloanal anastomosis. However, these patients usually maintain continence. Furthermore, neither excision nor preservation of the anal transitional zone has led to a functionally different result following this type of surgery. Considerable interest is seen in investigating the sensory component of the anal canal. In particular, two techniques have been described—mucosal electrosensitivity and temperature sensation. Currently, both of these modalities are largely investigational and their role in the clinical management of patients is unclear.

## BIOFEEDBACK

Biofeedback is a treatment whereby patients are trained to be more aware of and responsive to biological information provided to them. It has been increasingly used in the management of functional pelvic floor disorders, such as fecal incontinence, rectal pain, and obstructed defecation.

In the treatment of fecal incontinence, biofeedback attempts to improve both patient's awareness of their sphincter mechanism and the muscular function of this apparatus. Similarly, in patients with obstructed defecation, biofeedback is used to heighten their awareness of the sphincters so that they can be trained to consciously relax these muscles during evacuation. Hence, visual or auditory feedback of the muscular tone within the external sphincter or puborectalis complex is of importance. This input is generally provided through the use of manometry, balloon defecography, surface EMG, or intraanal EMG. Intrarectal balloon sensation training can be used separately or in combination with muscular training, particularly in those with fecal incontinence.

## CONCLUSIONS

No so long ago, anorectal physiology was considered a conglomeration of interesting but impractical investigations that provided novel but clinically irrelevant information. Currently, anorectal physiology is not only familiar to those who perform colorectal surgery but is available to most practitioners. Anorectal physiology provides useful data for both clinical decision making and prognostic information.

# 7

## Analgesia in Colon and Rectal Surgery

With the exception of pudendal nerve block and local infiltration of the anal and perianal areas, no specific analgesic technique is unique to the field of colon and rectal surgery. The method of performing a "field block" for hemorrhoidectomy is discussed in Chapter 8.

The severity of postoperative pain encountered in all surgical practice is often not adequately appreciated and, as a consequence, is frequently undertreated. The management of postoperative pain is often difficult, because of the obvious variation in analgesic requirements, the variability of pathophysiologic interactions with different therapies, and, of course, individual subjective pain experiences. Recent concepts in the management of postoperative pain use the assessment of pain when moving, pain when in bed, and the worst pain during the day. One method for analyzing the efficacy of pain control has been the development of a so-called "visual analog pain score." Using this scoring method, patients relate the severity of pain they are experiencing to a scale of 1 to 10, where 1 is almost no pain, and 10 is the most severe pain they have ever experienced. Pain relief is then administered to control the patient's perception of pain as well as allow the patient to complete important activities (e.g., coughing, physical therapy).

A number of approaches are used to control pain. It has been demonstrated that epidural analgesia provides more effective pain relief than does either patient-controlled analgesia (PCA) or intramuscular analgesic administrations. Preoperative use of opioid medications causes tolerance to these drugs and increases postoperative consumption. In addition, preoperative pain and opiate use is generally associated with a greater degree of postoperative pain. This chapter contains discussions of the place of opioids and the use of epidural anesthesia in colon and rectal surgery.

### OPIOIDS

Opioids produce their effect by binding to specific receptors. These receptors, which are present in the limbic system, thalamus, striatum, hypothalamus, midbrain, and spinal cord, have been given various Greek letter identifications, based on their location.

| | |
|---|---|
| mu | analgesia, miosis, respiratory depression |
| kappa | analgesia |
| delta | analgesia, miosis, respiratory depression |
| sigma | excitation, dysphoria |

### Actions and Effects

In addition to their analgesic action, opioids have numerous other effects. These include respiratory and cough suppression, increased smooth muscle tone throughout the gastrointestinal tract, increased tone of the bladder sphincter impeding urination, and an effect on the endocrine system.

Nausea develops as a consequence of orthostatic hypotension or by direct stimulation of the chemotactic trigger zone in the medulla oblongata. Orthostasis can occur as a result of vasodilatation from the peripheral release of histamine or from the suppression of sympathetic outflow from the vasomotor medullary center.

Inhibition of the release of thyrotropin from the adenohypophysis leads to a decrease in thyroid hormone. Opioids can also produce hyperglycemia by stimulating receptors near the foramen of Monro or by releasing epinephrine, which can be associated with a decrease in the metabolic rates by about 10% to 20%.

The exception is meperidine (Demerol, Pethidine), which can cause excitation, seizures, and tachycardia, but with less increased smooth muscle tone in the gastrointestinal tract. The relative potency of the various opioids are summarized in Table 7.1.

### Metabolism

Opioids are primary metabolized by the microsomes in the endoplasmic reticulum of the liver by hydrolysis, oxidation, and conjugation with glucuronide. Metabolism also occurs in the central nervous system (CNS), kidneys, lungs, and placenta.

**TABLE 7.1.** *Analgesic equivalent potency conversion*

| Opioids | Intramuscular (mg) | Oral (mg) | Intravenous (mg) |
|---|---|---|---|
| Morphine | 10 | 40–60 | 10 |
| Codeine | 130 | 200 | — |
| Heroin | 5 | 60 | 5 |
| Hydromorphone | 1.5 | 7.5 | 1.0 |
| Levorphanol | 2 | 4 | 1.5 |
| Meperidine | 75 | 400 | 75 |
| Methadone | 10 | 20 | 10 |
| Oxycodone | 15 | 30 | — |
| Fentanyl | — | 500 μg | 100 μg |

## Mechanism of Action

All opioid receptors appear to function primarily by exerting inhibitory modulation of synaptic transmission in the spinal cord, the myenteric plexus, and the CNS. When located at a presynaptic terminal, these receptors act to reduce neurotransmitter release and, therefore, to decrease conductance. All appear to be linked to guanine nucleotide-binding regulator proteins (G proteins). Opioids regulate the so-called "transmembrane signaling system"—adenylate cyclase activity, ion channel activity, and the activity of phospholysasis or phosphoinositol.

Within the intestinal tract, enterocytes, themselves, may possess opioid receptors. The transfer of fluid and electrolytes into the intestinal lumen is inhibited, and enterocyte basal secretion decreases. Additionally, the stimulatory effects of acetylcholine, prostaglandin $F_2$, and vasoactive intestinal peptides are inhibited. The activity of opioids in the periaqueductal gray or in the spinal cord will also inhibit gastrointestinal activity as long as the extrinsic innervation to the bowel is intact. This may explain why agents with poor penetration of the CNS (e.g., paregoric) can produce constipation at subanalgesic dosages.

## Patient-Controlled Analgesia

In the postoperative setting, a PCA device is used primarily to administer opioids to alleviate pain. Usually, morphine, hydromorphone (Dilaudid), fentanyl, or meperidine is used. The goal of PCA is the more timely administration drug doses, thereby, of enhancing patient satisfaction. The choice of which agent to use is often made by the surgeon on the basis of his or her previous experience with the medications and sense of patient needs.

In initially programming a PCA device, a target hourly "safe" dose should be selected. Then, the "demand" and "interval time" can be set according to the $t\frac{1}{2}$ alpha distribution times and times to peak analgesia. The total analgesic administered per hour is dependent on the volume of distribution, acid-base status, plasma protein-binding capacity, ventilatory mechanics, cerebral blood flow patterns, presence of metabolic abnormalities (e.g., hypothyroidism), as well as a number of other subtle factors.

When a basal (continuous) infusion is used, it is not regulated by the patient and may predispose to the accumulation of side effects.

## EPIDURAL ANALGESIA

In a busy, postoperative acute pain service, continuous epidural infusions of local anesthetics at dilute concentrations, in combination with epidural opioids, are an effective means for treating pain. All epidural opioids will achieve some plasma systemic levels, depending on the lipophilic qualities of the drug. By using PCA epidural, patients can medicate themselves, within strictly controlled parameters, with a lower risk of overdose or side effects. Epidural analgesia appears to be associated with faster resolution of postoperative ileus because of the lower dose of opioid required.

Epidural analgesia appears to have the greatest potential to improve perioperative outcome and morbidity when patients at high risk undergo major operations. This has been demonstrated to be the case for perioperative cardiovascular morbidity, pulmonary complications (including pulmonary embolus), and infection.

## Epidural Opioids

Epidural opioids act both by venous absorption, to produce systemic plasma levels, and by dispersion to the cerebrospinal fluid (CSF). Their activity may be caused by direct binding at the mu receptor complex in the substantia gelatinosa, the direct binding onto nerve roots, or to the spread and assimilation of morphine through the CSF to the periaqueductal gray of the central nervous system (CNS). By means of synergistic activity between opioids and local anesthetics, the concentrations can be reduced, thereby minimizing motor blockade or total sensory blockade.

The incidence of perioperative increase in coagulation tendency has been shown to be concomitant with a decrease in venous and arterial thrombosis.

Onset of epidural opiate analgesia is directly related to the lipid partition coefficient. The higher the lipid solubility, the more rapid the onset of analgesia. The duration of analgesia is inversely related to lipid solubility, but it is also influenced by the rate of dissociation from receptors.

It is important to weigh the potential benefit of the superior analgesia obtained with epidural opioids against the greater invasiveness and the possible complications of respiratory depression, pruritus, nausea, and urinary retention. Alternatively, an intravenous infusion of opioids may provide similar analgesia, albeit not as satisfactory in some respects, but with a greater risk of respiratory depression and nausea.

## Complications of Epidural Analgesia

Complications of epidural analgesia, include toxicity and seizures, urinary retention, epidural abscess, inadvertent dural puncture, backache, and nerve root injury.

### *Urinary Retention*

Urinary retention is caused because the reduced sensation caused by the epidural affects the ability of the patient to detect the need to void. This allows excess stretch of the bladder, to a volume such that it is unable to contract and empty. Urinary catheters are generally necessary while the epidural is in place. After about 6 hours after removal of the epidural, it is usually safe to remove the urinary catheter, with full expectation that the patient will be able to void spontaneously.

### *Toxicity and Seizures*

Toxicity and seizures are problems related to incorrect positioning of the epidural catheter, which causes an inappropriately high concentration of the drug to affect the CNS.

### *Dural Puncture*

A dural puncture results in a spinal anesthetic, requiring a lower dose to gain the neural blockade required. The blockade will also be complete (motor and sensory) rather than just control of pain. The risk of meningitis is greater and, consequently, the catheter must be removed and not left *in situ* for postoperative pain management. Also, a dural puncture can cause an epidural headache. This generally resolves spontaneously with supine rest in bed. A blood patch may be required to seal the defect if conservative management fails to correct the problem.

### *Backache*

Backache is possible with any epidural or spinal type procedure. In those who have had previous back surgery, or are long-term sufferers of back pain, it is inadvisable to place an epidural catheter and risk aggravating the premorbid state.

### *Epidural Abscess*

Epidural abscess is a rare complication of epidural analgesia. A patient may complain of severe back pain, local tenderness, and fever, with the presence of leukocytosis. Subsequent myelography may demonstrate obstruction to flow.

### Epidural Hematoma

Epidural hematoma is probably the result of needle or catheter trauma to the epidural veins. In a healthy patient, bleeding is minimal and ceases rapidly.

Regional anesthesia is not recommended in the presence of thrombocytopenia, following the administration of antiplatelet agents, or in patients with a qualitative defect in platelets (e.g., an abnormal bleeding time). If anticoagulation is continued in the postoperative period, the potential movement of the epidural catheter with mobilization poses a risk for venous trauma and hematoma formation.

Low dose heparin therapy for deep venous thrombosis prophylaxis represents a controversial area for the use of epidural analgesia. Epidural analgesia should not be considered in the presence of intravenously administered heparin therapy. Because of a slight chance of trauma and bleeding with an indwelling catheter, even with the patient on a low dose or mini dose heparin, the anesthesiologist is well advised to decline placement and continuation of this technique. We use epidurals with patients on Coumadin (warfarin) and low dose heparin, but wait until normal prothrombin time before removing the catheter.

### Duration of Catheter Placement

The postoperative duration for epidural infusion depends on the analgesic requirements of the patient. In most instances, an epidural catheter is left in place for up to 7 days and longer if the epidural is replaced. However, studies have shown tunneled epidural catheters are generally safe.

### Summary

In summary, the use of epidural analgesics introduces risks that must be balanced against the benefits of early ambulation, fewer respiratory complications, and improved gastrointestinal motility. Overall, epidural analgesia has proved to be an extremely safe and effective technique.

# 8

# Hemorrhoids

Hemorrhoidal disease affects more than 1 million Americans per year. From the patient's perspective, the complaint of "hemorrhoids" represents the diagnosis for a host of anal problems—itching, a lump, pain, swelling, bleeding, and protrusion. It is as likely that an individual's symptoms are attributable to another cause as they are to hemorrhoids.

Hemorrhoidal veins are essentially normal parts of the human anatomy, and symptomatic hemorrhoids are one of the most common afflictions of Western civilization. The problem can occur at any age and can affect both sexes. It has been estimated that at least 50% of individuals above the age of 50 years have at some time experienced hemorrhoidal complaints. Whites are affected more frequently than blacks, and an increased frequency is seen in those of a higher socioeconomic status. It is also more common in rural than in urban areas. The condition is relatively rare in rural Africa. The following factors have been suggested to contribute to the development of hemorrhoids:

- Heredity
- Anatomic features
- Nutrition
- Occupation
- Climate
- Psychological problems
- Scnility
- Endocrine changes
- Food and drugs
- Infection
- Pregnancy
- Exercise
- Coughing
- Straining
- Vomiting
- Constrictive clothing
- Constipation

## ETIOLOGY AND ANATOMY

In 1975, Thomson, in his master's thesis based on anatomic and radiologic studies, introduced the term *vascular cushions*. According to this theory, the submucosa does not form a continuous ring of thickened tissue in the anal canal, but rather a discontinuous series of cushions; the three main cushions are found in the left lateral, right anterior, and right posterior positions (Fig. 8.1). The submucosal layer of each of these thicker regions is rich with blood vessels and muscle fibers, the latter known as the muscularis submucosa . These fibers, arising from the internal sphincter and from the conjoined longitudinal muscle, are important in maintaining adherence of mucosal and submucosal tissues to the underlying internal sphincter and in supporting the blood vessels of the submucosa. It is postulated that the cushions, by filling with blood during the act of defecation, protect the anal canal from injury. The muscularis submucosa and its connective tissue fibers return the anal canal lining to its initial position after the temporary downward displacement that occurs during defecation.

The anal cushions receive their blood supply primarily from the terminal branches of the superior hemorrhoidal artery and from branches of the middle hemorrhoidal arteries. These branches communicate with one another and with branches of the inferior hemorrhoidal arteries, which supply the lower portion of the anal canal. The superior, middle, and inferior hemorrhoidal veins, which drain blood from the tissues of the anal canal, correspond to each of the hemorrhoidal arteries.

The anchoring and supporting tissue deteriorates with aging, and this phenomenon becomes apparent in the third decade of life. This ultimately produces venous distension, erosion, bleeding, and thrombosis.

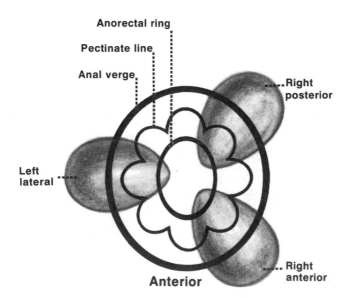

**FIG. 8.1.** The three primary hemorrhoidal groups.

The four major theories regarding the cause of hemorrhoids are as follows:

1. Abnormal dilatation of the veins of the internal hemorrhoidal venous plexus, a network of the tributaries of the superior and middle hemorrhoidal veins
2. Abnormal distension of the arteriovenous anastomoses, which are in the same location as the anal cushions
3. Downward displacement or prolapse of the anal cushions
4. Destruction of the anchoring connective tissue system

Hemorrhoids are not varicose veins. They are structures that are normally present but do not produce symptoms until the fibromuscular supporting tissue above the cushions deteriorates. This deterioration permits the cushions to slide, engorge, prolapse, and bleed.

Despite a vast literature on the subject of hemorrhoids, the pathogenesis remains controversial. Furthermore, a difference of opinion remains as to the definition of hemorrhoidal disease. The high prevalence of proctoscopic evidence of this pathologic entity and its weak relationship to symptoms suggest that perhaps these findings may be more a consequence of the aging process than truly a disease entity.

## Portal Hypertension and Rectal Varices

A number of studies have failed to demonstrate an increased incidence of hemorrhoids in patients with portal hypertension. However, rectal varices may be seen as enlarged portal-systemic collateral veins in these patients. This collateral circulation from the portal vein passes into the systemic circulation through the middle and inferior hemorrhoidal veins. In other words, hemorrhoids and rectal varices must be recognized as two separate entities, with no correlation between the presence of these varices and the severity of esophagogastric mucosal changes of portal hypertension.

It is essential to differentiate anorectal varices from bleeding hemorrhoids, because the treatment is so obviously different. Endoscopic ultrasonography and magnetic resonance imaging are noninvasive modalities for diagnosis and control after treatment.

Bleeding from varices can be treated by a transanal suture technique, by transhepatic inferior mesenteric venography and embolization, or by any one of the methods of portal-systemic shunting and decompression.

## PHYSIOLOGY

The anal sphincters of many patients with hemorrhoids demonstrate an abnormal rhythm of contraction and exert a greater force of contraction than those of asymptomatic control subjects. Whether this sphincter abnormality is a cause or an effect of hemorrhoids is not known. Objective anorectal manometric studies reveal increased anal canal pressure in patients with symptomatic hemorrhoids when they are compared with control subjects. However, ultrasonographic study of the anal canal reveals a clear image of the internal sphincter that is no different from that of controls. This absence of any significant differences in internal sphincter thickness between normal subjects and patients with hemorrhoids suggests that the high anal pressure observed in those with hemorrhoids is of a vascular origin. This elevated pressure usually returns to normal levels following hemorrhoidectomy.

## CLASSIFICATION

Hemorrhoids are classified by location (i.e., external, internal, or mixed) or by degree (i.e., first, second, third, and fourth). External hemorrhoids arise from the inferior hemorrhoidal plexus and are covered by modified squamous epithelium. They occur below the pectinate line and may become thrombotic and ulcerate. Internal hemorrhoids may prolapse, and they may be reducible or irreducible. This type of hemorrhoid occurs above the pectinate line and can ulcerate, bleed, and thrombose. They arise from the superior hemorrhoidal plexus and are covered by mucosa. Mixed hemorrhoids (i.e., external–internal) can be prolapsed, irreducible, thrombosed, or ulcerated. They arise from the inferior and superior hemorrhoidal plexus and their anastomotic connections.

In first-degree hemorrhoids, the veins of the anal canal are increased in number and size, and can bleed at the time of defecation. They do not prolapse but project into the lumen. Second-degree hemorrhoids present to the outside of the anal canal during defecation but return spontaneously to within the anal canal, where they remain otherwise. Third-degree hemorrhoids (i.e., internal and mixed) protrude outside the anal canal and require manual reduction. Fourth-degree hemorrhoids are irreducible and constantly remain in the prolapsed state.

### External Hemorrhoids

Two types of hemorrhoids are found at the external anal orifice. One occurs predominantly in the form of dilatation and engorgement of the veins beneath the skin, and the other is manifested as a thrombosis of these veins. When the clot forms, the patient becomes aware of its presence. The degree of pain depends on the size of the clot and the relationship it bears to the anal sphincters. A large clot will cause pain, but even if a clot is small, it can be uncomfortable if it lies within the anal musculature. Small, thrombosed hemorrhoids rarely ulcerate and bleed.

When the process spreads into external and internal tissue surrounding hemorrhoidal veins, considerable external swelling develops as edematous fluid fills the subcutaneous area at the anal margin. This can result in acute external and internal hemorrhoidal venous thrombosis and prolapse.

## External Tags or Skin Tabs

External tags or skin tabs, which are deformities of the external anal margin skin, occur as redundant folds. These may be the residual of prior thrombosed hemorrhoids that have become organized into fibrous appendages.

## Internal Hemorrhoids

The usual internal hemorrhoid is not evident on visual inspection of the anal area. When an individual strains, a bulging mass may appear that involves all or part of the anal canal. The full extent of pressure is exerted on the anorectal outlet only during defecation or straining. Therefore, a truly reliable examination should be made, preferably, with the patient seated on a commode.

## Thrombosed Hemorrhoids

Thrombosed hemorrhoids (i.e., clotted hemorrhoids) are seen most often in patients who (a) strain while defecating or when lifting heavy objects; (b) have frequent bowel actions, as with inflammatory bowel disease or malabsorption; or (c) sit for long periods of time. Theoretically, direct trauma to the area creates an inflammatory response, which leads to thrombosis. Additionally, Valsalva's action during straining can lead to protrusion, which, if irreducible, can precipitate this complication. Stasis of the blood flow during straining is another possible explanation.

## DIFFERENTIAL DIAGNOSIS

### Polyp, Adenoma, and Carcinoma

Sessile, polypoid (i.e., adenomatous) masses and true carcinomas, should be differentiated readily from hemorrhoidal tissue. Internal hemorrhoids uncomplicated by thrombosis, edema, prolapse, or other factors are usually easy to diagnose. Any anorectal abnormality that is readily palpable and may not be attributable to a thrombosis or recent injection therapy is not likely to be hemorrhoidal tissue. Biopsy and microscopic study of all suspected lesions are essential to establish the correct diagnosis.

### Hypertrophied Anal Papilla

A firm mass that seems to arise from an attached pedicle in the region of the dentate line most likely represents an hypertrophied anal papilla. Endoscopic study should establish the diagnosis with certainty by demonstrating that the pedicle arises from the dentate margin and that the entire lesion is invested by skin.

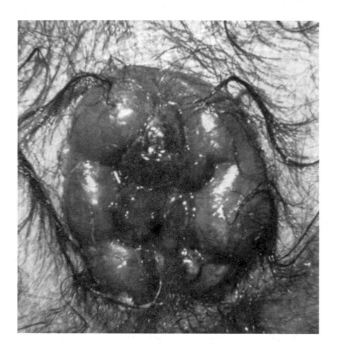

**FIG. 8.2.** Prolapsed, thrombosed hemorrhoids. These are irreducible and have an element of mucosal prolapse.

## Rectal Prolapse

Rectal prolapse can be either partial, involving only the mucosal layer of the rectal wall, or complete, involving the full thickness. Partial prolapse can affect either part or all of the circumference of the anal outlet. Differentiating prolapsed internal hemorrhoids from partial or mucosal prolapse can be somewhat difficult, but internal hemorrhoids are separated by sulci that radiate peripherally from the center of the anal outlet, whereas mucosal prolapse usually exhibits a more uniformly concentric protrusion. Partial rectal prolapse is not accompanied by evidence of inflammatory change. Usually, some element of mucosal prolapse is found when a circumferential rosette of hemorrhoids becomes irreducible and thrombosed (Fig. 8.2). Complete rectal prolapse should be readily distinguishable by its concentrically arranged mucosal folds, which are strikingly different from the radiating sulci separating prolapsed internal hemorrhoids.

### SIGNS AND SYMPTOMS

The most common presenting complaint of patients with hemorrhoids is bleeding. Usually occurring during or after defecation, it is exacerbated by straining and by frequent bowel actions. Blood can be evident on the paper, in the toilet bowl, or both. Occasionally, blood loss may be severe enough to produce a profound anemia. Pain is usually not caused by hemorrhoids, unless the hemorrhoidal vein is thrombosed, ulcerated, or gangrenous. Prolapse, is a common presentation of hemorrhoids.

Constipation is not a symptom of hemorrhoids, but defecation can be difficult when thrombosis or gangrene produces pain. Patients tend to avoid the toilet if hemorrhoidal symptoms are exacerbated by defecation; this can lead to refusal of the urge to pass stool and result in constipation or even obstipation.

## EXAMINATION

Physical examination should include proctosigmoidoscopy and anoscopy. Colonoscopy or a barium enema study must be performed in all patients who have rectal bleeding when the source is not readily apparent from these examinations. In patients above 50 years of age, an evaluation of the colon should be performed at some time, even if hemorrhoids are the apparent cause of the patient's symptoms. This can be deferred if an individual's symptoms preclude carrying out such studies at the time of the examination.

The incidence of bleeding attributed to hemorrhoids that caused anemia was found to be 0.5/100,000 population per year. Recovery from anemia after definitive treatment by means of hemorrhoidectomy is rapid. Failure to recover hemoglobin concentration should prompt further or repeated evaluation for other causes of the anemia.

## GENERAL PRINCIPLES OF TREATMENT

### Bleeding

Bleeding, if occasional and related to straining or to diarrhea, should be managed medically. Constipation can be controlled by appropriate dietary measures, a bowel-management program, stool softeners, laxatives, or a combination of these. Diarrhea or frequent defecation can be managed with antidiarrheal medications and diet. Attention should also be given to improvement of anal hygiene.

The use of commercial topical creams, lotions, and suppositories is worthy of comment. These preparations include Tucks pads and cream, Anusol cream and suppositories, Balneol lotion, PROCTOFOAM, and the most ubiquitous self-medication used by the average American for "symptomatic hemorrhoids," Preparation H. Preparation H is alleged to contain shark liver oil as well as a "skin respiratory factor" of unknown formulation that is supposed to improve wound healing. Preparation H probably acts essentially to soothe skin irritation and is as effective for this purpose as virtually any topical cream, lotion, or ointment. A number of other commercially available mechanical devices and products are used to facilitate cleansing of the anus (e.g., mini-bidets, Shower Mini, and Water-pic).

It is difficult to assess the actual efficacy of suppositories with regard to hemorrhoids. Because this anorectal disease is often self-limited, resolution may occur irrespective of this treatment. Furthermore, the physician cannot gainsay the psychological benefit that vigorous promotional effort of such products produces for the patient. Finally, the bullet-shaped suppository often used in the treatment of anal conditions cannot exert its primary benefit within the anal canal, as it must advance at least as far as the rectum. To be truly useful, a suppository should be hourglass- or collar button-shaped to maintain effective contact with the anal mucosa. Such a modification has yet to be produced.

If bleeding persists despite the aforementioned approaches, some form of interventional treatment should be considered

## Prolapse

Prolapsed hemorrhoids that return spontaneously or are manually reducible can usually be treated by an office procedure. Attempting reduction is important, because persistent prolapse predisposes the patient to thrombosis and gangrene. If the prolapse is irreducible or if an external component is present, an excisional approach, using either a local anesthetic or a surgical hemorrhoidectomy, may be indicated.

## Pain

If pain is caused by gangrenous, ulcerated, or thrombosed hemorrhoids, a surgical procedure is the best means of treatment. If hemorrhoids are associated with an anal fissure, hemorrhoidectomy should be considered and the fissure treated by internal anal sphincterotomy. A swollen, thrombosed external hemorrhoid that produces pain should be treated by local excision.

Few question that pain is considerably ameliorated by the application of heat, via sitz baths. Because patients often have elevated pressures, the lowering of resting anal canal pressure probably produces the observed symptomatic improvement.

## AMBULATORY TREATMENT

### Sclerotherapy: Injection Treatment of Hemorrhoids

Phenol (5%) in almond or vegetable oil is still the primary sclerosing agent used (in Great Britain) today; 3 mL is usually injected into each hemorrhoid site.

The combination of quinine and urea hydrochloride, widely used as a local anesthetic agent before the introduction of procaine, was associated with the development of fibrous tissue infiltration and sometimes sloughing at the site of injection. Sclerosants include sodium morrhuate and sodium tetradecyl sulfate (i.e., Sotradecol), but the safest continues to be phenol (5%) in vegetable oil. In essence, all the ambulatory, nonexcisional treatments of hemorrhoids produce fibrosis of the submucosa, thereby obliterating the redundant tissue.

## Indications and Contraindications

The nonprolapsing internal hemorrhoid is most amenable to injection treatment. Sometimes, a large, slightly protruding hemorrhoid can be successfully treated in this manner. Injection usually provides only temporary relief of symptoms when hemorrhoids are voluminous, contain a great deal of fibrous tissue, or require digital replacement after defecation. External hemorrhoids and internal hemorrhoids that are infected or contain thrombi should never be treated by injection. Tags, fistulas, tumors, and anal fissure are complicating conditions that contraindicate use of the injection method. Injection treatment should be limited to those individuals who have symptomatic hemorrhoids, especially bleeding, and in whom rubber band ligation cannot be tolerated.

## Technique

With the patient in the semi-inverted jackknife or left lateral (i.e., Sims') position, an anoscope is inserted and the anal canal observed (see Fig. 8.1). The point at which each injection is made, the amount of solution used, and the date of the injection should be recorded on the chart. The term *o'clock* should not be used to describe the location of the treatment or the location of the hemorrhoids.

The needle is introduced through the mucous membrane into the center of the mass of veins. No antiseptic is necessary. Care must be taken to avoid bringing the point of the needle into contact with the sensitive margin of the pectinate line. Unlike sclerotherapy for varicose veins, this technique requires that intraluminal injection be avoided.

After the needle is in position, 0.5 mL of sodium morrhuate, quinine, and urea hydrochloride, or Sotradecol, is slowly injected submucosally into each pile site. Alternatively, a 5% solution of phenol in almond, vegetable, or arachis oil can be used. A wheal should form, indicating that the injection was given in the proper plane. No more than 3 mL should be used for each treatment if a commercial sclerosant is being used. With the phenol solution, 3 mL may be injected in each pile site. All hemorrhoids should be injected at the first treatment session. If bleeding is not controlled by one complete injection treatment, alternative therapeutic approaches should be considered.

## Complications

### Sloughing

If sloughing follows the injection of a sclerosant, one or more of three errors are usually responsible:

1. The injection was too superficial.
2. Too much solution was injected into one area.
3. A second injection was made into a hemorrhoid too soon after the first.

Expectant management usually results in resolution without long-term sequelae. However, anal stricture can be a consequence of extensive tissue destruction.

### *Thrombosis*

Thrombosed hemorrhoids, whether internal, external, or both, are sometimes associated with the effects of sclerotherapy. With sloughing and thrombosis, treatment is conservative—sitz baths, analgesics, and topical anal creams.

### *Burning*

Burning in the anal canal is a late consequence of repeated sclerotherapy. The discomfort can be disabling, unremitting, and unresponsive to the usual local measures. Repeated injections are not recommended primarily because of this complication.

### *Abscess and Paraffinoma*

Submucous abscess and paraffinoma (i.e., oleogranuloma) have been reported, the latter after the use of oil-based sclerosing agents. These conditions are extremely rare, as is the complication of rectal perforation with retroperitoneal abscess.

### *Bacteremia*

Bacteremia following sclerotherapy has been reported in 8% of patients who undergo this procedure. Antibiotic prophylaxis is recommended for those individuals at an increased risk (e.g., valvular heart disease), although septicemia has not been reported in any such patients.

### Results

A single session of injection treatment using "adequate doses of sclerosant" (i.e., 3 to 5 mL) is as effective as multiple treatments but provides only short-term benefit for most individuals. Additionally, sclerosant therapy is less effective than a number of other options. One treatment should be sufficient; if symptoms persist, an alternative approach is indicated.

### Rubber Ring Ligation

Tissue necrosis and fixation can also be produced by rubber ring ligation. Any individual who has hemorrhoids manifested by bleeding, prolapse, or both is a candidate for this procedure. No anesthetic is required, but the rubber rings must be placed on an insensitive area, usually at or just above the dentate line. Skin tags or hypertrophied anal papillae cannot be treated by ligation because the patient would experience too much discomfort.

After a small cleansing enema has been given, complete proctosigmoidoscopy and anoscopy are performed. If the patient's history is suggestive of colonic disease, colonoscopy or barium enema examination is completed before any treatment of the hemorrhoids is considered. Explain to the patient the nature of the problem and the technique that will be used to treat it. Several treatments, spaced over 3- to 4-week intervals, may be required, depending on how many pile sites must be eliminated to alleviate the symptoms. Generally, I do not recommend multiple bandings in the first treatment session. Exceptions are usually made on the basis of patient insistence or convenience, lack of discomfort with the initial application, or the necessity of the patient traveling a considerable distance for subsequent therapy.

### Technique

All nonsuction instruments have the relative disadvantage of requiring two people to perform the procedure—one to maintain the anoscope or retractor in position, and the other to hold the ligator and grasping forceps. Alternatively, a suction hemorrhoidal ligator can be used that draws the hemorrhoid into the cup through suction and, therefore, does not require a grasping forceps. The most prominent hemorrhoid is treated first. It is grasped with the forceps (Fig. 8.3A) and pulled up through the drum of the ligator (Fig. 8.3B). If the patient experiences pain, a slightly more proximal point is selected, and this step is repeated. (If the patient is still very uncomfortable, the wise course would be to abandon this method of treatment and consider one of the alternatives.) The tissue is drawn into the drum until it is taut, and the trigger is released, expelling two rubber rings (Fig. 8.3C). Two rings are usually used, in case one breaks. When the rings are in place, the anoscope is withdrawn (Fig. 8.3D).

The patient rarely experiences pain so severe that removal of the rings is necessary; if required, however, this can be done by interposing the end of a conventional disposable suture-removal scissors or the application of a crochet hook. Other methods for removing the rings (e.g., cutting with a scalpel) tend to precipitate bleeding. Removal of the rubber rings can be accomplished with minimal trauma within a few minutes after application. If the patient returns at a later time because of pain, the associated edema precludes the possibility of safe removal. Adequate analgesic medication is the preferred option.

### Care Following Treatment

Bowel actions should be maintained without the patient straining. Appropriate dietary instructions, bulk agents, or a stool softener should be considered. Some bleeding may be noted initially and again when the rubber rings are dislodged.

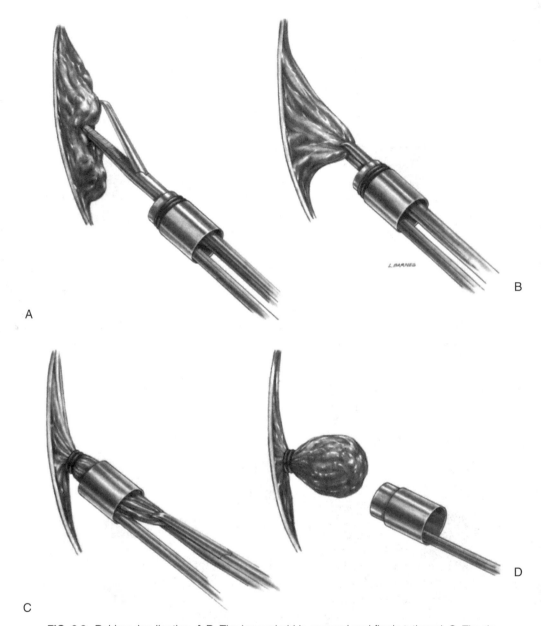

**FIG. 8.3.** Rubber ring ligation. **A,B.** The hemorrhoid is grasped and firmly tethered. **C.** The tissue is drawn into the drum. If the patient tolerates the maneuver, ligation can be performed with minimal or no discomfort. **D.** The two rubber rings are released.

One of the major advantages of rubber ring ligation is its convenience. The patient need not return at fixed intervals for further ligation. However, the patient should realize that if symptoms are not completely relieved, it is probably because other areas need to be addressed. Conversely, if the individual experiences complete relief after the initial ligation, therapy need not continue.

## Complications

A moderate sense of discomfort or fullness in the rectum can be anticipated for a few days, but complaints are usually minimal and can often be relieved by sitz baths and mild analgesics. Complications, occasionally seen after rubber ring ligation, can include the following:

- Delayed hemorrhage
- Severe pain
- External hemorrhoidal thrombosis
- Ulceration
- Slippage of the ligature
- Fulminant sepsis

### Delayed Hemorrhage

Late hemorrhage (i.e., 1 to 2 weeks after treatment) following rubber ring ligation occurs in approximately 1% of patients. This may be attributed to sepsis in the pedicle and can be a major bleeding problem requiring hospitalization, suture ligation, and transfusion. Increased bleeding, especially 7 to 10 days following ligation, warrants re-evaluation; it is, in fact, because of this complication that rubber ring ligation is relatively contraindicated in individuals who are on anticoagulants. An excisional option, sclerotherapy, or one of the other alternatives may be considered.

### Pain

A local anesthetic at the time of treatment may be a valuable adjunct if the patient is particularly apprehensive. Pain is much more likely to be a source of concern if multiple bandings are attempted. Pain that seems to worsen merits re-examination of the patient, especially if fever supervenes or a problem with micturition develops. Sepsis in the area can lead to gangrene or even death.

In the usual, uncomplicated scenario, sitz baths and adequate pain medication should be sufficient to relieve pain associated with rubber ring ligation. With respect to future management, it seems reasonable to conclude that if the patient tolerated the initial ligation poorly, other methods should be considered if additional treatments are required.

### Thrombosis

With ligation of internal hemorrhoids, the risk for subsequent thrombosis of corresponding external hemorrhoids is 2% to 3%. If thrombosis occurs, sitz baths and stool softeners are recommended. Occasionally, excision of the thrombosed hemorrhoid is required.

### Ulceration

Anal ulceration is a normal consequence of ligation. The rubber rings cause tissue necrosis, and they fall off in 2 to 5 days, leaving an ulcerated area. On rare occasions, a large ulcer, sometimes associated with a fissure, may be a troublesome complication. Treatment consists of sitz baths and perhaps a cortisone preparation; if the ulcer or fissure is persistent, internal anal sphincterotomy should be considered.

### Slippage

The rubber rings can slip or break at any time, but this usually happens after the first or second bowel movement. Breakage can be caused by a defective rubber ring—the reason to use two rings—but more commonly is caused by tension produced by the large bulk of tissue that has been ligated. The use of a mild laxative can help prevent passage of a hard stool, thereby, it is hoped, avoiding precipitous dislocation of the rings. Repeated ligation of the same pile site can be safely performed 3 to 4 weeks after the initial procedure.

### Sepsis

Aside from the normal sloughing that occurs from tissue necrosis, sepsis following rubber ring ligation had been virtually unknown before the past 15 years. Only a few cases have appeared, yet there seems to be a characteristic scenario of events. Young male patients seem to be at the greatest risk, with complaints of perineal pain, scrotal swelling, and difficulty urinating, which mandates emergency evaluation.

The cause of this potentially devastating complication is unclear, but some have suggested that these individuals may be in an immunocompromised state. A more likely explanation is failure to recognize a septic process as the cause of the patient's "hemorrhoid" symptoms. Obviously, alternative causes of anorectal complaints, especially pain, should be sought before embarking on rubber ring ligation.

Findings on physical examination can include fever, perineal edema, scrotal edema, perineal ulceration, cellulitis, or frank gangrene. Rectal examination may reveal a boggy, edematous anal canal that is exquisitely tender. Computed tomography of the pelvis can be useful, especially to demonstrate thickening of the rectal wall or any extrarectal pathology.

Treatment requires massive antibiotic therapy, vigorous debridement, and possibly hyperbaric oxygen treatment. A colostomy may be necessary. Reportedly, only a few individuals have survived this complication, and those who have were recognized early and treated aggressively.

### Error in Diagnosis

A theoretic disadvantage of rubber ring ligation and all the nonexcisional methods for treating hemorrhoids is that no pathologic specimen is obtained. Invasive epidermoid carcinoma or other tumor occasionally has been reported in an excised hemorrhoid specimen (perhaps 1% of cases). In the rare instance of its occurrence, such a lesion will obviously be missed.

### Results

Evaluation at 1 month will demonstrate 96% to be symptom free. Bleeding to a slight degree will be noted in 3%, but not require specific treatment. Bleeding to a significant degree may be expected in 1%. Only 2% of all patients treated have complications severe enough to interfere with daily activity.

Long-term assessment (5 years) of the value of rubber ring ligation as a treatment for hemorrhoids reveals that most patients (75% to 90%) consider themselves cured or greatly improved; however, only 44% are completely free of symptoms. The best results are obtained in patients who had grade I hemorrhoids. The effectiveness of treatment does not depend on the number of hemorrhoids ligated. Perhaps the most meaningful finding is that a single treatment can achieve satisfactory results. If more than three sessions are required to control symptoms, the procedure should probably be abandoned and hemorrhoidectomy performed.

Studies demonstrate that rubber ring ligation is far superior to sclerosing agents. Better long-term results, significantly more effective management of symptoms of protrusion, and greater likelihood of control of bleeding can be anticipated with this method of treatment.

## Cryosurgery

Cryosurgery is based on the concept of cellular destruction through rapid freezing followed by rapid thawing. The treatment of hemorrhoids by this technique has been advocated as painless, effective, and especially recommended for those patients who are medically unable to undergo general anesthesia.

### Technique

The following protocol is recommended by most authors:

1. The procedure is explained, and the patient is advised of the probability of profuse drainage and considerable swelling. If necessary, an intravenous

injection of a sedative is administered, and a local anesthetic is usually recommended.

2. The patient is placed in either the left lateral or prone jackknife position. The fingers, a plastic vaginal speculum, or a modified plastic proctoscope are used to isolate one primary hemorrhoidal plexus at a time. (A metal instrument is not used because it would conduct cold.) A water-soluble jelly is used to achieve good contact between the cryoprobe and the hemorrhoid.

3. The cryoprobe is applied. The tissue freezes around the tip. Thus, the distance between the tip and the outer border of the ice ball equals the depth of the ice ball. This allows the surgeon to determine visually how much tissue is being destroyed. Only that tissue encompassed within the ice ball allegedly will undergo irreversible cellular destruction. Changes at the boundary between the ice ball and normal tissue are reversible, and theoretically, no true cellular destruction occurs.

Theoretically, both internal and external hemorrhoids can be treated in one operation. The tip of the cryoprobe is placed in the center of either the internal or external hemorrhoidal plexus and remains there until the tissue to be destroyed is enveloped by the ice ball. The period of freezing varies according to the cooling power of the probe. With a liquid nitrogen probe at −196°C or a liquid nitrous oxide probe at −89°C, the application time is about 2 minutes per hemorrhoid area. The greater the vascularity of the hemorrhoid, the greater the cooling power required to freeze it. Therefore, the liquid nitrogen probe is more effective for large hemorrhoids than is the nitrous oxide probe. When an adequate amount of tissue has been frozen, the probe is switched off, rewarmed, and detached from the hemorrhoid; each plexus, in turn, is treated the same way.

### Care After Treatment

Considerable swelling and edema occur within 24 hours of the procedure, but they do not interfere with normal bowel function and elimination. Drainage usually starts several hours later; it is fairly heavy for the first 3 to 4 days but decreases during the following 2 to 3 weeks. Patients are instructed to use some form of sterile pad and to change the pad several times a day during the first 3 to 4 days.

Two to three hours after freezing, the tissue becomes swollen and erythematous. Within 72 hours, pale spots appear on the surface, and these coalesce to form irregular patches by the fourth day. By the fifth or sixth day, the whole hemorrhoidal area is pale; black, gangrenous areas may then appear. Gangrene is usually complete between postoperative days 7 and 9. Thereafter, the hemorrhoid begins to disintegrate and should come away completely by the 18th postoperative day, leaving, it is hoped, a normal-appearing anus.

## *Results*

When cryosurgical hemorrhoidectomy was first introduced, it was claimed to be painless, anesthetic-free, and effective for external tags and hypertrophied papillae. Since that time, reports have confirmed that it is not painless—local or general anesthetic is suggested by almost all observers—and that it is less effective, and in many ways ineffective, for the treatment of hypertrophied anal papillae and skin tags. For internal hemorrhoids, rubber ring ligation is superior to cryosurgery. It is quicker and cheaper and requires no anesthetic. For the external component or hypertrophied papilla, excision after local infiltration rapidly removes the offending tissue. Complete healing takes place in 7 to 10 days. Cryosurgical destruction requires the use of expensive equipment and is time-consuming to perform—some authors recommend hospitalization or an outpatient setting. Also, it results in profuse drainage and sometimes delayed healing. True, the initial postanesthetic pain may be somewhat less than with surgical hemorrhoidectomy, but this pain usually can be controlled with a mild analgesic.

Cryosurgery would appear to add nothing to the treatment of hemorrhoids that is not available by other means at lower cost, at greater efficiency, with fewer complications, and with as good if not better results.

## Infrared Coagulation

In 1979, infrared coagulation was first described as a method for the treatment of hemorrhoids. The apparatus produces infrared radiation and is focused by a photoconductor. It was developed as an offshoot of laser technology, but it is not a laser. Infrared light penetrates the tissue to a predetermined level at the speed of light and is converted to heat. The amount of tissue destruction can be regulated by direct visualization and by adjusting the pulse setting on the instrument.

### *Technique*

A 1-second or 1.5-second pulse is usually used in the treatment of hemorrhoids, with the probe applied at the same site where the physician would normally inject. The radiation causes protein coagulation 3 mm wide and 3 mm deep. The manufacturer recommends the application of three to five pulses to the normal mucosa proximal to the hemorrhoid, above the dentate line, and in a semicircular pattern around the apex of the hemorrhoid, but not directly over the pile. Following coagulation, the tissue appears white. Over the next week a dark eschar forms, ultimately leaving a slightly puckered, pink to red scar. One area can be treated at a time or all evident hemorrhoids can be ablated at once. Additional treatments may be repeated every 2 weeks if necessary. Although, reportedly, the procedure can be done without a local anesthetic, particularly if the coagulator is applied above the pectinate line, infiltrating the area with 0.5%

bupivacaine (Marcaine) is often recommended. Of course, if an external tag is to be treated, a local anesthetic is required.

### Results

Comparison of photocoagulation and rubber ring ligation in the treatment of hemorrhoids demonstrates no difference in the symptomatic outcome between these two groups up to 1 year following the procedure. A higher incidence of bleeding and pain is noted following banding, but additional outpatient procedures were more frequently encountered with photocoagulation. Photocoagulation and injection sclerotherapy are also considered comparable, although the injection group required fewer additional treatments. Comparison studies of the use of infrared coagulation and of bipolar diathermy (BICAP; see *Bipolar Diathermy* below) revealed no significant difference in rate of complications and number of treatments required. In a three-armed report involving the infrared technique, the heater probe, and the Ultroid device (Microvasive, Watertown, Massachusetts [see below]), it was concluded that all three methods are effective modalities for first- and second-degree hemorrhoids

### Ultroid

The Ultroid device is another tool used for the ambulatory treatment of hemorrhoids. It is a monopolar, low-voltage instrument that includes a generator unit, an attachable handle, single-use sterile probes, a grounding pad, and a nonconductive anoscope. Some have commented that it is confusing to have two electrodes, yet the instrument is not bipolar. The company contends that the mode of action of this device is not thermal but rather is a consequence of the production of sodium hydroxide at the negative electrode.

### Technique

By means of the nonconductive anoscope, the probe tip is placed at the apex of the hemorrhoid, above the dentate line. The amperage is slowly increased to the level of patient tolerance as the probe is inserted into the hemorrhoid. The probe is left in position for approximately 10 minutes, or until the "popping" sound ceases. Once the treatment has been completed, the current is gradually decreased to zero. Failure to do this will result in pain on removal of the probe. One site is usually treated per session, usually because of time constraints and the fact that the patient does not usually appreciate a prolonged anoscopy.

### Results

The results are comparable with those of other techniques, but the time required for treatment is a particular disadvantage. Also, the operator is required to hold the probe still for a long period of time.

## Bipolar Diathermy

As with photocoagulation, BICAP is a method of treating hemorrhoids that is designed to produce tissue destruction, ulceration, and fibrosis by the local application of heat. The disposable Circon ACMI (Santa Barbara, CA) BICAP hemorrhoid probe uses bipolar RF current to coagulate the blood vessels. The principle of action is the passage of current through tissue as it travels between adjacent electrodes located at the tip of the probe. The touted, perhaps theoretical, advantage of this technique over other methods (e.g., monopolar coagulation, laser coagulation, or photocoagulation) is that the BICAP device maintains a short current path, thereby producing a limited depth of penetration even after multiple applications.

### Technique

With the use of a disposable, nonconductive anoscope, the side of the probe tip is applied directly and firmly to the hemorrhoid above the dentate line. The generator, which is used on the infinity setting, is activated by a foot switch. A white coagulum approximately 3 mm deep is produced. All hemorrhoids are treated in one session, and no local anesthetic is usually required.

### Results

A number of controlled trials have been published comparing BICAP with other ambulatory methods in the management of hemorrhoids, demonstrating it to be essentially equally effective. Rates and types of complications are also similar.

## Lord's Dilatation

In addition to the ambulatory methods of treatment for hemorrhoids that have been discussed, another procedure (i.e., anal dilatation) should be included in this category.

In 1968, Lord reported a method he had devised for the treatment of hemorrhoids. He based his approach on the hypothesis that increased anal canal pressure contributes to the hemorrhoid problem, and that dilatation reduces this pressure, thereby ameliorating the condition. Although this method requires a general or spinal anesthetic, hospitalization can often be limited to a 1-day stay, or the patient can be discharged from an ambulatory care facility or similar surgical center.

### Technique

The patient is placed on the left side and given an intravenous anesthetic. A constriction to the outlet, which Lord believes is present in all patients with third-degree hemorrhoids, is identified.

Two fingers of one hand are pulled upward, and the index finger of the other hand presses downward to feel the constriction. The aim is to dilate the lower part of the rectum and anal canal gently and firmly until no constrictions remain. It is an "ironing out" process that is carried out by a circular movement through all four quadrants. Tearing should be avoided. During the procedure, eight fingers are inserted as high as they will reach, actually dilating not only the anal canal, but also the rectal ampulla. Not all rectums and anal canals can be dilated safely to this extent, and Lord cautions that it is much better to do too little than too much.

As dilatation is achieved, an assistant inserts a sponge, usually by means of a ring forceps. The sponge presses on the walls of the lower part of the rectum and anal canal, and is apparently used to reduce the risk for postoperative hematoma formation. The sponge is left in place for 1 hour, and the patient is discharged when alert.

### *Postoperative Care*

The patient is instructed on the insertion of a dilating cone, which can be used as required for anal symptoms, but researchers wonder whether it is vital to the success of the method. Under normal circumstances, the patient should take 2 or 3 days off from work and be seen after 2 weeks. If free of symptoms at that time, the patient is discharged.

### *Results*

Lord claims that less pain and postoperative morbidity occur after dilatation than after hemorrhoidectomy. He states that his method does not cause urinary retention, deep vein thrombosis, postoperative bleeding, or fecal impaction. The patients are free of pain during defecation, operating room time is saved, and the hospital stay is greatly shortened. Still, in Lord's opinion, rubber ring ligation is the treatment of choice for most hemorrhoid problems, and dilatation should be used as an alternative to surgical hemorrhoidectomy. However, he suggests that hemorrhoidectomy should be considered when hypertrophied papillae and external tags are present.

The procedure does result in a significant lowering of pressure following dilatation compared with that occurring in conventional hemorrhoidectomy. At 5 years, 75% of patients can be expected to be free of symptoms or greatly improved following dilatation.

A prospective study was carried out on 50 patients with hemorrhoids treated by the Lord method and followed for at least 4 years. Of 36 individuals who were free of symptoms, 19 still had evidence of anal congestion but no distinct hemorrhoids, and 4 subsequently underwent a standard hemorrhoid operation for persistent prolapse and bleeding.

Older patients who underwent anal dilatation occasionally reported control problems, so it is recommended that Lord's procedure be limited to those younger than 55 years of age.

*Comment*: Failure to deal with tags and papillae, and the risk for incontinence, especially in patients above 60 years of age, should preclude the application of this technique. Recognize that sphincter stretch inevitably must attenuate the external sphincter as well as the internal.

## TREATMENT OF THROMBOSED HEMORRHOIDS

### External

The patient with thrombosed external hemorrhoids usually presents with a painful, tender mass (Fig. 8.4), and may report that the lump appeared following a bout of constipation or diarrhea. An important predisposing factor for the development of recurrent thrombosed hemorrhoids is spending too much time on the toilet.

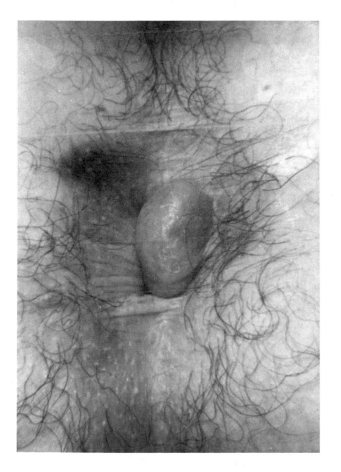

FIG. 8.4. A thrombosed external hemorrhoid.

If the problem has been present for more than 2 or 3 days, the discomfort usually has begun to subside and medical management should be offered. This consists of sitz baths and stool softeners. A mild analgesic may be recommended. The mass will usually resolve in 7 to 10 days. If ulceration or rupture has occurred, or if the patient is seen within 48 hours, it is usually advisable to excise the lesion. Certainly, if the pain is severe, excision is preferred.

## Technique

The hemorrhoid should be excised, not incised. Making a small incision and shelling the clot out like a pea from a pod often results in recurrent hemorrhage into the subcutaneous tissue and clot re-accumulation (Fig. 8.5). The area is infiltrated with a local anesthetic. The commercially prepared bupivacaine solution is acidic and it is often associated with extreme burning pain on instillation. Adding 1 mL of 8.4% sodium bicarbonate solution, *United States Pharmacopeia*, to 9 mL of bupivacaine with epinephrine markedly lessens the discomfort associated with the injection.

The underlying hemorrhoid is excised, as is a wedge of skin (Fig. 8.5). Bleeding is controlled with pressure, topically applied epinephrine, or electrocautery. Another option is Monsel's solution, a chemical styptic agent (ferric subsulfate). A pressure dressing is used.

## Postoperative Care

The patient is instructed to keep the pressure dressing on for a few hours. By this time there is usually some discomfort, and the dressing is then removed. If bleeding occurs, it can usually be controlled by the application of direct pressure on the wound with a cloth or compress. A small dressing or pad can be used to avoid soiling clothing. Twice-daily sitz baths are recommended until the wound heals (i.e., 7 to 10 days). A mild analgesic and a topical anesthetic cream may be of benefit.

## Internal

In addition to the aforementioned factors that can cause thrombosis of external hemorrhoids, prolapse with inadequate reduction can cause thrombosis of internal hemorrhoids. As a result, stasis develops within the vein and thrombosis occurs.

The treatment of thrombosed internal hemorrhoids is not as straightforward as that for external hemorrhoids. Fortunately, however, pain is not as frequent a complaint. Excision of a thrombosed internal hemorrhoid, however, requires instrumentation and a more extensive local infiltration. Suture is necessary for hemostasis, because the application of adequate direct pressure is virtually impossible.

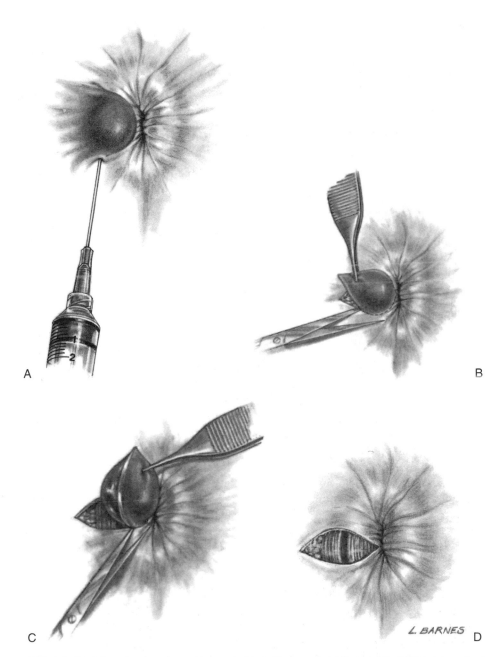

**FIG. 8.5.** Excision of a thrombosed hemorrhoid. **A.** The area is infiltrated with 0.5% bupivacaine in 1:200, epinephrine. **B,C.** The thrombosis is excised with the underlying vein and with a wedge of skin. **D.** Skin edges are sufficiently separate to permit adequate drainage, thereby preventing re-accumulation of a clot.

As operative intervention for the acute problem is rarely indicated, sitz baths are recommended, as well as a mild systemic analgesic and a topical anesthetic cream or suppository. A stool softener is also advisable. If the patient has concurrent extensive hemorrhoids, tags, hypertrophied papillae, or associated anal fissure, a surgical approach is usually advocated.

## TREATMENT OF GANGRENOUS, PROLAPSED, EDEMATOUS HEMORRHOIDS

The patient who presents with severely disabling gangrenous hemorrhoids requires emergency medical measures and, ideally, surgical hemorrhoidectomy within 24 hours. Pain, swelling, bleeding, foul-smelling discharge, and difficulty defecating are common presenting complaints. Of prior hemorrhoidal difficulties, prolapse is the most frequent. Proctosigmoidoscopic and anoscopic examination reveal edematous, thrombosed, irreducible hemorrhoids (see Figs. 8.2 and 8.5).

### Technique

In the office, a perianal field block is established using an alkalinized solution of 0.5% bupivacaine (Marcaine) with 1:200,000 epinephrine, and adding to this solution two 1-mm ampules of hyaluronidase (300 NF units of Wydase). A subcutaneous circumanal wheal is infiltrated in the edematous hemorrhoidal tissue (Fig. 8.6). Four deep injections are made in the intersphincteric groove in each quadrant to effect paralysis of the sphincter mechanism and to create total perianal anesthesia. After a few minutes' wait to allow the medication to take effect, direct massaging pressure is applied with a sterile pad to reduce the hemorrhoidal mass. A pressure dressing is used, and the buttocks are taped.

Ideally, the patient is admitted to the hospital on an emergency basis, and a hemorrhoidectomy is performed the following day. With reduction maintained, the patient is usually comfortable, and an adequate, safe operation can be performed with less edema than would be present without reduction.

### Results

Historically, the concept of surgical hemorrhoidectomy in the presence of thrombosed, ulcerated, gangrenous hemorrhoids was considered unwise because of the risks for pyelophlebitis, perianal sepsis, hemorrhage, and the subsequent development of anal stricture. However, with the application of proper surgical technique, the complication rate should be minimal. Operation for prolapsed and strangulated hemorrhoids in the acute stage should be safe and effective, comparable with that of elective operation for chronic hemorrhoidal complaints

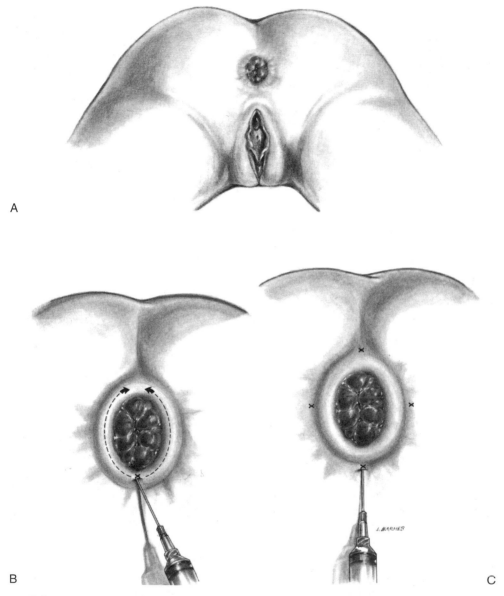

**FIG. 8.6.** Method of establishing a perianal field block. **A.** The patient is placed in the prone (i.e., jackknife) position. **B.** A subcutaneous perianal wheal is raised. **C.** Deep injections are made at four sites to effect further anesthesia and paralysis of sphincter muscles.

## SURGICAL HEMORRHOIDECTOMY

Surgical hemorrhoidectomy should be considered when the anorectal architecture has been severely and irreversibly compromised (e.g., in the presence of an external component, ulceration, gangrene, extensive thrombosis, hypertrophied papillae, or associated fissure.

### Preoperative Preparation

The most important preoperative measure is a small-volume enema the morning of the operation. Vigorous mechanical cleansing by means of laxatives is counterproductive. The patient should be able to defecate as soon as possible after the operation, yet be empty of stool that might encumber the surgeon during the procedure.

No antibiotics are indicated. Minimal intravenous fluids should be administered before induction of anesthesia, and the patient should be encouraged to void before the procedure. A small area may be shaved in the operating room if the situation warrants.

### Surgical Approaches

Inserting a dry sponge into the rectum and withdrawing it is an excellent way to demonstrate hemorrhoidal tissue, tags, papillae, and the extent of redundant mucosa. Whenever possible, a bridge of intact skin and mucosa should be left between excised hemorrhoidal sites to avoid subsequent stricture formation. This is particularly important when operating for acute, edematous, or gangrenous hemorrhoids.

### *Closed Hemorrhoidectomy or Ferguson Hemorrhoidectomy*

The patient is placed in the prone jackknife position with the buttocks taped apart. Having the patient in the lithotomy position is awkward for the assistant, because considerable suturing is required when the primary closure technique is used. Although the lateral decubitus position is recommended by the Ferguson Clinic group to avoid the need for spinal anesthesia or sometimes endotracheal intubation, this position is also very inconvenient for the assistant.

The anus is infiltrated with a solution of approximately 20 mL of 0.5% bupivacaine in 1:200,000 epinephrine. The infiltration technique minimizes any bleeding, and the anatomic plane between the hemorrhoidal mass and the underlying internal sphincter muscle is clearly delineated. Furthermore, by using local anesthesia and the aforementioned field block technique, perhaps with supplementary intravenous sedation while the medication is administered, no other anesthesia is necessary. Alternatively, a general, caudal, or spinal anesthetic can be used.

A Hill–Ferguson retractor placed in the anal canal reveals the extent of the hemorrhoids. Some surgeons like to place an anchoring suture in the rectum corresponding to the site of the hemorrhoid, but I prefer placing only a clamp to incorporate the skin tag and hemorrhoid that will be excised (Fig. 8.7). Excision can be performed with a scalpel or scissors or by electrocautery. The incision should be carried well beyond the anal verge, removing the external hemorrhoidal plexus and exposing the subcutaneous portion of the external sphincter muscle (Fig. 8.8). The incision is then carried into the anal canal; the internal sphincter muscle is carefully dropped away from the plane of dissection. Bleeding is avoided when the dissection is outside the hemorrhoid and medial to the internal sphincter. When the entire hemorrhoid pedicle has been mobilized, a suture ligature of absorbable material is placed. The pedicle is suture-ligated, and the hemorrhoid is excised (Fig. 8.9). Any residual, small internal or external hemorrhoids should be removed by means of a forceps and fine scissors (Fig. 8.10). This maneuver will minimize the possibility of delayed symptoms from hemorrhoidal veins that have been left behind. Hemostasis can be achieved with electrocautery.

The wound is closed completely with a continuous suture, using the same stitch as for ligation of the hemorrhoid pedicle (Fig. 8.11). When the mucocutaneous junction is reached, the skin is closed in either a subcuticular fashion or

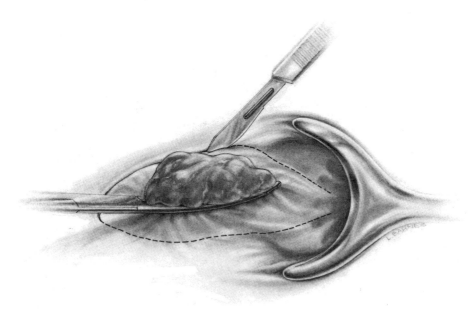

**FIG. 8.7.** The hemorrhoid is identified and grasped with a clamp. The area for excision is outlined by a *broken line.*

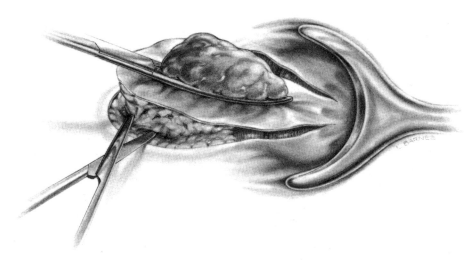

**FIG. 8.8.** After the area for excision is outlined, the hemorrhoidal plexus is removed from the underlying subcutaneous portion of the external and internal sphincters.

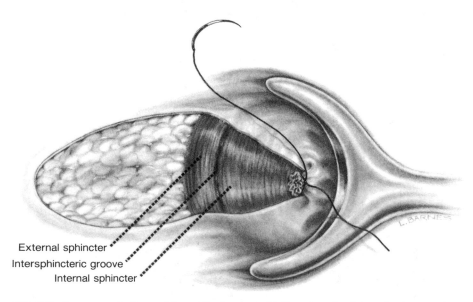

External sphincter •
Intersphincteric groove •
Internal sphincter •

**FIG. 8.9.** Open wound after excision of the hemorrhoid. No external or internal veins remain.

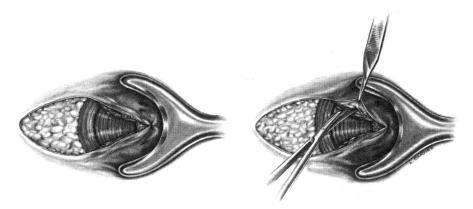

**FIG. 8.10**. Residual hemorrhoids are removed by undermining the mucosa.

by a continuous simple suture. In like manner, the remaining pile sites are excised, ligated, and primarily closed (Fig. 8.12). Aside from the cosmetic appearance of the wounds, the fact that the physician can close all incisions and maintain the retractor in place implies that the anal canal opening is adequate, and the physician need not be concerned about the subsequent development of a stricture.

The wounds are cleansed, and povidone-iodine ointment and a small dressing are applied. A bulky pressure dressing is avoided; no packing is used.

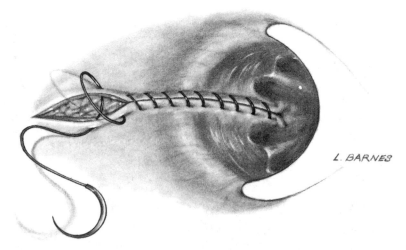

**FIG. 8.11.** The wound is primarily closed.

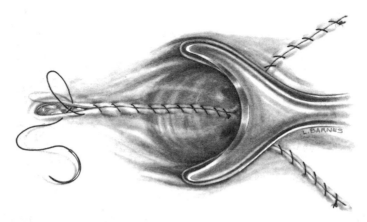

**FIG. 8.12.** Completed closed (i.e., Ferguson) hemorrhoidectomy. With a Hill–Ferguson retractor in place, no anal canal narrowing can occur.

### Hemorrhoidectomy and Sphincterotomy

If a fissure is present, an internal anal sphincterotomy is undertaken in the left lateral pile site by dividing the lower one third of the internal anal sphincter. I do not routinely use sphincterotomy, although some surgeons believe that this procedure reduces complaints of pain.

### Open Hemorrhoidectomy

Modifications of a closed or open hemorrhoidectomy are myriad. When hemorrhoids are gangrenous or circumferential, or when closure of wounds cannot be carried out with even a narrow retractor in place, an open technique at one, two, or all of the pile sites may be indicated. Certainly, the open hemorrhoidectomy is quicker to accomplish.

With an open technique, the procedure is identical to that described for the Ferguson operation with ligation of the hemorrhoidal pedicles, except that the operation ends at this point. Hemostasis is established with electrocautery. Alternatively, one or two sites may be left open, closed, or partially closed. Good results are possible with a combination of approaches.

### Submucosal Hemorrhoidectomy or Parks Hemorrhoidectomy

In the submucosal hemorrhoidectomy described by Parks, the mucosa of the anal canal and rectum is incised, and the hemorrhoidal tissue beneath is removed. The mucosa is then re-approximated. The goal of this method is to excise all the hemorrhoidal tissue without injuring the overlying squamous and columnar epithelium. The main potential advantage of this procedure is that the wounds allegedly heal more quickly, with reduced induration and scarring and less likelihood of the development of a stricture.

## Technique

A self-retaining anal (i.e., Parks) retractor is usually recommended, primarily by surgeons in the United Kingdom; however, virtually any conventional anal retractor can be used. A solution of 0.5% bupivacaine or lidocaine in 1:200,000 epinephrine is injected into the submucosa and the hemorrhoidal mass (Fig. 8.13A).

The skin incision starts outside the anus and is carried around the forceps holding the anal skin, removing a minimal amount of anal canal mucosa (Fig. 8.13B). The anal canal is undermined by scissors dissection to expose the hemorrhoidal tissue. The mucosa is elevated off of the hemorrhoidal vessels (Fig. 8.13C). The upper limit of the dissection should be about 4 cm above the mucocutaneous junction. The external and internal sphincters are identified as the hemorrhoidal mass is elevated and stripped off the internal sphincter to what is considered an adequate level (Fig. 8.13D). The hemorrhoidal mass is transfixed (Fig. 8.13E) and the hemorrhoid is excised. The flaps of the mobilized anal canal mucosa are re-approximated, and the underlying internal sphincter is incorporated with the sutures to prevent dislodgement (Fig. 8.13F). The skin can be left open or closed.

## Results

No meaningful results are yet available on the submucosal hemorrhoidectomy operations.

### Whitehead Hemorrhoidectomy

The Whitehead hemorrhoidectomy is rarely used by surgeons today because of the complications of stricture and ectropion, but the procedure that frequently results in these complications is not truly the one that was exactly described by the author. As originally recommended by Whitehead, the mucosa was sutured to the anal canal above the level of the pectinate line, but later surgeons misinterpreted this description and anchored the mucosa to the skin at the anal verge (Fig. 8.14). All too often, the suture line dehisced, and the wound was left to granulate and heal by second intention. More commonly, a mucosal ectropion, the so-called "wet anus" or "Whitehead deformity," was the consequence (Fig. 8.15).

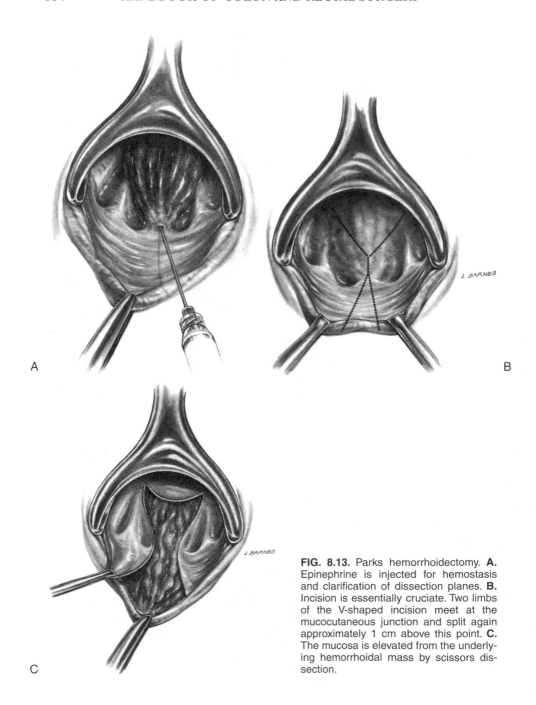

**FIG. 8.13.** Parks hemorrhoidectomy. **A.** Epinephrine is injected for hemostasis and clarification of dissection planes. **B.** Incision is essentially cruciate. Two limbs of the V-shaped incision meet at the mucocutaneous junction and split again approximately 1 cm above this point. **C.** The mucosa is elevated from the underlying hemorrhoidal mass by scissors dissection.

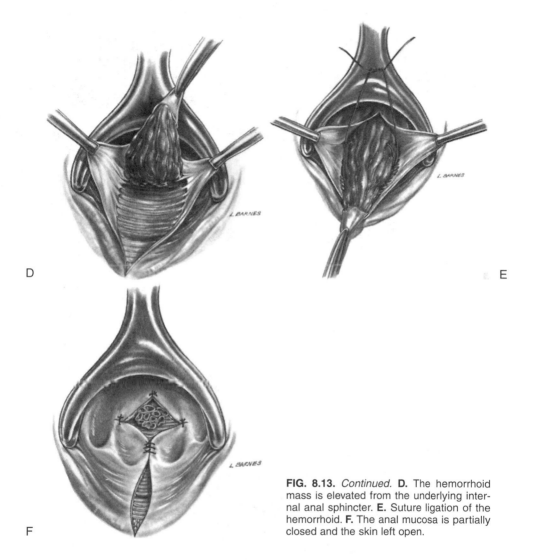

D

E

F

**FIG. 8.13.** *Continued.* **D.** The hemorrhoid mass is elevated from the underlying internal anal sphincter. **E.** Suture ligation of the hemorrhoid. **F.** The anal mucosa is partially closed and the skin left open.

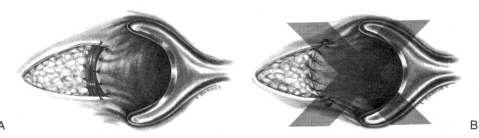

A                                                                          B

**FIG. 8.14.** Whitehead hemorrhoidectomy. **A.** Proper mucosal anchoring to the underlying internal sphincter. **B.** Improper anchoring can lead to ectropion.

## Results

Whether the physician simply anchors the cut edge of the rectum to the underlying internal sphincter, or combines an amputative hemorrhoidectomy with advancement of the perianal skin into the anal canal, the results should be satisfactory. Clearly, the mucosa should never be anchored to the skin outside the anus. Urinary retention occurs in approximately 33%, and a 5% incidence of hemorrhage and a 10% incidence of late complications (i.e., stenosis, ectropion, and incontinence) have been reported.

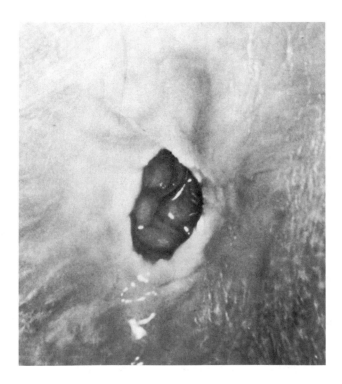

**FIG. 8.15.** Whitehead deformity. Note mucosal ectropion that developed after excision of the anal canal, the characteristic "wet anus."

## *Laser Surgery*

The three most common surgical lasers are the carbon dioxide, argon, and Nd:YAG. The different wavelengths of their light produce characteristic tissue effects that determine their usefulness in surgery. The carbon dioxide laser primarily cuts and is awkward to use endoscopically. Conversely, the argon laser coagulates surface vessels well, whereas the noncontact Nd:YAG can be used with deep vessels. Both, however, are limited by their unsatisfactory cutting qualities. A distinct advantage is the fact that Nd:YAG light will pass through optical fibers and, therefore, can be used through the operating channel of most endoscopy equipment.

### *Technique*

Use of the laser requires special training and precautions. Because the light is invisible, the operator must wear goggles to protect the eyes. After administration of a local anesthetic, with the patient in the prone position and with a Hill Ferguson retractor in place, the laser beam is aimed directly onto the surface of the pile. A red pilot light, provided by low-power laser, permits precise focusing of the therapeutic beam. The handle is moved while the laser beam destroys the tissue until the treated area is covered by a white membrane. Internal and external hemorrhoids are treated similarly.

### *Results*

Narcotic pain medication is necessary for the first few days, and healing usually occurs in about 1 month. The early and late complication rates are not significantly different from those of conventional surgical hemorrhoidectomy. Because of the increased cost of the laser, there is a significant price differential in using laser surgery.

### General Principles of Care Following Hemorrhoidectomy

The dressing is removed the evening of the operation, and 20-minute warm sitz baths are commenced. A small dressing helps to prevent soiling of garments.

The patient is discharged if able to void. Discharge medications include an analgesic, a bulk laxative, a stool softener or stimulant laxative if necessary, and cream and pads for the dressing regimen.

The patient is not seen until 3 or 4 weeks after discharge, at which time the wounds are usually healed.

### Complications of Surgical Hemorrhoidectomy

To avoid the pitfalls of hemorrhoid surgery, conscientious effort is required, not only with respect to meticulous surgical technique, but also with regard to a compulsive approach to postoperative management. Below is a partial list of the potential problems of surgical hemorrhoidectomy:

Pain
Urinary retention
Urinary tract infection
Constipation
Fecal impaction
Hemorrhage
Infection
Anal tags
Mucosal prolapse
Mucosal ectropion
Rectal stricture
Anal fissure
Pseudopolyps
Epidermal cysts
Anal fistula
Pruritus ani
Fecal incontinence
Recurrent hemorrhoids

### Pain

Although pain is not actually a complication of surgery, it is nonetheless the single most important reason why patients avoid hemorrhoidectomy.

Much emphasis has been applied to the management of pain in the hemorrhoidectomy patient, not only because of the pain itself, but because of the role it plays in urinary symptoms. Narcotic pain medicines are the mainstay of treatment for as long as necessary (usually several days). Toradol (ketorolac tromethamine) use has also been advocated in anorectal surgery, because it is effective in reducing pain and urinary retention. It is an effective adjunct to narcotic pain medication, and, in some instances, may supplant the need for narcotics entirely.

### Urinary Retention

Urinary retention, which is the most common complication following hemorrhoidectomy, occurs in as many as 20% of patients. Factors often held responsible include the following:

• Spinal anesthesia
• Rectal pain and spasm
• High ligation of the hemorrhoidal pedicle
• Rough handling of tissue

- Heavy suture material
- Numerous sutures
- Fluid overload
- Rectal packing
- Tight, bulky dressings
- Anticholinergics
- Narcotics

Generally, the incidence of urinary retention is not felt to be altered by the prophylactic administration of Urecholine (bethanechol chloride). Prophylactic α-adrenergic blockade has failed to prevent this complication, as has the administration of an anxiolytic agent.

Pain and fluid overload are the primary factors that cause urinary retention. If pain medication is inadequate, the patient cannot relax the sphincter mechanism sufficiently to urinate—it simply hurts too much. Fluids must be limited. The minimal intravenous infusion necessary is given during the operation, and the infusion is terminated in the recovery room. If hospital regulations require that an intravenous line be maintained, a heparin lock will suffice. Oral fluids are restricted until the following morning. Finally, patients are not routinely catheterized; this is carried out only when the bladder is distended or the patient complains, and then only after examination by a physician. In the morning, with the commencement of sitz baths, most patients will void who have not already done so. Once the nursing service has been educated not even to inquire about voiding, the incidence of retention and the associated complication of urinary tract infection will be significantly reduced.

If catheterization is necessary, it should be performed with a balloon catheter. If the residual urine is determined to be greater than 500 mL, the catheter should be left in place for 24 hours, because it is unlikely that the patient will be able to void subsequently. Conversely, with a residual of less than 500 mL, the catheter can be removed with a reasonable expectation that spontaneous urination will occur.

Local anesthesia is associated with a significantly lower incidence of urinary retention when compared with spinal anesthesia.

### Urinary Tract Infection

Urinary tract infection is usually a direct consequence of catheterization for urinary retention. The most common offending organisms are coliform bacteria. Appropriate antibiotics and catheter removal usually result in rapid resolution, but chronic infection, cystitis, and pyelonephritis can be late sequelae

### Constipation

Constipation after anorectal surgery must either be relieved effectively or prevented, because if untreated, it can lead to fecal impaction—a matter of special concern in this group of patients. Despite this concern, as long as 72 hours may elapse after operation before a laxative agent is first administered. Factors that contribute to this lag include the effects of analgesic medications given before or after the operation, the effects of anesthesia, and local physiologic dysfunction resulting from surgical manipulation, bedrest, and the patient's fear of painful defecation. A history of irregular bowel function and colonic hypomotility can complicate the problem further.

A stimulant laxative should be given on the evening of the operation and continued in increasing doses until defecation occurs. After the second postoperative day with no bowel action, a gentle tap water enema should be considered.

## Hemorrhage

Massive hemorrhage that occurs in the recovery room is always the result of a technical error and can usually be attributed to improper or inadequate ligation of the hemorrhoid pedicle. This most commonly occurs if the pedicle is simply hand-tied rather than suture-ligated. Such a complication requires emergency surgical intervention. Management of active bleeding after hemorrhoidectomy includes submucosal injection with 1 to 2 mL of 1:10,000 adrenaline, direct pressure with a finger or gauze, the use of topical epinephrine, or suture ligation.

Delayed hemorrhage (i.e., 7 to 14 days postoperatively) is probably the result of sepsis in the pedicle. This occurs in approximately 2% of hemorrhoidectomies. Patients may experience renewed slight bleeding, the passage of clots, or massive hemorrhage. Bleeding at 1 week or more following surgery after the patient has previously ceased bleeding warrants examination. Treatment varies from expectant management to in-hospital observation, transfusion, and resuture. Delayed hemorrhage usually is not a preventable complication.

## Infection

It seems surprising that there is not a higher incidence of septic complications following the operation. However, despite the presence of potentially virulent organisms (e.g., clostridia, anaerobic streptococci, bacteroides, and *Escherichia coli*), septic problems are uncommon. It has been hypothesized that the major venous drainage of the rectum, by passing through the superior hemorrhoidal veins into the portal system, is cleared of organisms by the reticuloendothelial system of the liver. This hepatic clearance, by effectively removing the bacteria released into the circulation, may be important in minimizing the impact of rectal colonic flora in the systemic circulation and may be the reason why infection is an uncommon complication after hemorrhoidectomy. Furthermore, as sitz baths are a routine part of the postoperative care, most skin problems (e.g., cellulitis, abscess) would be treated in an essentially prophylactic manner.

## Anal Tags

Anal tags can interfere with proper cleansing of the anus and thus lead to skin irritation. They usually can be avoided by excising redundant skin at the time of operation. More often, tags are the result of the manner in which the wounds heal, perhaps analogous to keloid formation in other incision sites. Bothersome tags can be excised as an office procedure if symptoms warrant.

## Mucosal Prolapse

Inadequate removal of redundant or mobile rectal mucosa at the time of hemorrhoidectomy can result in mucosal prolapse. Patients may complain of a lump that requires manual reduction. Problems with mucous discharge and pruritic symptoms are common.

Treatment usually consists of rubber ring ligation of the prolapsed mucosa. If extensive or circumferential involvement seems to exist, conduct the examination while the patient strains on the toilet in order to look for procidentia.

## Ectropion

Because the mucosa is more mobile than the perianal skin, the tendency for mucosal descent is greater than the likelihood of the skin ascending to reline the denuded anal canal (see Fig. 8.15). If redundant mucosa above the site of the excised hemorrhoid tissue is not properly anchored to the underlying internal sphincter, the mucosa can heal outside the anal verge (see Fig 8 14). If the entire anal canal is removed and the cut edge of the rectum is sutured to the perianal skin, the characteristic Whitehead deformity may be produced. If the mucosa is anchored to the skin in one or more quadrants, a partial ectropion may result. Ectropion can lead to mucous discharge, skin irritation, and pruritus ani. An ectropion that is evident in only one quadrant can be treated simply. As long as no stricture is present, a simple excision and transverse suture of the rectum to the underlying internal anal sphincter will suffice. The open wound should heal without the mucosal extrusion. An alternative approach is to perform an anoplasty.

## Anal Stricture

A considerable area of mucosa and anoderm may be denuded when the physician attempts to remove extensive, encircling hemorrhoids. If hemorrhoids are present in many areas, only minimal sections of intact, elastic anal tissue may be left following excision. With progressive healing, fibrous scar tissue can proliferate and contract the anorectal outlet. When healing is complete, a narrow, foreshortened stenotic orifice may remain.

As with ectropion, anal stenosis is a preventable complication. If adequate skin bridges are preserved, the risk for reducing the circumference of the anal canal is minimized. However, in the presence of gangrenous hemorrhoids, distortion of the anal canal, chronic fibrosis, chronic fissure, external tags, and hypertrophied anal papillae, extensive removal of the anal canal is often necessary to accomplish an adequate hemorrhoidectomy. Under these circumstances, the surgeon has two options: either compromise on the amount of tissue removed and accept the consequences of patient complaints of residual disease, or consider the possibility of performing an anoplasty at the time of hemorrhoidectomy.

An attempt must be made to preserve skin bridges; even one bridge is better than none. If because of sepsis, sloughing, or radical surgery (not treated by anoplasty) the potential for stricture formation becomes manifest, daily digital examination of the rectum is advisable while the patient is still in the hospital. It is probably worthwhile to advise the patient concerning insertion of a dilator twice daily after hospital discharge. Weekly office visits are also suggested. Prevention of anal stricture when there is legitimate justification for concern is the only indication for frequent digital examinations and the use of a dilator. If the wound heals without a stricture, digital examination and the use of a dilator can be discontinued, usually within 6 to 8 weeks. However, if a healed, fixed stricture develops, I prefer to perform an anoplasty rather than to have the patient use a dilator indefinitely.

## Anoplasty

Anoplasty is a procedure whereby perianal skin is moved to cover a defect in the anal canal. This defect is usually the result of an operative procedure, such as excision of a portion or all of the anal canal, hemorrhoidectomy, excision of an anal fissure, or excision of a lesion of the anal canal. Anoplasty can be performed to correct an anal stenosis or, coincidentally, with repair of a rectovaginal fistula or with sphincteroplasty for sphincteric injury. The following list summarizes the indications for this procedure:

Anal stricture
   Congenital
   Inflammatory (e.g., fistula, abscess)
   Trauma: operative (e.g., hemorrhoidectomy, fissurectomy, pull-through procedure, excisional procedures); accidental
   Disuse caused by laxatives, enemas, chronic diarrhea
   Coincident with excision of anal lesions
   Ulcer
   Tumor
Coincident with reconstructive anorectal operations
   Rectovaginal fistula repair
   Anterior fistula in women
   Sphincter repair
   Congenital anomaly (e.g., imperforate anus, ectopic anus)

Anal stricture can be one of the most disabling complications of anal surgery or anal disease. Stenosis can occur as a consequence of a number of conditions:

- Benign and malignant tumors
- Inflammations, especially Crohn's disease
- Congenital anomalies (e.g., ectopic anus and imperforate anus)
- Abuse of laxatives
- Trauma, especially surgical trauma

However, overzealous hemorrhoidectomy continues to be the most common reason why patients require an anoplasty.

### Symptoms, Findings, and Differential Diagnosis

The most troublesome complaint of patients with anal stenosis is difficulty with defecation. Constipation, obstipation, painful bowel movements, narrow caliber of the stool, abdominal cramping, and bleeding are frequently associated symptoms. The fear of fecal impaction or pain usually causes the patient to rely on daily laxatives or enemas.

Physical examination readily reveals the problem. It may be impossible to perform a digital examination, or only the small finger may be tolerated. Proctosigmoidoscopy and anoscopy will require narrow-caliber instruments. With any question concerning the cause of the stenosis or the possibility of a proximal lesion, a barium enema or colonoscopy should be performed if such examinations are technically possible. Sometimes, it is difficult to distinguish true stenosis with tissue loss from the sphincter spasm associated with an anal fissure. Administration of a local anesthetic may be helpful, but occasionally a general anesthetic may be required. The anesthetic abolishes the spasm associated with an acute fissure but will not produce an increased luminal diameter in a patient with true stenosis.

It is important to ascertain the cause of the stricture to determine proper therapy. Inflammatory bowel disease is an absolute contraindication to anoplasty, and obviously a malignant process must be treated by extirpation. Perhaps the most useful diagnostic tool is an accurate history. If the patient associates the onset of the problem with prior hemorrhoidectomy or with electrocoagulation of anal condylomata, the condition will be appropriately treated by an anoplasty. Conversely, with no such history in someone with long-term laxative abuse, correction of the stricture may produce anal incontinence. This problem occurs when sphincter muscle wasting accompanies an anal stricture, a consequence of passing small, narrow bowel actions over many years. Mineral oil is notorious for producing stenosis, probably because the lubricated stool fails to dilate the anal canal.

Symptoms present from birth imply a congenital etiology. Most common is an anteriorly situated ectopic anus, usually at the orifice of the vagina in female patients. A hooded anus and anorectal atresia are also congenital lesions that can produce stenosis, despite treatment early in life.

### Medical Treatment

As mentioned, the conservative management of anal stenosis includes laxatives, suppositories, dilatation, and enemas. These approaches can effect defecation, but they do not specifically treat the cause of the problem—a narrowed anal canal diameter. A dilator may tear the canal; a complication from its use can precipitate the need for surgical intervention.

### Surgical Treatment

#### Excision of Eschar and Sphincterotomy

The classic surgical treatment of anal stricture is lysis and excision of the eschar, transverse suture of the rectal mucosa to the underlying internal sphincter, and sphincterotomy. Furthermore, the term *anoplasty* should be limited to the procedures that actually replace the anal canal with new skin.

*Technique.* When the stricture is excised or lysed with a 29-mm (medium-size) Hill–Ferguson retractor inserted, the cut edge of the rectum can be sutured to the underlying internal anal sphincter in a transverse fashion, thereby widening the anal canal (Fig. 8.16 A,B). If the lumen is still inadequate, the same maneuver can be performed on the opposite side (Fig. 8.16C).

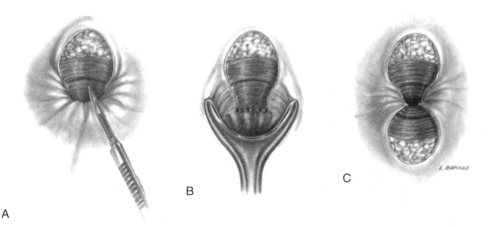

A    B    C

**FIG. 8.16. A.** Lysis of the anal stricture permits insertion of a 29-mm Hill–Ferguson retractor. **B.** The rectum is sutured to the underlying internal anal sphincter. **C.** Further widening can be done on the opposite side.

This is a perfectly acceptable technique that will yield satisfactory results if sufficient skin bridges remain. However, if this is not the case, frequent digital examinations must be performed or dilators used to prevent restricturing. As with sphincterotomy or sphincter stretch, this operation does not create a new anal canal lining with sensory-bearing mucosa. However, this procedure, or even sphincterotomy alone, may be adequate for a patient with a mild degree of narrowing. For more profound stenosis, a formal anoplasty should be performed to treat the basic problem—loss of anal canal tissue.

### Anoplasty for Minimal Stenosis

Esoteric anoplastic maneuvers should be reserved for loss of anal canal tissue, but even mild anal stenosis can be treated by skin replacement. A small advancement flap (Y-V) may be useful for stenosis accompanying chronic posterior anal fissure.

*Preoperative Management.* A complete mechanical preparation, and broad-spectrum systemic antibiotics are suggested. A cleansing enema before surgery is important.

*Operative Technique.* The patient is placed in the prone jackknife position on the operating table with the buttocks taped apart. Spinal, caudal, general endotracheal, or local anesthesia can be used. The stricture or fissure is incised (Fig. 8.17A), and an internal anal sphincterotomy is performed (Fig. 8.17B). A full-thickness flap of skin is elevated in the posterior midline (Fig. 8.17C). A 29-mm Hill–Ferguson retractor is kept in place for the entire operation to maintain the adequacy of the lumen. If the canal can be reconstructed with the retractor in place, the anal opening will be adequate.

Incisions are carried proximally for 5 to 8 cm. Care must be taken to avoid creating a narrow pedicle that might compromise the blood supply to the apex of the flap. Mobilization over the sacrum is unnecessary for this degree of anal canal defect. The full thickness of the skin is sutured to the rectal mucosa and to the underlying internal anal sphincter with interrupted long-term absorbable sutures. The completed repair is shown in Figure 8.17D. The external aspect can be left open if tension is produced by closure, or the entire wound can be closed primarily. This technique is simple and useful for stricture associated with an anal fissure. However, if more than 25% of the circumference of the anal canal needs to be covered, another anoplastic approach is indicated.

A so-called V-Y or island flap anoplasty is another option for the management of mild anal stenosis or the treatment of a limited mucosal ectropion. The full thickness of perianal skin is mobilized and advanced into the anal canal to create a new lining (Fig. 8.18). Care must be taken to preserve the blood supply to the graft. A similar modification has been termed the "house advancement flap." Its theoretic advantages are that (1) it provides a broad skin flap for the entire length of the entire anal canal, and (2) it provides primary closure of the donor

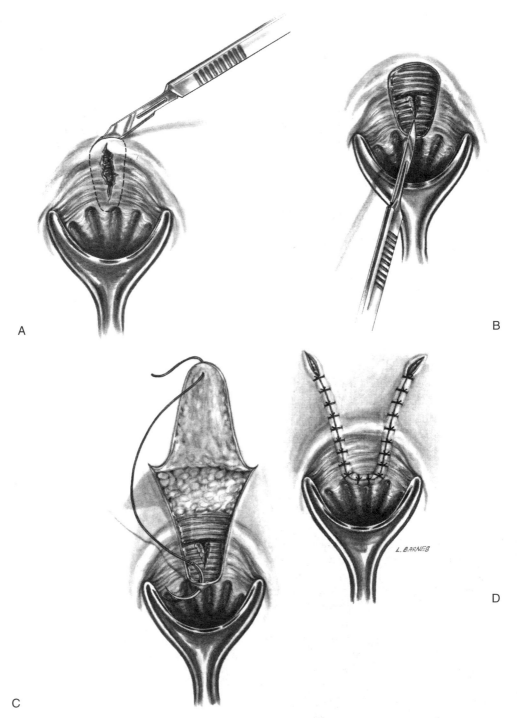

**FIG. 8.17.** Anoplasty for chronic anal fissure with minimal stenosis. **A.** *Dashed line* shows planned incision. **B.** An internal anal sphincterotomy is performed. **C.** The skin flap is elevated. **D.** The flap is advanced and sutured to the rectum.

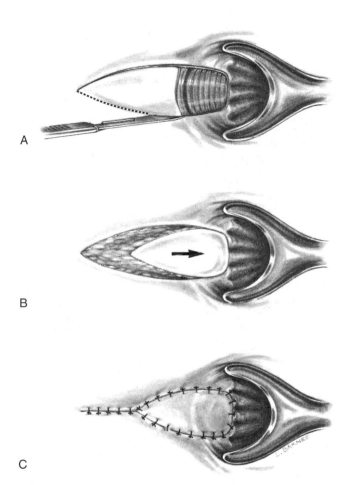

**FIG. 8.18.** V-Y anoplasty. **A.** The skin is mobilized. **B.** The pedicle of skin is advanced. **C.** Primary closure is completed.

site. The word *house* denotes the schematic representation of a house in terms of the way the flap is created. The technique is illustrated in Figure 8.19.

*Postoperative Management.* In all operations involving an anoplasty, an antibiotic, usually a cephalosporin, is given parenterally for 2 to 5 days, depending on the extent of the reconstruction. No attempt is made to prevent bowel action postoperatively, because only a small graft is created in anoplasty for mild stenosis. The patient is permitted a regular diet supplemented by a bulk laxative containing psyllium or a stool softener. Showers are permitted, but sitz baths are not recommended. Simple cleansing of the wound is all that is required, as infection is unusual. Rarely is it necessary to probe under the skin flap to evacuate a hematoma or purulent collection, but even under these circumstances the viability of the graft is usually not compromised. The patient is discharged when a bowel movement occurs and is then seen weekly or every 2 weeks until the wounds heal, usually in 5 to 6 weeks.

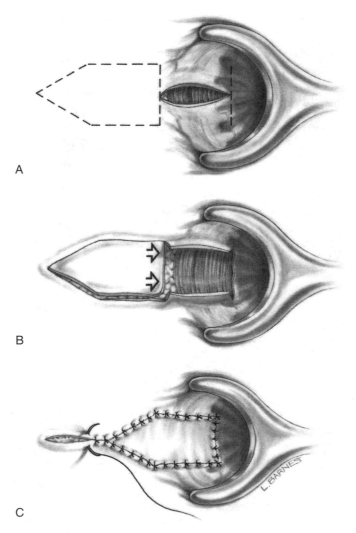

**FIG. 8.19.** House advancement flap for anal stenosis. **A.** A longitudinal incision is made later-ally for the length of the anal canal. **B.** After the wound edges are undermined, the incision assumes a rectangular shape. **C.** The completed house flap is advanced, lining the entire length of the anal canal, and sutured into place. (From Christensen MA, et al. "House" advancement pedicle flap for anal stenosis. *Dis Colon Rectum* 1992;35:201.)

### Anoplasty for Moderate Stenosis

When a greater area needs to be covered than can be accomplished with a sin-gle advancement flap, sufficient skin can often be obtained by performing bilat-eral advancements in the right lateral and left lateral positions. This will permit resurfacing of up to 50% of the anal canal circumference.

*Operative Technique.* The patient is placed in the prone jackknife position with the buttocks taped apart. A local anesthetic is not advised because of the extensive infiltration required and its associated discomfort. The full thickness of the skin is sutured to the cut edge of the rectum and the underlying internal sphincter with long-term absorbable sutures. This effectively increases the diameter of the anal canal.

*Postoperative Management.* It is usually advisable to confine the bowels after this procedure, because of the extent of the skin coverage attempted. This is accomplished with diphenoxylate hydrochloride (Lomotil), up to eight tablets a day; codeine, up to 240 mg daily; and deodorized tincture of opium, up to 80 drops a day. Sitz baths are withheld; the wounds are cleansed with an antiseptic such as povidone-iodine four times daily.

After 3 days, medications are discontinued, and a regular diet, supplemented with a bulk laxative and stool softener, is instituted. Some small separation of the wound may occur, but satisfactory healing with an adequate anal opening is anticipated. The patient is discharged when bowel function has returned, and usually is seen every 10 to 14 days until complete healing has taken place.

### Anoplasty for Severe Stenosis or for Major Coverage of the Anal Canal

The plastic maneuvers described above are useful for minimal or moderate problems of skin coverage. However, if 50% or more of the anal canal needs to be reconstructed, a rotation flap of skin should be considered. Conditions that may necessitate this maneuver include stricture secondary to radical hemorrhoidectomy, concomitant tissue loss with excision of an anal canal lesion, and mucosal ectropion. This last problem may be seen not only following the so-called Whitehead hemorrhoidectomy (see Fig. 8.15), but also after an abdominal-anal pull-through procedure. Another indication for this operation is to correct the "keyhole" deformity that can be seen after excision of an anal fissure or excision of a fistula.

Generally, rotation flaps are more effective for covering skin defects than are advancement flaps. Graft viability and suture line tension are much less likely to be issues of concern if the former technique is employed.

*Operative Technique.* The patient is placed in the prone jackknife position, and the buttocks are taped apart. In most instances, a single rotation flap will provide adequate skin. After excision of the scar, an outline of the incision is made, the flap is elevated and rotated medially, and the wound is closed, primarily with interrupted long-term absorbable sutures (Fig. 8.20).

In the correction of the Whitehead deformity or when the entire anal canal must be replaced, a bilateral rotation flap (S-plasty) must be performed. Spinal, caudal, or general endotracheal anesthesia is used; a locally administered anesthetic is not advised. The anal canal is incised posteriorly, and the lower portion of the internal sphincter is divided. The anal canal is incised further to permit insertion of a Hill–Ferguson retractor.

A full-thickness flap of skin is elevated, and the incision is begun in the midline and carried laterally in a curvilinear fashion for approximately 8 to 10 cm.

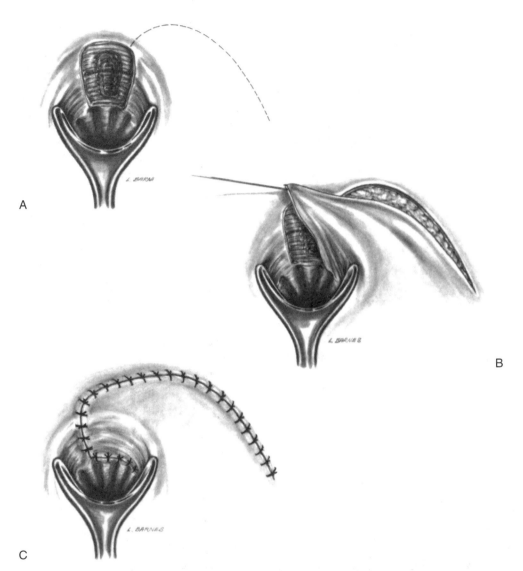

**FIG. 8.20.** Correction of keyhole deformity. **A.** The scar is excised; note the outline of the skin flap (*dashed line*). **B.** The skin flap is mobilized and rotated medially. **C.** The wound is primarily closed.

A longer length can be obtained by incising further laterally and, eventually, somewhat medially. Care should be taken to avoid necrosis; a thick flap that includes subcutaneous tissue is preferred. As mentioned, more than one flap is rarely required, as a new anal canal along one half of the circumference is more than adequate. However, if the entire anal canal needs to be reconstructed, as is necessary with the Whitehead deformity (in which all the mucosa must be excised completely, denuding the anal canal), a similar incision is performed on the opposite side. Hemostasis is effected with electrocautery. The wound is irrigated with saline solution, and the skin is rotated medially and sutured to the rectum and to the underlying internal sphincter with long-term absorbable sutures (Fig. 8.21). The mucosa tends to protrude readily; therefore, it is important to excise any redundant rectal mucosa. After the new mucocutaneous junction has been completed, continuous subcuticular 3-0 long-term absorbable or interrupted simple sutures of similar material are used, and the wounds are closed completely by mobilizing a full-thickness flap of skin cephalad and laterally. If too much tension still remains, the easiest alternative is to leave the lateral aspect open to granulate. Grafting by using split-thickness skin from the thigh may be done, but this is rarely indicated.

*Postoperative Management.* The bowel-confining regimen described previously is carried out for 3 days. Systemic antibiotic coverage is continued during this time. Rarely, a hematoma or an abscess will develop underneath one of the flaps. By insertion of a hemostat between the sutures, evacuation of the collection usually can be achieved without compromising the graft.

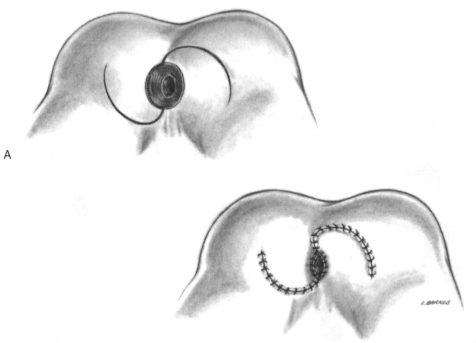

A

B

**FIG. 8.21.** Anoplasty is used for severe anal stenosis or for significant loss of anal canal tissue. **A.** The skin flaps are outlined; the eschar has been excised. **B.** The flaps are rotated and sutured to the rectum and underlying internal sphincter. The Hill–Ferguson retractor is not shown.

An anal stenosis of long duration or a Whitehead deformity usually results in an attenuated sphincter mechanism. With a widely patent anal orifice, discharge of mucus and incontinence for flatus or even for feces can occur during the initial few weeks after the operation. It is therefore advisable to start a regimen of perineal strengthening exercises to be performed 10 to 15 times a day. Significant improvement in control can take many weeks, but relatively normal continence should be achievable, except in the patient who has an anal stenosis with an atrophied sphincter. These individuals should be carefully selected before an anoplastic operation is considered; if surgery is felt to be advisable, a less-than-generous opening should be created. The patient needs to be forewarned that incontinence is a possibility.

### Internal Pudendal Flap Anoplasty

Another option for reconstructing the anal canal has been recently introduced—internal pudendal flap anoplasty. In a solitary case, this procedure was used when extensive coverage was required concomitant with excision of Paget's disease of the anus. This flap is based on the terminal branches of the internal pudendal vessels.

### Foreskin Anoplasty

An interesting operation has been described by Freeman for the treatment of mucosal ectropion—the foreskin anoplasty. The procedure, which obviously implies the availability of a prepuce, uses the foreskin to provide a full-thickness skin graft to the anal canal. Freeman reported his experience with six children in 1984, but no further publications have been noted since this initial report.

### Anoplasty with Sphincteroplasty

In restorative procedures of the anal sphincter mechanism, the skin often must be mobilized concomitantly to effect an adequate repair. Anoplasty with sphincteroplasty has been used for ectopic anus, perineal body reconstruction, and management of rectovaginal fistulas and other obstetric injury. The anoplasty described in Chapter 13 is most useful in women with ectopic anus, rectovaginal fistula, or sphincter injury.

### Results of Anoplasty

It is extremely difficult to interpret the results of the various anoplastic maneuvers. No controlled studies are available on the comparative advantages and disadvantages of the various anoplastic procedures; however, almost any approach will at least improve the patient's symptoms. However, the methods described for plastic reconstruction of the anal canal and perianal skin should be used only in selected individuals. Routine application for the uncomplicated hemorrhoidectomy, fissure operation, or fistula repair is inappropriate. However, with anal stenosis, mucosal ectropion, sphincter injury, rectovaginal fistula, obstetric injury, or tissue loss, one of these procedures should be extremely effective in ensuring a successful result.

## Rectal Stricture

Stricture of the rectum, a rare sequela of hemorrhoidectomy, usually is misdiagnosed as an anal stricture. The complication is caused by vigorous high ligation of the hemorrhoid pedicles that strips the rectal mucosa in several areas. It is most likely to occur if the patient has an element of prolapse or a laxity of the rectal mucosa. As with virtually all complications, prevention is the best approach. Care must be taken to avoid gathering a mass of rectal lining into the ligatures.

Management of this complication may require dilatation, either with Young's dilators if the stricture is distal, or a Hegar's dilator if the stricture is higher. Operative lysis may be necessary, possibly including either advancement of the rectal mucosa or proctoplasty.

## Fissure or Ulcer

An anal fissure can develop in a patient who has a contracted anorectal outlet after hemorrhoidectomy. Usually, the fissure is situated posteriorly. Repeated trauma from defecation results in laceration of the eschar, which can become a chronic, painful anal ulcer. Such postoperative fissures may respond to conservative management (e.g., laxatives, enemas, suppositories, topical creams such as cortisone) and dilatation. However, often an additional procedure is required, most commonly an internal anal sphincterotomy. Excision of the ulcer concomitant with the sphincterotomy may be of benefit, but some form of anoplasty may ultimately be required to increase anal canal circumference.

## Pseudopolyps

Hemorrhoidectomy usually requires ligation of the stump of the hemorrhoid. Tissue strangulation will take place at the site of ligation, resulting in sloughing of the stump. This leaves a defect that heals by granulation, the end result of which may be a pseudopolyp. Another possible contributing factor is a foreign body granuloma, which can be a consequence of the prolonged presence of suture material. This can be manifested by an edematous, polypoid, or sessile tumor at the site of the suture. Pseudopolyps can be excised with a local anesthetic or be electrocoagulated.

## Epidermal Cyst

In rare instances, some months after hemorrhoidectomy, asymptomatic inclusion cysts may appear in the anal canal or in the immediate perianal region. Their origin has been attributed to retention of keratin elements, hair particles, or exfoliated squamous epithelial cells in the wound. If these cysts are bothersome, they can be removed by local excision.

## Anal Fistula

Anal fistula is an unusual complication of hemorrhoidectomy, occurring in approximately 1% of patients. The fistula is inevitably low and subcutaneous, not transsphincteric or even intersphincteric unless the finding is coincidental. Fistulotomy, the appropriate treatment, can often be accomplished in the office.

## Pruritus Ani

Most causes of pruritus ani are related to diet or are caused by overaggressive attention to anal hygiene. However, pruritic symptoms following hemorrhoidectomy are not unusual and may actually have an anatomic basis. A mucosal ectropion or Whitehead deformity, for example, can produce mucous discharge, which can contribute to the pruritus. With a specific anatomic abnormality, anoplasty may be advisable. The medical management of pruritus ani is discussed in Chapter 19.

## Fecal Incontinence

Fecal soilage or incontinence following hemorrhoidectomy, although infrequent, is not as rare as the physician might expect. A possible explanation is the loss of anal canal sensation, resulting from removal of sensory-bearing tissue and its replacement by scar.

Almost all patients who have impairment of fecal control following hemorrhoidectomy are elderly. If a careful history is taken, it will probably reveal that many of these individuals have experienced some soilage before the operation, although the procedure may have exacerbated the problem. This is often the case when the patient has some degree of mucosal or rectal prolapse, and it is a particular concern in women. Special care should be taken when performing this operation in the older age group; it is important to avoid unnecessary sphincter stretch or sphincterotomy.

## Recurrence

Most patients who complain of recurrent hemorrhoids usually are describing skin tags or have pruritic symptoms. However, in some cases true hemorrhoidal veins have developed, which have become symptomatic after an assumed complete hemorrhoidectomy. The "recurrence" consists of veins that, either because of their normal appearance at the time of hemorrhoidectomy or in an effort to preserve adequate mucosal bridges, were left undisturbed. With increased pressure or collateral circulation developing over the years, dilatation occurs and symptomatic hemorrhoids result.

Because of this potential problem, all hemorrhoidal veins should be removed at the time of the surgical procedure. Tunneling out minute vessels from the underlying mucosa and debriding all veins over the external sphincter are important prophylactic maneuvers (see Fig. 8.10). When recurrent piles become symptomatic, ideal treatment should be by an outpatient procedure, usually rubber ring ligation or office excision.

### Retroperitoneal Air

A solitary case of retroperitoneal air following hemorrhoidectomy was reported by Kriss et al. The patient had been receiving steroids for rheumatoid arthritis, so this medication may have played some part in its occurrence. The authors suggest that air was introduced either during the dissection or subsequently, when the patient coughed or strained. A third explanation, not offered by the authors, is the possibility that this complication was unrelated to the operation. The patient responded well to nonoperative management.

## Results of Surgical Hemorrhoidectomy

Few contemporary studies evaluate the results of hemorrhoidectomy.

Meta-analysis involving a total of 18 trials to assess whether any method of hemorrhoid treatment has been demonstrably superior allowed the following conclusions to be drawn:

- Hemorrhoidectomy was found significantly more effective than manual dilation, with less need for further therapy.
- No significant difference was observed in the incidence of complications.
- Hemorrhoidectomy was found to be associated with significantly more pain.
- Patients undergoing hemorrhoidectomy had a better response to treatment than those treated with rubber band ligation.
- Hemorrhoidectomy was associated with more complications than rubber band ligation.
- Rubber band ligation was better than sclerotherapy in the treatment of all grades of hemorrhoids.

## HEMORRHOIDS IN INFLAMMATORY BOWEL DISEASE

Exacerbation of hemorrhoidal complaints is not at all uncommon in patients with inflammatory bowel disease

Any procedure performed on the anus or perianal skin in patients with inflammatory bowel disease should be limited to the minimal maneuvers that will effectively treat the patient's complaint. Definitive or extensive surgical treatment of any anorectal problem in such individuals could result in delayed healing or nonhealing, with greater disability to the patient than before the operation. Occasionally, when disease is quiescent and sepsis, fistula formation, and scarring are not present, bleeding or protrusion of hemorrhoids might reasonably be treated by rubber ring ligation.

## HEMORRHOIDECTOMY IN THE HIV-POSITIVE PATIENT

Although not clearly documented by statistics in the literature, definitive surgical hemorrhoidectomy in patients who are human immunodeficiency virus (HIV) positive is probably contraindicated only in those patients in whom full blown acquired immunodeficiency syndrome (AIDS) has developed. HIV-positive patients are clearly living longer and more normal lives, with the advent of better antiviral medications, and unless in the end stages of the disease, should be expected to heal completely most of the time.

## HEMORRHOIDECTOMY DURING PREGNANCY

As mentioned earlier in this chapter, women are often troubled by hemorrhoidal complaints during the latter part of pregnancy. Most such problems can be treated adequately by bowel management (e.g., laxatives, stool softeners) and by sitz baths. A thrombosed hemorrhoid can be excised in the usual way. No clear-cut answer is found for the question of what should be done when a pregnant woman has a sufficiently profound complication that surgical hemorrhoidectomy appears to be the best recourse. Procedures performed under local anesthetic would probably be safe, but general or systemic anesthetics are avoided if possible to minimize the potential risk to the unborn child.

# 9

# Anal Fissure

An anal fissure, a common anorectal condition, constitutes a cut or crack in the anal canal or anal verge that can extend from the mucocutaneous junction to the dentate line. It can be acute or chronic, and can occur at any age (it is the most common cause of rectal bleeding in infants), but is usually a condition of young adults. Both sexes are affected equally; however, an anterior fissure is much more likely to develop in women than in men (only 1% of those in men are anterior fissures). Still, 90% of fissures are found posteriorly in women.

## ETIOLOGY AND PATHOGENESIS

Generally, anal fissure has been attributed to constipation or to straining at stool. Increased risk is noted with frequent consumption of white bread, sauces thickened with a roux, bacon, and sausage. Decreased risk is associated with raw fruits, vegetables, and whole-grain bread. Risk is not related to coffee, tea, or alcohol.

Anal fissure can also be a consequence of frequent defecation and diarrhea. It can be associated with nonspecific inflammatory bowel disease. If suspicion arises, biopsy, stool culture, serology, and gastrointestinal evaluation may be indicated. When anal fissure occurs in an aberrant location, especially laterally, entertain the possibility of ulcerative colitis or Crohn's disease.

Why the fissure is most commonly located in the posterior anal canal is controversial. The explanation may be found in the structure of the external sphincter. The lower portion of this muscle is not truly circular, but consists of a band of muscle fibers that pass from posterior to anterior and split around the anus. The anal mucosa, therefore, is best supported laterally and is weakest posteriorly. The decreased anterior support in women may account for the greater occurrence in this location in women than in men. Another theory implicates the blood supply to the area. The posterior commissure is less well perfused than other areas of the anal canal; hence, ischemia may be an important etiologic factor in anal fissure, especially in the posterior location. It has also been proposed that

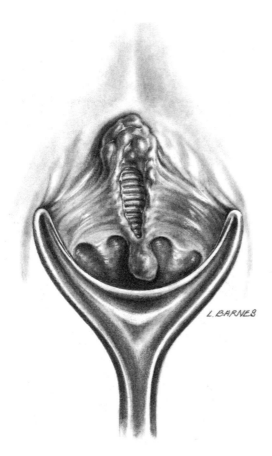

**FIG. 9.1.** Chronic posterior anal fissure with skin tag and hypertrophied anal papilla. Note fibers of the internal anal sphincter at the base of the wound.

ischemia of the anal canal mucosa might be the cause of pain and the failure of fissures to heal spontaneously.

Why some fissures heal spontaneously and others become chronic is an unresolved question. Ischemia, infection, or lymphatic obstruction secondary to persistent inflammation may be responsible. A characteristic skin tag (i.e., sentinel pile) can develop distally, whereas proximally, a hypertrophied anal papilla may be seen. Another observation is that the internal anal sphincter muscle fibers are often easily seen at the base of the open wound (Fig. 9.1).

## PHYSIOLOGIC STUDIES

Manometric testing will reveal that resting pressures are elevated in these patients with anal fissure. Following sphincter stretch, a moderate fall in pressure can be demonstrated, but will return virtually to normal by the eighth postoperative day. It has been suggested, therefore, that the therapeutic effect of sphincter stretch is not related so much to reduction in anal pressure as to prevention of the spasm. Others have concluded that the primary abnormality in fissure is persistent hypertonia affecting the entire internal sphincter.

If the rectum is distended by a balloon, internal sphincter relaxation (an expected response) is followed by a marked and prolonged contraction above the initial baseline. This reflexly stimulated sphincter spasm may be involved in the cause of anal fissure.

Anal canal ultrasonography can be important in identifying unrecognized obstetric sphincteric injuries before performance of internal anal sphincterotomy. Although this study might be difficult to perform in the presence of an acute, painful fissure, one might consider identifying such individuals before surgical creation of a second sphincter defect.

## HISTOPATHOLOGY

Nothing in particular is histologically diagnostic of an anal fissure. If the lesion is excised and submitted for pathologic examination, usually only typical, nonspecific inflammatory changes and fibrosis throughout the internal sphincter are observed.

## SYMPTOMS

The characteristic complaints of a patient with an acute anal fissure are pain and bleeding. The pain usually occurs with, and immediately after defecation. Usually, the pain ceases in a few minutes, but it can persist for hours. The pain of anal fissure can be differentiated from that of proctalgia fugax in that the latter condition produces discomfort that is usually not related to bowel action. Also, the patient with a fissure feels the discomfort in the anal area; the pain of proctalgia fugax is higher and more deep-seated. The other anal condition that commonly produces pain is a thrombosed hemorrhoid, but with this complaint, the patient also reports feeling a lump.

Bleeding is usually minimal and frequently occurs only on the toilet paper, but sometimes blood will be seen in the bowl. It is not uncommon for patients to report no evidence of bleeding.

Patients with a long-standing (i.e., chronic) anal fissure will present with a different symptom complex, including a lump representing the sentinel tag, drainage or discharge from the open wound, pruritus, or a combination of several symptoms. Bleeding may or may not be present, and pain is usually mild and frequently absent. Problems with micturition and dyspareunia occasionally accompany the symptoms of both acute and chronic fissure.

The patient often relates that constipation is the antecedent event, but once pain develops, the fear of the act of defecation and refusal of the call to stool can exacerbate this problem. This anxiety leads to fecal impaction, particularly in children and in the elderly.

## EXAMINATION

### Acute Fissure

The patient history is usually so characteristic that the diagnosis can be easily established. The open wound can often be seen by inspection or gentle retraction of the perianal skin. If the buttocks cannot be pried apart to view the area, the presence of an acute anal fissure is a virtual certainty. Under such circumstances, appropriate treatment should be initiated without more specific confirmatory evidence.

If desired, examination can still be possible after the application of a topical anesthetic. Palpation usually demonstrates a spastic anal sphincter or tight anal canal and will exacerbate the patient's discomfort. The open wound is often not evident by the examining finger in a patient with an acute anal fissure; usually no fibrosis is present and the cut is relatively superficial.

Anoscopic examination, if possible, confirms the location of the fissure. The ability to perform this examination, however, may reflect the chronicity of the problem. Ideally, proctosigmoidoscopic examination should be carried out before any surgical procedure to establish that the rectum is not involved by inflammatory bowel disease.

### Chronic Fissure

A fissure is defined as chronic when it has become a clearly recognized, well-circumscribed ulcer. Examination of the patient with a chronic anal fissure usually reveals the characteristic sentinel pile, which can become large (i.e., 3 to 4 cm). Digital examination reveals the presence of the fissure, induration, and fibrosis. A hypertrophied anal papilla often can be felt at the apex of the ulcer and can be mistaken for a tumor (see Fig. 9.1).

Anoscopy frequently can be accomplished without difficulty, as pain is not usually severe. However, scarring can result in narrowing of the anal canal, and it may be necessary to use a narrow-diameter anoscope. Characteristically, the internal anal sphincter fibers are clearly seen at the base of a chronic anal fissure.

Occasionally, the base of the fissure may become infected and form an abscess that may discharge as a fistula. This fistula is superficial when it occurs. Examination may reveal an external opening, virtually always in the midline, usually no more than 1 or 2 cm distal to the skin tag. Purulent material may be noted. A probe passed from the external opening emerges at the distal end of the fissure; usually, the internal anal sphincter is not traversed.

## TREATMENT

### Medical Management

Patients with a history suggestive of anal fissure of relatively recent onset are usually successfully treated by conservative measures (e.g., stool softeners, bulking agents, a high-fiber diet, and sitz baths). Preparations containing mineral oil are not advised because of difficulty in cleansing the area following defecation. Suppositories also are not recommended, because they do not act effectively within the anal canal. Inserting any one of a number of proprietary creams and ointments in the area, with or without a local anesthetic, may offer some transient relief. To prevent recurrence, the patient should be encouraged to continue with the diet, perhaps also with the addition of a bulk laxative agent, even after symptoms have resolved.

Injection of a long-acting local anesthetic can give temporary relief and may permit examination, but its use on an ambulatory basis is impractical. Anal dilators should not be used. Periodic reports have surfaced in the literature concerning sclerotherapy with the use of a local anesthetic. The technique is recommended for those symptomatic patients who do not respond to conservative management.

Chen et al. reported the topical use of Solcoderm in the treatment of anal fissure with a statistically significantly better healing rate with the drug at 1 month (84% vs. 28%) and at 1 year (84% vs. 44%). Others have used glyceryl trinitrate ointment, a nitric acid donor that contributes to internal anal sphincter relaxation. Topical glyceryl trinitrate provides rapid, sustained pain relief in individuals with anal fissure. Healing occurs in 45% to 70% of patients, but headache is a common complaint, and may reduce patient compliance. Additionally, recurrence rates appear to be approximately 25%, and may require repeat therapy or alternative treatments. Oral nitrates have also been suggested, which may result in fewer headache symptoms.

In 1993, Jost and Schimrigk reported injecting botulinum toxin type A into the anal sphincter as a new mode of treatment for anal fissure. The toxin acts by binding to the presynaptic nerve terminal at the neuromuscular junction, preventing the release of acetylcholine presynaptically and, thus, blocking transmission. Sphincter spasm is relieved by nonpermanent chemical denervation of the muscle that, in many cases, lasts long enough to allow the fissure to heal (80% to 85%). The major disadvantage of the procedure is the relatively high cost of the toxin. Transient continence problems have been reported, but appear to resolve spontaneously as the toxin effect wears off over several weeks.

### Surgical Management

The treatment for fissure-in-ano refractory to nonoperative therapy is internal anal sphincterotomy. Both closed and open techniques are suitable in an outpatient setting with general, regional, or local anesthesia. Antibiotic prophylaxis should be considered in any patient at risk for infection.

The operative approach to the treatment of anal fissure depends on both symptom duration and the physical findings. For an acute anal fissure without a tag, hypertrophied papilla, or significant hemorrhoids, the two procedures that have been advocated are sphincter stretch and internal anal sphincterotomy. For chronic anal fissure with an external component, or when the condition is associated with symptomatic large hemorrhoids, excisional therapy is the preferred option.

### *Sphincter Stretch*

Sphincter stretch can be carried out with a local anesthetic, but a brief general anesthetic is preferable, and an ambulatory surgical facility is optimal. The patient is placed in the lithotomy position; sterile draping is unnecessary (Fig. 9.2). The index finger of one hand is inserted into the rectum, followed by the

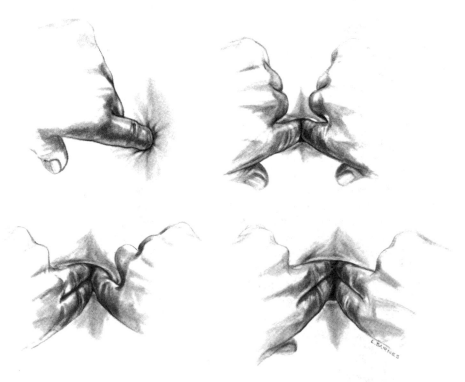

**FIG. 9.2.** Proper approach to performing a sphincter stretch. Male patients may require an anteroposterior stretch, because of the limitations of a narrow outlet and close approximation of the ischial spines. Female patients should always undergo a lateral stretch.

index finger of the opposite hand. Gentle, lateral retraction with each finger commences for approximately 30 seconds. The long finger is inserted and then the other long finger. With four fingers in place, the anal canal is stretched (massaged) cautiously for 4 minutes. In men, it is easier to stretch the sphincter in the anteroposterior plane because of the narrowness of the pelvic outlet. Sphincter stretch in women, however, should always be performed in the transverse plane. Narrowness is not a concern, but disruption of anterior sphincteric support is a real possibility.

## Results

Sphincter stretch is a reasonably effective procedure for the symptomatic relief of anal fissure, with cure rates of 93% to 94%. Disruption of some of the external sphincter fibers is a possibility in from 2% to 28% of patients. It can lead to complications related to control, usually for flatus alone but occasionally for feces, or swelling. Therefore, sphincter stretch should be applied to younger patients only; it is probably contraindicated in individuals above 60 years of age because of the likelihood of incontinence problems. Remember that sphincter stretch stretches both the external and internal sphincters. Impairment of control, therefore, is an inevitable consequence; it is simply a matter of to what degree the patient will be affected.

## *Internal Anal Sphincterotomy*

The internal anal sphincter is the continuation of the distal portion of the circular muscle of the rectum. Its length is essentially equal to that of the anal canal. Distally, it can usually be felt medial to the intersphincteric groove outside the anal verge. The subcutaneous portion of the external sphincter lies lateral to the groove.

The internal sphincter maintains the anal canal in the closed position; action is involuntary. The external sphincter is a striated muscle. The external sphincter and the levator ani are the muscles involved in voluntary control. Complete division of the internal anal sphincter is possible without creating significant impairment of fecal continence.

### *Technique*

The procedure of internal anal sphincterotomy has classically been performed in the posterior midline. Although this approach usually cures the condition (93%), it has been associated with the complication of the so-called "keyhole deformity," a high incidence (34%) of impairment for flatus and a 15% incidence of difficulty controlling feces.

In 1969, Notaras reported a technique used to perform an internal anal sphincterotomy in a closed fashion in the lateral position, resulting in a 6% incidence of fecal soiling. The procedure can be performed in the office using a local anesthetic or in an ambulatory surgical facility using a short-acting general anesthetic.

The patient can be placed in stirrups, in the left lateral position, or in the prone jackknife position. The fissure is infiltrated as well as the site for insertion of the knife—either the right lateral or left lateral position. A narrow anal retractor is used for the procedure if a local anesthetic is used. The intersphincteric groove is usually easily felt (Fig. 9.3), and the knife blade is inserted into the left lateral aspect (Fig. 9.4A). A theoretic advantage is seen in cutting on the right side, because the hemorrhoid sites are usually in the anterior and posterior positions. The tip of the blade is angled medially (Fig. 9.4B), pointing just above the dentate line, and the lower one third to one half of the internal anal sphincter is divided. When the knife is seen beneath the intact anal mucosa, it is withdrawn. The side of the finger is then used to break any residual sphincter fibers (Fig. 9.4C). If the physician pushes with the fingertip, there is a tendency to tear the mucosa, which can lead to bleeding and, possibly, the subsequent development

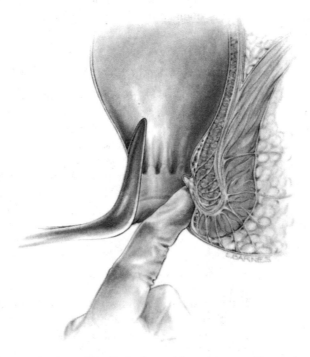

**FIG. 9.3.** Digital examination to identify the intersphincteric groove. The novice should practice palpating the groove on a number of asymptomatic patients before embarking on closed sphincterotomy. The location of the groove can be variable. The finger can be used to protect the external sphincter as the knife blade is inserted.

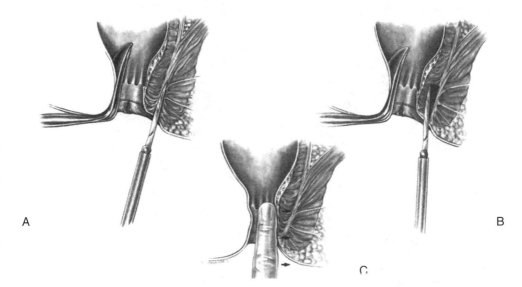

A                                                                                                                         B

C

**FIG. 9.4.** Lateral internal anal sphincterotomy using the closed technique with retractor. The patient is in the lithotomy position. **A.** A knife is inserted into the intersphincteric groove. **B.** The lower one third to one half of the internal sphincter is divided. **C.** The residual fibers are broken with the finger.

of a fistula. If bleeding occurs at the wound puncture site, it can be readily controlled by a few moments of direct pressure. If a tag or papilla is present, it can be removed by excision with a scissors or electrocautery. No dressings are required, and the patient is discharged when alert.

An alternative approach is to undertake the operation without a retractor in place. The index finger senses the knife blade beneath the anal mucosa, and the side of the finger is used to break the residual internal anal sphincter fibers. A third variation of the lateral sphincterotomy is the open technique, where a small, radial incision is made laterally at the lower border of the internal sphincter and intersphincteric groove (Fig. 9.5). Alternatively, a curvilinear incision outside the anal verge can be used. Because of the open wound and the possibility of bleeding, it is important to infiltrate the area with a local anesthetic containing epinephrine solution. The distal internal sphincter is grasped with forceps and bluntly freed. The lower one third to one half is divided with a scissors. The wound is closed with absorbable suture material, and a small dressing is applied.

## Postoperative Care

Sitz baths and a mild analgesic are the only postoperative measures advised. Pain is often less than that experienced preoperatively; most patients resume their normal activities within 48 hours.

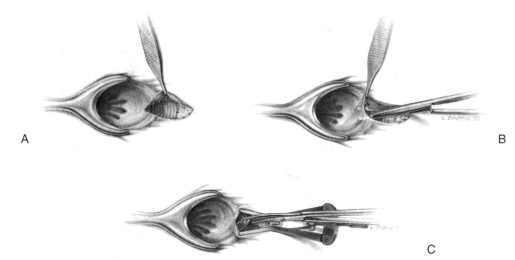

**FIG. 9.5.** Lateral internal anal sphincterotomy using the open technique with the patient placed in the lateral or the prone (i.e., jackknife) position. **A.** A radial incision is made across the intersphincteric groove. A narrow Hill–Ferguson retractor is in place. **B.** The internal sphincter is separated from the anoderm by blunt dissection. **C.** The internal sphincter is divided. The wound may be closed or left open.

## Complications

Surgery for anal fissure is associated with a number of complications, most of which are preventable by using judicious surgical technique and by being familiar with the anorectal anatomy.

Ecchymosis is frequently noted around the entrance wound if the closed technique is used, but this is of no concern. A massive hematoma is usually the result of failure to apply adequate pressure to the site. Hemorrhage, which is extremely rare, is much more likely to occur with the open procedure. Suture ligation may be required.

Perianal abscess occurs after 1% of closed internal anal sphincterotomies. It is virtually always associated with an anal fistula. This presumably is the result of penetration of the mucosa of the anal canal by the knife blade. It is surprising that this complication is not seen more frequently, because the anal canal mucosa must be breached more often than is believed. Treatment requires drainage of the abscess, identification of an internal opening (if present), and fistulotomy. Fortunately, the fistula is always low, provided the sphincterotomy divided only the internal anal sphincter.

Anal incontinence following a properly performed internal anal sphincterotomy should be extraordinarily rare. However, it is not that unusual for a patient to experience soilage of underclothes and incontinence for flatus. Because of their shorter anal canal, this is a particular problem in some women, as an internal anal sphincterotomy in the lateral position frequently divides more of the sphincter in women than it does in men. Therefore, caution should be exercised, especially in patients with prior obstetric trauma and in those with an ectopic anus. A keyhole deformity is a troublesome consequence of posterior fissure excision and internal anal sphincterotomy performed in the posterior midline. The resultant defect can produce symptoms of mucous discharge, pruritus, and soiling of the undergarments. When standard cleansing methods are unsatisfactory, the deformity is treated by anoplasty.

## Results

The two issues concerning long-term results are incontinence and recurrence or persistence. Fecal incontinence (i.e., the complete loss of bowel control) should not occur following sphincterotomy, because the internal anal sphincter has only a small role in maintaining anal continence. Most series report the incidence of soilage or incontinence to flatus in the range of 3% to 12%.

Between 95% and 100% of fissures should heal after proper application of the aforementioned methods. If the fissure fails to heal by conservative therapy (e.g., sitz baths, stool softeners), repeated sphincterotomy, during which a more generous portion of the internal sphincter is divided, is the appropriate treatment. If healing still does not take place, the patient should have gastrointestinal studies to identify the possibility of concurrent inflammatory bowel disease.

No significant difference in healing rate or morbidity is seen between the open and closed methods. Anal fistula occurs in 1% to 2%. An abscess occurs in 2% to 3%. When strict criteria for evaluation of morbidity are used, minor complications occurred in 35%. Consider the possibility of underlying inflammatory bowel disease in any patient whose wound fails to heal following surgery.

## CHRONIC ANAL FISSURE

Chronic anal fissure usually produces symptoms of pain and bleeding, but the pain is not as severe as that with an acute fissure. Frequently, the patient's symptoms are attributable to secondary changes (e.g., the presence of a lump). Other common complaints include mucous discharge, soiling of the underclothes, and pruritus. If the patient is concerned primarily with the pruritic symptoms, cleansing the area with warm water following defecation is usually helpful. Many patients believe that itching is caused by a lack of cleanliness, and they vigorously scrub the area with soap and water; this only serves to exacerbate the problem. Avoiding coffee, alcoholic beverages, smoking, and spicy foods will also have an ameliorative effect. If discharge is a problem and surgery is not considered appropriate, or if the patient refuses surgery, a ball of cotton can be placed at the anal opening and changed as necessary to avoid soiling underclothes and exacerbating pruritic symptoms.

### Surgical Treatment

The classic operative approach for chronic anal fissure is excision and internal anal sphincterotomy in the posterior position, but it carries the risk of a keyhole defect developing. Alternatively, the sphincterotomy can be performed in the lateral position. Unless the edges of the fissure are extremely fibrotic, removal of the tag and papilla by snipping with scissors should suffice. The underlying internal anal sphincter should not be incised.

### Results

Reports of the treatment of chronic anal fissure by lateral internal anal sphincterotomy are similar to those of acute anal fissure, with 94% to 100% experiencing complete healing, and results appear similar for open and closed techniques. Fecal soilage may be a slightly more common problem in those undergoing posterior midline sphincterotomy.

### Chronic Anal Fissure with Stenosis

Difficulty with defecation secondary to narrowing of the anal canal from chronic fissure can occasionally occur. The problem is more commonly seen, however, when excess anal canal mucosa is removed at the time of hemorrhoidectomy. Stenosis and fissure may supervene. Conservative medical management with stool softeners and a dilator is often advised, but an anoplasty can also provide good results.

### Anal Fissure and Hemorrhoids

When a patient has an anal fissure and a sufficiently convincing hemorrhoid problem to warrant surgical treatment, a hemorrhoidectomy and a sphincterotomy should be performed concurrently. The sphincterotomy should be carried out laterally, usually at the site of the left lateral pile.

### Anal Fissure and Crohn's Disease

If the fissure is ectopic, extends proximal to the dentate line, is particularly broad-based, or is especially purulent, the association with underlying inflammatory bowel disease must be considered. A history of diarrhea or abdominal pain is highly suggestive. When doubt exists about the cause of the condition, intestinal evaluation should be performed before a definitive surgical procedure is considered. It may be worthwhile to perform a small biopsy of the anal area. Other conditions can produce an anal fissure or ulcer, but the differential diagnosis usually poses little problem. Anal canal carcinoma, carcinoma of the anal margin, and tuberculosis all exhibit more extensive changes than a solitary anal fissure. Conservative (i.e., medical) treatment is the prudent course. The resultant surgical wound often tends to be indolent, more symptomatic than the original condition, and can be so debilitating that it precipitates the need for a diversionary procedure. Still, a number of published studies testify to a high rate of healing when internal anal sphincterotomy is performed, even in the presence of active Crohn's disease.

## Anal Fissure in the Homosexual Population

Anal fissures are common among male homosexuals, presumably as a consequence of traumatic anal intercourse. However, a number of anal and perianal ulcers occur in these individuals that can pose a problem in differential diagnosis. (The causes of such lesions have been reported to include syphilis, *Chlamydia, Haemophilus ducreyi*, cytomegalovirus, herpes simplex virus, human immunodeficiency virus (HIV), squamous cell carcinoma, non-Hodgkin's lymphoma, and Kaposi's sarcoma.) Because a high index of suspicion is necessary for diagnosis of these conditions, any fissure or perianal ulcer should be cultured and a biopsy performed in this group of patients. Individuals who are HIV positive with no identifiable associated etiology may be helped with aggressive debridement or intralesional steroid therapy. Sphincterotomy for uncomplicated fissure can be performed with the expectation of healing if symptoms warrant and if medical management has been unsuccessful.

# 10

## Anorectal Abscess

### ETIOLOGY

Anorectal abscess, an acute inflammatory process, often is a manifestation of an underlying anal fistula. Abscess can result from either specific or nonspecific causes. Specific causes include the following:

- Foreign body intrusion
- Trauma
- Malignancy
- Radiation
- Immunocompromised state
- Infectious dermatitides (e.g., suppurative hidradenitis)
- Tuberculosis
- Actinomycosis
- Crohn's disease
- Anal fissure

Anorectal abscess can also occur after anal operations (e.g., hemorrhoidectomy and sphincterotomy). The cause of nonspecific anorectal abscess and fistula is believed to be plugging of the anal ducts; this is known as the "cryptoglandular" theory. Between 6 and 10 of these glands and ducts, located around the anal canal, enter at the base of the crypts. Parks, in a histologic review demonstrated that (a) one half of all crypts are not entered by glands; (b) the ducts usually end blindly; and (c) the most common direction of spread is downward into the submucosa. Of particular interest is Park's observation that in two thirds of the specimens, one or more branches enter the sphincter, and in one half, the branches cross the internal sphincter completely to end in the longitudinal layer. However, he found that no branches crossed into the external sphincter. The implication is that infection of the duct can result in an abscess that can spread in a number of directions and can lead to the subsequent development of anal fistula.

Abscess can also be attributed to a defect in the dorsal portion of the cloacal membrane, which fuses with the hindgut during week 7 of gestation. In essence, then, contemporary theory implies that fistula-in-ano is the result of a congenital predisposition.

A congenital etiology has received further support by several other authors. One theory holds that an excess of androgens can lead to the formation of abnormal glands in utero, and that these abnormal glands are predisposed to infection. It has also been suggested that migratory cells from the urogenital sinus of the primitive hindgut become locally displaced and entrapped. Because fusion in females is less extensive, this might explain the greater incidence of fistula in males.

## AGE AND SEX

Abscess and fistula occur more commonly in men than in women, approximately 2 to 1. Two thirds of patients are in the third or fourth decade of life. The highest incidence is in the spring and summer.

Infants younger than 2 years of age represent a different spectrum of the disease when compared with older children and adults. An overwhelming male predominance with abscess and with concomitant anal fistula is noted (in excess of 85%). However, the distribution in older children tends to resemble that seen in adults.

## TYPES OF ABSCESS

Four presentations of anorectal abscess (Fig. 10.1) have been described:

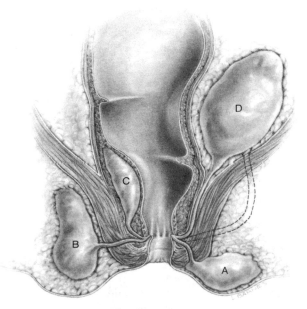

**FIG. 10.1.** Infection of the anal duct can present as an abscess in a number of locations. **A.** Perianal. **B.** Ischiorectal. **C.** Intersphincteric. **D.** Supralevator.

1. Perianal
2. Ischiorectal
3. Intersphincteric (i.e., submucosal)
4. Supralevator

It is important to distinguish among these presentations, because the cause, therapy, and implications for the presence or subsequent development of each differ.

## Perianal Abscess

Perianal (i.e., perirectal) abscess is identified as a superficial, tender mass outside the anal verge. It is the most common type of anorectal abscess, occurring in 40% to 45% of cases. The patient usually presents with a relatively short history of painful swelling that may be exacerbated by defecation and by sitting. Fever and leukocytosis are uncommon.

Physical examination reveals an area of erythema, induration, or fluctuation. Proctosigmoidoscopic examination may be difficult to perform because of pain, and even when it can be accomplished, it is usually unrewarding. Occasionally, however, anoscopic examination demonstrates pus exuding from the base of a crypt or at the site of a chronic anal fissure.

### *Treatment*

The American Society of Colon and Rectal Surgeons has established guidelines for the treatment of abscess and anal fistula:

ACUTE SUPPURATION (ABSCESS)
Presentation and Management
An abscess should be drained in a timely manner; lack of fluctuance is not a reason for delay in treatment. If the abscess is superficial, it may be drained in the office setting using a local anesthetic. If the patient is too tender to permit examination and drainage, then these measures should be undertaken in the operating room. Antibiotics may have a role as adjunctive therapy in special circumstances, including valvular heart disease, immunosuppression, extensive cellulitis, or diabetes. Location of the abscess should be documented. If possible, anoscopy should be performed to reveal the primary site of infection. Patients should notify the physician if pain recurs after abscess drainage.

When only erythema is present with no apparent mass, the surgeon may be misled into believing that incision and drainage will not be beneficial. Despite the absence of fluctuation or significant induration, an abscess is usually present. The procedure is easily undertaken in the office with a local anesthetic. A hypodermic needle inserted into the region of induration is a simple diagnostic test. If purulence is present, a small incision is made using a local anesthetic. The pus is drained, an iodoform gauze wick is placed, and a dressing is applied. The patient is instructed to remove the dressing and the drain in 24 hours while taking a sitz bath. Baths three times daily are advised, and the patient is reexamined in 7 to 10 days. At this time, proctosigmoidoscopic and anoscopic examinations are performed. If an external opening persists and a fistula tract is identified, a definitive procedure is indicated

### Antibiotics

In the patient who is at increased risk (e.g., with diabetes mellitus, valvular heart disease, or a compromised immune system), broad-spectrum antibiotics are suggested.

### Microbiology

Antibiotics are usually unnecessary, but culture does have some benefit in determining the likelihood of a fistula. If the culture demonstrates no bowel-derived organisms (i.e., skin bacteria), the chance of a subsequent fistula is virtually nil. Conversely, if enteric organisms are identified, the probability of the presence of a fistula is increased.

### Synchronous Fistulotomy

A fistula with an internal opening may be seen at the time that the abscess is drained. If the internal opening is low-lying, the surgeon can elect to perform fistulotomy at the same time the abscess is drained to avoid the need for a second procedure.

Anal fistula is usually not recognized at the time of drainage of a perianal abscess. If a simple, low-lying fistula is seen, I recommend making an incision of the tract if it can be easily accomplished at that time. In my experience and in accordance with my preference, the patient usually undergoes drainage as an office procedure; discomfort often precludes a more thorough evaluation and the ability to perform definitive fistulotomy. However, if an individual is to have a regional or general anesthetic, concurrent fistulotomy is an appropriate plan.

### Ischiorectal Abscess

Ischiorectal abscess may present as a large, erythematous, indurated, tender mass of the buttock, or may be virtually inapparent, the patient complaining only of severe pain. This type of abscess is seen in 20% to 25% of patients. Pus is almost always present. Needle aspiration will usually resolve the issue. Proctosigmoidoscopy and anoscopy are deferred because of the patient's discomfort, although the physician should keep in mind the possibility of a carcinoma or other colorectal condition producing this manifestation. Adequate rectal evaluation at some point is mandatory.

### *Techniques of Drainage*

Drainage of ischiorectal abscess requires some planning, because the condition is usually a consequence of a transsphincteric fistula. Most patients with this type of abscess will require a subsequent fistula procedure. It is important, therefore, to drain the abscess by creating an external opening as close to the anal verge as is possible. The abscess cavity can be entered and adequate drainage established without attacking the point of presentation or the most fluctuant area.

The technique for drainage of a large ischiorectal abscess differs little from that for a small, perianal abscess. Neither necessarily requires a general anesthetic or vigorous operative manipulation. After administration of a local anesthetic, a small incision is made and the pus is evacuated. The cavity is irrigated and an iodoform gauze wick inserted (not vigorously packed in). A dressing is applied, and the patient is instructed to take sitz baths. The patient removes the drain in 24 to 48 hours and is seen again in 1 week, at which time proctosigmoidoscopic and anoscopic examinations are performed.

### *In-Hospital Drainage*

Several factors can contraindicate draining an ischiorectal abscess as an office procedure. First, a general, spinal, or caudal anesthetic may be required because of patient insistence or because the patient is unable to tolerate the manipulation associated with a local procedure. Second, the surgeon may not have adequate office facilities; contamination of the examining room certainly limits its use for a time. Finally, an ischiorectal abscess should not be drained in the office when the patient is septic, except as a preliminary to hospitalization. Sometimes systemic antibiotics and more vigorous irrigations than are possible with an office procedure are needed.

In-hospital drainage follows essentially the same procedure advocated for office treatment. The incision should be minimal and medial. Irrigation with saline or an antiseptic solution is followed by insertion of a small drain or wick. Administration of an anesthetic also permits proctosigmoidoscopy and anoscopy, which may help to identify a specific cause for the abscess and localize an internal opening.

A simple way to determine the presence of an internal opening before drainage is to pass an anoscope while compressing the mass. Pus may be seen to exude from the crypt. If an opening is identified, its presence is noted for subsequent definitive treatment, usually any time after 2 weeks. I do not advocate fistulotomy of a transsphincteric fistula synchronously with drainage of an ischiorectal abscess.

Once started, antibiotics are continued for 48 hours. Drainage is the definitive therapy, and the patient almost invariably becomes afebrile within a few hours after the procedure.

## Deep Postanal Abscess

A transsphincteric fistula may present as an abscess in the deep postanal space (Fig. 10.2). This space is deep to the external sphincter and inferior to the levator ani muscle. Patients often complain of severe rectal discomfort. The pain may radiate to the sacrum, coccyx, or buttock, or display a sciatic distribution. Sitting may exacerbate the pain; defecation may be impaired and a fecal impaction may be present. The symptoms can mimic proctalgia fugax, coccygodynia, or lumbosacral strain. A helpful finding that implies the true nature of the problem is that the patient is frequently febrile. Someone with posterior rectal pain and tenderness of relatively short duration (i.e., <48 hours) that is continuous rather than intermittent and is not affected by position must be suspected of harboring an infection in the deep postanal space.

### *Examination*

Physical examination may be unrevealing except for exquisite posterior rectal tenderness. Frequently, the diagnosis is missed, and the patient is sent home with instructions concerning sitz baths and perineal exercises and told to take an analgesic. Eventually, the abscess will present at the skin or drain spontaneously, clearly establishing the diagnosis. A high degree of suspicion, therefore, may be

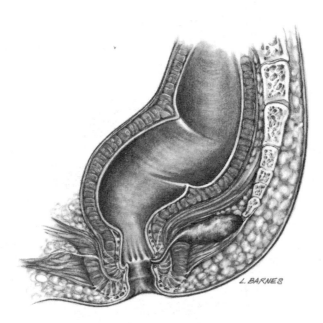

**FIG. 10.2.** Deep postanal abscess originating from a posterior crypt. Drainage is effected through an incision from the internal opening to the coccyx.

required if appropriate treatment is to be initiated. An attempt at aspiration between the rectum and coccyx in the midline may prove diagnostic. If an extrarectal mass is felt, the differential diagnosis includes presacral cyst, teratoma, chordoma, and a host of rare inflammatory and neoplastic conditions. Be aware of the fact that postanal infections can communicate with the ischiorectal fossa on either side. The presentation, therefore, may be that of bilateral ischiorectal abscesses, also known as a "horseshoe abscess."

### Treatment

Management requires drainage of the deep postanal space, a procedure that cannot be accomplished adequately with only a local anesthetic. Invariably, an internal opening in the posterior midline is identified at the time of drainage.

The best access to the deep postanal space to effect drainage was initially described by Hanley (see Chapter 11). He advocated placing a probe in the primary opening in the posterior midline and making an incision over the probe toward the tip of the coccyx. This incision bisects the superficial and subcutaneous external sphincter, and decompresses the cavity. Counterincisions can be made to drain the ischiorectal fossae if necessary (e.g., in the horseshoe abscess). Packing is advised and should be left in place for 24 to 48 hours.

### Intersphincteric Abscess

Intersphincteric abscess was initially described by Eisenhammer, who subsequently subdivided it into a high type and a low type. The condition arises from an infected crypt in the anal canal, and the infection burrows cephalad to present as a mass within the lower part of the rectum. It dissects in the intersphincteric plane (not under the mucosa), although it is frequently mistakenly called a "submucous" abscess. Intersphincteric abscess represents between 2% and 5% of perirectal abscesses.

The patient usually complains of rectal or anal discomfort, which can be exacerbated by defecation. A sense of fullness is often felt in the rectum. Pus or mucous discharge may be noted. The individual may or may not be febrile.

Rectal examination may reveal a tender submucosal mass, which may not be readily apparent by anoscopy or proctosigmoidoscopy. The condition can be confused with thrombosed internal hemorrhoids, but visual examination should distinguish the deep purple or black hemorrhoid from an abscess. The surface is edematous and indurated. An anal fissure is associated with the abscess in about 25% of patients. Pus from the associated crypt should leave no doubt to the nature of the lesion.

### Treatment

Treatment requires a general, caudal, or spinal anesthetic. This is *not* an office procedure. A Hill–Ferguson retractor or other appropriate anal retractor is inserted. The abscess is excised through the internal sphincter, removing the associated crypt-bearing area. Finally, the cut edge of the rectum and the underlying internal sphincter are sutured for hemostasis, leaving the wound open for drainage. No packing is required. The patient is discharged and advised to take a stool softener and sitz baths. Healing usually takes place within 3 to 4 weeks; no further procedure is required.

## Supralevator Abscess

Supralevator abscesses are relatively rare, comprising less than 2.5% of abscesses in most series. Pain in the perianal area and buttocks are the most common presenting complaints. Most patients are febrile and demonstrate leukocytosis.

Most individuals have a pelvic inflammatory condition (e.g., Crohn's disease, diverticulitis, salpingitis) or have had recent abdominal or pelvic surgery. Supralevator abscess may also occur as a cephalad extension of a transsphincteric or intersphincteric abscess (see Fig. 10.1).

### *Treatment*

The cause of the abscess determines the therapy: transrectal or transvaginal drainage for abscess caused by pelvic sepsis and external drainage for abscess secondary to transsphincteric fistula. To perform transrectal drainage when an internal opening is present at the level of the crypt is an invitation to disaster. Similarly, draining an abscess to the perineum when a communication is present above the levatores can result in a high extrasphincteric fistula. Effective treatment mandates an understanding of the cause of the septic process. To accomplish this, an appreciation of the history is helpful. More important, however, is to evaluate the situation by using an anesthetic, to attempt to identify an internal opening at the level of the crypt. If such an opening is found, the drainage procedure should be external; if absent, drainage probably should be internal (Fig. 10.3).

### *Internal Drainage*

For *internal drainage*, the patient is optimally placed in the prone position if the abscess is located anteriorly, or in the lithotomy position if the abscess is situated posteriorly. However, because the drainage procedure can be performed relatively quickly and anesthesiologists are disinclined to place patients face down, the lithotomy position is generally favored.

After aspiration, an incision is made into the cavity, either sharply with a knife or bluntly with a curved clamp. A de Pezzer (i.e., mushroom), Malecot, or Foley catheter is inserted into the cavity and delivered through the anal verge. The opening is made small enough for the catheter to remain in position without the need for suturing. The drain is removed in 24 to 48 hours.

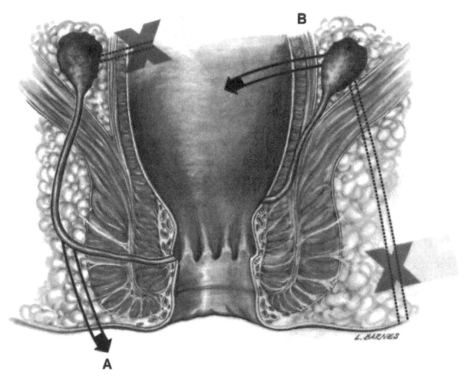

**FIG. 10.3.** Methods of drainage for supralevator abscess. **A.** Perineal drainage secondary to transsphincteric fistula. **B.** Transrectal drainage from pelvic sepsis. Unfortunately, the clearly defined possible scenarios illustrated do not necessarily facilitate decision making in individual cases.

In women, whenever possible, an anterior abscess should be drained transvaginally through the posterior cul-de-sac. Drainage is technically easier to perform, and the patient is more comfortable if the intact anal sphincter is avoided.

Despite the aforementioned suggestions and admonitions, the physician may credibly argue that drains are probably unnecessary. Once the abscess has been effectively evacuated, the cavity usually collapses and heals rather quickly.

### External Drainage

If *external drainage* is deemed appropriate, the patient is placed in the prone jackknife position. A larger external wound is required than for other abscesses because it is imperative to drain the supralevator collection adequately. The incision should be located as medial as possible. The supralevator space can be packed, or a Foley, de Pezzer (i.e., mushroom), or Malecot catheter can be placed in the cavity and left for 24 to 48 hours. Irrigation through the catheter may also be considered.

## Results

Essentially, little if any meaningful data are found in the literature on the results of surgery following drainage of supralevator abscesses. Definitive fistula surgery should probably best be undertaken during a subsequent hospitalization.

## TYPES OF INFECTION

### Necrotizing Infection

Anorectal abscess can cause severe necrotizing infection and death. Perineal gas gangrene (i.e., Fournier's disease) can also develop, and even tetanus following drainage of anorectal abscess has been reported. Delay in diagnosis and treatment—a week or more in most cases—and associated diseases (e.g., diabetes, obesity, malignancy, acquired immunodeficiency syndrome [AIDS], tuberculosis) are contributing factors. Treatment requires antibiotics, nutritional support, wide debridement, adequate drainage, and usually a colostomy.

### Anal Infection in Hematologic Disease

Abscess, fistula, and perirectal infections are commonly seen in patients with hematologic abnormalities (e.g., leukemia, granulocytopenia, lymphoma). These problems represent 3% to 8% of hematology admissions. The incidence in granulocytopenia, defined as a polymorphonuclear neutrophil count of less than 500/mm$^3$, has been reported to be 11%. One half of the patients die within 1 month of diagnosis, most of septic complications. In a study of more than 200 individuals with acute leukemia, perirectal infections developed in 7.9%.

#### Symptoms and Findings

Patients usually present with anal pain, but fever, septicemia, and shock may also be evident. Usually, neither fluctuation nor pus is present. Urinary retention, peritoneal signs, and infection of the genitalia are common. Of interest is the fact that cultured organisms may differ significantly from those usually identified with uncomplicated perirectal septic processes.

#### Treatment and Results

The prognosis closely correlates with the response to management of the underlying hematologic disorder. Conservative treatment (e.g., antibiotics, sitz baths, radiotherapy) is usually advised for those with leukemia if the disease is poorly controlled. Surgical drainage under such circumstances may result in fulminant sepsis and death. Patients with agranulocytosis who undergo operative intervention had slow wound healing, prolonged hospitalization, and a higher mortality rate when compared with patients who received antibiotics alone. Although some controversy exists concerning management options in these patients, a nonoperative approach is generally recommended.

### Perianal Infection Following Bone Marrow Transplantation

Perianal infection is a rare complication of bone marrow transplantation. Large series demonstrate perianal infections following transplants to occur in approximately 2.5%. The management of this complication is essentially the same as that described for patients with hematologic diseases. In general, perianal wound healing is not prolonged in those undergoing surgical drainage for infection following bone marrow transplantation.

### Anal Infection in AIDS

Patients with AIDS are extremely susceptible to opportunistic infections in the anorectal area. Colorectal manifestations of AIDS is discussed in Chapter 20.

# 11

## Anal Fistula

More surgeons' reputations reportedly have been impugned because of problems with fistula operations than from any other operative procedure. Complications of fistulectomy are myriad; they include fecal soilage, mucous discharge, anal incontinence, and recurrent abscess and fistula. The surgeon who has the opportunity to treat the patient initially is the one most likely to effect a cure, limit morbidity, and minimize disability.

### SYMPTOMS

The most frequent presenting complaints of patients with an anal fistula are swelling, pain, and discharge. The first two symptoms usually are associated with abscess when the external or secondary opening has closed. Discharge can be from the external opening or patients may report it as mucus or pus mixed with the stool. Most patients with fistula have an antecedent history of abscess.

Anal fistula can be confused with suppurative hidradenitis and pilonidal sinus; it can be secondary to anal or rectal carcinoma, or associated with specific and nonspecific inflammatory bowel disease.

### CLASSIFICATION

See list below, adapted from Parks AG, Gordon PH, Hardcastle JD. A classification of fistula-in-ano. *Br J Surg* 1976;63:1.

Intersphincteric
   Simple low track
   High blind track
   High track with opening into rectum
   High fistula without a perineal opening
   High fistula with extrarectal or pelvic extension
   Fistula from pelvic disease
Transsphincteric
   Uncomplicated
   High blind track

Suprasphincteric
  Uncomplicated
  High blind tract
Extrasphincteric
  Secondary to transsphincteric fistula
  Secondary to trauma
  Secondary to anorectal disease (e.g., Crohn's)
  Secondary to pelvic inflammation
Combined
Horseshoe
  Intersphincteric
  Transsphincteric

Complex fistulas are those other than intersphincteric and low extrasphinc-teric fistulas. They are more difficult to treat than conventional fistulas and are associated with increased risk of recurrence, as well as a greater likelihood for impairment of control. Most authors generally describe the following five types of fistulas:

1. Submucous
2. Intersphincteric (Fig. 11.1)
3. Transsphincteric (Fig. 11.2)
4. Suprasphincteric (Fig. 11.3)
5. Extrasphincteric (Fig. 11.4)

The *submucous fistula* is a misnomer; see the discussion in Chapter 10.

An *intersphincteric fistula* passes through the internal sphincter, then through the intersphincteric plane to the skin. Occasionally, an extension is observed to proceed cephalad in the intersphincteric plane (i.e., high blind tract), but this is of no consequence to the therapeutic decision making. Only the most superficial or subcutaneous portions of the external sphincter can be divided when per-forming a fistulotomy. The incidence of this fistula when compared with the oth-ers varies between 55% and 70% and is the most common of the fistula mani-festations.

A *transsphincteric fistula* passes through both the internal and external sphincters before exiting to the skin. The level of the tract determines how much of the sphincter is to be divided and, therefore, the risk of impairment for bowel control. This type of fistula is observed in 20% to 25% of most series. Occa-sionally, a supralevator extension of a transsphincteric fistula is identified (Fig. 11.5). Treatment requires recognition of this condition, curettage, irrigation, and packing of the supralevator extension. Under no circumstances should the exten-sion be drained into the rectum.

The incidence of a *suprasphincteric fistula* is probably in the range of 1% to 3%. This fistula starts in the intersphincteric plane, passes to a supralevator loca-

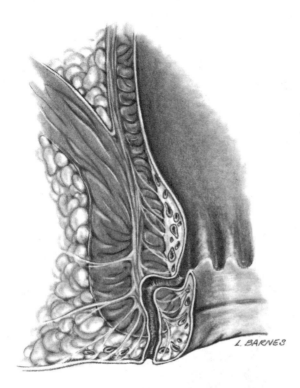

**FIG. 11.1.** Intersphincteric fistula. The tract passes through the internal sphincter and in the intersphincteric plane.

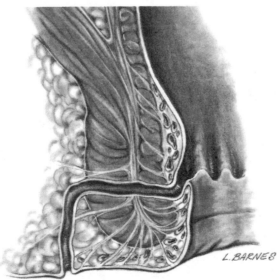

**FIG. 11.2.** Transsphincteric fistula. The tract passes through both the internal and external sphincters, into the ischiorectal fossa, and to the skin.

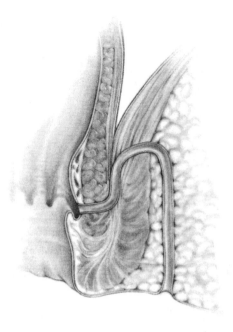

**FIG. 11.3.** Suprasphincteric fistula. The tract courses above the puborectalis muscle, after initially passing cephalad as an intersphincteric fistula. It then traverses downward through the ischiorectal fossa to the skin.

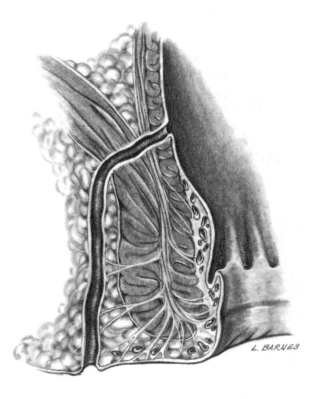

**FIG. 11.4.** Extrasphincteric fistula. The internal opening is above the level of the levator ani muscle, and the tract passes to the skin deep to the external sphincter in the ischiorectal space.

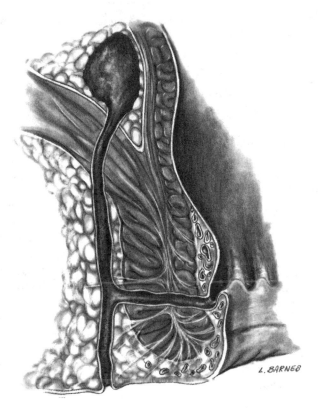

**FIG. 11.5.** Transsphincteric fistula with supralevator extension. Drainage of the extension into the rectum is contraindicated.

tion, and ultimately tracks between the puborectalis and the levator ani muscles to end in the ischiorectal fossa.

An *extrasphincteric fistula* is that with a supralevator internal opening with a tract that passes through the entire sphincter mechanism as it exits at the skin. It is usually a consequence of trauma (e.g., foreign body, surgical manipulation, impalement), Crohn's disease, or pelvic inflammatory disease. It can also develop when a supralevator abscess or transsphincteric fistula with supralevator extension ruptures spontaneously into the rectum. This type of fistula represents approximately 2% to 3% of fistulas, but in practices that have many individuals with inflammatory bowel disease, the incidence could be higher.

## PRACTICE PARAMETERS FOR TREATMENT

Practice parameters for the treatment of a number of colorectal conditions established by the Standards Practice Task Force of the American Society of

Colon and Rectal Surgeons also include recommendations for the evaluation and treatment of fistula-in-ano.

## IDENTIFICATION OF FISTULA TRACT

### Goodsall's Rule

When the external opening lies anterior to the transverse plane, the internal opening tends to be located radially. Conversely, when the external opening lies posterior to the plane, the internal opening is usually located in the posterior midline (Fig. 11.6).

The posterior course can result from a defect in fusion of the longitudinal muscle and the external sphincter in the posterior midline. A transsphincteric fistula, therefore, is more likely to occur in this position; the tract can then dissect into one or both ischiorectal fossae.

Although the rule is relatively consistent, exceptions are occasionally seen.

This rule is not a substitute for meticulous technique, clear identification of the tract direction, and ascertaining the internal opening location.

Usually, only one external or secondary opening is seen. Most commonly, fistulas pass into the intersphincteric plane; however, with transsphincteric fistulas, multiple openings can develop from communication with the deep postanal space and from the ischiorectal fossa—the cause of the so-called "transsphincteric horseshoe fistula."

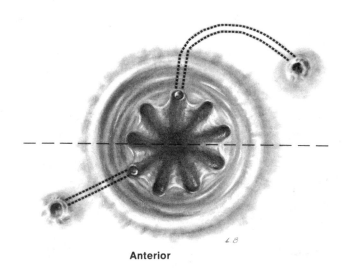

**Anterior**

**FIG. 11.6.** Typical courses of fistula tracts according to Goodsall's rule.

## Physical Examination and Endoscopy

Careful palpation may reveal the thickened tract entering the anal canal if the fistula assumes a relatively superficial position. This finding is most characteristic of an intersphincteric fistula. Bidigital examination, placing the thumb on the outside and the index finger within the anal canal, may also help to reveal the course of the tract. Failure to identify the tract by palpation implies that it is deep and, therefore, more likely to be a transsphincteric fistula. Anoscopic examination may demonstrate purulent material exuding from the base of the crypt. By gentle probing with a crypt hook or malleable probe, the presence of the tract may be confirmed. Occasionally, the tract will pass subcutaneously for a considerable distance and end in the perineum, scrotum, labia, or thigh. Failure to identify the internal opening does not mean that it has closed, however. Angulation or narrowing of the tract may preclude the possibility of adequate evaluation; excessive manipulation will cause considerable discomfort to the patient. Under these circumstances, examination under an anesthetic is required to adequately delineate the course of the tract.

## Passing a Probe

Passage of a probe can be attempted from both the external and the internal openings. A stenotic or sharply angulated area within the tract may preclude complete passage from either end. The probe should never be forced, merely gently maneuvered.

## Traction on the Tract

Theoretically, if a small portion of the tract is mobilized from the secondary (i.e., external) opening and traction applied, an indentation or dimpling will be evident at the level of the crypt—the site of the internal opening. The variable and often curvilinear course of more complex fistulas lessens the potential benefit of this method for tract identification.

## Injection Techniques

### *Dye*

If a substance such as methylene blue or indigo carmine is injected through the tract, the dye may appear in the rectum, confirming the patency of the tract and its communication with an internal opening. The problem with such agents is that the surgeon may have only one opportunity to visualize the internal opening before the material stains the entire mucosa.

## Milk

Milk can be used to identify the tract and the internal opening; sterility is not required. A DeBakey olive-end needle or an ordinary polyethylene intravenous catheter can be used to inject the milk while an anoscope is in position in the rectum. The milk can be wiped away without staining the tissue, permitting repeated attempts to inspect the internal opening. Failure to demonstrate communication with the internal opening implies stenosis of the tract, but if the milk is seen in the submucosa of the anal canal, even without escaping into the lumen, the associated crypt-bearing area should be excised with the presumption that the internal opening has closed.

## Hydrogen Peroxide

Hydrogen peroxide injection is probably the best means for identifying the internal opening. The liberated oxygen may be seen to bubble through the internal opening. The pressure created by the gas may be sufficient to penetrate even a stenotic tract and pass into the anal canal. Tissue staining does not occur.

## Fistulography

Fistulography, the radiologic delineation of a fistula tract with a water-soluble contrast agent, is generally thought to be of limited value. The technique is simple. The patient is placed on the x-ray table, usually in the left lateral position, and a small-bore catheter is inserted into the external opening. A few milliliters of water-soluble contrast material are injected, and films are taken in several projections.

Fistulography can be of particular value in those selected individuals (a) with no identifiable internal opening, (b) with suspected or known Crohn's disease, and (c) who have undergone a prior unsuccessful fistula operation. Unfortunately, many of the patients in this category will not benefit from the procedure, because no internal opening will be evident.

## Anal Endosonography

As with ultrasonography in the evaluation of rectal cancer, endoanal ultrasound has been suggested for imaging pathologic abnormalities in the anal canal and perianal region. This technique is an accurate and minimally invasive method for delineating the relationship between fistula tracts and the anal sphincter mechanism as well as identifying deeper areas of sepsis.

Particular problem areas, however, include specific internal opening sites and differentiation among abscess cavities, granulating tracts, and scars. Hydrogen peroxide enhances the contrast, resulting in a simple, effective, and safe method for improving the accuracy of endoanal ultrasound assessment for this condition.

## Magnetic Resonance Imaging

Another study recently introduced in an attempt to avoid the consequences of a missed internal opening at the time of surgery is magnetic resonance imaging (MRI). Dynamic contrast-enhanced MRI (DCEMRI) had a sensitivity of 97% and a specificity of 100% in the detection of anal fistulas. Furthermore, DCEMRI was able to identify more secondary tracts and was more accurate in identifying complex fistulas than either rectal examination alone or surgical exploration. The true place of this investigation awaits further trials and additional experience by other investigators.

## Additional Studies

Gastrointestinal evaluation, in addition to rigid or flexible sigmoidoscopy, is generally unnecessary for patients with conventional anal fistula. However, in the presence of known or suspected inflammatory bowel disease, colonoscopic examination and a small bowel series are strongly encouraged.

## PRINCIPLES OF SURGICAL TREATMENT

The management of anal fistula by division or "laying open" the tract was initially described by John of Arderne in the 14th century. With minor variations, this is the method most commonly used today. Failure to cure the patient is usually the result of either timorousness or temerity. The surgeon who traces the tract from the external opening to the level of the crypt but cannot pass the probe into the anal canal and subsequently desists from excising the crypt-bearing area is being too timid. In this situation, it is reasonable to assume that the crypt opening has sealed and that it is, indeed, the source of the fistula. Alternatively, if the surgeon identifies the internal opening but is reluctant to lay it open because of fear that it is too high, that decision may jeopardize the opportunity to cure the patient. The fistula will persist, and the subsequent procedure will be performed without the security of knowing that the observed internal opening occurred as a natural consequence. With few exceptions (e.g., Crohn's disease, a history of trauma), the surgeon should be able to open the tract at the time of the initial operation without fear of causing fecal incontinence. With persistent doubt about the safety of dividing at the internal opening, a seton can be used (see below).

Conversely, if the tract is only partially identified (i.e., not to the level of the crypt), and an assumption is made regarding where the opening should be and an artificial internal opening is created, the surgeon is being too aggressive. The opening and the tract can be bypassed completely. When confronted with a persistent fistula following such an ill-conceived maneuver, both the natural and the artificial internal openings must be considered.

The aforementioned injection techniques confirm the presence of the fistula and the internal opening. They do not, however, identify the course of the tract. If a probe can be passed, it is only necessary to incise down onto it. However, if this cannot be accomplished, the dissection must be carried out slowly and meticulously, following the epithelialized tract until it communicates with the anal canal.

A fistula operation should always be performed with electrocautery. Identification of the tract requires a dry operative field. In such a vascular area, no better means exists for maintaining hemostasis than this technique.

## Fistulotomy Versus Fistulectomy

Another source of controversy has been whether to perform fistulectomy or fistulotomy. Healing times were significantly shorter when the fistula was laid open in comparison with excision, whereas recurrence rates were comparable. However, a small portion of the tract can be removed for pathologic examination, especially if concern about the possibility of Crohn's disease (see below) exists.

## Office Fistulotomy

Office fistulotomy can be done synchronously with drainage of an abscess if the internal opening is low and intersphincteric. It can also be performed in the office as an interval procedure after abscess drainage. Local anesthesia or a field block is usually adequate. For most patients, however, definitive fistula surgery under optimal conditions should be performed in the operating room with a general, spinal, or caudal anesthetic. With the exception of some complex fistulas or those requiring concomitant sphincter repair, the operation can usually be done on an ambulatory basis.

The Standards Task Force of the American Society of Colon and Rectal Surgeons has recommended practice parameters for fistula surgery on an ambulatory basis. Their conclusions are as follows:

A fistula, fistula with abscess or a fistula associated with limited anorectal pathology may be treated on an outpatient basis if, in the judgment of the operating surgeon, it is safe to do so.

Fistulas involving adjacent organs or structures (e.g., rectovaginal, recto-urethral or horseshoe) often require more extensive surgery, and inpatient postoperative care is usually needed.

Fistulas associated with extensive cellulitis or abscess or additional anorectal pathology may require inpatient care, especially if intravenous antibiotics are necessary.

## SURGICAL APPROACHES

### Treatment of Conventional Fistula

After the external and internal openings have been identified, the tract is incised. Continuity of the epithelial lining confirms the completeness of the operation, and granulation tissue is removed by curettage. A portion of the tract can be excised and sent for pathologic examination. The external portion of the incision is widened relative to the size of the opening in the anal canal, because skin tends to heal more rapidly than does the anal mucosa. If this procedure is not performed properly, delayed healing of the anal canal may result. The cut edges of the anal mucosa and the underlying internal anal sphincter can be over-sewn with absorbable suture to effect hemostasis. The wound is otherwise left open and gently packed. The dressing is removed that evening or the next day, and sitz baths are commenced. Vigorous mechanical cleansing of the wound is encouraged, either by means of a washcloth or with a gauze pad. The use of a Water-Pic device or comparable irrigating equipment has definite merit in post-operative wound management. The principle is to be as rough as possible, main-taining the wound in a well-debrided and clean state. An office visit is recom-mended approximately 10 days later and every 1 to 2 weeks thereafter until healing has taken place. Less frequent appointments may be appropriate for indi-viduals with simple fistulas if the patient understands the need for and is com mitted to vigorous cleansing.

If a large portion of the external sphincter must be divided, consider primary sphincter repair or, possibly, seton division (see *Seton Division*). One situation, however, should always be considered for either reconstruction or another alter-native to limit sphincter injury—an anterior fistula in a woman. When a fistula occurs anterior to the transverse plane in a woman, surgical treatment inevitably will create some degree of impairment for control. To minimize the disability, sphincter reconstruction should be attempted at the time of fistulotomy. Another alternative for managing such a problem is to use a seton or to close the internal opening with a sliding endorectal flap, such as that recommended for rectovagi-nal fistula repair and high-level anal fistulas (see below). External drainage completes the repair.

### Treatment of Horseshoe Fistula

Horseshoe fistula can be intersphincteric or transsphincteric. It is so called because it is composed of multiple external openings joined by a subcutaneous U- or horseshoe-shaped communication (Fig. 11.7). The arms of the U are directed anteriorly, and the internal opening is in the posterior midline. Rarely, a horseshoe fistula presents with the opposite configuration; that is, the internal opening is in the anterior midline, and the arms of the U are directed posteriorly.

Treatment of this condition has evolved to be much less radical than has often been described. The classic procedure required identification of the tracts and internal opening, and unroofing or excision of each of them (Fig. 11.8). This inevitably resulted in a huge, gaping wound, which required a prolonged healing time. Disability after this operation can last for many months.

In 1965, Hanley described a conservative approach to the management of horseshoe fistula that limited the number and extent of the incisions. Excision of

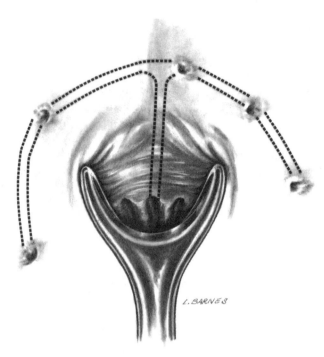

**FIG. 11.7.** Diagrammatic representation of a horseshoe anal fistula. The internal opening is in the posterior midline.

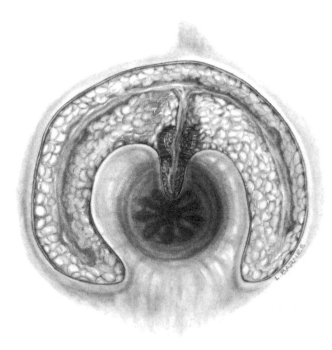

**FIG. 11.8.** Classic treatment of horseshoe fistula requires excision of all openings.

the internal opening along with establishing adequate external drainage should effect cure. If the internal opening has been removed, the external openings will close. Most surgeons have successfully adopted this approach to the treatment of horseshoe anal fistula.

The deep postanal space must be entered, curetted, and irrigated if the fistula is transsphincteric. This involves incision of both the internal sphincter and a portion of the external sphincter. It is then necessary only to unroof the external openings, curette the tracts, and drain the wound (Fig. 11.9). The cut edges of the anal canal and underlying internal sphincter are sutured to effect hemostasis. The deep postanal space is packed with iodoform gauze, and a dressing is applied.

When the fistula is approached in this way, healing is rapid, and the risk of functional impairment to the anus from scarring and deformity is lessened considerably. Length of disability is markedly reduced.

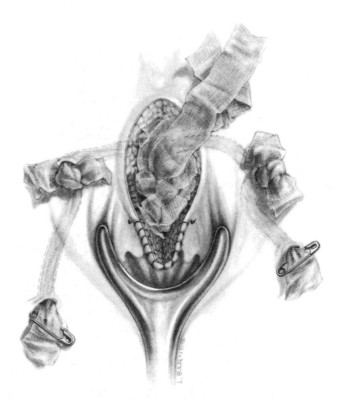

**FIG. 11.9.** Treatment of horseshoe fistula-in-ano requires unroofing in the posterior midline to adequately drain the deep postanal space. The external openings are individually drained, with curettage only of the underlying tracts. Packing is placed through each opening and in the deep postanal space.

Postoperatively, the packing is removed in 24 to 48 hours, and the patient is begun on sitz baths. Weekly office visits are recommended until the wounds have healed.

### Treatment of Suprasphincteric Fistula

The management of suprasphincteric fistula, which is comparable to that of other complex fistulas, includes endorectal advancement flap, primary closure and drainage, and seton division. In general, fistulotomy can be accomplished distal to the internal opening by dividing the lower portion of the internal and external sphincter. The cephalad component, including the internal opening, is treated by means of seton division (see below).

### Treatment of Extrasphincteric Fistula

When the internal opening is thought to lie above the levatores, division of the tract can result in fecal incontinence. If the puborectalis sling is completely divided, anal incontinence will surely ensue. When doubt exists as to the level of the internal opening, a seton can be used as a diagnostic tool. This involves placing a heavy suture through the tract and out the anal canal, which can be facilitated by passing the material through the eye of a probe. The suture is loosely tied, and no further procedure is undertaken at this time.

When the patient is alert, rectal examination is performed. While the patient alternately tightens and relaxes the sphincter, the seton can be felt to be above or below the levatores. If it is below, a fistulotomy can be performed safely. Conversely, if the internal opening is above the level of the levatores, an alternative procedure must be undertaken. A number of possible operative approaches exist for the treatment of extrasphincteric fistula.

### *Seton Division*

Seton division was described by Hippocrates in the fifth century BC, in his medical works known as the *Hippocratic Collection*. His concepts are still applicable today for the management of difficult fistula problems. It is certainly the simplest of the methods available for the treatment of extrasphincteric fistula, and probably produces results comparable to the more esoteric approaches, at least with respect to cure rates. Bowel control, however, may be less satisfactory when compared with other options.

The principle involved in the use of the seton as a therapeutic tool is analogous to that of a wire cutting through a block of ice. The ice is still adherent after division by the wire. Theoretically, by tightening the suture and permitting it to cut through over a number of days or weeks, the resultant inflammatory response keeps the sphincter muscle from retracting and separating.

If a seton is used, the skin and anal canal mucosa between the openings first must be incised before the suture is passed. Some surgeons prefer doubled no. 2 silk, but other alternatives are elastic bands (e.g., vessel retractor tapes) or a ¼-inch Penrose drain. The seton is securely tied, usually with moderate tension. Another method of securing and tightening the seton involves the use of a so-called "hangman's knot" (Fig. 11.10). Alternatively, multiple setons can be inserted, initially, securing only one. As each cuts through, another one is tied. If an elastic band or Penrose drain is used, it is necessary to secure the drain to itself with a ligature, thereby creating similar tension.

The patient is reexamined 1 week later. By that time, the suture has either loosened or, if minimal tissue has been incorporated, passed by necrosing through the residual muscle. Following injection of a local anesthetic into the sphincter, a second suture can be used. If an elastic band has been used, it can be twisted or stretched and retied at a higher level. Two weeks later the seton has usually eroded out. If not, the fistulotomy can be completed in the office, because usually little tissue remains to be divided. However, a third insertion can be performed.

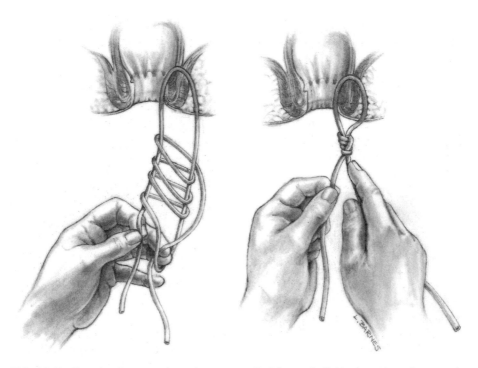

**FIG. 11.10.** Securing the seton in such a manner that it permits tightening using a hangman's tie. (Adapted from Loberman Z, Har-Shai Y, Schein M, et al. Hangman's tie simplifies seton management of anal fistulas. *Surg Gynecol Obstet* 1993;177:413.)

## Long-Term Seton Drainage

The concept of seton drainage without definitive fistulotomy has been applied to the management of extrasphincteric fistulas in patients with Crohn's disease for some time (see below). However, some individuals have used this approach in the management of low transsphincteric and intersphincteric anal fistulas. This permits continuous drainage of the fistula, thereby preventing recurrent abscess formation. The suture will either cut through the anal and perianal skin on its own, or the surgeon can perform fistulotomy at a subsequent operation. The mean duration of the presence of the seton is in excess of 1 year. This is certainly a disadvantage in that the patient must contend with the situation for a prolonged period of time. Still, the recurrence rate is only 3.7%, and less than 1% of patients experience problems with bowel control.

## Fistulotomy with Sphincter Repair

Complete division of an extrasphincteric fistula is a hazardous undertaking. Although direct repair can be performed immediately, breakdown is common. It should still be considered, however, as an alternative technique for the treatment of high-level fistulas, and, as mentioned, in the management of transsphincteric anterior fistulas in women.

The entire tract is divided. The epithelial lining is excised and the wound irrigated. A layered closure is performed using long-term absorbable sutures, closing the rectal wall and reconstructing the sphincter muscles. The ischiorectal fossa is widely drained externally. A protective colostomy is strongly suggested if fistulotomy with sphincter repair is contemplated.

This operation is usually reserved for patients who have had multiple failed attempts to cure the fistula. The decision to embark on this approach should be made by someone who has a special knowledge of anorectal anatomy and considerable experience with complex fistula surgery.

## Internal Opening Closure and Extrasphincteric Tract Drainage

Closure of the internal opening and drainage of the extrasphincteric tract is less destructive of tissue than fistulotomy with sphincter repair, but the procedure is also technically difficult to perform. More importantly, the operation rarely seems to be successful. The procedure involves debridement and closure of the internal opening through a transanal approach. External drainage is widely established, and the supralevator area is vigorously curetted, irrigated, and packed. A concurrent colostomy is advisable to enhance the possibility of a successful outcome. Another option that conserves the sphincter mechanism in high anal fistula is to do the same operation with primary closure through the intersphincteric plane. This has been described by the St. Mark's Hospital group (Fig. 11.11). In their operation, the entire tract is excised through this approach and the defects in the sphincter muscle that are produced as a consequence of tract removal are primarily closed.

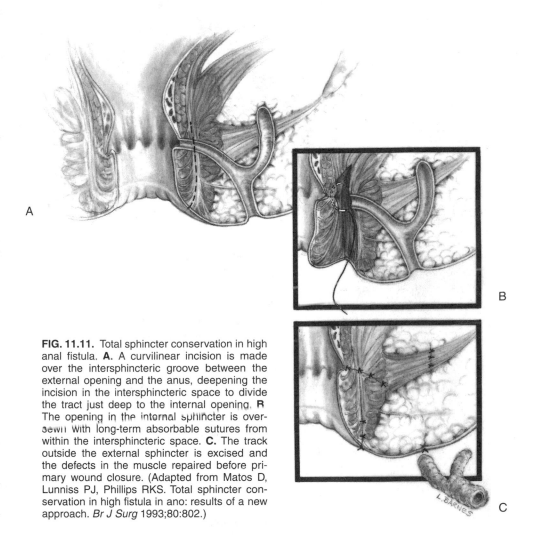

**FIG. 11.11.** Total sphincter conservation in high anal fistula. **A.** A curvilinear incision is made over the intersphincteric groove between the external opening and the anus, deepening the incision in the intersphincteric space to divide the tract just deep to the internal opening. **B.** The opening in the internal sphincter is over-sewn with long-term absorbable sutures from within the intersphincteric space. **C.** The track outside the external sphincter is excised and the defects in the muscle repaired before primary wound closure. (Adapted from Matos D, Lunniss PJ, Phillips RKS. Total sphincter conservation in high fistula in ano: results of a new approach. *Br J Surg* 1993;80:802.)

Whereas these authors report a failure rate of approximately 30%, they conclude that, if the operation is successful, continence is better than after other approaches. As opposed to fistulotomy with sphincter repair, closure of the internal opening and drainage of the extrasphincteric tract is less likely to cause harm to the patient; however, extrasphincteric fistulectomy with endorectal mucosal advancement is the approach to use if this type of procedure is contemplated.

### *Extrasphincteric Fistulectomy with Endorectal Mucosal Advancement*

The concept of endoanal or endorectal mucosal advancement has evolved into three principal methods: vertical or tongue flaps, semilunar lip flaps, and circumferential tubal or sleeve flaps (Fig. 11.12).

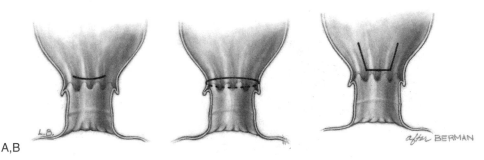

A,B
C

**FIG. 11.12.** Endorectal mucosal advancement. **A.** Semilunar flap. **B.** Tubal or sleeve flap. **C.** Vertical or tongue flap. (Adapted from Berman IR. Sleeve advancement anorectoplasty for complicated anorectal/vaginal fistula. *Dis Colon Rectum* 1991;34:1032.)

The incision begins distal to the internal opening; the flap is mobilized and the scar excised. The method used for flap construction is a matter of opinion. Some suggest an oblique incision, but this risks ischemic necrosis at the apex. Others prefer mobilization in a circumferential fashion, incorporating as much as 50% of the rectum. The dissection can be facilitated by means of infiltration with a dilute epinephrine solution. It is the general contention that mucosa alone is not adequate, and that muscularis is also needed. Others believe that the flap should be the full thickness of the rectal wall to limit the likelihood of dehiscence. The internal opening, which is closed separately, can be sutured to a portion of the overlying muscularis.

Management of the external portion of the tract is a matter of some controversy regarding "coring out" versus simple debridement. The application of a sleeve advancement for individuals who have even more extensive fistula problems has been suggested.

### Use of PMMA Beads

Polymethyl methacrylate (PMMA) beads (Septopal) have been suggested in the management of complex anal fistulas. In patients in whom more traditional approaches have failed, gradual removal of the beads with closure of the internal opening results in healing. The bead material, used in the management of osteomyelitis, consists of a polymer impregnated with gentamicin sulfate and zirconium dioxide as a contrast medium.

### Other Techniques

Other approaches that can be used to manage an extrasphincteric fistula depend on its cause. These may include low anterior resection, abdominosacral resection, and transsacral excision. Rarely, a diverting colostomy alone will permit spontaneous healing, but it is reasonable to consider either a concomitant ileostomy or colostomy when attempting repair. This is especially true if a stoma is contemplated in the event of failure. When the patient has minimal symptoms, expectant management (i.e., using a small dressing and sitz baths), draining an abscess when it occurs, and inserting a small drain or seton in the tract may offer adequate palliation of symptoms (see below).

### Results of Surgery for Anal Fistula

The three primary criteria for determining success or failure of fistula surgery are the following:

1. Recurrence
2. Delayed healing
3. Incontinence

A few generalizations can be made in interpreting the published results:

* The more complex the fistula, the higher the internal opening.
* The more sphincter that is divided, the longer it takes to heal, and the greater the likelihood of recurrence and risk of fecal soilage.

The most likely cause of recurrence, however, is the failure of the surgeon to identify and adequately excise the internal opening.

### Results of Surgery for Conventional Fistula

Generally, recurrence rates vary from 4% to 10%, with missed internal openings at the initial surgery accounting for most such recurrences. Certainly, those individuals with high openings, posterior openings, or fistula extensions are at increased risk of recurrence. Factors associated with recurrence include complex type of fistula, horseshoe extension, lack of identification or lateral location of the internal fistulous opening, prior fistula surgery, and even the surgeon's experience level.

Besides the issue of recurrence, the other major concern is incontinence, which reportedly is between 10% and 50%. Typically, the symptoms are loss of control for gas and occasional mild soilage. Frank fecal incontinence is rare.

### Results of Surgery for Extrasphincteric Fistula

#### *Advancement Flap*

The advancement flap technique results in recurrence rates of 13% to 29%. Healing seems more rapid than with other methods; less tissue destruction occurs; and postoperative discomfort is minimal. Certainly, bowel control should be optimal when compared with the other methods. If recurrence develops, it is still possible to redo the repair without necessarily expecting deterioration of function.

### Seton Division

None who were treated with a cutting seton (13 patients) developed a recurrence. Minor instances of incontinence developed in 5% to 55% of those treated by two-stage fistulotomy or by cutting seton.

Major fecal incontinence requiring the use of a pad occurred in 5%, with recurrent fistulas identified in 3%.

### Results of Surgery for Horseshoe Fistula

Using the Hanley technique, as described above, resulted in recurrence rates of 7% to 18%. It may be advisable for more frequent use of a seton to promote drainage and to avoid premature closure.

### Management of Skin Defects

The use of skin grafting to treat defects in the skin that may occur following fistula operations is generally not encouraged. Advancement or rotation flaps may be more appropriate when scarring produces sufficient symptoms to warrant anoplasty. The methods of sphincter reconstruction to correct problems with fecal incontinence are discussed in Chapter 13.

### DUAL ANAL FISTULAS

Rarely, a patient presents with two anal fistulas, each with separate external and internal openings (an incidence of ~2% to 4%). Treatment of simultaneous low-lying fistulas consists of identifying the external and internal openings and performing fistulotomies in the standard fashion. This condition should be easily distinguished from horseshoe fistula, because the latter presentation is associated with only one internal opening.

### ANAL FISTULA AND CROHN'S DISEASE

Fistula and abscess are among the most difficult manifestations of Crohn's disease to manage (see Chapter 30). Anal fissures, fistulas, and abscesses occur as complications in 22% of cases. This is more common with colonic inflammation (52%) than with small bowel involvement (14%).

### Clinical Features

Lesions in patients with Crohn's disease tend to be chronic, indurated, and cyanotic, but are often painless unless an abscess is present. Skin irritation is frequently noted, which may be caused by diarrhea rather than by intrinsic disease of the anus. The fistula may be low-lying, with an internal opening at the level of the crypt. More commonly, however, the fistula is associated with a deep ulcer, and the internal opening may either be inapparent or found in a supralevator location.

## Treatment

The presence or absence of symptoms is the important criterion that determines therapy. Many individuals with fistulas are relatively asymptomatic; approximately 25% of patients in one series did not even require specific treatment. It has been suggested that metronidazole (i.e., Flagyl) can produce symptomatic improvement in some patients with perianal disease, but no irrefutable proof indicates that fistulas are likely to close with continued therapy (see Chapter 30).

When anal fistula occurs as a complication of the condition, it is important to distinguish between anal Crohn's disease with fistula, and Crohn's disease of the intestinal tract and a coincidental fistula-in-ano. This distinction is critical, because the fistula procedure can be performed with relative safety in a patient with Crohn's disease in whom the disease does not involve the anus, provided that the abdominal condition is quiescent. A definitive fistula operation that is undertaken in the presence of active inflammatory bowel disease, however, is hazardous. The resulting wound may be a greater management problem than was the original condition. Another important precaution is to evaluate the entire gastrointestinal tract before embarking on surgery for suspected anal Crohn's disease.

In the presence of known anal Crohn's disease, it may be possible to ameliorate the patient's condition and to relieve the discomfort associated with anal abscess and fistula without performing a definitive fistulotomy; however, superficial cryptoglandular fistulas can be successfully treated by this method. Simple incision and drainage is obviously appropriate for treating perianal and ischiorectal abscesses. As with abscess in the absence of Crohn's disease, the incision should be made as medial as possible. Long-term, continuous drainage can be facilitated by insertion of a Pezzer (i.e., mushroom) or Malecot catheter or by the application of seton drainage. Another method of treating patients with Crohn's disease is to establish adequate drainage of the internal opening. This is best accomplished by excising the internal opening and the underlying internal anal sphincter in the same manner described for the treatment of intersphincteric abscess. The external opening can then be unroofed, and drainage can be established between the external sphincter and the external opening. Although not a conventional fistulotomy, this procedure provides complete drainage of the fistula on either side of the external sphincter. However, because this lesion frequently heralds the onset of intestinal manifestations, the most prudent course of action is to incise and drain the abscess when it becomes symptomatic.

A third alternative is to use a rectal mucosal advancement flap. To attempt a definitive repair, this is the safest method for treating anterior fistulas in women, extrasphincteric fistulas, and high anal canal fistulas.

Obviously, proctectomy will cure the fistula. Many individuals will be served best by removal of the rectum.

### Results of Treatment of Fistulas in Crohn's Disease

With proper selection, more than 90% of fistulas in Crohn's disease heal following definitive fistulotomy. Success correlates with the absence of rectal disease and quiescence elsewhere in the gastrointestinal tract. Most authors agree that medical treatment or a minimal surgical procedure is preferred for complex fistulas, high transsphincteric fistulas, or extensive or active inflammatory bowel disease. Proctectomy is ultimately the best option in this latter group of patients. Conversely, most concur with the position that in carefully selected patients, definitive fistulotomy is a relatively safe procedure.

With respect to advancement flap, it seems clear that the procedure is justifiable in this group of patients. Primarily, it gives them short-term improvement without precipitating the need for more radical surgery.

*Comment*: In analyzing the results of treatment for anal fistulas associated with Crohn's disease, much confusion can result from the plethora of approaches employed, as well as the varied presentations of the condition. Thus, the physician may be intimidated to the extent of recommending only the most general of principles concerning management. These principles may be summarized as follows:

Absence of symptoms: no treatment

Active Crohn's disease: systemic treatment and surgical drainage, or long-term drainage only

Quiescent Crohn's disease with anal and rectal sparing: fistulotomy

Superficial, intersphincteric, and low transsphincteric fistulas: definitive fistulotomy

Complex fistulas: drainage with consideration given to mucosal advancement flap as the preferred operative alternative

### ANAL FISTULA AND CARCINOMA

Rarely, carcinoma can develop in a chronic anal fistula. Fewer than 150 cases are reported in the literature. Long-standing, chronic inflammation in the region of the anal glands is felt by some to lead to malignant degeneration. Tumor mass, bloody discharge, and mucin secretion are suggestive of the presence of an underlying tumor.

Differential diagnosis includes anal canal carcinoma (e.g., epidermoid, cloacogenic) with fistula, carcinoma of the rectum with fistula, suppurative hidradenitis with malignant degeneration, and carcinoma arising in an anal duct. Carcinoma of the colon has also been reported to seed into a preexisting fistula. This observation certainly corroborates the opinion that the entire colon should be evaluated when a perianal malignancy is identified. The importance of histologic examination of all tissues recovered from an anal fistula in an individual who is suspected of harboring a tumor is obviously extremely important.

Potentially curative treatment usually requires abdominoperineal resection, perhaps with preoperative chemoradiation therapy (see Chapters 23 and 24).

## ANAL FISTULA IN INFANTS AND CHILDREN

The anomaly of a congenital anal fistula without an imperforate anus is rare, representing less than 1% of anorectal malformations. As mentioned, an overwhelming male predominance is seen in infants with abscess, and concomitant anal fistula is noted in more than 85%. The embryologic basis for this congenital malformation in a normally placed anus remains speculative and may not be the same for the two sexes. In the experience of Duhamel, the onset of the condition in 70% was in the first 10 months of life, most arising in the first month (22%). Presenting symptoms and signs include diarrhea, inguinal adenopathy, and proctitis. The fistula is usually simple, with a tract running directly between a crypt and the external opening. In children, fistulas are almost always superficial and intersphincteric. Again, in Duhamel's experience, multiple fistulas are fairly common, but these consist of separate tracts. Treatment consists of identification of the tract by one of the means described above and standard fistulotomy.

# 12

## Rectovaginal and Rectourethral Fistulas

### RECTOVAGINAL FISTULA

Rectovaginal fistula is not usually a manifestation of anal fistula, because it is rarely a consequence of cryptoglandular infection. The condition most commonly occurs following trauma, especially obstetric injury. Of all normal deliveries, 5% result in episiotomy-associated third- and fourth-degree lacerations. Of the fourth-degree lacerations, 10% disrupted after primary repair.

In addition to obstetrically related causes, other etiologic factors related to the development of rectovaginal fistula include the following:

- Inflammatory bowel disease—the second most frequent cause
- Carcinoma
- Radiation
- Diverticulitis
- Foreign body
- Penetrating trauma
- Infectious processes
- Congenital anomalies
- Pelvic, perineal, and rectal surgery, especially vaginal hysterectomy
- Anorectal ergotism

### Symptoms and Classification

Patients often complain of passage of flatus, feces, or pus from the vagina. Depending on the cause, location, and extent of the problem, the woman may also have difficulty controlling flatus and feces per rectum.

I prefer to categorize the fistula on the basis of its level in the anal or rectal opening: anal, low rectal, or high rectal. The equivalent gynecologic classification is low, mid, and high vaginal. The location of the fistula is important, because it will determine the appropriate operative approach.

A low fistula is usually readily apparent on inspection or anoscopy. Usually, little difficulty exists in identifying the tract and passing a probe, but the tone and contractility of the muscle above the fistula should be carefully studied. A mid-rectal (mid-vaginal) fistula is also relatively easy to visualize, particularly when attempting to pass a probe from the vagina to the rectum. A high fistula can be difficult to diagnose, especially if the opening is small. This type is usually a complication of diverticulitis or of hysterectomy. It can also develop as a consequence of an anastomotic leak following anterior resection.

## Evaluation

Physical examination should include both rectal and vaginal evaluation. Proctosigmoidoscopic examination and gastrointestinal contrast studies are indicated, especially if doubt exists concerning the cause of the fistula. With high fistulas, proctosigmoidoscopic examination seldom demonstrates the opening, but gentle probing at the apex of the vagina often permits identification of the defect. Barium enema examination may show opacification of the vagina. A biopsy should be done if the fistula is secondary to radiation injury to determine the presence or absence of tumor.

If the patient's symptoms are characteristic, but the fistula cannot be confirmed by one of the aforementioned means, two other approaches are worth attempting. One procedure is to place the patient in the lithotomy position and insert a proctoscope in the rectum. With the woman in a slight Trendelenburg position, the vagina is filled with warm water. Air is then insufflated through the proctoscope; if bubbles are seen in the vagina, the diagnosis is confirmed. Another alternative is to give the patient a methylene blue small retention enema and leave a tampon in the vagina. The tampon is removed after 1 hour to see if the blue color appears on it.

Depending on the cause of the fistula, it may be appropriate to evaluate the proximal colon before definitive repair. This is usually readily accomplished by means of either colonoscopy or barium enema examination. Occasionally, however, it may be difficult to advance the endoscope above the fistula site, and contrast medium may preferentially pass completely out of the vagina. Under these circumstances, a combination of guide wire passage of the instrument, placement of a Foley catheter above the communication, or both will facilitate proximal evaluation.

## Treatment

As suggested, the treatment of rectovaginal fistula depends on its location and cause. High rectovaginal fistulas, which are approached transabdominally, involve a bowel resection if colon or rectal disease precipitated the communication. If the fistula occurred secondary to hysterectomy, it may suffice to separate the bowel from the vagina, close the opening, and interpose omentum, a peritoneal flap, or fascia. For mid and low rectovaginal fistulas, a number of operative approaches have been advocated, including transvaginal, perineal, transanal, and transsphincteric. One operation that should not be done, even for anovaginal or introital fistulas, is simple fistulotomy. Dividing the perineum, even for relatively superficial fistulas, causes some degree of impairment of fecal control. The following is a summarization of the various operative alternatives:

Perineal
    Fistulotomy alone
    Fistulotomy with muscle repair: anoplasty
    Interposition (e.g., bulbocavernosus—labial flap [Martius])
Transanal
    Repair in layers
    Repair in layers with sliding flap: anterior rectal wall; internal sphincter
Transsphincteric (Mason)
Transvaginal
    Repair in layers: with sliding vaginal flap (Warren); with interposition
Abdominal
    Simple closure: with interposition
    Resection (low anterior, pull-through, abdominosacral, coloanal): with interposition
    Colostomy

The following discussion is confined to low and midlevel fistulas. Operations that require an abdominal approach are similar to those performed for other conditions; these are discussed in Chapters 22 and 23. Those associated with radiation injury are addressed in Chapter 28.

All patients should be placed on a bowel preparation as if for colon resection. Broad-spectrum perioperative antibiotics are also suggested. A Foley catheter should be inserted before surgery and kept in place as long as is reasonable or convenient. Standard vaginal antiseptic preparation should be performed at the time of surgery.

### *Techniques for Performing Anal and Low-Rectal Fistula Repairs*

Any attempt at repair must primarily address the anal or rectal opening, even though the fistula may have arisen from a vaginal source. Many surgeons and all gynecologists prefer to repair a rectovaginal fistula using the transvaginal approach. This is not recommended, because the high-pressure zone is in the rectum. If the repair of the rectal opening is satisfactorily accomplished, it is not necessary to deal with the vagina. Conversely, no matter how meticulous the technique is when performed through the vagina, if the rectal closure does not remain secure, failure will result.

In the anal canal or low-rectal fistula that occurs secondary to obstetric trauma, I prefer to perform a perineal operation with a concomitant anoplasty and sphincteroplasty. The reason I believe this to be necessary is that the condition is usually the result of an ectopic location—anterior displacement of the rectum. Many of these patients will have significant impairment of feces control even if they do not actually have a rectovaginal fistula. To effect a satisfactory repair, reconstruction of the perineal body is required and, to accomplish this, an anoplasty is preferred. One method of transvaginal repair is illustrated in Fig. 12.1.

General and colon and rectal surgeons, in recent years, have tended to use the endorectal advancement flap technique to repair anal or low-rectal fistulas. This is the same approach described in Chapter 11 for fistula-in-ano. It is much more likely to be successful for low rectovaginal fistulas than for anovaginal fistulas,

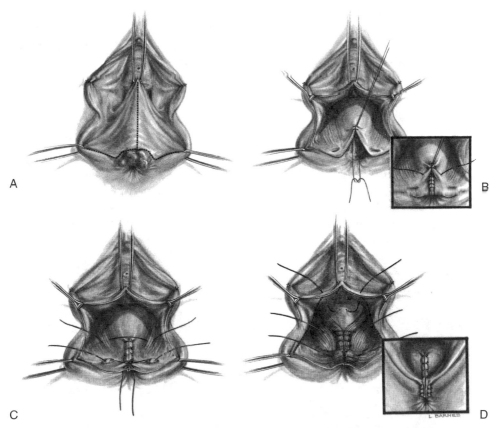

**FIG. 12.1.** Repair of complete perineal body disruption with or without rectovaginal fistula. **A.** Incisions in the posterior vaginal wall and perineum are indicated (*dotted lines*). **B.** Repair of the anterior rectal wall. A second layer is placed through the muscularis (*inset*). **C,D.** The external sphincter and levator ani are sutured together. The wound is primarily closed (*inset*). (Adapted from Howkins J, Hudson CN. *Shaw's textbook of operative gynecology*, 4th ed. Edinburgh: Churchill-Livingstone, 1977.)

however. A sleeve advancement technique for complicated anorectal and recto-vaginal fistulas is felt to be particularly useful for individuals in whom the fistulas encompass an extensive portion of the anal or rectal wall or in those with multiple internal openings.

### Techniques for Performing a Mid-Rectal Fistula Repair

A mid-rectal (i.e., mid-vaginal) fistula is the most difficult type to repair satisfactorily. The condition is often a consequence of tumor or of radiation injury—hence, the poor results of treatment. For convenience, the operation is often performed transvaginally, but a transanal or transcoccygeal approach may be more advantageous. The principles of excision, layered closure, and endorectal advancement flaps are illustrated in Chapter 11 and in Fig. 12.2.

A transcoccygeal (i.e., transsacral) alternative is shown in Fig. 12.3. This technique is essentially that described in Chapter 23 for the management of certain types of rectal tumors. The approach is also useful for closure of a rectourethral fistula (see later). Other options advocated by various authors include interposition of gracilis muscle, fascia lata, or fat.

### Use of Fibrin Glue

Fibrin has been used to seal surgical openings for almost a century. With the development of microsurgical techniques, a fibrin sealant system has come into application, particularly in Europe. It has been used primarily in orthopedics but is finding utilization in other fields. By combining autologous fibrinogen in cryoprecipitate with reconstituted bovine thrombin, the final stage of the coagulation cascade is reproduced, resulting in a fibrin seal. Complete healing is reported in 50% to 60% of cases.

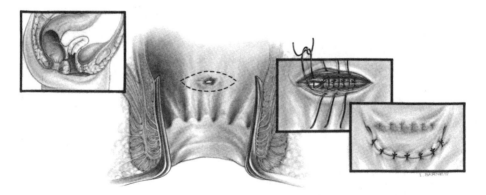

**FIG. 12.2.** Transanal repair of a low to mid-rectovaginal fistula. The importance of the location is that it permits a layered closure with mucosal advancement. If the high-pressure zone in the rectum is successfully repaired, a vaginal approach or vaginal closure is unnecessary.

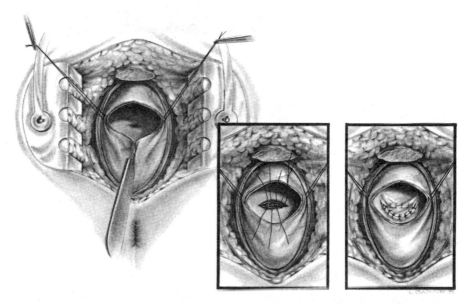

**FIG 12-3.** Transcooooygeal repair of rectovaginal or rectourethral fistula. The so-called "Kraske operation" permits excellent exposure for low- or mid-rectal fistulas. Through a posterior proctotomy, the fistula site is identified and repaired by suture closure and mucosal advancement.

## Results

So many surgical options and causes of fistulas exist that, at best, only generalizations can be made. The transanal approach with endorectal advancement flap, the most popular method for treating this complication today, results in primary healing in 75% to 100%, according to many authors.

Patients who undergo the combined procedures are almost always continent, whereas approximately 50% of those not having either sphincteroplasty or perineal body reconstruction with an endorectal advancement flap report impairment of control. It would appear that the emphasis on the importance of perineal body reconstitution is justified (see Chapter 13). Persistence of rectovaginal fistula after failed repair should not be managed by advancement flap.

### Rectovaginal Fistula in Crohn's Disease

One of the most challenging problems in patients with Crohn's disease is the management of rectovaginal fistula. Certainly, rectovaginal fistula is more frequently associated with granulomatous colitis than with small bowel disease. This complication may ultimately require a diversionary procedure or a proctectomy; diversion alone, however, is unlikely to cure the condition. The endorectal advancement flap is probably the only definitive surgical option that should be considered if fistula repair is to be attempted. Besides the obvious, the major advantages of this approach are that no sphincter is divided; continence is not impaired; there is no perineal wound with which to contend; and rarely is the underlying condition exacerbated.

Technical considerations that should be implemented in the endorectal advancement flap procedure include the following:

- Use the prone jackknife position.
- Ensure precise anatomic definition of the fistula.
- Infiltrate with epinephrine to facilitate dissection and minimize bleeding.
- Make the advancement flap thick, which may necessitate taking a portion of the internal sphincter.
- Mobilize without creating tension.
- Perform excision, curettage, and watertight closure, with closure of the defect in muscularis.
- Consider temporary fecal diversion.

### *Results*

Several factors adversely influence the outcome of the advancement flap procedure: an internal opening higher than 2 cm from the dentate line; active Crohn's disease elsewhere; severe proctitis; and persistent or undrained sepsis in the rectovaginal septum (long-term drainage should be performed initially). However, with proper patient selection, successful results are possible.

Many patients with rectovaginal fistula with Crohn's disease are managed nonsurgically, and those who do come to the operating room have proctectomy in one third to one half of cases. Keep in mind, however, that occasionally rectovaginal fistula is seen in individuals with ulcerative colitis. However, for patients with Crohn's disease, the preferred method of repair is the endorectal advancement flap. With this technique, a success rate of 60% to 70% should be expected, and a recurrence rate of around 30%.

### Rectovaginal Fistula after Radiotherapy

Rectovaginal fistula after radiation therapy presents a particularly difficult management problem (see Chapter 28). However, some patients are seen for whom repair can produce satisfactory results.

Individuals with this condition often have a history of having had radiotherapy many years previously, usually for carcinoma of the cervix. In more recent years, such a complication may be the result of radiation treatment for cancer of the anal canal, rectum, or bladder. Most of these patients present with a fistula above the sphincters, usually in the mid or upper rectum.

In a patient with a history of malignancy, it is imperative to establish whether the patient has evidence of recurrent disease. Obviously, reconstruction is contraindicated under such circumstances. Complete evaluation by means of multiple biopsies, radiologic investigation including computed tomography (CT) scan, and hematologic studies is required. The genitourinary tract should also be investigated.

### Techniques and Results

A number of operative approaches to the repair of radiation-induced rectovaginal fistula have been described. Optimally, normal, nonradiated tissue should be brought to the area. This would involve a resection, such as the pull-through operation, coloanal anastomosis, bowel interposition, or an abdomino-transsacral resection

Layered closure has also been used successfully, along with the sartorius muscle and the gracilis muscle interpositions. The endorectal advancement flap is probably a poor choice; because the radiated bowel inevitably would be used if the patient were not a candidate for reconstruction, a diversionary procedure is indicated.

## RECTOVAGINAL CYST

Benign cysts of the vagina, especially inclusion cysts, are extremely common. These are usually located near the introitus or in episiotomy scars. Other cystic lesions that may appear in the area are Gartner's duct cysts, endometriosis, adenosis, and vaginitis emphysematosa. Occasionally, an inclusion cyst can present in the rectovaginal septum. The lesion is often asymptomatic, but it can be associated with constipation, mucous discharge, and, if ulcerated, rectal bleeding. Most patients complain of a swelling or mass in the vagina, accompanied in some by stress incontinence, dyspareunia, dysfunctional uterine bleeding, or a history of episiotomy or vaginal lacerations.

Physical examination usually reveals a mass in the rectovaginal septum, but endoscopy will fail to identify a mucosal abnormality. The size of the cyst can be variable ($\geq 7$ cm in diameter), but most are smaller than 2 cm.

Most of these lesions are simple inclusion cysts, but in one third of reported cases in one series, they were of Müllerian origin. However, others have reported a higher incidence of the Müllerian type than the epidermal inclusion cyst. Other cysts reported include Gartner's duct type, Bartholin's duct type, and endometriotic type.

Most of these lesions are excised transvaginally, but if the cyst seems to be extending into the submucosa of the rectum, transanal excision is warranted.

## RECTOURETHRAL FISTULA

Rectourethral fistula, fortunately, is a rare condition. It is most frequently encountered as a complication of prostatectomy, especially when done via the perineal route. Occasionally, it is also seen as a sequela of radiation therapy for carcinoma of the bladder or prostate. Trauma, infection, and Crohn's disease are more unusual causes. Even in the adult, a congenital anomaly may be the cause. Thompson reported the Mayo Clinic experience over a 30-year period: 36 rectourethral fistulas; 14 followed prostatectomy, 6 occurred after trauma, 3 were associated with Crohn's disease, and 4 resulted from other causes; and 9 patients had malignant fistulas. Although no distinction was made between the symptoms of rectovesical and rectourethral fistulas, 90% had urinary tract infections, and 83% reported urine issuing from the rectum. More than one half of the patients noted pneumaturia and fecaluria. Bleeding through the rectum implied a malignant process. Cystoscopy established the diagnosis in 84% of patients; proctoscopy was of value in 70%.

## Treatment

Many approaches have been used to treat rectourethral fistula, including (a) abdominoanal pull-through with perineal repair; (b) abdominal operation with interposition of appropriately tailored omentum; and (c) a transanal approach in which the rectum and sphincters are divided posteriorly, the fistula then closed in layers, and the rectum reconstructed.

Transrectal mucosal advancement has been performed in patients with such fistulas, with and without fecal diversion. Selected patients with rectourethral fistula and Crohn's disease, who have relative sparing of the rectum, may be treated by a rectal advancement flap. The perineal approach, with advancement of the rectal mucosa, has also been used, as has the transcoccygeal route. Resection with J-pouch coloanal anastomosis is another potential choice.

In patients with unresectable malignant disease, a diversionary procedure is the treatment of choice. If the tumor is resectable, a pelvic exenteration is the optimal course of action. For benign conditions, successful repair requires long-term catheter or suprapubic drainage of the urinary tract.

In the nonradiated patient, I prefer either a transanal or transcoccygeal approach, with sliding rectal advancement flap. I cannot overemphasize, however, the importance of using the services of a urologist with a particular proficiency and interest in performing reconstructive urologic procedures.

## ANTERIOR PERINEAL SINUS OR CYST

Congenital cysts of the genitoperineal raphe are extremely rare. Two theories concerning their cause have been proposed:

1. Infolding of dermal elements at the time of closure of the genital folds
2. Outgrowth of epithelial cells in the raphe after the genital folds have closed.

Patients complain of perineal discharge, irritation, and pain; recurrent infection is common. Differential diagnoses include epidermal cyst, hidradenitis, and anal fistula.

Male predominance (87%) and midlife presentation (mean age, 44 years) characterize these individuals. The lesions usually occur along the median raphe. Treatment consists of excision of any nodules with laying open of the sinus tracts. A recurrence rate of 15% has been reported.

# 13

# Anal Incontinence

## INCIDENCE

Reports of the incidence of incontinence are limited. One study surveyed a total of 2,570 households comprising almost 7,000, with an overall incidence of anal incontinence of 2.2%. Of those, 30% were above 65 years of age, and approximately two thirds were women. Independent risk factors included female sex, advancing age, poor general health, and physical limitations.

## ETIOLOGY

### Causes of Fecal Incontinence

Trauma
    Surgical (e.g., fistulectomy, fistulotomy, hemorrhoidectomy, sphincterotomy, sphincter stretch, pull-through operations, low anastomoses)
    Obstetric
    Accidental (e.g., war injury, social injury)
Colorectal disease (e.g., hemorrhoids, rectal prolapse, inflammatory bowel disease, malignant tumors)
Congenital anomaly (e.g., spina bifida, myelomeningocele, imperforate anus, Hirschsprung's disease)
Neurologic disease
    Cerebral (e.g., tumor, vascular accident, dementia, trauma)
    Spinal
    Peripheral (e.g., diabetes mellitus, multiple sclerosis, pudendal nerve injury)
Miscellaneous
    Laxative abuse
    Diarrheal condition
    Fecal impaction
    Encopresis

### Surgical Trauma

Fistula surgery is the most common cause of fecal incontinence. Varying degrees of control impairment are seen, even after what is considered proper division of a portion of the sphincter muscle (see Chapter 11).

Internal anal sphincterotomy performed for anal fissure can also produce partial anal incontinence (see Chapter 9).

Sphincter stretch for anal fissure or manual dilatation as a treatment for hemorrhoids should be abandoned, as this procedure is associated with uncontrolled tearing of the sphincter muscles, resulting in the risk of fecal incontinence.

Partial incontinence can be a late complication of hemorrhoidectomy, such as is performed during the Whitehead hemorrhoidectomy, with the risk of rectal mucosa prolapse. This discharge of mucus or incontinence for flatus can also be associated with bowel resections designed to preserve the anal sphincter (e.g., low anterior resection, the various pull-through procedures, coloanal anastomosis, abdominosacral resection).

### Obstetric Trauma

Anal incontinence caused by obstetric injury is uncommon. Most injuries to the anal sphincter following delivery are recognized and repaired by the obstetrician, usually by layered closure. Occasionally, however, because of sepsis, hematoma, or suture breakage, the repair will separate. This can lead to impaired control of flatus or feces and be associated with a fistula between the anus or rectum and the vagina (see Chapter 12).

Even women without overt injury following vaginal delivery are subject to an increased risk of impairment for fecal control. Physiologic studies on postpartum women have shown that multiparity, forceps delivery, increased duration of the second stage of labor, and high birthweight can lead to pudendal nerve damage and to sphincter atrophy. This is especially true in the situation of an ectopic anus (see *Management of Obstetric Injuries*).

### Accidental Trauma

Trauma to the perineum can injure the sphincter mechanism. Treatment depends on the degree of injury, and the amount of sepsis involved (see later).

### Colorectal Disease

Incontinence for flatus or feces can be associated with anorectal disease (e.g., hemorrhoids, fissure, fistula), even without surgical intervention. Rectal prolapse causes stretching of the sphincter and attenuation of the pudendal nerves. Management is definitive treatment of the prolapse (see Chapter 17) with an expectant outcome. Other conditions that can be associated with incontinence include nonspecific inflammatory bowel disease (e.g., ulcerative colitis and Crohn's disease), malignant conditions, and infectious and parasitic diseases.

### Congenital Anomaly

Congenital incontinence can be caused by spina bifida, meningocele, myelomeningocele, aganglionic megacolon (i.e., Hirschsprung's disease), and surgery to correct anorectal malformations (e.g., imperforate anus; see Chapter 18).

### Neurologic Disease

Neurologic diseases can affect bowel control; they include diabetes mellitus spinal cord injury, spinal cord tumor, and cauda equina lesions, which can produce incontinence by denervation of external sphincter and levator ani muscles.

Idiopathic (i.e., neurogenic) incontinence is the term used to describe denervation injury to the sphincter muscle that occurs for no apparent cause. Habitual straining at defecation, nerve entrapment, the preprolapse state, and the syndrome of the descending perineum have all been implicated.

### Laxative Abuse

One of the nonsurgical causes of fecal incontinence is laxative abuse. Over a period of years of their use, the muscle can atrophy, because the sphincter is not stretched by a normal stool. Any attempt to repair the sphincter in a patient with such a history and cause of incontinence will be unsatisfactory.

### Diarrhea

Diarrhea can be associated with fecal incontinence, even if the patient has a normal sphincter.

### Fecal Impaction

Fecal impaction frequently is associated with incontinence, probably on an overflow basis. Treatment may require manual disimpaction, enemas, and laxatives. After the impaction is cleared, prevention consists of the establishment of a proper bowel management program. This may be supplemented by colonic irrigations and perineal strengthening exercises (see *Nonsurgical Treatment*).

### Encopresis

Encopresis, or psychogenic soiling, is defined as the passage of formed or semiformed stool in a child's underclothes (or other inappropriate places) that occurs regularly after the age of 4 years. It is essentially an involuntary evacuation of the bowel not caused by organic factors. Encopresis is at least four times more common in boys than in girls and is analogous to enuresis as it pertains to urinary incontinence.

Behavioral factors that may contribute to the problem include the following:

- Excessive parental attention to toilet habits
- Laxative use
- Harsh or lax toilet training methods
- Fear of the toilet or the loss of feces
- Desire for attention
- Family or personal stress

The goal is to establish a practical time for defecation and, ultimately, a spontaneous bowel evacuation habit. Treatment is usually directed toward bowel management, stress reduction, and child and family psychological counseling. The use of laxatives, enemas, and dietary regimens are recommended, as well as encouraging the child to sit on the toilet for 10 minutes twice daily at the same time each day. Uridine-5-triphosphate has been suggested to have some limited success.

## PHYSIOLOGIC AND ANATOMIC BASES OF CONTINENCE

The neuromuscular control for fecal continence has been the subject of considerable investigation and debate (see Chapter 6). See Chapter 1 for a discussion of the anatomy of this region. In essence, two concentric cylinders—an internal one composed of smooth muscle, and an external one composed of striated muscle—control continence. The internal sphincter is the continuation of the distal portion of the circular muscle of the rectum. The internal sphincter is maintained in a state of near maximal contraction at all times and provides approximately 85% of the resting tone of the anal canal. Its major reflex response to rectal distention is relaxation.

The external anal sphincter is part of a composite muscle encircling the anal canal that enables voluntary control of continence. It has been arbitrarily divided into three parts: subcutaneous, superficial, and deep. The distinction between the three parts of the external sphincter is of little practical importance.

As with the internal sphincter, the external sphincter is also in a state of contraction; however, its major reflex response to stimuli is contraction. The degree of external sphincter contraction varies with alterations in intraabdominal pressure and posture. Resting activity can be supplemented by voluntary contraction, which is accompanied by a marked rise in electrical action potentials and a substantial increase in recorded intrasphincteric pressure. Because of fatigue, maximal voluntary contraction can be maintained only for about 50 seconds.

## PHYSIOLOGY OF DEFECATION

Mechanical and physiologic retentive forces in the rectosigmoid normally maintain the distal rectum in an empty and collapsed state. As feces accumulate in the rectum, the bowel wall muscle relaxes, allowing distention and accommodation of the enlarging fecal mass. Sensory receptors within the anal canal determine the nature of the luminal contents, whether flatus, liquid, or solid stool. Threshold stimulation of the afferent nerve endings is reached, and involuntary precipitation of the anal reflex occurs, enabling the rectum to empty. Successive functional segments of colon coordinate their activity to produce a mass peristaltic wave above the fecal mass. Concomitantly, the distal part of the intestine and the internal sphincter relax, and the external sphincter contracts. If elimination is to proceed, voluntary inhibition of external sphincter contraction occurs.

If a voluntary effort is required to defecate, intraabdominal pressure is increased by both closure of the glottis and contraction of the muscles of the pelvic floor (resisting the forward movement of stool and closing the lumen distally). At the end of defecation, when straining is discontinued, the pelvic floor rises to its normal position and again obliterates the lumen. A rebound contraction of the anal sphincter occurs; this has been termed the "closing reflex."

## EVALUATION OF THE PATIENT

### History

To determine the appropriate therapy for the patient with anal incontinence, probably the single most important criterion is the cause of the problem. Patients who have sustained loss of sphincter function through injury, whether surgical, obstetric, or accidental, are those most amenable to reconstructive efforts. However, those who are incontinent because of disease are generally poor candidates for reconstruction. In this group of patients appropriate counseling (e.g., dietary, exercise, bowel management) may be the most efficacious mode of therapy.

Requisite information should include an accurate bowel-function history (onset, duration, and related factors, frequency, medications), neurologic information (including any sensory loss), obstetric history in female patients, and, of course, the degree of impairment for control—whether for flatus, loose stool, or formed movements. Probably the Wexner score is used most commonly to objectively assess the degree of fecal incontinence.

### Physical Examination

In the absence of a history of trauma, a comprehensive medical evaluation is frequently suggested, but it is rarely illuminating. Usually, inspection and palpation reveal the information that will dictate the therapy. Spreading the buttocks enables the determination of whether the anus is patulous, which implies either a loss of sphincter muscle or neurologic impairment, evidence of a perineal tear or obstetric injury, or other scars or deformities.

By palpation, the resting tone of the sphincter can be assessed, and by asking the patient to "tighten up," the degree of contractility can be evaluated. A defect in the sphincter muscle can also be perceived. In neurologic conditions, including lesions of the spinal cord and cauda equina, normal tone may be apparent; however, if gentle traction is applied to any segment of the anorectal ring, it is followed by gaping of the anal canal. Some authors have demonstrated that an informed history and a digital examination are as reliable as manometric investigations.

Impaired sensation to touch or to pinprick implies that surgical repair efforts will be compromised.

Although proctosigmoidoscopy, colonoscopy, and barium enema examinations are important studies in the evaluation of any patient with a colorectal problem, they are usually unrewarding in someone who complains of fecal incontinence. Conversely, defecography as it is used to diagnose the preprolapse condition may be helpful (see below and Chapters 6, 16, and 17).

## Physiologic Studies

Renascent interest has arisen in physiologic evaluation of the gastrointestinal tract (see Chapters 2 and 6).

### Electromyography

Electromyography has been largely replaced by pudendal terminal motor nerve latency testing, except when identifying anal muscle at the time of reconstruction, particularly in those with imperforate anus.

### Nerve Conduction Studies

Pudendal and perineal nerve stimulation techniques assess the distal motor innervation of the external anal sphincter and periurethral striated sphincter muscles. The method consists of stimulating the pudendal nerve on either side of the pelvis and measuring the latency to the onset of the electrical response in the muscle. The application of pudendal nerve terminal motor latency (PNTML), which is discussed in Chapter 6, is a useful test; if findings are abnormal, it will predict a worse outcome.

### Anorectal Manometry

Anorectal manometry can be undertaken by a number of methods (e.g., open-tipped or closed-tipped catheters, perfused catheters, macroballoons, and microballoons; see Chapter 6). In the United States, the most common type is the open-tipped, perfused catheter, whereas in the United Kingdom the microballoon is preferred. Methods are discussed in Chapter 6.

### *Computerized Vector Manometry*

With three-dimensional computerized vector manometry, the computer can construct a three-dimensional anal pressure vectorgram from the data obtained by manometry and allow the anus to be viewed from all perspectives. Whether this new modality, which provides a still more accurate assessment of the sphincter mechanism, merely permits better information, but leads to a more appropriate therapeutic approach in the individual patient is the unanswered question.

### *Applications*

Anorectal manometry has been found to be a useful tool for the preoperative and postoperative evaluation of patients who have problems with constipation or incontinence, whether caused by any of the following:

- Hemorrhoids
- Anal fissure
- Anal fistula
- Rectal prolapse
- Perineal descent
- Sigmoidorectal intussusception (i.e., the preprolapse condition)
- Procidentia
- Encopresis
- Sphincter-saving operations
- Obstetric injury
- Congenital anomalies (e.g., Hirschsprung's disease)

Additionally, the procedure is of value in assessing rectal compliance. With this investigation, objective assessment of the subjective digital conclusions can be ascertained. Whether the additional information is necessary, is debated.

### *Anal Sensation*

The role of anal canal sensation in maintaining continence is an issue that has stimulated considerable debate. Some have proposed that temperature changes influence anal canal function. Others feel the change is too small to be detected by the anal canal mucosa.

### *Rectal Sensation*

Rectal sensation has been thought to play a part in the mechanism for maintaining bowel control, but it is poorly understood. Currently, its application is uncertain.

## Proctometrography or Ampullometrography and Defecometry

A proctometrogram (i.e., ampullometrogram) is a procedure applied to the rectum that is analogous to the cystometrogram as used for evaluating bladder response to filling. Rectal distensibility, compliance, sensation threshold, and maximal tolerance can be determined by continuous, controlled fluid inflation with a balloon probe or microtransducer in place. This technique is the best method for measuring rectal compliance, but the role of abnormal or decreased rectal compliance in the cause of fecal incontinence is not always clear.

## Balloon Proctography or Topography

A balloon filled with barium or other radiopaque substance can be inserted into the rectum and used to evaluate pelvic floor and sphincter function during contraction and during straining. Defecography, a better test, is preferred by most.

## Defecography and Cineradiography or Videoproctography

Defecography is a physiologic study where the rectosigmoid is filled with thickened barium suspension, and the patient is asked to defecate while sequential radiographs are taken in the lateral projection. Fluoroscopic examination supplements the permanent films. Cinedefecography (i.e., video/proctography) provides a means for assessing the speed of evacuation as well as a dynamic recording for subsequent review and analysis. Both studies can illustrate functional disturbances of defecation such as may be seen in rectal prolapse, solitary rectal ulcer, and the preprolapse and in the postoperative review of children with anorectal malformations.

## Scintigraphic Defecography

Some have proposed scintigraphic defecography as an alternative investigation. Three radioactive technitium-99m ($^{99m}$Tc) markers are placed over the subject's pubis, lumbosacral junction, and coccyx. An artificial stool is made by adding water containing 100 MBq of $^{99m}$Tc to oat-porridge to form a mixture of stool-like consistency. This is then introduced into the rectum. Dynamic images are then acquired every 5 seconds for 30 seconds during rest, and then patients are instructed to evacuate with image acquisition continued every 5 seconds for up to 10 minutes.

Investigators are then able to demonstrate objective data on anorectal dynamics. The benefit of this investigation over defecography is debated.

## Anal Endosonography

In addition to Chapter 6, anal endosonography is discussed in Chapter 11 as it has been applied to the evaluation of patients with anal abscess and fistula.

With this technique, high-resolution images of the sphincter muscles can be achieved. Defects appear as amorphous areas of varying echogenicity that interrupt the normal striated pattern.

Most recommend endoanal ultrasound for all patients with fecal incontinence to detect occult sphincter defects, thereby demonstrating a surgically correctable condition.

### Magnetic Resonance Imaging

Magnetic resonance imaging has been used for a host of indications, including evaluation of sepsis and tumors in the anus and rectum. Recently, the application of high-resolution imaging of the anal sphincter mechanism has been successfully achieved by means of an endoanal coil.

## NONSURGICAL TREATMENT

The treatment of anal incontinence should always be directed to the cause. Patients who attribute their incontinence to trauma are the optimal candidates for repair. However, despite the potential appeal of surgical intervention, many individuals can be adequately managed by noninvasive means. Certainly, medical treatment should be offered to those (a) who have no antecedent history of trauma; (b) for whom the potential benefits are problematic; (c) who are felt to be at risk for surgery; and, obviously, (d) who decline an operation.

### Bowel Management Program

The aim of a bowel management program is to establish a routine for defecation that is safe, convenient, and dependable. Ideally, the bowel can be reeducated to empty regularly and at a predictable time. The following recommendations are made to help ensure that the patient will be clean and that minimal restrictions will be necessary because of the fear of fecal incontinence.

- Make certain that the patient maintains a well-balanced diet with sufficient fiber and adequate fluid intake (2,500–3,000 mL/d).
- Establish a workable time for defecation. Ascertain the patient's prior bowel habit and plans for an optimal schedule. Take advantage of the gastrocolic reflex that occurs 20 to 30 minutes after meals to stimulate defecation.
- Start the training regimen after the rectum is empty; disimpact if necessary, and give enemas until the returns are clear.
- Insert a suppository, such as glycerine or bisacodyl (i.e., Dulcolax). The suppository should be inserted at the same hour every day or night during the first week of the program.
- Instruct the patient to massage the abdomen from right to left and top to bottom several times, beginning 15 to 20 minutes after insertion of the suppository; having the patient bend forward and strain may also be helpful.

• Stool softeners, constipating medications, bulk laxative preparations, or even stimulant cathartics can be given if necessary.

## Perineal Exercises

In 1950, Kegel suggested an exercise regimen that appeared to be demonstrably beneficial in the medical treatment of both fecal and urinary incontinence. Since then, a number of papers have been published attesting to the validity of this method. A simple exercise of this type is to pretend to hold in a bowel movement and to count to 15. This can be performed 15 or 20 times a day, while walking down the street, riding in a car, or sitting in a chair—whenever the patient thinks of it. However, a more effective approach is to combine the exercise program with biofeedback, a method for reinforcement.

### *Operant Conditioning or Biofeedback*

Biofeedback training appears to be of specific value in the treatment of fecal incontinence in the elderly, as opposed to suboptimal results obtained by sphincter exercises without biofeedback. Biofeedback therapy has also been successfully applied to the management of refractory excessive stool frequency and incontinence following anterior resection and total colectomy.

The results of biofeedback therapy can deteriorate over time. Therefore, it has been suggested that it may be useful to reinitiate biofeedback therapy in some individuals, particularly if they report recurrence or deterioration of their situation.

A number of electronic home biofeedback systems have appeared on the market in the United States in recent years. One is the Dobbhoff Anorectal Biofeedback (Biosearch Medical Products, Inc., Somerville, NJ). This consists of a silicone anorectal probe and battery-charged monitor with color illumination to indicate the patient's response. It is an excellent tool for instructing patients on the correct method of performing perineal strengthening exercises as well as to use in the training of individuals troubled with obstructed defecation (see Chapter 16).

## Electrical Treatment

An electrical device applies a tetanizing stimulus to the anal sphincter and pelvic floor through a plug-shaped electrode. Electrical current causes contraction of the anal musculature, possibly with the result of gradual buildup in sphincter tone and contractility. Although perineal strengthening exercises would undoubtedly accomplish the same goal, electrical stimulation, particularly in a patient who is unable to perform such exercises, offers some improvement in selected patients.

## Anal Plug

A plug, with a balloon is inserted into the rectum through a simple valve mechanism; it can be inflated and deflated with a 30-mL syringe. This device may have a valid place in the treatment of selected patients with anal incontinence.

## SURGICAL TREATMENT

Successful surgical repair of incontinence requires an understanding of the underlying pathophysiology, and only those patients who have lesions amenable to reconstruction should be selected.

The two primary methods of surgical treatment of anal incontinence are direct repair of a localized sphincter defect, and repair designed to supplement the sphincter mechanism.

### Surgical Options in the Management of Incontinence

Among the surgical options used to manage incontinence are the following:

Anorectal muscle repairs
    Apposition of sphincter muscles
    Overlapping of sphincter muscles
    Reefing of sphincter muscles
    Postanal pelvic floor repair (i.e., Parks' procedure)
    Narrowing of the anal canal
    Use of perineal muscles other than the anal sphincter
    Pubococcygeus repair
Use of other muscles
    Gluteus
    Vastus internus
    Adductor longus
    Gracilis
Anal encirclement procedures
    Fascia lata
    Thiersch operation using wire, Teflon, Marlex, catgut, Mersilene, Dacron-impregnated Silastic, Silastic to create an artificial sphincter
    Artificial Bowel Sphincter
Colostomy

No one perfect incision exists for all sphincter repairs. A curvilinear incision outside the anal verge is commonly used. This usually provides adequate exposure of the underlying muscle if a direct repair is required. However, if additional skin coverage is needed to close a defect, a concomitant anoplasty may be necessary (see Chapter 8).

The three standard operations for repairing the injured sphincter are apposition, overlapping, and reefing (i.e., plication). Each method has its advocates, but no one of these procedures can be consistently used with success. In principle, the surgeon usually attempts to repair the external sphincter muscle, puborectalis sling, or both. If difficulty arises in identifying viable muscle, a Peña muscle stimulator can be helpful.

Repair of the sphincter in incontinent patients is most successfully approached after operative or nonoperative trauma and is best accomplished as soon as possible after the injury. Repair can be carried out many months after the original trauma with expectation of a good result. However, with disuse, with its resultant loss of muscle tissue, a lesser outcome is possible.

## Preoperative Preparation

All patients undergoing reconstructive anorectal surgical procedures should be prepared as if for colonic resection (i.e., a vigorous oral cathartic regimen). Systemic antibiotics should be administered approximately 1 hour before operation and for a varied duration postoperatively, depending on the nature of the procedure and the amount of contamination.

Some patients undergoing anorectal surgery may already have a colostomy. Under no circumstances should a colostomy be closed at the time of reconstruction. The requirement for creation of a colostomy at the time of repair is a matter of the surgeon's judgment. A generally safe rule might be, the more extensive the reconstruction, the more one should consider a diversion.

## Postoperative Care

Postoperatively, depending on the extent of the reconstruction and the risk of breakdown, the patient can be placed on a bowel-confining regimen. This consists of a clear liquid diet with the following medications: codeine (60 mg), diphenoxylate (Lomotil; two tablets), and deodorized tincture of opium (15 drops), each four times daily. The wounds are cleansed three times daily with a topical antiseptic solution. After 3 to 5 days, the medications are discontinued and a regular diet is instituted.

## Direct Sphincter Repair

In the acute emergency trauma situation, initial treatment usually consists of debridement of nonviable tissue, removal of foreign material, open drainage, and, often, proximal colostomy with distal washout (see Chapter 14). Depending on the extent of injury, especially that of associated trauma, reconstructive sphincteric surgery may be deferred. However, any attempt to appose the sphincter muscle, even in such adverse circumstances, should be ameliorative.

## *Results*

It is difficult to evaluate the relative merits of different operations for the treatment of fecal incontinence. Generally, the best results are obtained if direct sphincter repair is possible. Good results in up to 70% are reported. If little or no residual sphincter is present, an attempt at resuture is unlikely to be successful. In this situation, alternative approaches should be used.

## Sphincter Repair in Crohn's Disease

Even in Crohn's disease, highly selected patients should be considered for direct sphincter repair, with a good outcome expected.

## Obstetric Injuries

The incidence of anorectal complications following vaginal delivery has been reported to be approximately 5%. Perhaps 10% of these will fail repair at the time of delivery and require subsequent revision or reconstruction.

A word of caution concerning episiotomy. Although rectovaginal fistula and fourth-degree perineal injuries are uncommon complications of vaginal delivery, be wary of performing episiotomy in the midline if the woman is recognized to have an ectopic anus, that is, if the anus is anteriorly displaced toward the vagina. This is a congenital variation seen in approximately 10% of women.

## *Technique of Repair*

Often, rectovaginal fistula repair requires a concomitant sphincter reconstruction (see Chapter 12). How the approach is effected depends on the location of the openings and the cause of the problem. For a fistula between the vagina and the anal canal, I prefer performing the repair through a transperineal approach, with a concomitant anoplasty. For a higher level fistula, the option of mucosal advancement should be considered (see Chapter 12), although it still is possible to approach the fistula through the perineum. For still higher fistulas, either a mucosal advancement or an abdominal operation is suggested. As implied, most women with rectovaginal fistula harbor an ectopic anus. To achieve the best functional results, the perineal body should be reconstructed.

The patient is placed in the prone jackknife position. A cruciate incision is made across the perineal body, and full-thickness flaps of skin are developed. A Hill–Ferguson retractor is kept in the anal canal for the entire operation to maintain adequacy of the lumen while the muscle repair is completed. The rectovaginal septum is infiltrated with 0.5% bupivacaine (Marcaine) with 1:200,000 epinephrine, which aids in hemostasis and facilitates the dissection. The rectum is separated from the vagina, and the fistula tract, if present, is identified. The cephalad limit is reached, and a plication of the levator ani muscle is carried out anterior to the rectum. This reefing usually requires three or four long-term absorbable sutures (e.g., no. 1 Vicryl or Dexon). The redundant mucosa, including any fistula, is excised from the vagina and the rectum. The external sphincter muscle is reapproximated in one or two layers, using the same suture material. It can be difficult to identify the residual external sphincter, but the Peña stimulator can be used if there is a question of location. The final step in the operation is to advance and interdigitate the two triangular flaps of skin.

*Comment*: Generally the results of anal sphincteroplasty with or without anoplasty in the delayed management of anal incontinence as a consequence of obstetric injury are good. The one exception appears to be in those patients who harbor concomitant pudendal neuropathy. In order that the patient can make a reasoned decision and have realistic expectations concerning the results of reconstructive surgery, PNTML is strongly recommended. It has been our experience, however, that irrespective of the results of this study, patients who have significant impairment for bowel control will opt for a repair even though the prognosis may be suboptimal.

### Postanal Pelvic Floor Repair or Parks Repair

Postanal pelvic floor repair is a procedure that has been largely abandoned in the treatment of fecal incontinence.

### Operations for Supplementing the Sphincter Mechanism

When sufficient residual sphincter is available, direct repair usually produces satisfactory results. However, if muscle tissue has been lost, whether as a result of trauma or disuse, such an approach is usually unsuccessful. In these instances, surgical reconstruction designed to create an artificial sphincter may have some merit.

### Gracilis Muscle Transposition

Gracilis muscle transposition is a procedure that has been most efficacious for those who had become incontinent as a result of trauma or as a consequence of a congenital anomaly, usually when other sphincteroplastic approaches had failed. Patients who have a history of diarrhea are poor candidates, and those with neurologic impairment generally do less well. Individuals with bowel management problems are poorly suited to this procedure because it is difficult to train the bowel to defecate on command in these patients.

### Neuromuscular Stimulation of the Gracilis Muscle (Dynamic Graciloplasty)

Dynamic graciloplasty has improved outcome because of the use of an implantable stimulator. This has produced histologic changes in the transposed muscle, with an increased percentage of type I slow-twitch, fatigue-resistant fibers. Reports indicate that up to 70% of patients have improved anal continence with this advance. Failures were attributable to poor muscle contraction, perforation of the anal canal during stimulation, infection at the stimulator or lead site, and, of course, incontinence, soiling, and intractable constipation.

## Gluteus Maximus Transposition

Gluteus maximus transposition is a procedure of historical interest only.

## Artificial Sphincter Approaches

Those with a bowel management problem (i.e., constipation, diarrhea) or those with sensory impairment are poor candidates for reconstruction by artificial sphincter. Such patients should be considered for one of the following approaches.

### *Anal Encircling Procedure or Thiersch Procedure*

Anal encircling (i.e., Thiersch) procedures were originally advocated for the management of rectal prolapse (see Chapter 17), but Gabriel recommended its application for the treatment of anal incontinence.

A simple but generally less satisfactory alternative to the transposition of the gracilis or gluteus muscle for supplementing the sphincter mechanism is to implant a Dacron-impregnated Silastic sheet as a prosthesis encircling the anus.

Complications of the procedure include infection, stricture, fecal impaction, persistent incontinence, and pain. This procedure and the artificial urinary sphincter are the basis for the development of the artificial bowel sphincter.

### *Prosthetic Implantation*

We recently participated in a multicenter trial using the artificial bowel sphincter. We had a 40% explantation rate (secondary to sepsis, erosion), but of those who successfully used the device, all were grateful for the improvement in fecal control. Other institutions have had a similar success rate, but an explantation rate as low as 10%. The role of this device in the future is still uncertain.

### Pudendal Neurolysis

Shafik described treatment of anal incontinence in those individuals who have pudendal nerve injury through pudendal nerve decompression.

This is a unique concept, and as of this writing no reports have been made from other individuals or institutions.

## Colostomy

The performance of a colostomy in a patient with fecal incontinence is thought generally to be an admission of failure, but it should not be regarded as such. Fecal diversion is virtually always the optimal choice for a patient confined to a nursing home or to a convalescent facility. Perhaps more frequently than for those with any other condition discussed in this text, persons with fecal incontinence need to be willing partners in the decision-making process.

### *Continent Colonic Conduit*

A colonic conduit, which incorporates an intussuscepting valve to manage fecal incontinence and disordered evacuation through an antegrade irrigation technique, has been described. No appliances are required. The few reports that have been made are all encouraging.

### *Closing the Colostomy*

When to close a colostomy that has been placed prior to reconstruction of the anal sphincter is often a difficult decision. When making this decision, consider the physiologic studies discussed above. We rely on physical examination, the presence of healed wounds, and, in this litigious society, informed consent.

*Comment*: Anal incontinence as a consequence of trauma is optimally treated by direct sphincter repair with or without puborectalis plication. If this fails or if inadequate residual muscle remains with which to accomplish a repair, a muscle transposition or an artificial bowel sphincter should be considered. Colostomy should be the last recourse in the management of patients with anal incontinence.

# 14

## Colorectal Trauma

Most of the literature on penetrating abdominal wounds in general, and colonic injury specifically, has come from experience on the battlefield. However, many of the classic dicta concerning management are not necessarily appropriate today, even with the high-velocity injuries that occur in the civilian population.

The colon is injured in from 15% to 39% of penetrating abdominal wounds. It is expected that this will continue to be a pervasive problem in our society because of the frequency of motor vehicle accidents and the ready availability of firearms, especially in the United States. Considerable controversy remains concerning the appropriate management of colorectal injuries. As with all aspects of the management of acute surgical illnesses, appropriate judgment, skill, and common sense are requisites.

### HISTORY

For centuries, colon injuries were untreatable and virtually always resulted in the victim's death. The decision about nonoperative intervention was made simply because such injuries were virtually always fatal, regardless of the method of treatment. Furthermore, such a noninterventionist approach was probably based on the fact that surgeons had no good idea of what to do when confronted with such a problem.

Following World War II, with combat-learned techniques, exteriorization of the injured segment and the use of colostomy became the standard treatment for all colorectal injuries. However, some considered civilian injuries different from those of combat and, therefore, in certain circumstances, primary repair was considered an appropriate alternative. Today in the United States, a victim of penetrating abdominal trauma is frequently transported to the hospital within a few minutes following injury. Sophisticated radiographic equipment is readily available, as well as the obvious intravenous fluids, blood, blood products, and antibiotics. Furthermore, a surgical team, even if not present, can be assembled in a relatively short period of time. Under these conditions, it is little wonder that the mortality rate for civilian colorectal injuries is now less than 5%.

Over the past 30 years, numerous articles have been published on primary repair. Stone and Fabian reported in 1979 on a randomized trial of patients meeting so-called "good-risk criteria." Patients with colonic injury who were felt to be good risks were randomly allocated either to a primary repair or to a colostomy. Fewer septic complications were observed in the former group. In fact, some feel that primary anastomosis is safe for most patients who require colon resection for severe injury.

## ETIOLOGY AND EVALUATION

### Penetrating Trauma

Most colon injuries result from penetrating wounds to the abdomen. Of all such wounds, 20% are associated with injury to the large bowel. Septic morbidity is a real danger because of the combination of fecal spillage, soft-tissue injury, and bleeding—all of which predispose to subsequent infection. Furthermore, gunshot wounds to the colon are typically associated with more tissue destruction and result in an increased number of associated injuries in comparison with stab wounds. Because gunshot wounds to the abdomen are associated with intraabdominal injury in 95% of cases, little argument is seen against the requirement for laparotomy. This is in contrast to stab wounds of the abdomen, for which the associated intraabdominal injury rate is only approximately 50%. Still, some issues are clear; all hypotensive patients or those with signs of peritoneal irritation should undergo laparotomy. Conversely, individuals who harbor wounds that do not penetrate the anterior fascia can be treated on an ambulatory basis.

The real controversy surrounds the management of patients who are stable and without signs of peritoneal irritation in whom the wound penetrates the anterior fascia or peritoneum. Options include the following:

- Immediate exploratory laparotomy
- Diagnostic peritoneal lavage
- Close evaluation with serial abdominal examinations
- Laparoscopy

Over the last decade, laparoscopy has been used to evaluate patients with penetrating abdominal trauma. Several authors have suggested that in stable patients with penetrating trauma and no clinical evidence of intraperitoneal injury, laparoscopy effectively and safely detects those with peritoneal penetration.

### Blunt Trauma

Blunt trauma to the abdomen is associated with colonic injury in fewer than 5% of cases. Mobile segments of the colon (e.g., cecum, transverse colon, and sigmoid colon) are more susceptible to injury, although other areas of the bowel can be affected. The use of seat belts seems to be a predisposing factor. These individuals have a high incidence of gastrointestinal injuries and, in addition, associated lumbar spinal injuries.

The same principles of treatment as those discussed with respect to penetrating injuries apply here, but be aware that delay in diagnosis is one of the major concerns. Certainly, in conjunction with associated injuries, this is one of the important predictors of morbidity and mortality.

## *Diagnosis*

Peritoneal lavage, computed tomography of the abdomen, and abdominal ultrasonography are all useful adjunctive measures for evaluating patients with blunt injury. Of the three, peritoneal lavage is the most sensitive.

Although the returns may be grossly positive with stool or blood, or microscopically positive with blood, patients who have small perforations or mesenteric vascular injuries may not demonstrate an abnormality until a few hours following the injury.

Results of computed tomography and ultrasonography can be difficult to interpret. Certainly, the presence of free fluid without liver and spleen injury is worrisome, as is the presence of mesenteric edema or a hematoma.

*Abdominal ultrasonography* will not detect an injury to the colon unless sufficient fluid or blood is present. Some authors feel this investigation can be used as the initial method for diagnosis of blunt abdominal trauma.

Nolan et al. opine that physicians should entertain the possibility of mesenteric injury in all patients presenting with blunt abdominal trauma, even if few clinical findings are initially present or computed tomography fails to demonstrate a definitive abnormality or injury. Blunt injury, in particular, requires a high degree of suspicion to minimize the likelihood of missing significant intraperitoneal trauma.

## Surgical Management

### *General Principles*

Once the decision has been made to perform an exploratory laparotomy, the abdomen is entered through a midline incision. As with all operations in the abdomen, a midline incision is recommended. It is important to preserve the area overlying the rectus muscles, in case a stoma should be required (see Chapter 31). Initial efforts are directed toward identifying and controlling any source of bleeding. An attempt should be made to contain spillage of intestinal contents by using atraumatic clamps and sponges. Following control of hemorrhage and sources of contamination, a thorough search is made for all possible sites of injury. The entire gastrointestinal tract and mesentery are carefully inspected.

Special attention should be given to the number and location of all wounds. Usually, the bowel has an even number of openings, which is compatible with a typical through-and-through injury pattern. However, when an odd number of wounds appears to be the case, make a great effort to look for the "missing hole." The bowel should be carefully re-inspected, especially the region adjacent to the mesentery, where breaches of the bowel wall may be hidden. Once the injuries have been identified, then proceed with the repair.

When primary repair is attempted, care must be taken to avoid narrowing the lumen; therefore, this is often accomplished in a transverse fashion. When the colon is destroyed or its blood supply is compromised, resection is required. If diversion of the fecal stream is required, either the injured segment is brought out to the abdominal wall or a proximal portion of bowel is selected as a colostomy or ileostomy. Meticulous attention should be given to creating a satisfactory stoma. Generally, the skin wound should be left open or sutures placed for delayed primary repair. Approximately 50% of all primarily closed wounds that are associated with emergency surgery for trauma become infected. The presence of concomitant shock, soft-tissue injury, and fecal contamination creates an environment unlike that of elective colon surgery, one that is much more conducive to the development of overwhelming sepsis.

### Operative Treatment

Operative treatment choices are summarized below:

Operative alternatives for treating penetrating colonic injury
    Simple closure
    Resection with primary anastomosis
    Resection with proximal diversion
    Intracolonic bypass (i.e., Coloshield)
    Exteriorization with repair
    Exteriorization of injury site

A wide variety of operative techniques are available for managing the injured colon. However, each can be classified as one of three primary approaches: fecal diversion, primary repair, or exteriorization repair. Each approach has merit, with considerable support in the literature.

### Exteriorization Repair

Exteriorization repair is a hybrid of primary repair and fecal diversion in which the colon wound is repaired and brought out to the abdominal wall. Subsequently, if the enterotomy closure breaks down, it is then matured into a standard ostomy. However, if it heals, it is then replaced into the peritoneal cavity. Although a number of investigators have recommended this type of approach, conversion rates to an ostomy range between 21% and 50%. This is considerably higher than the incidence of clinically significant leak rates associated with primary repair.

Exteriorization repair does not completely preclude the possibility of intraabdominal sepsis. Breakdown with abscess or fecal fistula is still possible once the bowel is returned to the abdomen. This approach has been generally abandoned and, consequently, is not recommended.

### Fecal Diversion Versus Primary Repair Versus Resection and Primary Repair

Mandatory colostomy, even today, is conceptually attractive because it eliminates or minimizes the complications associated with the creation of an anastomosis. In 1951, primary repair was proposed as an alternative to colostomy formation. Since then, vigorous debate surrounds the management of colonic injuries. Recently, Murray et al. proposed resection and primary anastomosis for those with severe colonic injuries. Variables that affect these decisions are summarized as follows:

Factors predisposing to increased morbidity and mortality
  Increased age
  Associated organ injury
  Multiple blood transfusions
  Left colon injury
  Preoperative shock
  Gross fecal contamination
  Delay in initiating therapy
  Extensive colonic injury
  Questionable viability of the bowel
  Requirement for more than one suture line to effect repair

These risk factors can also be assessed by the Colon Organ Injury Scale (CIS) (Table 14.1), and the Abdominal Trauma Index (ATI). ATI is a method of quantifying the risk of complications following penetrating abdominal trauma. The index is calculated by scoring the severity of injury to each intraabdominal organ system on a scale of 1 to 5. This number is then multiplied by the risk factor (1 to 5) for complications within each organ system. Organ systems that have a high potential for complications following injury (e.g., the duodenum, pancreas,

TABLE 14.1. *Colon organ injury scale*

| Grade | Type of injury | Description of injury |
| --- | --- | --- |
| 1 | Hematoma | Contusion or hematoma without devascularization |
| 2 | Laceration | Laceration <50% of circumference |
| 3 | Laceration | Laceration ≥50% of circumference without transection |
| 4 | Laceration | Transection of the colon |
| 5 | Laceration | Transection of the colon with segmental tissue loss |
|   | Vascular | Devascularized segment |

or colon) are assigned risk factors of 5. The sum of the individual organ scores is then added together to obtain the final ATI score. Patients with a score of greater than 25 have a 50% or greater chance of complications.

## Retroperitoneal Trauma

Retroperitoneal trauma usually affects both the intraperitoneal anterior and retroperitoneal posterior walls. It must be emphasized that the retroperitoneum must be inspected when an intraperitoneal hole is found or whenever the wound is in the flank or the back. Colostomy is always required for such an injury.

### *Strategies to Prevent Infection*

The combination of soft-tissue injury, hypotension, and fecal contamination provide all the elements necessary for infection (a nutritive medium, a susceptible host, and the presence of bacteria). Careful and vigorous debridement is mandatory. When the debridement has been completed, the remaining tissue should be uninjured, well vascularized, and clean. In addition, planned reoperation for further debridement and irrigation must be considered.

Wounds should be managed either by delayed primary closure or by dressing changes with healing to take place by secondary intention.

No prospective, randomized clinical trial has compared the use of prophylactic antibiotics with that of a placebo following colonic injury. However, data certainly support the use of such drugs in this circumstance. Based simply on the principles of effective use of antibiotics in other clinical settings and the diverse colonic flora, a nontoxic drug directed at gram-negative aerobes and anaerobes should be administered as soon as possible after the injury. The tissue level should be high at the time the skin incision is made to ensure maximal effectiveness. Generally, it is unnecessary to continue the antibiotics after 24 hours. Prospective, double-blind, randomized trials have demonstrated that 5 days of antibiotic therapy is not superior to 24 hours of therapy. If intraoperative bleeding is a problem or the operation is longer than two drug half-lives, the antibiotics should be re-administered intraoperatively. Prolonged use of antibiotics may be associated with superinfection, resistant organisms, and pseudomembranous colitis (see Chapter 33).

It has been demonstrated that a statistically significantly increased risk for infection is associated with increased age, injury to the left colon, the administration of a greater number of units of blood or blood products, and associated organ injury. Another factor that may be associated with an increased risk for the development of infection is hypothermia. Another issue that has stimulated some interest is the presence of a retained foreign body—specifically the missile. Some authors have discovered that after a bullet passes through the colon, a retained foreign body is frequently the source of postoperative abscess. Generally, removing the bullet is relatively easy to accomplish. Therefore, it is recommended to take whatever additional time is reasonably necessary to remove the retained missile, especially if it has passed through the colon or rectum.

The value of nutritional support and whether enteral or parental supplementation is more efficacious has been considerably debated. Two randomized trials have reported on the use of jejunostomy followed by immediate enteral feeding. Fewer abscesses and pulmonary infections were noted in the enteral feeding groups. Another trial compared a standard elemental formula with one enhanced with arginine, omega-3 fatty acids, and glutamine (immune-enhancing diet). The immune-enhancing regimen was associated with a statistically significantly reduced incidence of infections when compared with the standard regimen. The use of early enteral feeding is strongly recommended, except for those individuals with severe hypotension or prolonged ileus. The placement of a small-bore feeding jejunostomy has itself been associated with a low complication rate.

## Results

Stone and Fabian performed a randomized, controlled study of primary closure versus exteriorization in patients with perforating colon trauma. During a 44-month period, 268 individuals with colon wounds underwent an operation. Excluded were those with (a) profound preoperative shock; (b) blood loss in excess of 20% of estimated normal volume, with more than two intraabdominal organ systems injured; (c) significant fecal contamination; and (d) patients in whom the surgery was begun more than 8 hours following the injury. The authors concluded that primary suture of colon wounds could be safely performed in selected patients if they met the criteria outlined.

Another randomized, prospective study undertaken by Chappuis et al. involved 56 patients who were managed by primary repair or by resection in one group or diversion in the other. The authors concluded that independently of associated risk factors, the complication rates were similar. Burch et al. reviewed more than 700 patients with civilian colon injuries. They disagree with those who maintain that suture closure should not be performed in the presence of shock. They believe that simple suture of small wounds may be the most appropriate therapy to minimize blood loss and to save time. They believe that primary repair should be the mainstay for the treatment of most civilian injuries. Most concur that with judicious selection, trauma in this population can be treated by primary repair with debridement and closure or resection.

Although the principle of primary repair for the management of colonic injuries is liberally applied, it is important to recognize that serious concerns exist if the use of colostomy is entirely discarded. Patients who require colonic resection because of trauma to the bowel itself or disruption of the blood supply deserve special consideration. The injuries are much more complex and frequently involve other organs.

Flint et al. reviewed their experience with colonic injury to ascertain whether their intraoperative classification could permit the assessment of patients and the determination of an appropriate choice of operative procedure. Grade 1 injuries were characterized by minimal contamination and the absence of other organ involvement. These wounds were managed by primary closure (i.e., suture closure of the perforation). Grade 2 injuries implied through-and-through perforation with moderate contamination, and grade 3 injury indicated severe tissue loss, devascularization, and considerable contamination. The authors advocated either exteriorization with or without colostomy or resection with colostomy for the last two groups. One of 25 patients classified as grade 1 died; no complications occurred in this group of patients. In 116 patients with a grade 2 injury, the mortality rate was 2% and the complication rate was 20%. With a grade 3 injury (16 patients), four deaths (25%) occurred and a complication rate of 31% was seen.

Stewart et al. noted in their experience at the Regional Trauma Center in Memphis, Tennessee, reviewing primary resection without a stoma, even in individuals with destructive or devitalized wounds, that the leak rate in 43 patients so treated was 14%, much higher than had been anticipated. Specific risk factors identified were multiple blood transfusions and preexisting medical illness. The anastomotic breakdown rate in those without either risk factor was 3%, in comparison with 42% for those who had received more than 6 U of transfused blood or had a preexisting medical condition. Interestingly, the amount of contamination or the presence of associated injury did not appear to increase the chance of breakdown. The leak rates and septic complication rates were identical when anastomosis between the ileum and the colon was compared with a colocolonic anastomosis (see earlier discussion). The mortality rate for anastomotic breakdown was 40%.

Murray et al. reviewed 140 patients who required resection for severe colonic injury at the Los Angeles County Hospital. Of these, 80% had primary anastomosis, whereas 20% had a colostomy created. They found no significant differences in the complication rate for abscess, wound infection, fascial dehiscence, and the number of deaths when comparing colostomy formation, ileocolic or colocolic anastomoses. Also, no difference was noted in anastomotic leak rates between ileocolic and colocolic anastomosis. However, a 29% mortality rate was found for the seven patients who developed a left-sided anastomotic leak. Conclusions were that because of fewer anastomotic leaks, only hypotension on admission and an ATI score of greater than 25 were considered as risk factors for the development of anastomotic complications. The authors recommended that caution should be exercised when performing anastomoses in the presence of these risk factors.

### Conclusions

Many surgeons have concluded that the physiologic status of the patient at the time of the anastomosis appears to be the best predictor for anastomotic success or failure. Therefore, colostomy is strongly recommended for patients at high risk with destructive colonic wounds. When contamination and associated organ injury are minimal, primary closure or resection and anastomosis can be safely performed. With extensive colonic trauma, vascular impairment, multiple organ involvement, gross contamination, and multiple blood transfusions, it is probably wiser to resect and perform a diversionary procedure. Many factors, however, enter into decision making, so that despite the above counsel and the various classifications that have been proposed to aid the surgeon, the choice of therapy ultimately rests on the surgeon's personal experience and judgment.

## Anorectal Trauma

Injuries to the anus and rectum can result from various surgical procedures (e.g., obstetric, gynecologic, and urologic), proctosigmoidoscopy, ingestion of foreign bodies, and blunt and penetrating injuries to the perineum. Additionally, trauma can be secondary to pneumatic injury, vacuum toilet, sexual assault, insertion of enema nozzles and thermometers, bull horn injury, and even suicide attempts by rectal administration of corrosives. Anorectal trauma has been classified into the following groups:

- Intraperitoneal perforations
- Retroperitoneal perforations
- Subperitoneal perforations
- Incomplete perforations
- Perineal injuries

### Symptoms

In unsuspected rectal trauma, the usual complaint is rectal pain. This can be delayed for several hours to several days following the initial injury. Abdominal pain is an ominous sign, because it implies peritonitis. Rectal bleeding with a history of trauma suggests a mucosal tear, at the minimum.

### Examination

Physical examination should include digital rectal examination and careful palpation of the perineal area. In female patients, a vaginal examination should be performed. Asking the patient to "tighten up" the sphincter muscle may help evaluate the efficacy of its mechanism. Anoscopic and proctosigmoidoscopic examination should be performed, although care must be taken to avoid extending the injury. Rectal irrigation may help to facilitate visualization.

### Diagnostic Studies

Whenever anorectal trauma is suggested, take care not to underestimate the possible gravity of the injury. A high index of suspicion must be maintained to establish the nature of the patient's complete injury and initiate proper therapy. This is particularly true for avulsion injuries of the perineum and for gunshot wounds of the abdomen. The mortality rate can approach 100% if an untreated rectal injury continues to provide a source for sepsis. Barium enema examination is contraindicated if rectal injury is suspected; a water-soluble technique should be used. Obviously, the presence of intraperitoneal gas implies a perforated viscus.

Urinalysis should be routinely performed to detect the possible presence of hematuria. If blood is identified, obtain a urethrocystogram. It is also important to remember that failure to recognize an extraperitoneal perforation of the rectum is as potentially lethal as failure to identify an intraperitoneal perforation.

Peritoneal lavage can be misleading in these patients, giving false-negative results in those who have sustained isolated rectal, retroperitoneal, or rectosigmoid perforation.

### *Treatment*

As with colon trauma, the location, cause, length of time since the injury, and association with other organ involvement will dictate the appropriate therapeutic option. If rectal injury is suspected, broad-spectrum antibiotic therapy should be initiated within as quickly as possible, preferably not longer than 6 hours after the incident. It has been demonstrated that the results of surgical treatment are improved if antibiotics are given as early as possible. It is often difficult to identify the site of injury to the rectum at the time of laparotomy. A hematoma, if present, should be carefully assessed. Some have suggested infusing methylene blue through a Foley catheter inserted into the rectum while occluding the proximal bowel with the finger. Minor to moderate injuries of the anus below the level of the levator ani muscle can be treated by debridement, suture, drainage, antibiotic therapy, tetanus prophylaxis, and close observation. Intravenous fluid replacement and restriction of oral intake are advised. An elemental diet may be implemented for several days until the patient's condition is felt to have stabilized.

Injuries above the levators should be treated according to the principles listed below.

Principles of Managing Patients with Rectal Trauma
    Perineolithotomy position
    Management of concomitant injuries
    Debridement
    Complete proximal diversion
    Removal of foreign body, if any
    Drainage of presacral space
    Distal rectal washout
    Repair of rectal injury, if appropriate
    Primary sphincter repair, if possible

External wound drainage

Broad-spectrum antibiotics

The principles of management are summarized by the mnemonic "three *Ds*"—diversion, distal irrigation, and drainage. Copious irrigation of the distal segment with normal saline solution is performed until the returns are clear. Drainage is established by entering the presacral space following division of the anococcygeal ligament.

Whether to perform a direct sphincter repair as part of the initial management is a matter of some debate, because no meaningful statistics are available. Of course, every effort must initially be directed to saving the patient's life; therefore, it is not surprising that most articles place little or no emphasis on sphincter reconstruction. An important principle to remember, however: endeavor to preserve sphincter muscle if vigorous debridement of the perineum is required. Subsequently, marking the ends with nonabsorbable sutures facilitates the identification of the cut muscle. Direct repair should also be performed with sufficient time and satisfaction with the viability of the tissue. Delayed reconstruction should be considered in accordance with the principles outlined in Chapter 13. Finally, the likelihood of septic complications is reduced if perineal skin wounds are left open to heal by second intention or closed in accordance with a delayed primary repair technique.

Most surgeons recommend closure of the stoma when the patient has completely recovered—usually in 3 to 4 months.

In the absence of major bleeding from perineal and rectal lacerations, patients with profound hypotension resistant to massive intravenous fluid and blood administration must be considered to have intraabdominal bleeding or an expanding pelvic hematoma. For patients with persistent hypotension and a nondistended abdomen, pelvic arteriography and embolization of any bleeding vessel are recommended before a laparotomy is performed. Ligation of the hypogastric arteries is not felt to be the optimal approach to the management of bleeding from pelvic fractures.

### Complex Perineal Injuries

Complex wounds to the perineum, with or without pelvic fracture, present a considerable challenge to the surgeon. Early death is usually a consequence of bleeding and pelvic sepsis, whereas pulmonary embolism and multiple organ failure are the causes of late demise in these individuals. Often, associated is extensive soft-tissue injury. An organized approach is essential to prevent complications following these devastating wounds. The principles are summarized in Table 14.2. As discussed, colostomy with distal irrigation is, of course, essential, as is aggressive soft-tissue debridement, often by means of frequent examinations under anesthesia. This approach greatly reduces the incidence of pelvic sepsis. Although it is imperative to remove all nonviable tissue, every effort

**TABLE 14.2.** *Complex perineal wounds: management guidelines*

Resuscitation with hemorrhage control
Identification and treatment of associated injuries
Fecal diversion (consider feeding jejunostomy at same time)
Urinary diversion for complex urologic injuries
Aggressive initial debridement with pressurized pulsatile irrigation
Immediate fracture fixation
Early enteral nutrition
Daily intraoperative debridement
Wound coverage with skin graft as soon as feasible
Deep venous thrombosis prophylaxis

should be made to preserve the anal sphincter mechanism. Debridement of the muscle should be conservative. As stated, repair should be delayed under these circumstances. Pay particular attention to the prevention of deep venous thrombosis, as pulmonary embolism is a frequent cause of morbidity and mortality, especially following pelvic injury with fracture.

### Gunshot Wounds to the Buttocks

Gunshot wounds to the gluteal region warrant special consideration, because this type of injury often poses a challenging diagnostic and therapeutic dilemma. The question is whether it represents pure soft-tissue injury—that is, injury unrelated to the colorectal area—or whether concern that associated bowel problems are present. Velmahos et al. identified 59 consecutive patients with wounds of the buttocks during a 1-year period at Los Angeles County, University of Southern California Medical Center. The buttocks were defined as the body area confined between the posterior superior iliac spines superiorly, the gluteal folds inferiorly, and the projection of the midaxillary lines laterally. Superficial wounds and those tracking away from the retroperitoneum were excluded. The postulate of the study was that clinical examination is a safe and reliable tool for triaging individuals with these types of injuries. Essentially, it was felt that patients could be managed selectively on the basis of clinical findings alone. Based on these observations, approximately one third (19) had surgery, with all but two individuals found to have significant intraabdominal injuries. The remaining 40 patients (two thirds) were successfully observed. No injuries were missed or diagnoses delayed. The authors concluded that clinical examination is a safe method for selecting patients with gunshot wounds to the buttocks for nonoperative treatment. Authors have proposed that sigmoidoscopy can be performed *selectively* in individuals who have sustained a gunshot wound to the buttocks when the possibility of involvement of the rectum is in doubt. This recommendation stems from the fact that no rectal lacerations were missed.

## CONCLUSIONS AND RECOMMENDATIONS

The history of colorectal wound injuries and their management is fascinating, but has often been surrounded by controversy. However, recent prospective, randomized, controlled trials have helped to clarify what should be the appropriate management for most patients. It is certainly clear that recommendations can be made for the treatment of nondestructive colon wounds. Unfortunately, the data are less conclusive for more extensive wounds and for rectal injuries.

In summary, all uncomplicated colon wounds can be safely managed by primary repair. Destructive or devitalized colonic injuries require resection and, therefore, have a higher leakage rate if an anastomosis is attempted. These should be selectively managed. Primary anastomosis without diversion should be reserved for *good-risk, healthy individuals who do not have associated significant hemorrhage.*

Extraperitoneal rectal injuries are managed preferentially by fecal diversion, distal irrigation, and presacral drainage. Although the data concerning drainage are somewhat less clear, this approach certainly minimizes the risk for pelvic sepsis and is associated with a very low morbidity rate.

# 15

# Management of Foreign Bodies

Foreign materials can be ingested accidentally (e.g., swallowed dental bridge, nail, screw, paper clip, toothpick, chicken bone), or intentionally (e.g., in psychiatric or prison populations). Occasionally, a physician may be responsible for the introduction of a foreign body that requires special efforts to remove. Once an item passes beyond the pylorus, it usually can be eliminated without difficulty. One area of relative hindrance to passage, however, is the terminal ileum. Erosion can occur, which can lead to perforation, abscess, and fistula formation. Risk factors that increase the probability of foreign body perforation include inflammatory bowel disease, adhesions, diverticular disease, Meckel's diverticulum, tumors, and hernias.

Those patients who are at risk for foreign body ingestion have been categorized into four main groups:

1. Children up to 5 years of age who accidentally ingest a foreign body (e.g., buttons, coins)
2. Adults who present with food impaction, often related to being edentulous
3. Individuals who have accidentally or deliberately ingested a foreign body
4. Individuals attempting to profit from drug smuggling (i.e., "mules"—also known as "body packers" or "body baggers"). Rupture or impaction can lead to fatal drug toxicity.

The list of objects that have been removed from the rectum is virtually endless (e.g., light bulbs, catheters, pens and pencils, glass tubes, candles, vibrators, bottles, deceased gerbils, and jars).

## EVALUATION

Individuals present with a host of complaints, including rectal bleeding, anorectal pain, and difficulty with micturition. Embarrassed, apprehensive, and uncomfortable, many deny ill doing, often claiming to have fallen on the foreign body, which miraculously disappeared beyond their reach.

It is important to evaluate the patient's abdomen for signs and symptoms suggestive of peritoneal irritation. An indwelling catheter may be necessary with any concern about urinary retention. Inspection and palpation of the anal canal and rectum may reveal the foreign body. An x-ray film of the pelvis will demonstrate the contours of any radiopaque foreign material. Also seek to identify any unsuspected second foreign body.

## MANAGEMENT

Extracting foreign bodies from the rectum has become virtually epidemic. The presence of these objects in the rectum or colon poses particular difficulty in management. Some surgeons have suggested several principles to consider in this situation.

1. More damage is generally inflicted on the anorectum by a forceful attempt to remove a foreign body than by the original insertion.
2. Never attempt to remove a foreign body unless the patient's anal sphincter is fully relaxed by local, spinal, or general anesthesia.
3. Never attempt to extract a foreign body using instruments in an uncooperative patient, because a sudden move can precipitate tearing or perforation.
4. Large foreign bodies are preferentially removed in the operating room under a spinal or general anesthetic.
5. Following retrieval of the object, meticulous endoscopic examination should be undertaken and repair effected for any associated lacerations.
6. Rectal perforation, whether intraperitoneal or extraperitoneal, requires a diverting stoma.
7. Senile patients with a patulous anus can usually have foreign bodies removed without an anesthetic. Thermometers are the most frequently encountered foreign objects in this age group.

With these principles in mind, the following protocol has been recommended for management:

1. Immediate attempt at colonoscopic extraction if the foreign body is associated with bleeding or obstruction
2. Plane abdominal radiograph for nature and location
3. Barium enema for difficult-to-localize, suspected, or known radiolucent foreign body
4. Serial radiographs to follow progression
5. High-fiber diet, bulk laxative, mineral oil (no cathartics)
6. Enemas before the procedure to enhance visualization
7. Broad-spectrum antibiotics before the procedure
8. Colonoscopic extraction if the object fails to progress on serial radiographs during 48 hours
9. Observation for 24 hours after removal

In general, the removal of foreign bodies located within the rectum can be attempted as an outpatient procedure or in the emergency department, as long as the patient is cooperative. Conversely, foreign bodies located above the rectum, and in patients who are uncooperative, removal should be attempted in the operating room, where the administration of glucagon, spinal anesthesia, or general anesthesia assists in relaxing the sphincter, which greatly facilitates the removal of a rectal foreign body. Alternatively, a colonoscopic removal can be attempted if deemed appropriate. However, if symptoms of peritoneal irritation develop, removal will require laparotomy and colotomy.

A number of techniques have been suggested to remove objects from the rectum, including the use of blunt hooks or sponge holders, bimanual manipulation, and the use of a nasogastric tube as a lasso. A Foley catheter is particularly useful for a hollow body, such as a jar. It is crucial that once the presence of a foreign body has been determined, it be removed under adequate anesthesia to avoid the possibility of further injury. This is of particular concern if the object is glass. If a laparotomy is required, attempt to "milk" the foreign body down into the field of vision of the perineal operator; hence, the perineolithotomy position should be used. If injury to the rectum has occurred, the previously discussed principles apply. If the object cannot be removed transanally, a colotomy should be undertaken. In the controlled situation, without fecal contamination, no colostomy is performed.

# 16

## Disorders of Defecation

### CONSTIPATION

Chronic idiopathic constipation and abdominal pain are among the most common reasons for patients to solicit medical advice. In the United States alone, the cost of over-the-counter laxatives for 1991 was in excess of $400 million. This chapter addresses a number of conditions associated with bowel evacuation problems, the presenting complaint of which is often constipation.

### Physiology (see also Chapter 2)

The two primary functions of the colon are absorption and propulsion. The bowel absorbs water, certain electrolytes, short-chain fatty acids, and bacterial metabolites. The basic motility activities of the colon are slow net distal propulsion, extensive kneading, and uniform exposure of its contents to the mucosal surface. Material in the bowel is moved along a pressure gradient, with the rate and volume related to the pressure differential, the diameter of the tube, and the viscosity of the contents. The length and diameter of the colon tend to favor prolonged contact between the contents and the absorptive mucosa, which increases the amount of water removed and, as a consequence, may yield hard stools.

Three types of contractions are usually attributed to the colon (see Chapters 2 and 6):

1. Individual phasic contractions of short and long duration
2. Organized groups of contractions
3. Special propulsive contractions

Individual phasic contraction is the basic unit of contractile activity throughout the gastrointestinal tract. Short-duration contractions last less than 15 seconds, and long-duration contractions last 40 to 60 seconds. Individual phasic contractions are highly disorganized in both time and space; they are effective in mixing, kneading, and carrying out slow distal propulsion. The special propulsive contractions (i.e., giant migrating contractions) provide the strong propulsive force required for defecation and for mass movements. Despite what might appear to be a straightforward concept, considerable controversy exists about the relative merits of the physiologic techniques used to assess the pathophysiology of the various processes and conditions.

Even today, we do not fully understand how all the elements of the colon (i.e., morphology, innervation, function) integrate to produce organized movement of intestinal contents. Furthermore, both the normal range of colorectal motor activity and its variations in disease have yet to be clearly defined.

The process of evacuation of feces consists of two stages. The *first stage* is involuntary, during which the contents are gradually propelled into the rectum. This is the total effect of short-duration, long-duration, and giant migrating contractions. The *second stage* is the act of defecation, during which feces are expelled. When the process goes awry, an organized approach is needed to evaluate and treat this extraordinarily commonplace symptom, if appropriate therapy is to be instituted. A number of specific studies, especially physiologic investigations, should be considered. Some of these have also been discussed in Chapter 13. It may be useful to review the sections on physiologic studies in Chapters 2, 6, and 13 to obtain a better perspective of these two, often interrelated, conditions.

Disorders of defecation can be divided into three categories: (a) those with motility (i.e., transit) problems; (b) those with obstructed defecation (e.g. anismus); and (c) those with irritable bowel syndrome (see Chapter 26).

## Etiology

A number of diseases can be associated with chronic constipation and even megacolon. First, establish whether the patient is taking any of a host of drugs that can produce constipation (see Chapter 3). The bowel symptoms and the radiologic findings of colonic dilatation may completely resolve after the medication has been discontinued. An abbreviated summary of the causes of and conditions associated with constipation follows:

Dietary
    Low intake of fiber (consider poor dentition, poverty)
    Poor intake of fluid
Functional
    Depression
    Confusion
    Inadequate toilet facilities
    Immobility
    Psychosis
    Encopresis
Medications
    Anticholinergics
    Antidepressants

    Narcotics and opiates
    Iron
    Bismuth
    Antiparkinsonian drugs
    Antacids (e.g., aluminum)
    Antihypertensives (e.g., diuretics, ganglionic blockers, calcium-channel blockers)
    Anticonvulsants
    Ion-exchange resins
    Bulk laxatives without adequate hydration
Endocrine, Metabolic, and Collagen–Vascular Diseases
    Hypothyroidism
    Hypoparathyroidism
    Diabetes mellitus
    Hypokalemia
    Chronic renal failure
    Pregnancy
    Hypopituitarism
    Porphyria
    Scleroderma
    Amyloidosis
    Hypercalcemia
Neuromuscular Disorders
    Cerebral
        Cerebrovascular accident
        Parkinson's disease
        Intracranial tumor
    Spinal
        Cauda equina lesion
        Myelomeningocele
        Trauma (e.g., cord injury)
        Multiple sclerosis
        Tertiary syphilis
    Peripheral
        Diabetes mellitus
        Autonomic neuropathy
        Chagas' disease
        Hirschsprung's disease
        von Recklinghausen's disease
        Stimulant laxative abuse
        Vincristine
    Functional
        Outlet obstruction (i.e., anismus, obstructed defecation, spastic pelvic floor syndrome)

Colonic Inertia
  Slow-transit constipation
  Intestinal pseudo-obstruction (Ogilvie's syndrome)

One final cause of an evacuation problem is massive colonic dilatation suggesting an obstructed cause. Intestinal pseudoobstruction (i.e., colonic ileus) has come to be known as "Ogilvie's syndrome." The condition is discussed later in this chapter.

## Clinical Presentations

A plethora of clinical presentations encompass the broad clinical diagnosis attributed to the symptom of constipation. These can include such severe abdominal signs and symptoms as to mimic an acute abdominal catastrophe. More commonly, however, patients simply complain of an inability to defecate. At least 80% of these patients are women.

Chronic, severe constipation is usually defined as bowel movements less frequent than once in 5 days, with symptoms persisting longer than 18 months. Irrespective of the duration of symptoms, constipation is generally regarded as fewer than three bowel movements per week in an individual on a standard diet containing 19 g of fiber daily. No evidence should be seen of intestinal obstruction, and intestinal transit time should be prolonged (see *Bowel Transit*).

An important complication of constipation, especially in the elderly, is fecal impaction, but the proximate cause of many other symptoms, complications, and diseases can be directly attributed to or associated with the inability to evacuate normally. These include the following conditions:

- Fecal incontinence
- Spurious diarrhea
- Urinary retention
- Mental disturbance and anxiety
- Arrhythmias
- Syncope
- Autonomic dysreflexia
- Pneumothorax
- Hypoxia
- Hypotension
- Dysfunctional labor
- Volvulus
- Stercoral ulceration
- Cecal perforation
- Hemorrhoids
- Anal fissure
- Rectal prolapse

Be aware, however, of the paradoxical situation in which diarrhea or fecal incontinence supervenes and the underlying problem is actually constipation with impaction. Although impaction as a cause of colonic obstruction is uncommon (1.3%), in selected populations (e.g., those in nursing homes or with spinal cord injuries), the incidence can approximate 50%.

Patients, usually women with severe idiopathic constipation, are characterized by extreme disability and by severe abdominal pain and distension. The syndrome often commences in infancy, childhood, or, more commonly, with menarche. An investigation found that constipated individuals had a greater volume and pressure of rectal distension for both sensation and sphincter relaxation, diminished basal and postmorphine motility indices in the distal rectum, delayed transit, and an empty rectum, even though severely constipated.

## Stercoral Ulcer

A hard, scybalous, inspissated fecal mass can produce an ulcerating lesion in the colon or rectum, which can then lead to perforation. The condition usually occurs in constipated, bedridden patients. It often presents as an isolated lesion in the rectosigmoid along the antimesenteric margin, but the lesions can be multiple.

In reviewing the literature, it is evident that the mortality rate associated with stercoral ulcer is high. This can be attributed to several factors, not the least of which are the morbidity and mortality associated with colonic perforation and peritonitis. Additionally, these patients often are elderly and have major medical problems that place them at an increased risk.

## Evaluation of the Constipated Patient

A thorough history of the constipated patient should be obtained, especially with regard to frequency of bowel actions, consistency of stools, and timing. It is important to note the existence of any associated pain, mucus, or blood; a sense of incomplete evacuation; and whether manual means are used to effect evacuation. Medical problems and medications must be identified (see earlier display and Chapter 3).

### *Physical Examination and Endoscopy*

Obviously, efforts must be made to eliminate a primary anal, rectal, or colon problem as the cause of this symptom. This includes abdominal and digital rectal examination, together with rigid or flexible sigmoidoscopy.

### *Rectal Biopsy*

Full-thickness rectal wall biopsy may be indicated in suspected cases of a form of Hirschsprung's disease (see later). Classically, the lack of ganglion cells has been felt to be diagnostic of the condition. However, in recent years, some authors have felt that in the short-segment form of the condition, biopsy is superfluous. It is important to include the muscularis propria to obtain an adequate specimen for interpretation, but the major problem with such a biopsy for distal disease is that ganglion cells can be normally absent in this location. With the understanding that difficulties may exist with respect to interpretation of biopsy specimens, the diagnosis can be made of short-segment involvement on clinical grounds supplemented by barium enema and manometry.

### Radiologic Studies

A plane film of the abdomen is strongly suggested in an individual with abdominal distension. Barium enema in these patients will often reveal a huge colon with considerable fecal residue or a markedly redundant bowel. Although this finding does not imply a specific cause of the problem, it indicates the magnitude of the anatomic abnormality and will inevitably influence the decision whether the patient is a candidate for surgical intervention.

Barium enema study performed for suspected short-segment Hirschsprung's disease does not show the decompressed rectum seen with classic Hirschsprung's disease; on the contrary, the rectum is dilated to the level of the aganglionic segment. The barium enema is usually the more rewarding study for colon evaluation in the constipated patient. This, in combination with defecography (see Chapters 6 and 17), constitutes our preferred initial investigation.

### Defecography or Evacuation Proctography

The method of performing defecography (i.e., evacuation proctography) is discussed in Chapters 6 and 13 and is further addressed in Chapter 17. Its particular value is in the diagnosis of two conditions—internal procidentia (i.e., the pre-prolapse condition) and obstructed defecation. Paradoxical puborectalis muscle contraction can be appreciated during an attempt at eliminating the thickened barium (see later), or internal prolapse may be seen. The implication of the latter condition in pudendal nerve injury and as the cause of fecal incontinence is discussed in Chapter 13. Other observations may include the presence of an enterocele, a rectocele, perineal descent, and the possibility of unsuspected incontinence. The defecogram cannot be used alone in therapeutic decision making, unless either of the two specific conditions is unequivocally identified.

### Bowel Transit

The most objective assessment of colonic transit is obtained by asking a patient to swallow three different types of radiopaque markers each morning for 3 days while taking no laxatives and being fully ambulatory. Another method for calculating colonic transit is discussed in Chapter 6. A simple approach is to have the patient take a capsule containing 24 radiopaque rings (Konsyl Pharma-

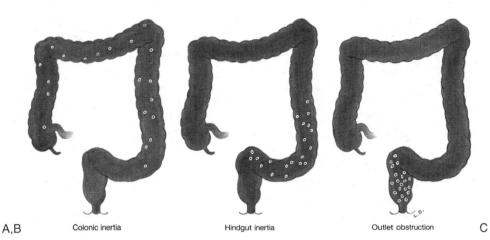

**A,B**            Colonic inertia                      Hindgut inertia                    Outlet obstruction            **C**

**FIG. 16.1.** Artist's representation of three types of radiologic appearances that might be seen with radiopaque rings on the plane abdominal x-ray film. **A.** Colonic inertia. Typical pattern of distribution throughout the colon. **B.** Hindgut inertia. Markers are clustered on the left side of the colon, but not limited to the rectum. **C.** Outlet obstruction. Markers are clustered in the rectum, a classic pattern indicating obstructed defecation.

ceuticals). Laxatives must be avoided. A plane abdominal radiograph is taken on the fifth day after ingestion. By the fifth day, 80% of the markers should have been eliminated and all should be passed by the seventh day.

Figure 16.1 identifies three patterns of abnormal distribution of these markers, which serve to illustrate a variety of pathophysiologic processes responsible for abnormalities of defecation. Obviously, the results of the transit study must be correlated with those of other investigations.

### Scintigraphic Studies

Radiopaque markers have been demonstrated to be extremely useful in distinguishing patients with normal and those with slow intestinal transit; in the latter group, however, they are not especially useful in identifying the precise region of delay. Scintigraphic studies are increasingly being used to evaluate intestinal transit in a quantitative, noninvasive manner. This investigation, however, does not influence the intervention undertaken when compared with the more simple marker transit study at this time.

### Anorectal Manometry

The value of anorectal manometry in the investigation of patients with fecal incontinence is discussed in Chapters 2, 6, and 13. Manometric studies have also been demonstrated to be useful for establishing the diagnosis of short-segment Hirschsprung's disease (see later), where a lack of the internal sphincter relaxation response, also known as the "rectoanal inhibitory reflex," is noted. The reflex can also be absent if resting anal canal pressures are low, as in some individuals with rectal prolapse and neurogenic fecal incontinence following low rectal excision.

### Electromyography

The role of electromyography (EMG) in the evaluation of patients with anal incontinence is discussed in Chapters 2, 6, and 15, but EMG of the external anal sphincter and puborectalis is another technique for establishing the diagnosis of paradoxical or inappropriate puborectalis contraction. Failure of inhibition of electrical activity during the act of defecation is pathognomonic for anismus. Most, however, would use a balloon expulsion test to make this diagnosis.

### Rectal Sensation

As mentioned in Chapter 15, rectal sensation is usually assessed by balloon distension. Investigators observed a raised threshold to electrosensory testing that suggested the presence of a rectal sensory neuropathy in severely constipated individuals. How these observations will affect the subsequent therapeutic choices remains to be explored.

### Analysis of Myoelectrical Activity

Myoelectrical activity of the colon can be assessed by means of sigmoidoscopic attachment of electrodes to the colorectal mucosa. Constipated individuals fail to demonstrate an increase in spiking activity under these circumstances, which suggests the possibility of a neurogenic defect as the cause of this condition.

### Pudendal Nerve Terminal Motor Latency

The importance of pudendal nerve terminal motor latency evaluation for patients with incontinence is discussed in Chapters 2, 6, and 15. Investigators of constipated individuals have concluded that unsuspected neuropathy is present in 24% of patients.

### Psychological Profiles

Some difference of opinion exists with respect to studies concerning the incidence of psychosocial disturbances in severely constipated women, especially those with slow-transit problems. Some authors have concluded that certain individuals may require a behavioral and psychological approach to the management of their constipation. In some centers, a standardized personality test (e.g., Beck

Depression Inventory, Minnesota Multiphasic Personality Inventory [MMPI]) is administered to every patient for whom a surgical alternative is considered. It is certainly appropriate to assess individually the psychosocial factors that may contribute to a given patient's complaints. This and thyroid function tests are probably the most often omitted, potentially helpful, studies in the evaluation of patients with intractable constipation.

## Medical Management

### *Diet, Exercise, Laxatives, Enemas, and Suppositories*

For most patients, the treatment of constipation includes appropriate dietary counseling, a regimen of activity, and often the use of laxatives, enemas, or suppositories (see Chapter 3). When no organic pathology is present or the condition does not lend itself to management by means of specific medical or surgical measures, the initial approach to the treatment of uncomplicated constipation is usually directed toward dietary measures. Generally, this consists of increasing fiber intake, especially whole-grain cereals (e.g., bran), fruits, and vegetables; an increase in the volume of fluid intake is also helpful. Exercise is also important in the treatment regimen.

Despite efforts at counseling constipated people to eat a proper diet, get a proper amount of activity, and not disregard the urge to defecate, many believe that they require laxatives. Breaking the laxative habit is especially difficult because of advertisements implying that it is unhealthful not to have a daily bowel action. However, some people benefit from and indeed require cathartics (see also Chapter 3). Table 16.1 illustrates the classification of cathartics based on the mechanism of action of the drug.

### *Stimulant Cathartics*

Stimulant cathartics produce their effect by local irritation or by action on Auerbach's plexus, which results in increased motor activity of the intestine. As with all cathartics, stimulants are contraindicated in the presence of intestinal obstruction or peritonitis and in the postoperative period after laparotomy, especially after bowel resection.

*Melanosis Coli.* The anthraquinone cathartics cascara sagrada and senna are usually responsible for melanosis coli. Proctosigmoidoscopic examination reveals the mucosa to be brown, deep purple, or black, broken into "small angular polyhedral designs by fine netlike striae of lighter shade, either yellow or brown." The pigment itself produces no symptoms.

Melanosis coli usually occurs in older age groups, as it takes years of laxative use or abuse to cause color change of the mucosa. Biopsy of the rectum will reveal the presence of pigment-laden macrophages in the lamina propria; these are what give the mucosa its characteristic color. When an individual

**TABLE 16.1.** *Classification of cathartics*

| Class | Drugs |
| --- | --- |
| Stimulant | Cascara sagrada |
| | Senna |
| | Danthron |
| | Phenolphthalein |
| | Acetophenolisatin |
| | Bisacodyl |
| | Castor oil |
| Saline | Magnesium sulfate |
| | Milk of magnesia |
| | Magnesium citrate |
| | Sodium sulfate |
| | Sodium phosphate |
| | Potassium phosphate |
| | Potassium sodium tartrate |
| Osmotic | Polyethylene glycol and electrolytes (*i.e.,* Colyte, GoLYTELY) |
| Bulk-forming | Plantago (*e.g.,* psyllium) seed |
| | Methycellulose |
| | Sodium carboxymethylcellulose |
| | Agar |
| | Tragacanth |
| | Bran |
| Lubricant | Mineral oil |
| | Dioctyl sodium sulfosuccinate |
| | Calcium docusate |

ceases to take the anthracene laxative, the pigment often disappears within 3 to 6 months.

### Saline Cathartics

Saline cathartics achieve their effect on the intestinal tract by the osmotic activity of a slowly absorbed salt ion. Water is retained in the small intestine when salts that contain magnesium sulfate, phosphate, or tartrate are ingested. The increase in volume causes the intestine to contract and to expel the contents. The latency period for action depends on the dose and usually varies from 3 to 6 hours.

Although saline cathartics are relatively safe, they can be dangerous in those with renal or cardiac disease.

One particularly valuable use of such a cathartic, however, is as an enema. This is especially useful in preparing for proctosigmoidoscopy, flexible fiberoptic sigmoidoscopy, and anal operations. Therapeutically, it can be effective for the treatment of a soft fecal impaction.

### Osmotic Cathartics

Osmotic cathartics are usually orally administered electrolyte lavage preparations for the colon (e.g., GoLYTELY, Colyte) delivered in the form of water-soluble components for reconstitution. Despite their ability to cleanse the colon rapidly and induce diarrhea, virtually no net ion absorption or loss occurs even though large volumes of fluid are ingested. Osmotic cathartics are usually used for bowel cleansing before colonoscopy, barium enema, or colon surgery. They are also useful in treating the severely constipated individual and are especially effective when combined with a volume enema.

### Bulk-Forming Cathartics

Bulk-forming cathartics are composed of synthetic or natural polysaccharides and cellulose derivatives that swell or dissolve in the intestinal tract without being absorbed. They act primarily by adding bulk to the stool. All bulk laxatives should be taken with adequate fluid. Their effect is much less dramatic and may become apparent only 12 to 72 hours after administration.

### Lubricant Cathartics

Lubricant cathartics lubricate the feces without stimulating peristalsis (e.g., after hernia repair and for patients with coronary artery disease). However, mineral oil is helpful in situations in which straining must be avoided but it has many side effects and contraindications. Granulomas can form at the site of the healing wounds. Aspiration of the ingested oil produces an often fatal lipoid pneumonia. Oil absorbed into the system can produce granulomas in the mesenteric lymph nodes, intestinal mucosa, liver, and spleen. Finally, although mineral oil produces a lubricated stool, its prolonged use can lead to atrophy of the anorectal sphincter mechanism, because it is not stretched when a greasy stool is passed.

Dioctyl sodium sulfosuccinate and other emulsifying agents can also be considered lubricant cathartics. They have been widely used in industry to facilitate the mixture of water and fatty substances and are often prescribed as a stool softener after anal surgery.

### Enemas

Enemas, although not truly laxatives, need to be considered as a therapeutic option in the management of the constipated patient. The many substances administered in this manner include tap water, soap suds, saline solution, vegetable oils, hydrogen peroxide, milk and molasses, and even champagne for certain special patients.

Several specific indications are found for the use of enemas:

- To evacuate the bowel before surgery, childbirth, a contrast radiologic study, or endoscopic examination
- To remove a fecal impaction—in conjunction with manual removal

- To rid the bowel of barium to prevent inspissation
- To stimulate bowel activity after certain surgical procedures
- To relieve certain colonic obstructions (e.g., an impaction proximal to a carcinoma of the rectosigmoid colon)
- To empty the distal bowel before certain operations, procedures, or studies
- To evacuate the bowel in patients with emptying problems, especially if caused by neurologic dysfunction

### Suppositories

Suppositories can contain glycerin, bisacodyl, dioctyl sodium sulfosuccinate, or senna, or they can release carbon dioxide. Manufacturers advocate their use whenever an enema is considered, but the relative efficacy of enemas versus suppositories is open to question.

### Pharmacologic Therapy (see also Chapter 3)

It is appealing to have an agent that acts specifically to enhance propulsive activity rather than as an intestinal irritant. Metoclopramide (Reglan) is a prokinetic agent that affects motility primarily in the upper gastrointestinal tract. Erythromycin, also a prokinetic agent, has little activity in the colon. Another, Cisapride, in a double-blind, randomized trial, is showing considerable promise in the treatment of motility disorders affecting the hindgut. Also, it has been shown to decrease the rectoanal inhibitory reflex threshold and the conscious rectal sensitivity threshold in constipated children. Newer prokinetic agents (prucalopride and SDZ HTF-919), which act via the 5-HT4 receptor, are currently in advanced clinical trials.

Somatostatin has been used to manage intestinal motility problems in individuals with scleroderma. Proponents have demonstrated that migrating complexes propagated at the same velocity and had two thirds the amplitude of the spontaneous complexes in normal subjects. Abdominal symptoms such as nausea, bloating, and pain were much reduced. Further experience with this new agent is awaited.

Trimebutine maleate has also been used to treat manifestations of functional bowel disease, including abdominal pain and constipation. This drug may be of value in the treatment of patients with chronic idiopathic constipation, provided that a careful pathophysiologic evaluation reveals a prolonged colonic transit time.

Methylnaltrexone, the first peripheral opioids receptor antagonist, has been used in trials of those with advanced cancer requiring methadone for pain control, in whom other therapies to control constipation have failed. All subjects receiving the drug had improved transit compared with none in the placebo group. No side effects and, in particular, no opioid withdrawal occurred.

Some investigators have used colchicine, a neurogenic stimulator of the gastrointestinal tract, in those with intractable constipation. Preliminary work shows promise, but larger, long-term studies are needed.

### Spastic Pelvic Floor Syndrome; Obstructed Defecation; Anismus

The spastic pelvic floor syndrome is one of nonrelaxation of the levator muscles during defecation. Authors have confirmed this by demonstrating, using defecography, an abnormal increase in the activity of the sphincter mechanism during evacuation.

The balloon expulsion test is a simple and inexpensive method used to evaluate a patient's ability to expel and retain stool. An ordinary latex toy balloon may be used, a Foley catheter, or one of the biofeedback devices mentioned in Chapter 13.

### *Treatment*

#### *Behavioral Medicine; Operative Conditioning; Biofeedback*

In Chapter 13, biofeedback is discussed as it applies to the management of patients with fecal incontinence. By positive or negative verbal reinforcement or by the use of a variety of devices, bowel control can be improved.

*Balloon Expulsion.* The same devices can be used to train individuals who are constipated, especially those suffering from so-called "obstructed defecation" (anismus). In biofeedback, patients watch a needle gauge or lights while trying to adjust their sphincteric responses to rectal balloon insufflation; in this way, they can learn to relax the sphincteric mechanism to expel the balloon.

Ho et al. reported the results of biofeedback treatment using the manometric biofeedback equipment described in Chapter 13. Of 56 patients, 90% were subjectively improved.

*Electromyographic Biofeedback.* Some advocate a treatment regimen of EMG biofeedback followed by simulation of the defecation process by rectal insertion of oatmeal porridge. They reported an 89% success rate at a mean length of follow-up of approximately 9 months.

*Manometric Anal Sphincter Probe Feedback.* Turnbull and Ritvo used biofeedback from a manometric anal sphincter probe in their patients. Follow-up of up to 4.5 years showed continued improvement in bowel function and abdominal symptoms.

#### *Biofeedback—Other Methods*

By use of an electrode plug, the patient records the muscular activity used at rest, during squeeze, and during straining to expel the plug. Subsequent sessions are directed toward attempting to control the activity of the sphincter mechanism during straining. A final step is the instillation of psyllium slurry (120 mL) to simulate an actual bowel movement.

*Comment*: It is not clear how long and how often biofeedback sessions are necessary, but all investigators seem to agree that booster treatments are suggested for those individuals who relapse. Ideally, training should be performed several times a day for 10 or 15 minutes at a time.

*Botulinum Toxin.* Investigators have used botulinum toxin in four individuals who had failed to respond to conventional biofeedback, all of whom improved, with no morbidity or mortality.

## Surgical Approaches

With the physiologic abnormality described as the spastic pelvic floor syndrome, it seems unlikely that subtotal colectomy or any other operative approach would be beneficial, unless the operation succeeds in overcoming the resistance of the spastic sphincters.

Maria et al. performed progressive anal dilation in 13 patients with anismus, using three dilators of 20, 23, and 27 mm in diameter. These were inserted every day for 30 minutes. At 6 months, significant improvement was seen in weekly mean spontaneous bowel actions from 0 to 6, and the number of patients with a need for laxatives decreased from 12 with a weekly mean of 4.6 to 2 patients who required them once per week. None was incontinent for formed stool and none experienced mucous discharge or fecal urgency.

*Comment*: The obvious questions posed are how aggressive to be in the medical management of the constipated individual, and at what point is surgical intervention warranted? Certainly, if the patient's symptoms are disabling or intractable despite the application of standard therapeutic measures, an alternative approach must be considered.

### *Treatment of Fecal Impaction*

Fecal impaction is a common finding in surgical patients. The diagnosis is not usually difficult to make, unless the impaction is beyond the reach of the examining finger. Even under these circumstances, the patient history and the plane abdominal radiograph are usually more than suggestive.

A number of complications are seen with fecal impaction, the most common of which is incontinence. Other, more serious potential sequelae include the following:

• Stercoral ulceration
• Large-bowel obstruction
• Perforation at some distance from the rectum, especially in the cecum
• Gangrene secondary to ischemia
• Autonomic dysreflexia

- Pneumothorax from straining
- Hypoxia
- Associated colorectal problems (e.g., hemorrhoids, rectal prolapse, volvulus)

Treatment usually requires manual disimpaction, laxatives, and large-volume or retention enemas. In the interest of patient safety and comfort, manual disimpaction ideally should be done in the operating room with intravenous sedation or a general, local, or regional anesthetic. When the bulk of the mass has been removed, a high colonic irrigation with isotonic salt solution is done by means of a large-bore catheter.

### Short-Segment, Adult, or Late-Onset Hirschsprung's Disease

Hirschsprung's disease (see Chapter 18) occurs once in 5,000 births; it is seen four times more often in boys than in girls. The clinical picture is of a physiologic intestinal obstruction caused by lack of peristalsis in the aganglionic segment. If the aganglionic segment is long, medical management is not possible, and a colostomy is performed proximal to the aganglionic segment. When the child achieves a weight of approximately 20 pounds, definitive surgery is performed in the form of an abdominoanal pull-through procedure or endoanal anastomosis (e.g., Swenson, Duhamel, Soave; see Chapter 18).

Occasionally, a child can reach several years of age or even adulthood with a mild form of Hirschsprung's disease (i.e., short-segment involvement) that involves 2 or 3 cm of distal rectum. This condition can cause symptoms of severe constipation or the inability to eliminate except by means of rectal stimulation and enemas. The diagnosis is based on clinical, radiographic, manometric, and histologic studies, all of which have been discussed.

### *Treatment*

Anorectal myectomy is the surgical treatment generally recommended for short-segment disease. This is essentially an extensive internal anal sphincterectomy. The internal anal sphincter is divided—or, ideally, partially excised—in the lateral position from the level of the dentate line, incorporating the muscularis of the bowel wall for a distance of approximately 8 to 10 cm.

Once the colon has become very dilated, anorectal myectomy alone will probably fail to ameliorate the complaint adequately, even if the problem initially was a consequence of short-segment disease. Such an individual will usually require a more extensive resection. Options include the other pull-through procedures (e.g., Swenson or Soave), and low anterior resection with coloanal anastomosis, with or without an intervening pouch; a Duhamel procedure; or even an ileal pouch-anal anastomosis.

## Results

The results of anorectal myectomy have been mixed, greatly depending on the length of the aganglionic segment; that is, the shorter the segment of involvement, the more successful the myotomy was in achieving a satisfactory result.

In those managed by the Duhamel procedure by some surgeons, 90% were felt to have had an excellent functional result. Others have used the Swenson procedure, anorectal myectomy, and a variety of bowel resections. Although the morbidity rate is low, the failure rate is up to 40%. Consequently, no obvious best choice of operation exists for Hirschsprung's disease, but anorectal myectomy, with or without low anterior resection, the endorectal pull-through, and the Duhamel procedure are all associated with relatively good long-term results. Because untreated short-segment disease inevitably leads to intractable symptoms and to megacolon, it is wise to recommend surgery as soon as the diagnosis is confirmed.

## Surgery in the Management of Constipation

### Resective Alternatives

If resection is to be performed as the definitive treatment for chronic idiopathic constipation, most or all of the colon must be removed. To remove some of the rectum could result in intractable diarrhea and probably fecal incontinence. Therefore, some form of restorative operation (e.g., ileal pouch-anal anastomosis procedure) would be necessary when rectal resection is considered. The technical aspects of all the resective approaches are discussed elsewhere: subtotal and total colectomy in Chapter 22 and restorative proctocolectomy in Chapter 29. As a last resort, ileostomy may be the best option in selected patients.

## Results

Pemberton et al. categorized patients as having slow-transit constipation, pelvic floor dysfunction, a combination of the two, or irritable bowel. Tailoring the treatment to the specific physiologic abnormality should result in the successful selection of those who would benefit from total colectomy and ileoproctostomy. With this approach, of those with slow transit constipation, up to 97% have been satisfied with the results of the surgery. Interestingly, in this series, no difference in the outcome was seen in patients with slow-transit constipation alone compared with those who also had pelvic floor dysfunction.

Others have reported an overall success rate of approximately 80%, with a mean follow-up period of 5 years in those treated by subtotal colectomy.

A report from Johns Hopkins stated that 88% of patients with generalized intestinal dysmotility had initial improvement; only 13% had prolonged relief with total colectomy. The authors concluded that two distinct types of colonic dysmotility exist: with and without generalized disease. Although they emphasize the importance of upper gastrointestinal physiologic studies to identify those individuals who will have a poor long-term response to total colectomy, most dispute the value of this finding.

## Antegrade Enemas

A number of operative techniques have been developed to facilitate the administration of antegrade washouts to empty the colon and to prevent soiling as well as to deal with constipation and the inability to evacuate. This usually involves the creation of an appendicocecostomy, which permits a channel that can be catheterized to allow colonic washouts. The procedure has also been used successfully in children who have undergone pull-through procedures for Hirschsprung's disease or other anorectal malformations.

## Continent Colonic Conduit

A continent colonic conduit has been described that incorporates an intussuscepted valve constructed from the sigmoid colon. Some authors have proposed constructing the conduit from transverse colon. Intubation of the conduit permits irrigation and evacuation in individuals with severe constipation.

*Comment*: Idiopathic constipation can be attributable to several conditions: slow transit, rectal inertia, short-segment Hirschsprung's disease, and outlet dysfunction (i.e., obstructed defecation). Patients can exhibit characteristics of more than one of these conditions.

These patients must be sorted in an organized way, according to the cause of their condition. Specific investigations must include anorectal manometry or some means to determine whether a person is suffering from obstructed defecation. Manometry is also useful in establishing the diagnosis of Hirschsprung's disease, although biopsy with special staining techniques is at least as valuable. Alternatively, balloon expulsion, commercially available biofeedback devices, and defecography should be able to confirm or exclude anismus satisfactorily. Transit studies to determine the presence of slow-transit constipation and the primary area of involvement are mandatory.

Our approach to treating the adult patient with megacolon in the absence of anorectal pathology is to perform a subtotal or total abdominal colectomy. Even if the rectum is abnormal, a dilated, atonic colon cannot be restored to normal function in these individuals. Unless a specific reason is seen to do otherwise, if the rectum is normal, we place the anastomosis approximately 15 to 18 cm from the anal verge. A lower anastomosis predisposes the patient to diarrhea and incontinence. Frankly, we have had no experience with the pouch procedures for this particular indication, but we would certainly consider this alternative in an individual with colonic ileus and evidence of short-segment Hirschsprung's disease. Using the criteria described, and applying the appropriate investigations in proper sequence and performing strict preoperative selection, the physician can arrive at a suitable recommendation and embark on the treatment that is most likely to produce a satisfactory functional result.

## INTESTINAL PSEUDOOBSTRUCTION; OGILVIE'S SYNDROME

Ogilvie's syndrome and intestinal pseudoobstruction are terms used to denote a condition in which patients appear to have signs and symptoms suggestive of intestinal obstruction without an evident mechanical source. As such, this condition is often seen in association with other diseases, occasionally complicating the postoperative course of patients who have had one of several types of operations, particularly abdominal surgery. The differential diagnosis includes Hirschsprung's disease, especially short-segment involvement; toxic megacolon in ulcerative colitis, and Crohn's disease; volvulus; fecal impaction; and a distal obstructing lesion. Predisposing factors include a virtual textbook of medical and surgical ills, including the following:

- Scleroderma
- Dermatomyositis
- Systemic lupus erythematosus
- Periarteritis nodosa
- Chagas' disease
- Myotonic dystrophy
- Multiple sclerosis
- Familial dysautonomia
- Psychotic disorders
- Hypothyroidism
- Diabetes mellitus
- Hypoparathyroidism
- Renal failure
- Renal transplantation
- Blunt abdominal trauma
- Orthopedic procedures
- Porphyria
- Amyloidosis
- Congestive heart failure
- Hypoxia
- Sepsis
- Lead poisoning
- Electrolyte imbalance
- Cesarean section
- Radiotherapy
- Certain medications
- Drug abuse

### Clinical Manifestations and Diagnosis

Presenting features of colonic ileus are abdominal distension, abdominal pain, constipation, and, occasionally, diarrhea. It is important to distinguish among severe idiopathic constipation, mechanical obstruction, and pseudoobstruction. Pseudoobstruction is basically a radiologic diagnosis, where endoscopy and contrast studies may be necessary to confirm that no mechanical factor is causing the condition. Computed tomography is usually unhelpful except to show the massively dilated bowel.

Chronic intestinal pseudoobstruction is manifested, as might be suspected, by recurrent signs and symptoms. Patients are often cachectic, with hypoactive or absent bowel sounds, and have a mildly tender, distended abdomen. Probably the most common cause is scleroderma. Associated conditions include scleroderma, familial visceral myopathies, and familial visceral neuropathies.

## Treatment and Results

### *Noninterventional Management*

Initial management should include restriction of oral intake, nasogastric intubation, and correction of any fluid or electrolyte abnormalities. It is imperative that specific problems (e.g., infection) be treated, if possible. Conservative treatment consists of the aforementioned measures of initial management plus gentle enemas, a rectal tube, and a decreased narcotic dosage.

### *Colonoscopy*

Colonic decompression by colonoscopy is thought to be the most effective therapeutic modality for selected patients with nonobstructive colonic dilatation. Care should be taken to visualize the lumen adequately and to insufflate minimal air.

### *Drug Therapy*

Another possible method of treatment is the use of ceruletide, a synthetically produced decapeptide that has been demonstrated to stimulate intestinal motility.

The prokinetic agent cisapride, mentioned previously, has also been used. It has been proposed by some as a helpful adjunct to management.

Intravenous neostigmine has been demonstrated to achieve adequate colonic decompression in most patients. Adequate monitoring is required while instigating this treatment.

### *Surgery*

In the patient with intestinal pseudoobstruction, surgical intervention should not be performed unless a genuine fear of impending cecal perforation exists. This is one of the few indications for performing a cecostomy. Generally, the operation is carried out by the standard open technique. Percutaneous cecostomy under computed tomographic guidance also has been used successfully as an alternative to surgical cecostomy for decompressing a massively dilated cecum.

Another suggestion is to perform percutaneous colonoscopic cecostomy, a technique analogous to that of percutaneous gastrostomy. Also, a technique of laparoscopically guided percutaneous cecostomy, using T-fasteners to retract and anchor the cecum to the anterior abdominal wall, has been described.

If the bowel is ischemic or perforated, resection with or without anastomosis is required in accordance with the principles discussed in Chapter 26. Results of resection are too apocryphal to submit for meaningful analysis.

## PROCTALGIA FUGAX; LEVATOR SYNDROME; LEVATOR SPASM

Levator spasm (i.e., levator syndrome) is a condition that occurs predominantly in women. Characteristically, the patient complains of severe, episodic, often agonizing discomfort within the rectum. The location of the pain distinguishes the condition from a thrombosed hemorrhoid or an anal fissure, problems that are often localized to the anal or perianal area. The pain, often on the left side, may awaken the individual from sleep, and is usually unrelated to bowel activity, although sometimes it is exacerbated by defecation. The discomfort usually lasts only a few seconds, but occasionally persists for several hours. The condition often occurs in patients who spend a great deal of time on the toilet, whether straining, with diarrhea, or reading the newspaper. Other predisposing factors that have been suggested include trauma from riding a long distance, childbirth, low anterior resection or pelvic surgery, anal surgery, spinal surgery, psychiatric disorders, irritable bowel syndrome, and the act of sexual intercourse. A hereditary predisposition has also been reported.

Physical examination is usually unrewarding, but sometimes a tender, spastic puborectalis muscle is felt, particularly on the left side. The characteristic discomfort may be duplicated when the physician presses on the sensitive area.

### Treatment

Primary treatment consists of instructions on bowel management and removing reading materials from the toilet. Also, encourage Kegel exercises to strengthen the perineal muscles and the use of muscle relaxants such as Levsin. If, however, these modalities fail to control the problem, an alternative in the treatment of the levator syndrome is the use of electrogalvanic stimulation (EGS) by means of a specially designed rectal probe.

In our experience, approximately two thirds of patients seem to benefit from three or more treatments of 1 hour each, spaced over weekly intervals. In an occasional individual, one session may suffice. About one third report no improvement.

## COCCYGODYNIA

Coccygodynia is part of the levator syndrome, or another manifestation of proctalgia fugax, but the pain is directed to the coccyx. This is probably caused by spasm of the pubococcygeal portion of the levator ani muscle. Classically, the pain is exacerbated when the person rises from a sitting position.

Treatment of this condition is the same as for levator spasm.

Coccygectomy has been offered as a method of treating coccygodynia, usually by orthopedic surgeons. In our opinion, this operation should not be performed for this condition unless the coccyx has been injured or is dislocated. Even under these circumstances, coccygectomy rarely alleviates the pain.

# 17

# Rectal Prolapse, Solitary Rectal Ulcer, Syndrome of the Descending Perineum, and Rectocele

## RECTAL PROLAPSE OR PROCIDENTIA

Rectal prolapse (i.e., procidentia) is an uncommon clinical entity that was recognized in antiquity, having been described in the Ebers Papyrus of 1500 BC. It usually occurs in persons at the extremes of life. The two types of presentation are (a) complete or full-thickness involvement of the bowel and (b) partial or incomplete involving prolapse of the mucosa only. The latter can be circumferential or can involve only a portion of the rectal mucosa.

### Anatomy and Physiology

The normal spine with its vertebral curves and the tilt of the pelvis serve to shift the weight of the abdominal organs forward, away from the pelvic floor, and cause the rectum to follow a serpentine course through the pelvis. The stability of the rectum is greatly aided by the support of the levator ani muscle. An extensive interweaving of the longitudinal fibers of the rectum with the levator fibers creates a stable attachment between the rectum and this muscle. This attachment provides a firm fixation to the pelvic floor, and is an important element in rectal stability (Fig. 17.1) The puborectalis sling functions by elevating the lower end of the rectum and tilting it forward toward the pubis, creating an acute anorectal angle and compressing the structures in front of the rectum to decrease the opening of the pelvic floor. Relaxation of the puborectalis sling results in descent of the pelvic floor, obliterating the anorectal angle so that the rectum becomes more vertical.

During the act of defecation, intraabdominal pressure is increased by contraction of the abdominal wall musculature and the diaphragm. Contraction of the

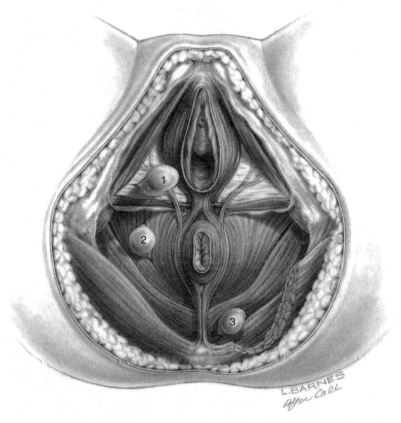

**FIG. 17.1.** Muscles of the pelvic floor showing fixation of the rectum to the levator fibers. Weaknesses in the floor can lead to herniation as is illustrated in several locations: (1) anterior perineal hernia through the urogenital diaphragm; (2) posterior perineal hernia through the levator ani muscle; (3) posterior perineal hernia between the levator ani and coccygeus muscles. (From Cali RL, Pitsch RM, Blatchford GJ, et al. Rare pelvic floor hernias: report of a case and review of the literature. *Dis Colon Rectum* 1992;35:604.)

levator ani muscle is inhibited, the puborectalis sling lengthens, and the pelvic floor descends, thereby obliterating the anorectal angle. The external sphincter muscle, which functionally forms a single unit with the puborectalis sling, relaxes at the same time. The rectum now occupies a vertical position, and the fecal mass is expelled by the contraction of the circular muscle of the rectum combined with the pressure from above. The rectum is held in place by fixation of the levator muscle anteriorly and by the various ligamentous structures laterally when the rectum is in a vertical position. The levator sling returns to its usual support position after defecation.

## Etiology

The precise cause of rectal prolapse is not thoroughly understood, but a number of factors, both congenital and acquired, seem to be implicated in the development of the condition. Possible predisposing influences and associated conditions are summarized below.

Poor bowel habits, especially constipation
Neurologic disease (e.g., congenital anomaly, cauda equina lesion, spinal cord
    injury, senility)
Female gender
Nulliparity
Redundant rectosigmoid
Deep pouch of Douglas
Patulous anus (i.e., weak internal sphincter)
Diastasis of levator ani muscle (i.e., defect in pelvic floor)
Lack of fixation of rectum to sacrum
Intussusception, possibly secondary to colonic lesion
Operative procedure (e.g., hemorrhoidectomy, fistulectomy, abdominoanal
    pull-through)

The unique pelvic anatomy, especially as observed at the time of laparotomy, is thought to play an important role in the cause of prolapse. A redundant rectosigmoid is often seen, as is a deep pouch of Douglas. Whether these are truly causative factors or merely frequently associated anatomic variables is a subject of considerable debate. Similarly, the patulous or weak sphincter mechanism, with diastasis of the levator ani muscle that produces a defect in the pelvic floor, seems more the result of the prolapse than its cause.

In infants, prolapse can be caused by a lack of skeletal support and by excessive intraabdominal pressures from above. In adults, prolapse can result from incomplete skeletal development. A free mesentery to the entire colon and rectum is a congenital anomaly that can undermine the support mechanism. Because of the complicated development of the levator ani muscle and its fixation to the rectum, anomalies of this muscle, including tenuous fixation to the rectum, can occur more often than is realized and may also contribute to instability of the rectum.

Intussusception has been postulated as the primary cause. What initiates the intussusception is not exactly clear, but over time the intussusception pulls the rectum farther from the sacrum as it descends, and eventually the bowel presents at the anal verge. Lack of fixation of the rectum to the sacrum can be observed at the time of laparotomy and with cineradiography. When the act of defecation is viewed by this means or by defecography, the sequence of events is confirmed. A so-called "colorectoanal intussusception" can occur, with a tumor acting as a lead point.

When compared with control subjects, those with rectal prolapse, mucosal prolapse, and solitary rectal ulcer have lower anal pressures, demonstrate a higher incidence of repetitive rectal contractions, and require lower threshold volumes to cause a desire to defecate.

It is hypothesized that the similarity of these observations suggests that the three disease entities share a common pathophysiology.

Rectal prolapse may be a consequence of a number of anorectal surgical procedures, but it is important from the perspective of treatment to distinguish between true procidentia and mucosal prolapse. Surgical injury to the puborectalis muscle, such as what might occur after anal fistula procedures and pull-through operations, also may be a predisposing factor. If a considerable portion of the sphincter has been divided, mucosal prolapse may be seen on the side of the injury.

Diseases of the nervous system and lesions of the cauda equina can contribute to rectal prolapse. Excessive pressure on the pelvic floor, particularly when related to attenuated muscle, is another causative factor.

Patients in psychiatric hospitals and nursing homes are not uncommonly afflicted with this otherwise rare condition. The reason for the frequency of mental disturbance is not clearly understood, but it may have something to do with a systemic degenerative process.

In adults, an overwhelming majority of rectal prolapses occur in women (90%). The peak incidence occurs in the sixth decade. Multiparity may be a possible causative factor, ranging from 39% to 58%. Such rates of nulliparity are much greater than would be expected from the general population. With the frequent occurrence of bowel management problems in this disease, the most likely candidate for rectal prolapse is a neurotic, constipated, childless woman.

## Clinical Features and Evaluation

The most frequent primary complaint is referable to the prolapse itself: three fourths of patients report the protrusion. Problems with bowel regulation and incontinence are also common presenting features. Almost one half of patients have a history of constipation. Significant bleeding is rarely seen unless the prolapse is massive or irreducible.

Fecal incontinence associated with prolapse is a frequent complaint. Some suggest that, because of stretch injury to pudendal and perineal nerves, loss of continence in individuals with rectal prolapse is secondary to the prolonged protrusion. Findings indicate that denervation causes pelvic floor weakness, with prolapse and incontinence in some patients; in others, however, prolapse occurs without detectable abnormality of the pelvic musculature.

Incontinence becomes more severe as the protrusion increases in degree. Dilatation of the canal by the mass results in further relaxation of the sphincter muscles and further prolapse. Mucous discharge can also become a problem. Protrusion can occur when lifting or coughing, not necessarily solely on defecation. Manual replacement eventually becomes necessary, and ultimately, the mass may protrude from the anus most of the time. Infrequently, the prolapse becomes incarcerated or even strangulated if it has occurred after excessive straining. Transanal evisceration of the small bowel through a rent in the protruding rectum has also been reported.

The duration of symptoms before the patient seeks specialized attention is often prolonged. This may be a reflection of the patient's psyche, but too often it represents failure of the family physician to recognize the entity and to recommend appropriate consultation. Usually, the diagnosis of a full-thickness prolapse presents no problem (Fig. 17.2); it can be associated with uterine descensus, uterine prolapse, or cystocele.

When symptoms are suggestive of rectal prolapse, having the patient sit on the toilet and bear down is often the only means by which rectal prolapse can be visualized.

An important part of the examination is to determine the tone and contractility of the sphincter mechanism. If sphincter tone is poor and the anus patulous, and if the patient is unable to contract the puborectalis sling voluntarily, functional results after repair of the prolapse may be suboptimal. On the other hand, if the patient has relatively good sphincter tone and contractility, good bowel control can be ultimately anticipated.

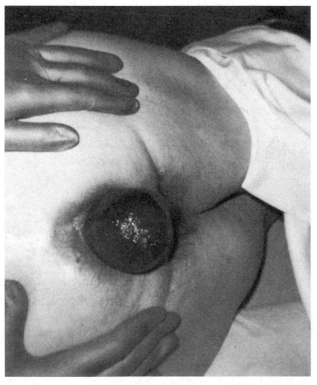

**FIG. 17.2.** Standard, full-thickness rectal prolapse or procidentia. (From Corman ML, Veidenheimer MC, Coller JA. Managing rectal prolapse. *Geriatrics* 1974;29:87.)

A thorough endoscopic examination is necessary in individuals with any anorectal complaint; this is particularly true in patients with rectal prolapse. It is important to specify the degree of prolapse and whether it is full thickness or mucosal. Occasionally, a polyp or carcinoma of the rectum or sigmoid colon may be the "lead point" for an intussusception. A high index of suspicion should be maintained, especially in a male patient who has no evidence of neurologic disease. Total colonic evaluation, either by means of barium enema or by colonoscopy, is mandatory, Flexible fiberoptic sigmoidoscopy or colonoscopy may reveal the straightened rectal segment and the intussusception if the examination is performed with the patient straining and in a sitting position. Likewise, cinefluorography can be helpful if the diagnosis is in question.

As in the evaluation of patients who have sustained obstetric injury and who are incontinent, pudendal nerve terminal motor latency (PNTML) study should be considered for individuals with procidentia. With associated pudendal neuropathy, the prognosis for improved bowel control following surgical repair of the prolapse is less favorable than if no conduction abnormality were present. Although the presence of pudendal neuropathy does not contraindicate repair, it is helpful to know this in advance to give the patient an understanding of the likelihood of resolution of the incontinence problem after cure of the prolapse.

## PREPROLAPSE, SIGMOIDORECTAL INTUSSUSCEPTION, INTERNAL INTUSSUSCEPTION OF THE RECTUM

As with rectal prolapse, women are overwhelmingly affected by preprolapse, sigmoidorectal intussusception, and internal intussusception of the rectum.

The patient may complain of a feeling of fullness or a lump inside the rectum. Symptoms can become exacerbated by prolonged periods of standing or sitting. Often, the individual experiences the perception of an obstruction when attempting to pass flatus or to have a bowel movement. A sensation may be felt of incomplete evacuation, and manual pressure used to eliminate is frequently reported. A number of patients complain that "something drops down and blocks the anal opening." Pain may be present in the perineal area with occasional sciatic or obturator radiation. However, the most frequent indication for an operation, according to one observer, is the complaint of incontinence.

Proctosigmoidoscopic assessment by an inexperienced examiner can be singularly unrewarding, especially if the prone jackknife position is used. Careful inspection of the mucosa may reveal an area of hyperemia and edema from 8 to 15 cm, and the bowel wall may appear to be thickened. Occasionally, an intussusception of the rectosigmoid may be perceived. With this history and with the proctoscopic findings described, a strong likelihood of preprolapse exists.

### Defecography

Radiologic study of the rectum by means of defecography is the most effective means for identifying the preprolapse condition and other defecatory disorders. Fluoroscopic and spot filming in the lateral projection is done with the patient sitting and straining. Much of the physiologic nature of defecation is lost when the patient lies down, as if for a standard barium enema examination.

The normal anorectal angle is $90.00° \pm 4.76°$ at rest and $111.00° \pm 5.02°$ during straining, but others suggest that this determination lacks clinical relevance. Besides intussusception and increased distance between the rectum and sacrum, defecographic abnormalities that can be observed include the following:

- Megarectum
- Unsuspected incontinence
- Abnormal anorectal angle
- Nonrelaxing puborectalis (i.e., obstructed defecation)
- Abnormal perineal descent (i.e., >2.5 cm)
- Mucosal prolapse
- Solitary ulcer
- Rectocele
- Enterocele

Findings suggestive of preprolapse include funnel-shaped configuration of the rectum, lack of fixation of the rectum to the sacrum, excessive rectosigmoid mobility, the formation of a "ring pocket," and, of course, a demonstrable intussusception. As with typical rectal prolapse, a redundant sigmoid colon with a wide, deep pouch of Douglas may be seen. Irrespective of the radiologic findings, however, be circumspect and do not attempt to over-interpret possible abnormalities.

Defecography has no real place in the evaluation of individuals with procidentia.

## Colpocystodefecography

Colpocystodefecography is a technique that combines vaginal opacification, voiding cystography, and defecography. It may be more useful than clinical evaluation for the diagnosis of preprolapse and enterocele.

## Results

Retrorectal sacral fixation in patients with internal prolapse has relieved symptoms with no resulting morbidity. The Delorme procedure appears equally useful, with relief of pelvic symptoms and of severe constipation. Late follow-up revealed sustained symptomatic relief in more than 70% of cases. Another alternative is reduction of rectal reservoir capacity by means of multiple rubber ring ligations or staple excision of the redundant mucosa. Polyvinyl alcohol sponge (i.e., Ivalon) abdominal rectopexy for internal prolapse has been used with mixed functional results. If obstructed defecation is part of the clinical presentation, this operation probably should not be offered. Suspension operations in patients with obstructed defecation caused by preprolapse resolves defeco-graphic abnormalities, but the patients are generally not completely relieved of their symptoms.

## SOLITARY RECTAL ULCER SYNDROME

Solitary ulcer of the rectum is an unusual condition. Unfortunately, the term is confusing, because the syndrome does not necessarily have to be solitary, nor does it have to be confined to the rectum; in fact, it can be polypoid rather than ulcerating. The condition is often confused with nonspecific inflammatory bowel disease, villous adenoma, colitis cystica profunda, and other inflammatory and neoplastic diseases affecting the colon and rectum.

### Etiology

The cause of solitary rectal ulcer syndrome is uncertain, but chronic constipation and fecal impaction may play a role. Patients who frequently resort to manual disimpaction can produce an inflammatory reaction, ulceration, and fibrosis, autoeroticism has been thought to be involved with many of these individuals, so much so that Turnbull suggested that the treatment of the condition should be bilateral long-arm casts. Additionally, the injudicious use of ergotamine suppositories has been reported to cause solitary rectal ulcer. Another possible mechanism is the failure of inhibition of puborectalis muscle contraction, which may result in a repeated desire to defecate and cause the persistent need to strain to pass stool. However, most observers believe that the solitary ulcer syndrome is a distinct clinical inflammatory manifestation that is associated with rectal prolapse or, more specifically, the preprolapse condition.

### Clinical Features

Solitary rectal ulcer syndrome is usually seen in women. Symptoms typically constitute various bowel complaints: constipation, diarrhea, passage of mucus, tenesmus, rectal bleeding, and proctalgia fugax. Classically, physical examination reveals an ulcer with hyperemic edges and surrounding induration. Alternatively, exophytic lesions may be seen. A combination of ulcerating and polypoid lesions is often noted on the anterior rectal wall, usually at a level of 6 to 8 cm.

### Histopathology

A number of characteristic features permit the pathologist to distinguish solitary rectal ulcer from other lesions. Inflammatory changes can consist of replacement of the normal lamina propria by fibroblasts arranged at right angles to the muscularis mucosae (Fig. 17.3). The microscopic appearance, however, is variable and can include loss of normal polarity of the glandular epithelial cells,

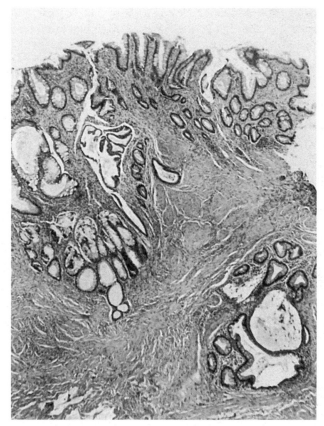

**FIG. 17.3.** Solitary rectal ulcer. Markedly hyperplastic muscularis mucosa separates a group of glands in the submucosa (*lower right*) from the overlying mucosa. Fibers of muscularis mucosa extend into and obliterate the lamina propria between crypts. (Original magnification ×40; courtesy of Rodger C. Haggitt, M.D.)

shortening of the crypts, mucin depletion, mucosal thickening, and inflammatory reaction in the submucosa. Many of the manifestations are those that have been described for patients with inflammatory bowel disease. Electron microscopic changes have also been identified; these include dense collagen deposition within the lamina propria as well as numerous fibroblasts.

## Physiologic and Contrast Studies

Anorectal physiologic evaluation of patients with solitary rectal ulcer has been reported. Defecography has frequently revealed an occult rectal prolapse. Other findings that have been noted include failure of the sphincter to relax on defecation, high intrarectal pressure, increased anorectal angle, perineal descent, and impaired sensation on balloon inflation of the rectum. It has been suggested that a high evacuation pressure can cause mucosal ulceration by exposing the rectal wall to a high transmural pressure gradient.

## Transrectal Ultrasound

Transrectal ultrasonography has been used in an attempt to understand the pathogenesis of solitary rectal ulcer syndrome. A thickened rectal wall is a common finding. Poor relaxation of the puborectalis muscle during straining is noted in three fourths of patients. The enlargement of the muscularis propria indicates a chronic mechanical load on the rectal wall and suggests that ulcerations are formed as a consequence of this phenomenon. Nonrelaxation of the puborectalis muscle can be an important element in the pathogenesis of this condition.

## Management

Treatment of solitary rectal ulcer syndrome is problematic. A high-fiber diet and bowel management instruction can ameliorate symptoms for many individuals. With the characteristic rectal abnormality, consider a trial of hydrocortisone enemas. Others have observed a marked reduction in symptoms through the use of sucralfate retention enemas; however, histologic changes persisted. Rarely, a colostomy is indicated for the treatment of massive rectal bleeding.

Because operations designed to treat rectal prolapse have been of benefit to patients with the solitary ulcer syndrome, a high index of suspicion for the presence of sigmoidorectal intussusception (i.e., preprolapse) should be maintained when the characteristic changes in the rectal mucosa are perceived. Anorectal physiologic evaluation, specifically defecography, is strongly encouraged under these circumstances.

## Results

In the experience of the Cleveland Clinic, intractable symptoms led to surgery in 60% of patients, with symptomatic improvement noted in more than two thirds of them. Further findings were that the optimal surgical procedure is still indeterminate, but rectopexy, local excision, and fecal diversion seem to achieve improvement in most patients.

## SYNDROME OF THE DESCENDING PERINEUM

When a healthy person increases intraabdominal pressure and relaxes the pelvic musculature, no significant change can be observed in the concavity of the perineum. However, in patients with chronic illness, malnutrition, and preprolapse, perineal descent may be observed, with the normal concavity being obliterated when the patient strains. In those with this syndrome, either the anal canal is situated several centimeters below a line drawn between the pubis and coccyx, or it descends 3 or 4 cm during straining. The perineal area can even descend 5 or 6 cm in some persons (Fig. 17.4).

A descending perineum is the result of injury to the pelvic floor muscles, especially the levatores. Patients usually complain of tenesmus, difficulty evacuating, and incontinence. The problem with bowel control lies in excessive straining with defecation, which stretches the pudendal nerves and results in anorectal muscular atrophy. Prospective studies to assess the correlation between perineal descent and pudendal neuropathy found no correlation, concluding that these may represent independent findings despite their being frequently observed in those with disordered defecation.

Treatment is usually directed toward bowel management (e.g., diet, laxatives, suppositories) and education (e.g., avoiding straining). When incontinence is the major complaint, restoration of the pelvic floor, with possible implantation of mesh, and resection or suspension of the rectum may be necessary. An alternative is to hitch the posterior wall of the rectum to the sacrum through a transcoccygeal (i.e., Kraske) approach (Fig. 17.5). The operation can be combined with reefing of the levatores muscles as well as an anterior perineorrhaphy. Unfortunately, almost irrespective of the various options that may be implemented, results are less than ideal. A possible exception to this is a new innovation for pelvic floor laxity (including enterocele, rectocele, and cystocele) by performing total pelvic Marlex repair. This complicated operation involves stripping the parietal and visceral peritoneum from the pelvis floor; separating the posterior vaginal from the rectum all the way down to the perineal body; and then implanting a trapezoid-shaped Marlex mesh with two additional strips—securing the

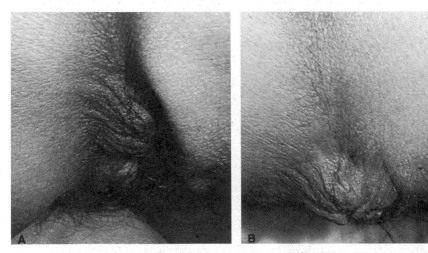

**FIG. 17.4.** Descending perineum (perineal descensus). **A.** At rest. **B.** During straining. (From De los Rios Margrina E. *Color atlas of anorectal diseases.* Philadelphia: WB Saunders, 1980.)

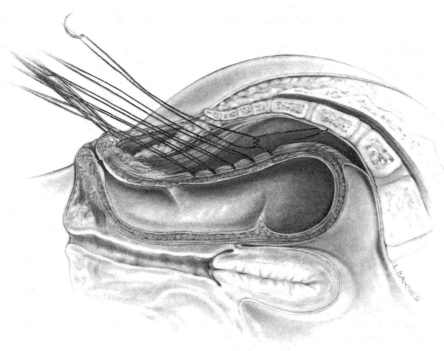

**FIG. 17.5.** A series of plication sutures are placed 1 cm apart in the posterior wall of the rectum. Sutures are then sewn individually to the anterior periosteum of the sacrum. (Adapted from Nichols DH. Retrorectal levatorplasty for anal and perineal prolapse. *Surg Gynecol Obstet* 1982;154:251.)

mesh at the introitus, at the adjacent endopelvic fascia, and to the upper sacrum. In addition, the Marlex is secured to Cooper's ligament on each side as part of the anterior fixation.

## DIFFERENTIAL DIAGNOSIS OF RECTAL PROLAPSE

Prolapsed hemorrhoids is the condition that most often misleads examiners into believing the problem is procidentia. A protruding mass of hemorrhoidal tissue tends to be lobular; a definite sulcus or groove is present between the masses of tissue and the perianal skin. With large hemorrhoids that have become edematous and thrombosed, the enlarged size frequently gives the incorrect impression that the entire rectal wall is protruding. However, with rectal prolapse, concentric rings of intact tissue are evident throughout the entire circumference.

Sometimes, the differential diagnosis includes a large rectal polypoid lesion prolapsing through the anus. The mass should be replaced and the rectum examined manually and endoscopically. A polypoid lesion is usually mobile and can be separated from the lower part of the rectum and anal canal by digital examination. Proctosigmoidoscopic examination should clarify any differential diagnostic problem.

The anal deformities associated with radical hemorrhoidectomy, fistula surgery, and pull-through procedures can produce an ectropion or mucosal prolapse, but should pose no difficulty in differential diagnosis. It is extremely important, however, to distinguish full-thickness prolapse from mucosal prolapse because treatment of the two conditions is decidedly different.

## Treatment of Rectal Prolapse

In general, partial or incomplete (i.e., mucosal) prolapse should be treated by an anal operation. If only one quadrant is involved, simple excision, leaving the wound open, may be all that is required. If the area involved is circumferential, excision with an S-plasty may be considered.

With respect to the management of acute, incarcerated (i.e., irreducible) rectal prolapse, a local anesthetic to paralyze the sphincters may effect reduction. Others suggest a spinal or general anesthetic. Placement of ordinary table sugar on the bowel mucosa can result in decreased edema and spontaneous or easily induced reduction from the desiccating effect; this is a well-recognized technique in the veterinary literature. Emergency resection is rarely indicated, usually because of gangrene.

If surgical treatment for incomplete or complete prolapse is contraindicated, or if the patient refuses an operation, a number of noninvasive approaches and limited office procedures can be used, as follows:

### *Nonoperative Treatment of Rectal Prolapse*

Adhesive strapping of buttocks
Manual anal support during defecation
Correction of constipation
Establishment of workable time and method of defecation
Perineal strengthening exercises
Electronic stimulation
Injection of sclerosing agent
Rubber ring ligation
Infrared coagulation

Although instructing the patient on proper bowel management and perineal exercises can be salutary and other methods offer some degree of palliation of symptoms, these measures cannot be expected to produce a cure.

More than 50 operations have been designed to treat complete rectal prolapse. Most are variations of a few basic modes of therapy and depend on the surgeon's concept of the anatomic defect. The options for treatment include narrowing of the anal orifice, obliteration of the peritoneal pouch of Douglas, restoration of the pelvic floor, resection of the bowel (by an abdominal, perineal, or transsacral approach), and suspension or fixation of the rectum to the sacrum or to other structures. Additional operations listed below combine one or more of these approaches.

## Modes of Surgical Therapy for Rectal Prolapse

Narrowing of the anal orifice
Obliteration of the peritoneal pouch of Douglas
Restoration of the pelvic floor
Resection of bowel
    Transabdominal
    Perineal
    Transsacral
Suspension or fixation of the rectum
    To the sacrum
    To the pubis
    To other structures
Combinations of two or more of the above

### General Principles

All patients having surgery for rectal prolapse should have a thorough mechanical cleansing of the bowel with an orally administered laxative and colonic irrigation the morning of the operation. Nonabsorbable, orally administered antibiotics should be ordered routinely whenever resection is contemplated or intrusion into the bowel is a possibility. Systemic, broad-spectrum antibiotics are advised during the perioperative period, especially if foreign material is to be implanted.

Postoperative care for abdominal operations is essentially the same as for any bowel resection. Intravenous fluid replacement is continued until flatus is passed. A progressive diet is instituted, and the patient is discharged when the bowels have functioned. A longer period of ileus may be observed when the physician operates for rectal prolapse than when the same procedure is undertaken for other disease processes in the rectosigmoid.

### Narrowing of the Anal Orifice

#### Thiersch Repair

In the older, poor-risk patient, many surgeons prefer to use the Thiersch operation. This procedure can be performed with a local anesthetic, making it a satisfactory technique for these individuals. In the classic operation, silver wire was placed into the perianal space to encircle and narrow the anus. Today, surgeons have abandoned the use of wire because of the complications of breakage and ulceration. Other materials, such as nylon, Mersilene, Dacron, polypropylene mesh (i.e., Marlex), Teflon, fascia lata, silicone rubber, Silastic, and Dacron-impregnated Silastic are used for the same purpose.

### Operative Technique

The patient is placed in the lithotomy position on the operating table, and the perianal area is prepared with an antiseptic solution. A local anesthetic can be used to infiltrate the area; however, for convenience, a general or spinal anesthetic may be more desirable. A small incision is made in the anterior and posterior positions, 1 cm outside the anal verge (Fig. 17.6A). The suture is passed from anterior to posterior on either side of the anus in the ischiorectal fossa (Fig. 17.6B). The knot should be buried posteriorly. A no. 16 or no. 18 Hegar dilator is an appropriate standard for determining luminal size. To avoid a bulky knot, suturing is required when using Mersilene tape; alternatively, a stapling device can be used to secure the tape. The two wounds are primarily closed with 3-0 or 4-0 long-term absorbable sutures.

### Postoperative Care

Frequent examinations are necessary to be certain that fecal impaction does not develop. Stool softeners, laxatives, suppositories, or enemas may be required. A topical antiseptic ointment, such as povidone-iodine (i.e., Betadine), is advised. Despite the relative simplicity of the operation, the difficulty with postoperative management implies that the procedure ideally should be performed on an inpatient basis. The patient is discharged when bowel function has been established.

### Complications

Complications are frequently seen with Thiersch and Thiersch-type repairs. Patients often complain of the sensation of "sitting on a lump." Tenesmus, a feeling of incomplete evacuation, and bowel-management difficulties are the rule rather than the exception. The implant can profoundly narrow the anal opening to the extent that removal becomes necessary. Wound infection is a common problem, the next most frequent reason for removal of the material. Finally, if the prolapse recurs, the rectum can become incarcerated and even strangulated. Recurrent prolapse following a Thiersch repair requires urgent evaluation and treatment. If for whatever reason—erosion, sepsis, or obstruction—the material must be removed, the operation can be performed again once the wounds have healed.

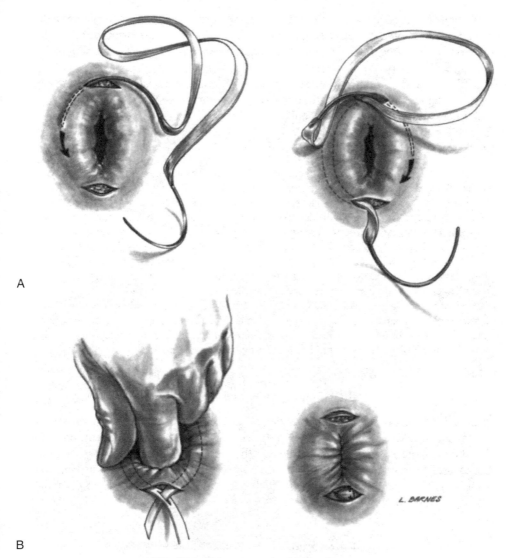

**FIG. 17.6.** Thiersch repair with Mersilene tape.

### Other Thiersch-Type Repairs

Other approaches have been advocated as alternatives to the Thiersch operation. Marlex, Mersilene, and polypropylene meshes have been used. Mersilene mesh, a woven polyester fiber, has been used as well. A Dacron-impregnated Silastic sheet has also been used. The operation is similar to that of any Thiersch approach. A strip is cut to 1.5 cm wide, with care taken to prepare it in such a way that it is elastic along its longitudinal axis. An overlap of 1 cm is created, and a linear stapler is used to secure it in place. All wounds are primarily closed. The particular appeal of this material is that it can stretch; on rectal examination, it simulates a normal sphincter.

Full-thickness prolapse has been treated by implanting Silastic rods. These (4 mm in diameter) are inserted through two small stab incisions. The two ends are secured by a self-locking plastic clip, which fixes the overlapping ends of the rod and secures them into place by a cable gun. These appear to provide adequate control of the prolapse in 70% of patients.

*Comment*: It can be stated without equivocation that procidentia has stimulated more ingenious efforts at surgical treatment than virtually any other condition. A multitude of other techniques and devices has been suggested with similar results. Evaluation of the long-term results of the classic Thiersch procedure (i.e., using wire) is absent from contemporary writings, and even the newer materials are often described with little more than case report experience. The Thiersch-type operations, in my opinion, should rarely be employed; in most circumstances, the complication rate is extremely high. Furthermore, the procedure does not cure the prolapse; it most certainly would recur if the material were removed. Finally, the operation serves only to exacerbate bowel management problems.

However, in certain limited situations, the Thiersch-type operation can be recommended. For example, with a patient who "cannot tolerate a haircut," it is a simple and reasonably safe alternative. And, for more convenient management of patients in nursing homes and psychiatric facilities, it is certainly appropriate to offer this suboptimal choice.

### Obliteration of the Pouch of Douglas

The Moschcowitz procedure was designed with the theory that the cause of rectal prolapse is a sliding hernia. The technique involves the placement of serial purse-string sutures into the floor of the pelvis to obliterate the pouch of Douglas. The recurrence rate, however, is close to 50%. The lack of success of others and the theoretic premise on which it is based would seem to imply that the procedure should be abandoned.

### Restoration of the Pelvic Floor

Restoration of the pelvic floor by reefing the levatores muscles and obliterating the pouch of Douglas was initially described by Graham in 1942. In subsequent writings, a number of authors have advocated this operation, either alone or in combination with other modes of surgical therapy. The procedure can be accomplished through the abdomen or the perineum, or after removing the coccyx or lower sacrum. Reefing the levatores transabdominally can be performed anterior or posterior to the rectum, although the latter may be technically difficult to accomplish. When it is employed with sacral fixation or resection, restoration of the pelvic floor is an unnecessary and often tedious maneuver that does not increase the likelihood of cure. If plication of the levatores was the sole method of treatment for rectal prolapse, the incidence of recurrence would be prohibitively high.

## Resection of the Bowel

### Anterior Resection

Anterior resection for the treatment of rectal prolapse has many advantages over other techniques, but it also has a number of potential concerns. One major advantage is the removal of the redundant sigmoid colon; this excess colon can pose a problem in some patients who are to have suspension or fixation procedures. A mobile sigmoid can predispose to torsion or to volvulus. Furthermore, those who have resection may have some bowel complaints ameliorated, especially constipation, if the redundant segment is removed. A sling operation, however, can worsen bowel symptoms.

The major disadvantage of resection is the possibility of an anastomotic leak, but this risk should be minimal. The technique for performing anterior resection of the bowel is described in Chapter 22. It is important to remember that when this operation is performed for prolapse, the rectum should be mobilized to the level of the lateral ligaments, but the anastomosis should be performed at or just below the sacral promontory (Fig. 17.7). Mobilization of the rectum in these patients can be accomplished easily. The broad, deep pouch of Douglas, with the lack of fixation of the rectum, expedites the dissection.

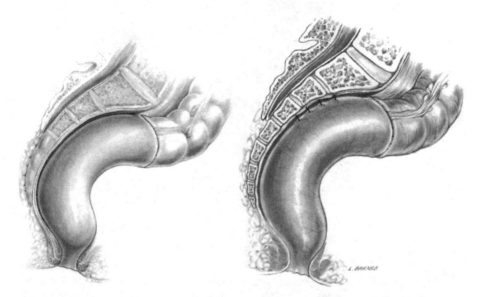

**FIG. 17.7.** Anterior resection is performed with anastomosis at or just below the sacral promontory. Sacral fixation can be performed with or without concomitant resection. Sutures are placed directly into the muscularis of the rectum and through the periosteum of the sacrum.

*Results*

Recurrence rates when anterior resection has been used range from 2% to 9%, and complications occur in 15% to 30%. Reportedly, the procedure has also been carried out successfully through a laparoscopically assisted approach.

Despite the success of this operation, dependence on adhesions to fix the rectum posteriorly is unpredictable. Therefore, some authors advise some form of rectal fixation when anterior resection is performed.

### *Anterior Resection with Sacral Fixation*

A modification of anterior resection to include fixation of the distal rectal segment to the sacrum has been suggested. The posterior rectal wall or intact lateral ligaments are secured to the sacrum with three or four heavy, nonabsorbable sutures; the redundant sigmoid colon is then removed (Fig. 17.8).

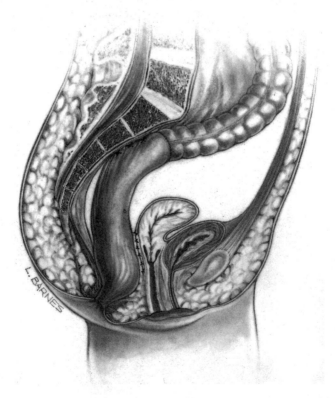

**FIG. 17.8.** The rectum is mobilized and elevated, with the lateral rectal stalks sutured to the periosteum of the sacrum. The endopelvic fascia anterior is also sutured to the rectum, with obliteration of the cul-de-sac. The excess peritoneum is excised. (It is believed that the authors no longer apply an anterior fixation—MLC.) (From Frykman HM, Goldberg SM. The surgical treatment of rectal procidentia. *Surg Gynecol Obstet* 1969;129:1225.)

## Results

Reported recurrence rates after the use of this modification of anterior resection range from 0% to 2 %. A particular concern when suturing the rectum to the presacral fascia is the possibility of causing severe bleeding. Because the results are so favorable without this added maneuver, it seems prudent to limit the risk. It is not surprising that, because most patients are constipated and are found to have a redundant sigmoid colon, anterior resection should yield optimal functional results.

### Perineal Resection

Perineal resection of the prolapsed segment, an operation that has been employed for nearly 100 years, appears to be a relatively simple means of addressing the problem; unfortunately, the relatively high rate of recurrence has dissuaded many surgeons from adopting this approach. It can, however, still be used in the rare instance of gangrene of the prolapsed bowel or when the patient cannot tolerate a laparotomy. Anastomotic leakage is still a concern, but with avoidance of tension on the suture line and attention to preservation of the blood supply, the risk should be minimal.

### Altemeier Operation

With the patient in the lithotomy position and an indwelling Foley catheter in place, the perianal area is prepared and draped. The prolapse is exteriorized, and its apex is grasped with clamps (Fig. 17.9A). A circumferential incision is

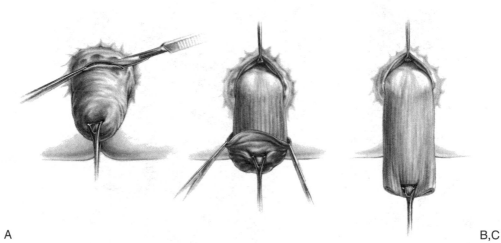

A

B,C

**FIG. 17.9.** Altemeier procedure. **A.** An incision is made circumferentially in the anal canal, just above the dentate line. **B,C.** The rectum is mobilized and completely everted.

made through all layers of the outer bowel wall just proximal to the muco-cutaneous junction (Fig. 17.9B). When the circumferential incision is completed, clamps are reapplied to the distal edge of rectum, and the prolapse is delivered as a single loop of exteriorized bowel (Fig. 17.9C). Any hernial sac located on the anterior surface of the bowel is identified and the peritoneal cavity entered (Fig. 17.10A). The redundant colon is delivered through the defect (Fig. 17.10B). The peritoneum is repaired using a continuous suture to obliterate the sac (Fig. 17.11).

A modification adopted for this procedure involves plication of the levator ani muscle. This maneuver seems to be associated with a lower incidence of recurrence and may have an ameliorative effect on the subsequent problems with bowel control. The levator ani muscles are identified and reefed anterior or posterior to the bowel by interrupted long-term, absorbable sutures (Fig. 17.12), which eliminates the large defect in the pelvic diaphragm. The redundant intestine is then divided in half by anterior and posterior incisions carried to the point of the proposed resection. The intestine is transected obliquely and progressively, completing the anastomosis of the intestinal wall to the anal ring in each quadrant (Fig. 17.13). Anastomosis is effected with an interrupted, long-term absorbable suture technique; no drains are used. In principle, ideally, the pelvic

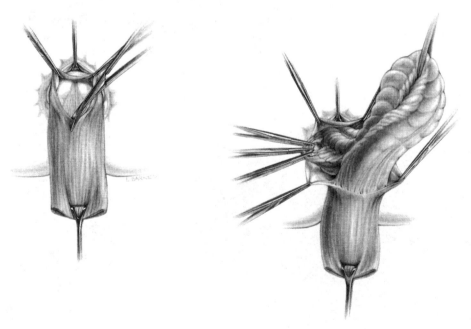

A

B

**FIG. 17.10.** Altemeier procedure. **A.** The peritoneal reflection is identified and opened. **B.** Any redundant bowel is delivered through the peritoneal defect.

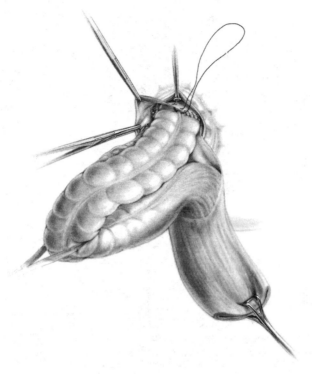

**FIG. 17.11.** Altemeier procedure. The peritoneum is closed, and the sutures are anchored to the bowel wall, as illustrated.

pouch is obliterated, the levatores plicated, and the redundant bowel resected. However, the rectum is not fixed to the sacrum.

### Results

Despite the successful experience of some authors, the relatively complex technique and the unfamiliar approach dissuade most surgeons from attempting this operation. Reported recurrence rates range from 3% to 10%.

A simplified approach to perineal rectosigmoidectomy without levator plication, using the circular stapling device has been described and results are similar.

### Delorme Procedure

The Delorme operation, less commonly used today, is another operative approach performed by the perineal route. With the patient in the lithotomy or the prone jackknife position, a circumferential incision is made 1 cm proximal

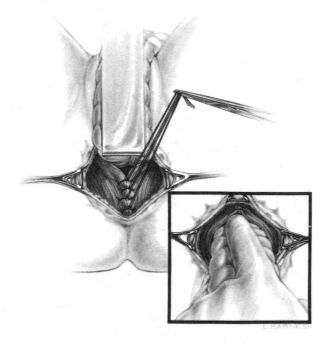

**FIG. 17.12.** Altemeier procedure. The levator ani muscle is reefed anteriorly or, as illustrated, posteriorly, with long-term absorbable sutures. Care should be taken to avoid narrowing the rectum. A finger should be able to pass easily through the defect (*inset*).

to the dentate line, similar to that for the Altemeier procedure (Fig. 17.14). Using electrocautery, the mucosa is stripped to the apex of the protruding bowel. Infiltrating the submucosa with saline or a dilute epinephrine solution can facilitate dissection. The redundant mucosa is excised, and the denuded muscularis is pleated longitudinally, collapsing the bowel like an accordion (Fig. 17.15). The edges of the mucosa are then sutured. Alternatively, the mucosa–muscularis layers can be directly reapproximated in a circumferential fashion with multiple interrupted absorbable sutures.

Complications from this operation are common; they include hemorrhage, hematoma, suture line dehiscence, stricture, incontinence, and, of course, recurrence.

### Results

Recurrence rates after the use of the Delorme procedure range from 7% to 22%. Additionally, one half to two thirds of patients experience some improvement in bowel control. Most surgeons are reluctant to consider this operation because of the cumbersome dissection and the relatively high recurrence rate when the procedure

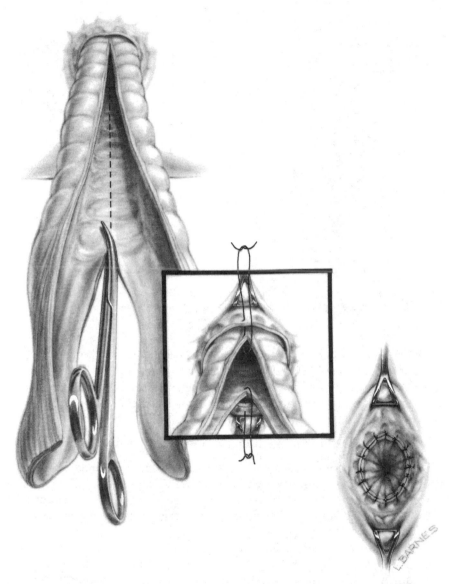

**FIG. 17.13.** Altemeier procedure. The redundant bowel is incised longitudinally and sutured in the anterior and posterior midline to the residual cuff of the anal mucosa (*inset*). After the redundant bowel is trimmed, interrupted sutures are placed between the anal canal and the underlying internal sphincter to the full thickness of the rectum.

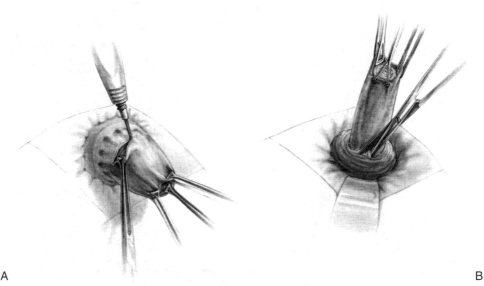

A
B

**FIG. 17.14.** Delorme procedure. **A.** The mucosa is circumferentially incised above the dentate line. **B.** Submucosal stripping is carried out as far cephalad as is possible.

is not performed with meticulous care. Even under the best of circumstances, the operation cannot possibly be as gratifying as the previously discussed Altemeier procedure for resecting a large prolapse. However, in the individual at poor risk, this approach appears to be acceptable in the hands of a competent surgeon.

### Combined Abdominal and Perineal Operation

The perineal operation is essentially the same as that described by Altemeier. The abdominal operation, however, is done several days later. Full mobilization of the rectum is carried out, and a plication of the ligamentous structures lateral to the rectum is performed. The pouch of Douglas is obliterated in the manner of Moschowitz.

This is an extensive operation requiring two major procedures. Although the belt-and-suspenders approach can be useful under some circumstances, simpler and equally reliable alternatives are found to this procedure. Furthermore, in recent years no reports on this approach have been published.

### Transsacral Resection

The transsacral operation uses the approach to the rectum described by Kraske for resection of rectal cancer (see Chapter 23). An incision is made overlying the sacrum and coccyx, and the latter is disarticulated and removed. The levator ani muscles are divided to expose the rectum. The peritoneum is incised anteriorly

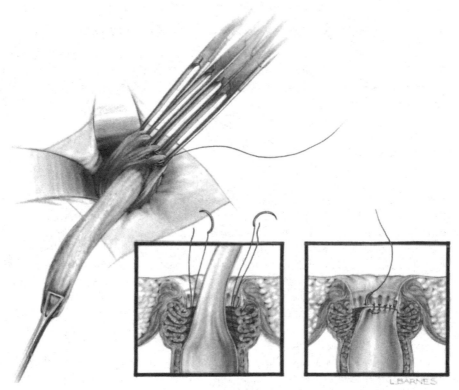

**FIG. 17.15.** The circular muscle of the rectum is prepared for suturing by the placement of serial Allis clamps. Plication is carried out using 2-0 long-term absorbable sutures. The insets illustrate the completed "anastomosis" after the redundant mucosa has been amputated. (Adapted from Berman IR, Harris MS, Rabeler MB. Delorme's transrectal excision for internal prolapse: patient selection, technique, and three-year follow-up. *Dis Colon Rectum* 1990;33:573.)

and the rectum fully mobilized. The redundant colon is liberated and delivered through the sacral wound. The levator ani muscles are approximated anterior to the rectum, the peritoneum is closed, and the redundant bowel is resected. After the anastomosis is completed, all wounds are primarily closed.

The theoretic advantages of this procedure are that the operation does not require a laparotomy and that the levator ani muscles are reconstituted, thus narrowing the defect in the pelvic floor. The pouch of Douglas is obliterated, and the rectum is secured posteriorly. The major disadvantage is that the patient has a painful sacrococcygeal wound that is subject to infection. The possibility of a fecal fistula is well recognized when this procedure is undertaken for other indications.

*Comment:* As with other procedures for the treatment of this condition, the esoteric, unfamiliar operation described above contraindicates its use for most surgeons, particularly in light of the simpler alternatives available for cure. Again, no reports have been published of its use in a number of years.

## Suspension or Fixation of the Rectum

### Teflon or Marlex Sling Repair, or the Ripstein Operation

Arguably, the most common surgical approach for the treatment of rectal prolapse in the United States today is the sling repair, a procedure that was described initially by Ripstein in 1965, and is sometimes called by his name. The sling is made out of Teflon, Marlex, or Gore-Tex.

### Technique

The patient is placed in the Trendelenburg position on the operating table, and a midline hypogastric incision is made. Exploration of the abdomen usually reveals the characteristic defect of redundant sigmoid colon, lack of fixation of the rectum to the sacrum, and a deep pouch of Douglas. The rectosigmoid is mobilized, the presacral space is entered, and the inferior mesenteric vessels carefully preserved. Mobilization of the rectum to the level of the levator ani muscle can be accomplished easily. This is a particularly important maneuver that facilitates adhesion or passive fixation of the rectum to the sacrum. Sutures can be placed into the periosteum of the sacrum approximately 1 cm to the right of the midline by using a one-half circle Mayo trocar-point needle. Three or four nonabsorbable sutures are used. The Teflon mesh (or Marlex or Gore-Tex) can be secured to the sacrum in one of three ways.

The Teflon mesh is trimmed to approximately 4 cm wide and secured in place along the right side of the sacrum. At this point in the operation, it is important for the assistant to maintain proximal traction while the mesh is anchored to the muscularis propria of the rectum. If the rectum is not under tension in a cephalad direction and if redundant rectum is left below the mesh, prolapse will recur. Nonabsorbable sutures are placed from the mesh into the rectal wall. After the mesh has been laid around two thirds of the bowel, the redundant material is appropriately trimmed so that it can be secured without tension. Sutures are then anchored in the sacrum on the left side and placed into the mesh. A defect of approximately 1 cm is present posteriorly. The remaining sutures on the left side are placed through the mesh and in the muscularis of the bowel.

Another method of securing the mesh is to place a single row of sutures into the midline of the sacrum. The middle of the mesh is sutured into place and the material brought onto either side of the rectum. With proximal traction maintained on the rectum, the mesh is anchored, leaving a 1-cm defect anteriorly. This is a simpler technique than the former, but it has the potential risk of leaving only a solitary row of sutures posteriorly with which to hold back the rectum.

A simpler modification for attaching the mesh to the sacrum has been proposed using a power fascial stapler to accomplish fixation expeditiously and with essentially no risk of inducing hemorrhage. Following suspension, it is not necessary to reperitonealize the floor of the pelvis. If hemostasis is secure, no pelvic drains are used.

## Management of Presacral Hemorrhage

If a presacral vein is entered, the ligature can be tied. All too often, however, the basivertebral vein exits directly from the bone, and massive hemorrhage can ensue. Application of direct pressure to the area with an abdominal pad will usually stop the bleeding. Dissecting the area in an attempt to visualize the bleeding point only adds to a potentially massive blood loss. A suggested alternative is to occlude the bleeding site with a titanium thumbtack inserted into the bone. Other methods have been described to deal with presacral bleeding, including the use of the an endoscopic stapling device, a Silastic tissue expander for tamponade, and pressure with a muscle fragment held into position over the bleeding area while indirect coagulation is performed through the muscle. Prevention, however, is the key; direct visualization of the presacral space by sharp dissection is less likely to tear the fascia, rather than the blunt, manual maneuver usually used.

## Postoperative Management

Postoperative management of Teflon sling repair is essentially the same as that for a bowel resection. An indwelling urinary catheter is recommended for several days. Patients are given intravenous fluids until bowel sounds develop and flatus is passed, at which time a progressive diet is instituted. The patient is discharged when the bowel has functioned

## Laparoscopy

Another proposed method of suspension is that of laparoscopic insertion and securing of the mesh. It will be interesting to see whether this technique will replace conventional laparotomy for the Ripstein operation. Certainly, if any colon operation lends itself to the principles of laparoscopy, it is this one.

## Results

Success rates for sling repair are generally reported to be above 95%. Complications are less common, occurring in 10% to 15%.

Sepsis is an unusual complication of Teflon sling repair; when it occurs, however, it is an extremely difficult problem to treat. Removal of the mesh inevitably becomes necessary, a technical tour de force that may eventuate in a bowel resection. It is primarily because of the risk of entering the bowel during some phase of the procedure that a full antibiotic and mechanical preparation is strongly suggested. If the lumen is breached, carry on with a resection rather than risk insertion of the foreign material in a contaminated field.

Bowel management and incontinence can remain persistent problems after the prolapse is corrected. Approximately one third of patients complain of difficulty in regulating bowel function after the repair, and 10% report incontinence or soiling. Of course, bowel function and incontinence problems are common complaints before surgical intervention. The habits of excessive straining to pass stool and dependence on laxatives are often long-standing and not remedied by anatomic correction of the prolapse. It is for this reason that I have become much more enthusiastic about the resection option.

Gordon and Hoexter, in a study based on a questionnaire sent to members of the American Society of Colon and Rectal Surgeons, acquired information on 1,111 Teflon sling repairs performed by 129 surgeons. The overall complication rate was 16.5%, with a recurrence rate of 2.3%. Complications seemed to be related primarily to applying the mesh too tightly around the rectum. The complication rate seems to diminish as the surgeon's experience increases.

## Late Complications

Barium enema examination shows the stenosis. Any narrowing can also be identified by proctosigmoidoscopy. Rectal stricture is uncommon, but may necessitate removal of the sling and possible resection of the bowel.

Other authors have confirmed that difficulties have arisen with Teflon as the suspension material. Gore-Tex is an ideal material, because of its inert properties and its porous structure, which allows tissue incorporation. Placing the sling posteriorly, leaving the anterior rectal wall free to distend may minimize the problem of stricture.

Constipation is not relieved by Teflon sling repair. On the contrary, abdominal pain, distention, and constipation can be exacerbated by the now-exaggerated redundancy of the sigmoid colon. Sigmoid volvulus has been reported to occur under these circumstances. In some individuals who present with obstructive symptoms relatively soon after the operation, faulty technique must be assumed. However, fibrotic reaction secondary to the mesh repair must also be considered as a possible contributing factor. In any patient with chronic constipation, particularly with a history of long-standing rectal prolapse, consider performing an anterior resection initially. At the very least, careful preoperative investigation of these individuals is needed to identify those who have associated disturbances of function (e.g., slow-transit constipation, obstructed defecation).

Recurrent rectal prolapse after Teflon sling repair usually is related to faulty surgical technique. The mesh may not be secured adequately to the presacral fascia or bone. In addition, as has been stated, when traction on the rectosigmoid is not maintained while the sling is inserted, the mesh will not be anchored sufficiently low on the rectum. The error is more likely to occur in a man whose pelvis is narrow and in whom mobilization and suture placement are more difficult. In our experience, a higher ratio of men to women is observed in the group of patients with this complication.

*Comment*: I believe that the Teflon sling repair should be abandoned in favor of anterior resection for all patients, but especially for men. Exceptions that come to mind are patients who develop a prolapse many years following an abdominal-anal pull-through operation. Because of the risk of devascularization of the lower rectal segment if resection is performed, a suspension operation is probably the better choice in this instance. Another exception is the patient who has severe diarrhea, especially if a subtotal colectomy had been performed. A suspension operation would be the preferred alternative.

## Ivalon Sponge Implant or the Wells Operation

Wells initially described the use of Ivalon sponge as a wrapping about the rectum in 1959. The Ivalon sponge implant operation basically consists of the implantation of a synthetic polymer around the rectum. After full mobilization of the rectum, the appropriately tailored sponge is sutured to the sacrum in the posterior midline, not unlike the modified Teflon sling operation. It is then wrapped around the rectum, leaving a defect in the anterior midline.

### *Results*

Follow-up study revealed nine mucosal recurrences—the incidence of recurrence is high, ranging from 3% to 20% for full-thickness prolapse and 24% to 35% for mucosal prolapse. A conscientious effort to fully mobilize the rectum, shorten the lateral ligaments, and excise the redundant peritoneum minimizes the recurrence rate. Despite the absence of recurrence, constipation (5%) and incontinence (20%) cause difficult management problems.

Although septic problems are not common, removal of the sponge can be difficult, particularly when the physician attempts to identify foreign material within an abscess cavity. Symptoms of this complication include sacral, coccygeal, or lower abdominal pain, pus per rectum, pus per vaginam, rectal discharge, and fever. The implant should be removed through the vagina or through the rectum if at all possible.

*Comment*: The apparent advantage of the Ivalon sponge implant operation is that fecal impaction has not been as great a problem. However, because the incidence of recurrence is greater than that generally reported for the Teflon sling repair and for resection, I would not adopt the technique for my patients. Of course, the fact that it is not approved for use in the United States makes the matter academic.

## Teflon Halter Operation

A unique approach to rectal suspension has been suggested by Nigro. He contends that the most important factor is the angulation and fixation provided by the pelvic floor musculature and that maximal support comes with contraction of the muscle as it lifts the lower rectum and tilts it forward toward the pubis.

The patient is placed in the Trendelenburg position on the operating table. A midline incision is made in the lower abdomen, and the rectum is mobilized in the same manner as that for a Ripstein or Wells repair. Care is taken to avoid injury to the inferior mesenteric vessels. The dissection is carried posteriorly down to the coccyx. The mesh is tailored (~4 cm wide by 20 cm long). The central portion is secured to the rectum with interrupted, nonabsorbable sutures. It is then sutured to the posterior and lateral walls of the rectum as low as possible.

The space of Retzius, in front of the bladder and close to the pubic rami, is opened. A long, curved clamp is placed into this space and directed downward and posteriorly to the presacral space. The mesh is then grasped and pulled forward to lie on the pubic bone. The same is done on the contralateral side. Each end is then secured to the pubic ramus with interrupted, nonabsorbable sutures. Graft length is determined by holding it to the pubic bone with just enough tension to prevent slack. The presacral space is left open, and the abdomen is closed without drainage. Postoperative care is essentially the same as that for the conventional operation.

### Results

Reports are few, but no mortality, operative morbidity, or recurrence was seen with a minimum follow-up of 6 months. Severe incontinence was corrected in all but one patient, and this person was improved. No problems with sexual function or urination ensued.

*Comment*: The utility of this operation is rather problematic. Dissection along the anterior pelvis places vital urinary and genital structures in jeopardy. If carried out in a woman of childbearing age, a subsequent pregnancy will require a caesarean section. If the procedure is performed in a male patient, impotence is much more likely to be a complication than if the conventional alternative is used. Its theoretic advantage with respect to continence is probably overrated.

### Fascia Lata Suspension (Orr)

In 1947, Orr described a suspension procedure by which the rectum is anchored to the sacrum with strips of fascia lata. The incidence of recurrent prolapse with this procedure was 3.6% to 8%.

### Nylon Suspension

A modification that employs strips of nylon for the same purpose has been described. A recurrent rectal prolapse was observed in 4.3%, with a minimum follow-up of 5 years.

### Suture Rectopexy

Perhaps the simplest abdominal approach to the treatment of rectal prolapse is rectopexy. This operation consists of mobilizing the rectum down to the levator ani muscle and securing the mesentery of the rectum and the muscularis to the sacral fascia or bone, which can be performed simply by using interrupted, nonabsorbable sutures. Recurrence rates are comparable to that of standard suspension procedures.

*Comment*: It is evident that fixation of the rectum to the sacrum by whatever means has a high success rate with a low morbidity and mortality. Although I have had no experience with the above techniques, their simplicity makes them appealing.

## Rectal Prolapse and Fecal Incontinence

As implied from the aforementioned studies, most patients will experience resolution of their incontinence difficulties once the prolapse has been adequately treated. This is not surprising, because in addition to the prolapse no longer stretching and attenuating the sphincter, median perineal descent during attempted defecation usually decreases, and the anorectal angle becomes narrowed.

A small group of people remains, however, for whom anal incontinence can be disabling, despite correction of the rectal prolapse. Furthermore, the more severe the prolapse, the worse the result.

*Comment*: The success of the operation from the surgeon's viewpoint, and, from that of the patient, depends on many factors, not the least important of which is the ability to improve bowel habits. Perineal strengthening exercises, dietary measures, stool softeners, even periodic enemas or suppositories may be advisable. Although laxatives are usually discouraged, patients often resume their use. The physician cannot expect to remedy the bowel problems of a lifetime, but with appropriate counseling, most patients will come to good terms with the condition.

## Recommendations

The varied operative procedures available for rectal prolapse can be confusing. Some of the maneuvers are relatively esoteric and can be performed successfully only by the few surgeons who have developed the specialized techniques. It is recommended, therefore, that the surgeon who is less experienced with rectal prolapse adopt one of the standard operations. A rectopexy or suspension procedure without resection can be performed safely with good results and low morbidity and mortality rates. Anterior resection, with or without sacral fixation, also offers an excellent cure rate and is familiar to most surgeons.

The Thiersch-type approaches should probably be reserved for those individuals who cannot tolerate laparotomy. The material chosen should be one of the commercially available synthetic products. Wire should not be used. The Silastic-impregnated Dacron prosthesis for this operation has some potential benefit, especially for the incontinent patient. Results of further studies are awaited.

## RECTAL PROLAPSE IN CHILDREN

Rectal prolapse in children is an uncommon disease that occurs primarily in Western countries—most frequently seen in infants with cystic fibrosis. The condition can be associated with any illness that causes diarrhea (e.g., amebiasis, giardiasis, worms); constipation; frequent cough, especially whooping cough; or malnutrition. These associated conditions are described in more detail below.

Diarrhea (e.g., amebiasis, giardiasis, ulcerative colitis, trichuriasis)
Constipation
Straining to urinate (e.g., phimosis)
Vomiting
Cough (e.g., pertussis)
Malnutrition
Cystic fibrosis
Polyp or tumor
Ehlers-Danlos syndrome
Myelomeningocele
Spina bifida
Hirschsprung's disease

Malnutrition is by far the most common predisposing factor for the development of rectal prolapse in infants and children in developing countries. Most of the reports in the current literature emanate from Africa and Asia. The reasons for this geographic distribution are probably attributable to the diarrhea, in addition to the loss of ischiorectal fat and the lack of support for the rectum experienced by children in these regions.

## Etiology

The cause of rectal prolapse in infancy may be related to the loose attachment of the mucosa to the underlying muscularis. In this age group, the rectal mucosa can be normally redundant. Other anatomic factors in the child which tend to predispose to the development of prolapse are the vertical course of the rectum, flat sacrum and coccyx, low rectal position in relation to other pelvic organs, and lack of levator support. Rectal prolapse is most common in children younger than 3 years of age, with the most frequent incidence being in the first year of life. In this age group, it is the mucosa that tends to prolapse, not the full thickness of the bowel. Most studies report an approximately equal gender incidence.

## Symptoms and Findings

Symptoms can include protrusion, bleeding, passage of mucus, diarrhea, constipation, abdominal pain, and those complaints that may be referable to the associated or predisposing condition. Findings include the protrusion, lax sphincter tone and contractility, and, often, malnutrition. The most common differential diagnostic condition is that of a juvenile polyp. Distinction between the two entities should not be difficult, however.

## Treatment

Treatment usually consists of medical management, with normal growth of the child producing a cure in most patients. However, children with severe malnutrition and those without access to quality medical care and nutritional support are less likely to have spontaneous resolution of the prolapse condition.

Medical management consists of manual replacement, with sedation if necessary; the knee-chest position may be helpful. Supporting the perineum during defecation is also beneficial, as well as having the child defecate in the recumbent position. It may be necessary to tape the buttocks to prevent the prolapse from recurring spontaneously. Stool softeners are suggested for constipation and paregoric for diarrhea.

Surgical treatment is advised for patients who are malnourished and for those who do not respond to medical management. Recommended procedures include the following:

Excision of the mucosal prolapse
Anal encirclement with Silastic or with catgut
Use of a sclerosing solution (e.g., 30% saline or 70% alcohol)
Packing of the presacral space with gauze or Gelfoam
Linear cauterization of the anorectum
Transsacral rectopexy with obliteration of the pouch of Douglas and puborectalis plication
Transcoccygeal rectopexy and puborectalis plication
Perineal proctosigmoidectomy
Transanal rectopexy with delayed suture removal

*Comment*: My limited experience with this condition in children is such that I believe that medical measures are almost always successful. For the infant or child who fails to respond, it seems that a minimal surgical approach is appropriate: perirectal injection with a sclerosing agent, presacral packing, an anal encircling operation, or linear rectal cauterization. All have been reported in large series to have excellent results with minimal morbidity. Whereas more extensive adult-type operations are undoubtedly successful, I cannot justify their application in children when I note the availability of simpler, safer, effective alternatives.

## RECTOCELE

Rectocele is not a prolapse nor is it a descensus, but it does represent one of those conditions that occurs as part of the pelvic laxity syndrome. In essence it is a hernial protrusion of part of the rectum into the vagina; it has also been referred to as a "proctocele" (Fig. 17.16). The condition is often associated with anterior pelvic laxity, leading to cystocele and cystourethrocele.

Repair is generally indicated when a rectocele is identified in a patient with the following symptoms:

Constipation
Rectal pain
Need to insert a finger into the vagina to effect evacuation
Stool pocketing
Protrusion
Requirement of cystocele repair

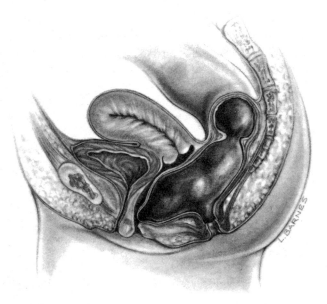

**FIG. 17.16.** Sagittal view of a typical rectocele deformity.

Careful preoperative investigations are important before surgically treating a rectocele because emptying difficulties are so frequently observed.

Parenthetically, it is interesting to note that rectocele is not consistently associated with any physiologic change apart from an increased frequency of pelvic floor descent. The success of the transanal or transvaginal repair is not influenced by the concomitant presence of perineal descent, internal prolapse, radiologic signs of anismus, or the size of the rectocele.

### Techniques

One operation that has been suggested is basically a mucosal excision in the anterior quadrant with reefing of the deep external sphincter and levator ani muscle (Fig. 17.17). An obliterative, deep-suturing technique is advocated as an expeditious (i.e., "6-minute") alternative to conventional rectocele repair. Others advocate a combined transvaginal–transanal repair. The combined procedure commences initially with a posterior colporrhaphy and then repositioning the patient in the prone-jackknife position. Mucosal redundancy is excised from the anterior rectal wall through a transanal approach, followed by a transverse plication of the muscular layer of the rectal wall as is described in Figure 17.17.

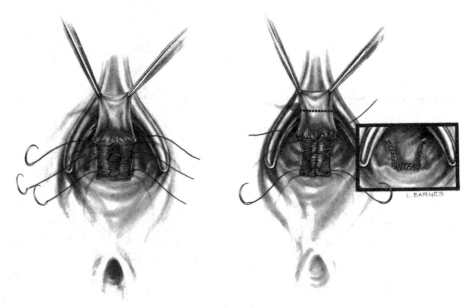

**FIG. 17.17.** Transanal rectocele repair. Plication in layers of the lax rectovaginal septum.

## Results

A number of large series reveal orocllcnt results of transanal operations, doopite an infection rate in excess of 5% and the occurrence of a few postoperative rectovaginal fistulas.

However, the procedures described above are not reasonable alternatives to conventional transvaginal surgery if the patient harbors a cystocele that requires repair. Limited application of a transanal technique to those symptomatic patients who have an isolated rectocele or who are undergoing an anorectal operation for another problem seems prudent.

# 18

# Pediatric Surgical Problems

In this chapter, the spectrum of three congenital anomalies that affect the anorectal area is discussed: aganglionosis, neuronal intestinal dysplasia (NID), and imperforate anus. In addition, a brief review of an acquired intestinal condition called "necrotizing enterocolitis" (NEC) is presented. Other diseases in the pediatric population are presented within the appropriate chapters of this text.

## CONGENITAL MEGACOLON OR HIRSCHSPRUNG'S DISEASE

### Pathophysiology and Embryology

Congenital megacolon is an anomaly characterized by partial or complete colonic obstruction associated with the absence of intramural ganglion cells. The aganglionic portion of the colon is always located distally, but the length of the segment varies. The so-called "typical" variation occurring in about two thirds of all patients is the one in which the aganglionic segment includes the rectum and much of the sigmoid colon. The long-segment variety, representing approximately 10% of the cases, is that in which the aganglionic portion may extend to any level between the hepatic flexure and the descending colon. Total colonic aganglionosis including a variable length of terminal also represents approximately 10% of the entire group. Some debate is seen to the existence of so-called "ultrashort" aganglionosis or short-segment Hirschsprung's disease (see Chapter 16). It is frequently misinterpreted as functional chronic constipation; its histologic confirmation is also a matter of some debate.

Typically, the aganglionic portion of the colon appears narrow when compared with the distended, proximal part. The aganglionic portion demonstrates absence of intramural, submucosal, and intermuscular ganglion cells with increased size and prominence of nerve fibers. The proximal, normally innervated portion of the colon is usually distended, and its wall is thickened because of muscle hypertrophy. Mucosal ulcerations are also frequently seen. Between these two areas is the so-called "transition zone," a cone-shaped portion of colon that is often histologically described as "hypoganglionic."

Congenital megacolon is believed to be a disease caused by an arrest in the craniocaudal migration of the neuroenteric ganglion cells from the neural crest into the upper gastrointestinal tract, down through the vagal fibers, and along the distal intestine.

## Incidence and Associated Malformations

The incidence of Hirschsprung's disease is in the range of 1 of 5,000 births. It also seems to be more common in whites. Although boys are much more frequently affected than girls, the long-segment manifestation is seen at least as often in girls. Inheritance patterns seem to be multifactorial. Approximately 5% to 21% of all individuals affected with Hirschsprung's disease have an associated congenital anomaly, particularly anorectal malformations.

Genetically, a deletion in the long arm of chromosome 10 has been found and seems to overlap the region of the *RET* proto-oncogene. Currently, however, the identification of the gene and the exact sequence of the DNA code still elude us.

## Clinical Manifestations and Differential Diagnosis

Infants suffering from Hirschsprung's disease usually become symptomatic during the first 24 to 48 hours of life. Occasionally, a child may have minimal or absent clinical manifestations during the first days or weeks and exhibit moderate, intermittent bouts of symptoms later in life (see Chapter 16)

Abdominal distention, delayed passage of meconium, and vomiting are the most frequent observations in patients. This triad of symptoms may be followed by a spontaneous or induced explosive, massive deflating passage of liquid bowel movement, and gas, which dramatically improves the baby's condition. This is followed by a period of hours or days of relative absence of symptoms, followed by recurrence of the same manifestations. When the abdomen is distended, the infant usually is very ill from sepsis, hypovolemia, and endotoxic shock. Ischemic enterocolitis with necrosis proximal to the aganglionic segment is the most serious complication. A mortality rate of up to 50% is seen during the first year of life.

The differential diagnosis includes any condition that causes intestinal obstruction in the newborn, probably the most frequent being the so-called "meconium-plug syndrome." The expulsion of a plug of meconium with resolution of symptoms and the absence of other signs characteristic of Hirschsprung's disease help establish the diagnosis.

Another condition that can lead to confusion in differential diagnosis is the small left colon syndrome. Barium enema demonstrates a narrow left colon to the level of the splenic flexure. Symptoms usually improve following this study and resolve after several weeks. The mother is frequently diabetic.

Other, nonsurgical conditions that can be confused with Hirschsprung's disease include hypothyroidism, adrenal insufficiency, and cerebral injury.

Patients who survive with inadequate treatment or with relatively mild symptoms ultimately develop the classic clinical picture initially described for this condition. These children suffer severe constipation with an enormously distended abdomen. The proximal colon is huge and full of inspissated fecal material. At this stage, the diagnosis can be confused with chronic constipation (e.g., colon inertia or megarectum). In the latter condition, children usually become symptomatic after the sixth month of life; they neither vomit nor become seriously ill. An important characteristic in this group of patients is overflow incontinence or encopresis, a constant, chronic soiling without evidence of neuromuscular disturbance (see Chapter 16). Rectal examination in these children reveals a severe fecal impaction just above the anal canal. Patients with Hirschsprung's disease can have an empty rectum, or examination may disclose only a small amount of feces.

## Diagnosis

### *Radiologic Studies*

A plain abdominal film of a neonate is not diagnostic. An enema examination performed with a dilute suspension of barium or, preferably, with water-soluble contrast material is the most valuable radiologic study for establishing the diagnosis of this condition.

No bowel preparation is required. The infant is placed in a lateral position, and a rectal tube is introduced to barely above the anal canal. Injection of contrast is optimally controlled by hand with a syringe. The introduction of a catheter beyond the limit of the anal canal will risk a misdiagnosis, because the tip may reach the distended colon and result in injection above the aganglionic portion. The dye is instilled until it reaches the distended portion of the intestine, at which point the study is terminated. Injection of excessive amounts of contrast material, especially barium, can produce further evacuation problems and impaction.

This study should reveal the presence of an extremely distended proximal colon, the transition zone, and a "contracted" distal rectosigmoid. Barium enema is less accurate in infants with very short aganglionosis or when the entire colon is involved. In instances of total colonic aganglionosis, a barium enema can reveal a short colon, with retraction of the hepatic and splenic flexures and straightening of the sigmoid.

### *Anorectal Manometry*

Normally, when the rectum is distended with a balloon, pressure in the anal canal falls because of internal sphincter relaxation. In infants with aganglionosis, this reflex is absent (see Chapter 6). This abnormal response has been interpreted as diagnostic for this condition. However, this test has several limitations, the primary one being the technical difficulty of evaluating the newborn. In my experience, this test is useful primarily for older children (see Chapter 16).

### Rectal Biopsy

Confirmation of the diagnosis is based on the absence of ganglion cells and the presence of an excess of nonmyelinated nerves in an adequate rectal biopsy. The specimen must be a full-thickness biopsy taken at least 1.5 cm above the pectinate line. This is performed by suction biopsy, which does not require an anesthetic.

Some would suggest the presence of large amounts of acetylcholinesterase in the mucosa and submucosa as a diagnostic alternative.

## Management

### Medical Treatment

Bowel irrigation with saline solution is a valuable procedure for the emergency management of distention and vomiting. However, it should not be a substitute for surgical intervention.

### Surgical Treatment

#### Preliminary Decompression by Colostomy

Colostomy remains the preferred method of initial management of congenital megacolon. It addresses the emergency situation and provides protection for the subsequent, definitive repair.

A right transverse colostomy is an effective and safe method for decompressing the colon in most infants with Hirschsprung's disease. However, many surgeons advocate the creation of the colostomy immediately above the transition zone. This alternative means that the colostomy must be pulled down at the time of the definitive repair, depriving the patient of the protection of a subsequent proximal diversion. Obviously, the advantage to this approach is that the child will require only a two-stage procedure, whereas a right transverse colostomy commits to a three-stage operation.

Other surgeons suggest a one-stage repair. This implies the performance of a primary pull-through operation in the neonate without a protective colostomy. The long-term effects of this approach, including the incidence of late constipation, enterocolitis, and fecal incontinence, remain to be seen.

### Definitive Operations

#### Swenson Procedure

With the child in the lithotomy position, the abdomen is entered through a Pfannenstiel, hockey-stick incision. Resection of the aganglionic portion of the colon is performed, including that of the most dilated portion of the bowel. The aganglionic area below the peritoneal floor is freed by precise dissection as close as possible to the rectal wall down to the level of the levator ani muscle. Anastomosis is effected by a conventional, transanal, hand-sewn technique. Because of the tedious pelvic dissection and the risk of anastomotic breakdown, most surgeons perform a Swenson operation only if the patient had previously undergone a protective colostomy.

### Duhamel Procedure

The Duhamel procedure was devised to avoid the extensive pelvic dissection required in the Swenson operation. This is accomplished by preserving the aganglionic rectum and dividing the bowel at the peritoneal reflection as distally as possible. The rectal stump is then closed. Normal (i.e., ganglionic) intestine, usually above the most dilated portion, is pulled through a presacral space that had been created by blunt dissection and an anastomosis between the colon. Then, the aganglionic rectum is created as wide as possible, and the rectal stump as small as possible, to avoid fecal accumulation.

### Soave Procedure

The Soave procedure is an ingenious and appealing operation, because the aganglionic rectosigmoid is removed by an endorectal dissection, theoretically minimizing the risk of the pelvic injury associated with the Swenson procedure. The normally innervated colon is passed through a rectosigmoid muscular cuff, using the Boley modification of a one-stage operation by effecting a primary anastomosis to the anal verge. No aganglionic segment of rectum remains, such as that which occurs with the Duhamel procedure.

### Results

The Soave operation with Boley modification is the procedure of choice.

### Surgical Management of Total Colonic Aganglionosis

When the diagnosis of total colonic aganglionosis is made, an ileostomy is required initially; the definitive operation is recommended after 1 year. At this time, the ileostomy is taken down and sufficiently mobilized to reach the perineum. The ganglionic terminal ileum is pulled down through the retrorectal (i.e., presacral) space as described for the Duhamel procedure. The next step, however, consists of creating a long, side-to-side anastomosis between the distal ileum and rectum, sigmoid, and descending colon up to the level of the splenic flexure. The proximal aganglionic intestine is excised.

Others have proposed a modification of the above technique. The first operation consists of an ileostomy; the second stage is a side-to-side ileo-ascending colon anastomosis. At the final stage, the terminal ileum, with the right colon as a free patch, is pulled down using any of the available techniques (i.e., Soave, Duhamel, or Swenson).

### *Total Intestinal Aganglionosis*

Reports from the Children's Hospital Medical Center at the University of Cincinnati, have described the management of the challenging problem of 16 neonates who presented with intestinal obstruction secondary to total (extending to the stomach) or near total intestinal aganglionosis confirmed at one or more leveling operations. Their operation included extending an antimesenteric myectomy from the ganglionic-aganglionic transition zone for variable lengths, the operative design being to create sufficient small bowel lengths to support life (a minimum of 40 cm). Of 10 survivors, 2 were totally gut nourished, 6 received from 20% to 80% of total calories enterally, and 1 received minimal enteral feeding.

### *Management of Short-Segment Aganglionosis*

The management of the "ultrashort" or "short segment" variant of aganglionosis is discussed in Chapter 16.

### *Neuronal Intestinal Dysplasia*

Recent evidence suggests that the disorders of bowel innervation and ganglion distribution are represented by a spectrum of conditions, including an entity known as "neuronal intestinal dysplasia." The implication of this observation is that the presence or absence of ganglion cells (e.g., as in Hirschsprung's disease) represents only a part of this spectrum.

The precise options for therapy have not been clearly established because of the lack of well-defined clinical, radiologic, and manometric findings.

## ANORECTAL MALFORMATIONS

### Incidence

It is reported that 1 of every 5,000 newborns will have an anorectal malformation. Male infants seem to suffer this condition more frequently than female infants.

### Embryologic Considerations

Anorectal defects probably develop during gestational weeks 4 to 12. The urinary, genital, and rectal tracts empty into a common channel, the cloaca. Ultimately, they are segregated by the urorectal septum during its craniocaudal descent, separating the cloaca into an anterior urogenital sinus and a posterior intestinal canal. Two lateral folds of the cloaca also move simultaneously toward the midline. The perineal mound appears to be the caudal extension of the urorectal septum, which develops into the perineal body. In men, the inner and outer genital ridges meet to form the urethra. In women, these ridges do not coalesce but form the labia minora and majora. Various types of failures in this process have been postulated to explain each of the anorectal malformations. The resulting defects constitute a spectrum that ranges from the most severe examples (e.g., caudal regression and persistent cloaca) to the more easily managed concerns (e.g., cutaneous fistula and low malformation in the male).

## Classification

A spectrum of malformation must be dealt with in cases of imperforate anus. Thus, in attempting to separate these groups of defects into categories, a risk exists of being arbitrary and artificial. Keep in mind the basic concept of a spectrum. With this cautionary note, the classification shown in Table 18.1 is considered practical and useful for therapeutic purposes. Another is the "Wingspread Classification" (Table 18.2). It has embryologic implications rather than therapeutic ones.]

## Basic Anatomy

The posterior sagittal approach used to repair anorectal malformations, in addition to managing tumors, rectal trauma, amebiasis, and rectal prolapse, permits conceptualization of the anatomic details of a normal man and a normal woman. The external sphincter is represented by a group of parasagittal muscle fibers. The levator ani and external sphincter blend and become indistinguishable, forming a funnel-shaped continuum of muscle. The portion of muscle located between the parasagittal fibers of the external sphincter and levator ani muscle is integrated mainly by vertical fibers that run parallel with the rectum, called the "muscle complex." The levator ani, muscle complex, and external sphincter are indivisible structures working in concert. In the upper portion of the funnel, horizontal fibers

**TABLE 18.1.** *Specific anomalies of the spectrum of anorectal malformations*

| Male | Female |
|---|---|
| Cutaneous fistula, NC | Cutaneous (perineal) fistula, NC |
| Anal stenosis, NC | Vestibular fistula, C |
| Anal membrane, NC | Vaginal fistula, C |
| Rectourethral fistula, C | Anorectal agenesis without fistula, C |
| Bulbar (prostatic), C | Rectal atresia, C |
| Rectovesical fistulav | Persistent cloaca (colostomy required), C |
| Anorectal agenesis without fistula, C | Complex malformations |
| Rectal atresia (colostomy required), C | |

NC, no colostomy required; C, colostomy required.

TABLE 18.2. Wingspread classification of anorectal malformations (1984)

| Male | Female |
|---|---|
| High | High |
| Anorectal agenesis | Anorectal agenesis |
| With rectoprostatic urethral fistula | With rectovaginal fistula |
| Without fistula rectal atresia | Without fistula rectal atresia |
| Intermediate | Intermediate |
| Rectobulbar urethral fistula | Rectovestibular fistula |
| Anal agenesis without fistula | Rectovaginal fistula |
| | Anal agenesis without fistula |
| Low | Low |
| Anocutaneous fistula | Anovestibular fistula |
| Anal stenosis | Anocutaneous fistula |
| | Anal stenosis |
| | Cloaca |
| Rare | Rare |
| Malformations | Malformations |

predominate and push the rectum forward; in the lower part of the funnel (i.e., muscle complex), vertical fibers predominate and elevate the anus. Because the parasagittal fibers meet together in front of the anus as well as posterior to it, contraction occludes the anus; this gives the fibers a circular appearance.

## Specific Defects in the Male

When discussing results of surgical treatment, it is imperative to compare only malformations with a similar potential for bowel control. Thus, rather than comparing groups of malformations, specific defects must be examined (Fig. 18.1).

### Cutaneous Fistula

Cutaneous fistula is a low malformation. The rectum has passed normally through much of the sphincter mechanism. However, the lowest part of the rectum is anteriorly deviated and ends as a perineal (i.e., cutaneous) fistula anterior to the center of the external sphincter. Frequently, the fistula tract lies immediately below a thin layer of skin, with the external opening somewhere in the midline from the anus to the ventral portion of the penis. Often, a midline, black, ribbonlike structure caused by meconium is perceived beneath the skin. The infant does not require further investigation and surgery without a colostomy can be performed. Prognosis is excellent, because the patient has all the necessary anatomic elements for maintaining fecal continence.

### Anal Stenosis

Anal stenosis is another benign defect, consisting of a ring of fibrous tissue located at the anal verge. From the external perspective, the anus appears normal; a Hegar dilator must be inserted to detect the malformation. Digital rectal

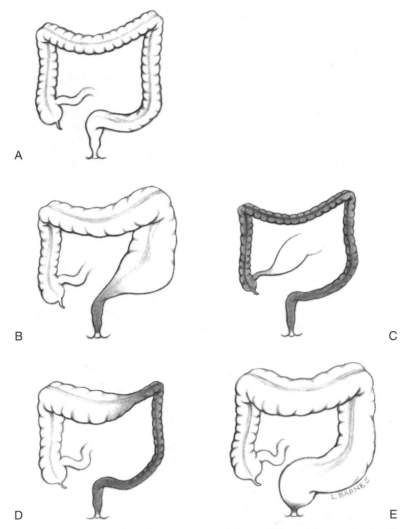

**FIG. 18.1.** Different presentations of Hirschsprung's disease according to the length of the aganglionic segment. **A.** Normal bowel. **B.** Typical involvement. **C.** Total colonic aganglionosis. **D.** Long-segment disease. **E.** Short-segment disease.

examination is impossible. The patient has difficult moving the bowels; the mother often describes a ribbonlike appearance of the feces. The patient can be treated either by surgery or by simple dilatation; a colostomy is unnecessary.

### *Anal Membrane*

Anal membrane is an unusual type of malformation. The infant presents with a thin membranous covering of the anus through which meconium can be seen.

The diagnosis can be made by mere inspection. A simple surgical procedure without a colostomy is indicated in these children.

### Rectourethral Fistula

Rectourethral fistula is the most frequent malformation seen in the male. Congenitally, the rectum descends through a considerable portion of the funnel-shaped muscle structure, but at some point it deviates anteriorly and connects with the urethra. Distal to the fistula site, the muscle structure becomes a solid mass, which is very thin laterally and situated very close to the posterior urethra. This muscle is usually of good quality. A patient with bulbar fistula usually has a better potential for continence because the rectum has already passed through a significant portion of the levator ani and muscle complex mechanism; the muscle quality is more satisfactory; and the sacrum has developed more normally. Higher malformations are more frequently associated with a poor sacrum, and consequently, poor innervation with a poor quality of muscle. The perineum in patients with rectourethral fistula usually exhibits a well-developed midline groove and an easily recognized anal dimple or fossette. These signs are usually indicative of good muscle development.

Occasionally, however, a patient with a rectourethral fistula, usually prostatic, has a poor sacrum and a poor-looking perineum with a "flat" or "round bottom" consisting of an absent anal fossette and a poor midline groove. All of these signs usually imply that the patient has poor striated muscle.

These infants require a posterior sagittal anorectoplasty (PSARP), preceded by a protective colostomy (see later).

### Rectovesical Fistula

In the case of a rectovesical fistula, the rectum usually opens at the level of the bladder neck. Levator ani muscle, muscle complex, and external sphincter are frequently underdeveloped. A very high frequency is seen of an association with abnormal sacrum, "flat bottom," and poor-looking perineum—all signs of poor prognosis for fecal continence. These infants must be treated with a colostomy, followed by PSARP and a laparotomy. In my experience, this group represents approximately 10% of the series.

### Anorectal Agenesis without Fistula

Anorectal agenesis without fistula is an unusual malformation. Even without a fistula, only a thin membrane separates rectum from urethra. Treatment consists of a protective colostomy followed by a PSARP.

### Rectal Atresia

Rectal atresia, an unusual malformation, appears much more frequently in females than in males. It consists of a complete (i.e., atresia) or partial interruption (i.e., stenosis) of the rectal lumen between the anal canal and the rectum. The distance between the rectal pouch and the anal canal in these patients is variable.

## Specific Defects in the Female

The characteristics of the striated muscle mechanism in female infants are similar to those described for males (Fig. 18.2).

### *Cutaneous or Perineal Fistula*

Cutaneous (i.e., perineal) fistula represents the most benign defect of the female spectrum. As with the male abnormality, the rectum traverses most of the sphincter mechanism, deviating in its most distal portion to communicate with the skin through a fistula located a few millimeters anterior to the center of the external sphincter. These infants have all the necessary elements for normal bowel control. A simple anoplasty (i.e., minimal PSARP) is sufficient to treat this type of malformation without the need for a protective colostomy. Treatment is indicated primarily for cosmetic and psychological reasons only.

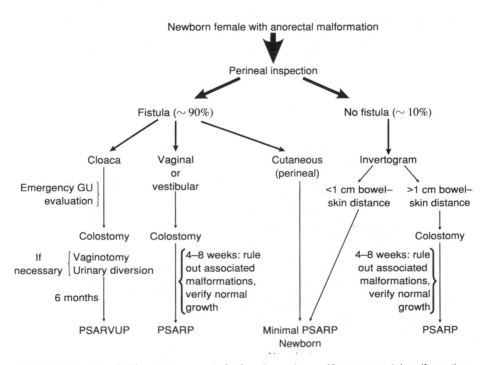

**FIG.18.2.** Algorithm for the management of a female newborn with an anorectal malformation. GU, genitourinary; PSARP, posterior sagittal anorectoplasty; PSARVUP, posterior sagittal anorectovaginourethroplasty.

### Vestibular Fistula

Vestibular fistula is the malformation most frequently seen in female infants. The bowel is anteriorly deviated at a higher level, opening immediately behind the hymen into the vestibule. The rectum and the vagina are opposed, with only a thin, common wall separating the two structures. Most patients have the potential for normal continence, a normal-appearing sacrum, adequate innervation, and a good-looking perineum.

Fecal diversion before performing a limited PSARP is the ideal management for this condition.

### Vaginal Fistula

Vaginal fistula is an unusual malformation in females. The rectum may open in the lower one half of the vagina or, as an even more uncommon manifestation, in the upper portion. The higher the malformation is, the shorter the common wall between the rectum and vagina. The higher the fistula, the greater the risks of an abnormal sacrum and a poor-looking perineum. Treatment consists of a diverting colostomy followed by a full PSARP.

### Anorectal Agenesis without Fistula

Anorectal agenesis without a fistula is also an uncommon malformation. The rectum is usually located approximately 2 cm above the skin. The rectovaginal septum is thin, and good residual muscle, good looking perineum, and well-developed sacrum are seen. Treatment consists of a diverting colostomy followed by a PSARP. The prognosis for potentially normal bowel control is excellent.

### Rectal Atresia

Rectal atresia is treated in the same manner for both female and male infants.

### Persistent Cloaca

Persistent cloaca represents the extreme in the spectrum of complexity of malformations in the female infant. With this anomaly, the rectum, vagina, and urinary tract meet and fuse together into a single channel. Inspection of the perineum in these infants reveals small genitalia. Meticulous examination discloses a single orifice at the urethral site with no evidence of vagina or rectum.

Persistent cloaca, itself, is represented by a spectrum of defects. Many infants have a double or septated vagina, with different degrees of septation or division of the uterus. Frequently, the vaginal opening into the cloaca is obstructed, with a resultant severe hydrocolpos. The common channel varies in length from 1 to 7 cm. This is considered an important indicator of the potential difficulty that will be encountered if an attempt is made to repair the defect. Lower, short cloacae, with good residual muscle and sacrum, are usually easier to repair. Longer cloacae are frequently associated with poor muscle and inadequate sacrum; they, therefore, have an unlikely potential for continence.

In managing this malformation, the treatment commitment is to achieve normal bowel control, normal urinary continence, and normal sexual function, as well as childbearing capacity. Success is more likely in children with a normal sacrum and an adequate vagina. These patients require a colostomy and often need some form of urinary diversion as well as vaginostomy for decompression of a hydrocolpos. After an appropriate interval, these procedures are followed by a posterior sagittal anorectovaginourethroplasty (PSARVUP).

## Associated Abnormalities

### Sacrum and Spine

The sacrum is frequently defective, with sacral vertebrae deformed or reduced in number, or short without the normal anterior concavity. Also, sacral anomalies are more frequently associated with a higher malformation.

### Urogenital Defects

Genital and urinary (GU) abnormalities are often associated with anorectal malformations in 20% to 40% of cases.

The most common GU anomaly encountered is renal agenesis. Other important associated defects include cryptorchidism, ureteral duplication, hypospadias, rotated kidney, neurogenic bladder, renal dysplasia, renal ectopia, megaureter, hydronephrosis, and ureterovesical obstruction.

Consequently, we perform renal and bladder ultrasound screening of all children born with imperforate anus before creating a colostomy or performing perineal surgery.

## Surgical Technique

### Colostomy

Diverting colostomy is considered an important step in the management of anorectal malformations. It is important to leave sufficient bowel length distally so that a safe pull-through operation is possible. A common error is to place the colostomy too far distally, interfering with the final reconstruction.

## Repair of Specific Defects in the Female

### Cutaneous Fistula

The rectum and vagina are dissected apart. Electrical stimulation will demonstrate that parasagittal fibers may be found on both sides of the fistula, but the anterior portion is usually devoid of muscle.

Vertical fibers and parasagittal fibers cross at two places, creating two corners that mark the limits of the new anus. The dissection does not reach the levator ani muscle. Tapering of the rectum is not required in these individuals. The rectum is then relocated within the limits of the muscle, and the perineal body is closed, bringing together the anterior limit of the muscle complex.

The posterior limit of the sphincter muscle is then sutured, incorporating part of the bowel wall to anchor the rectum and to prevent prolapse. An anoplasty is accomplished by suturing the rectum to the skin after trimming, preserving as much tissue as possible.

### Vestibular Fistula

The primary characteristic of vestibular fistula is that the rectum and vagina share a common wall distally. It is imperative that complete separation of both structures be achieved to obtain a successful repair. The size of the fistula orifice is variable. As a consequence, these infants may manifest different degrees of obstruction, although normal bowel movement patterns may be evident during the newborn period.

Surgical management of this malformation requires a completely diverting colostomy. Definitive repair can be delayed until the child is of sufficient size that the technical aspects are facilitated.

The child is placed in the prone position with the pelvis elevated. Electrical stimulation demonstrates the contraction of the external sphincter muscle considerably posterior to the fistula site. A "racket type" incision is made. Separating the rectum from the vagina can be assisted by injection of epinephrine solution into this wall. The sagittal incision extends into the muscle complex, and sometimes into the inferior portion of the levator ani. This procedure is called a limited PSARP, because the dissection usually does not extend to the coccyx and levator ani muscle. Mobilization of the rectum must be sufficiently adequate to permit relocation within the muscle complex and the external sphincter without tension. Tapering is usually not necessary with this malformation.

The anterior perineum is reconstructed with both anterior edges of the muscle complex approximated. The posterior limit of the muscle complex is also sutured together along with a portion of the posterior rectal wall, which reduces the likelihood of a subsequent prolapse. An anoplasty is then created within the limits of the external sphincter in the same manner as that described for cutaneous fistula.

Postoperative care requires only perineal cleansing and the use of bacitracin ointment daily for 1 week. Dilatations are begun 2 weeks following the procedure. The child can usually eat the day of the operation and is usually discharged the following day.

### Vaginal Fistula

The communication between rectum and vagina may be located in the lower part of the vagina (most frequent), or in the upper portion (very unusual). The lower the fistula is located, the longer is the common wall. The sacrum may demonstrate different degrees of dysplasia, and the muscles may be deficient.

These infants require a colostomy before repair. Management is similar to that described for the vestibular malformation, except that the levator ani may also need to be reconstituted.

Postoperatively, the patient can sit, walk, and be discharged the day after surgery.

### Atresia and Stenosis of the Rectum

With PSARP, a unique opportunity exists to repair atresia and stenosis of the rectum. This approach permits excellent exposure to the anomaly, and makes the repair truly simple. The operation usually requires a full PSARP, with a diverting colostomy a requisite before reconstruction.

### Persistent Cloaca

Management of the complex malformation of persistent cloaca requires a number of surgical maneuvers. The procedure is called posterior sagittal anorectovaginourethroplasty (PSARVUP).

The external sphincter, muscle complex, and levator ani are divided in halves. The rectum, including the common channel, is then opened exactly in the midline. Once the entire visceral structure has been opened, the rectal, the vaginal, and urethral orifices can be identified (Fig. 18.3). A Foley catheter is then

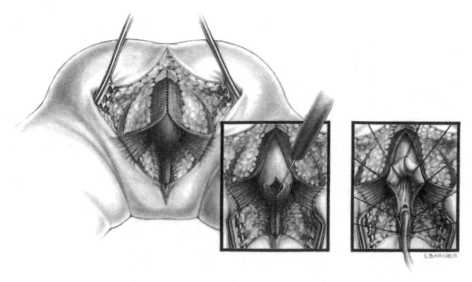

**FIG. 18.3.** Repair of persistent cloaca. Rectum and vagina are exposed; a catheter has been placed in the urethral orifice.

inserted through the urinary opening. Attempts to pass the catheter before opening the cloaca are usually unsuccessful, because of the inability to ascertain which opening was entered.

Because the rectum and vagina share a common wall, no natural plane for separation exists. A rectal submucosal dissection is commenced and continues cephalad to the point where the vagina and the rectum separate. No attempt is then made to separate the vagina from the urinary tract; rather, the entire urogenital sinus is dissected and mobilized. The wall of the urogenital sinus is divided completely, ventral to the vagina. This involves division of avascular fibrous ligaments attached to the pelvic rim. These ligaments must be divided to free the vagina, bladder, and urethra without the need for dividing the blood supply to these structures. The dissection continues circumferentially until enough length has been gained to connect the vaginal edges to the perineum. Thus, a urethral and vaginal opening of a near-normal appearance is created. The vaginal edges are then sutured to the skin or the labia of the perineum with the urethral opening located 5 to 8 mm from the clitoris.

A urinary catheter is usually left in place for approximately 10 days. Anal dilatations are started 2 weeks following the operation, as described for the other malformations.

Repair of these malformations represents the ultimate challenge in pediatric pelvic surgery and should be performed only by individuals who have considerable experience with this type of surgery.

## Repair of Special Defects in the Male Low Malformations: Cutaneous Fistula, Anal Stenosis, and Anal Membrane

Low malformations represent the most benign type of male anorectal defect. No colostomy is required with the reconstruction. The primary characteristic of patients with these anomalies is the location of the rectal fistula—immediately anterior to the center of the external sphincter. The surgical technique used for the repair is similar to that which has been described for cutaneous fistula in females.

### *Rectourethral Fistula*

Rectourethral fistula is the rectal anomaly most commonly seen in male patients. The fistula can be located at the bulbar level or at the prostate. Infants require a protective colostomy prior to reconstruction (i.e., full PSARP).

A Foley catheter is inserted, and a midsagittal incision is made from the middle portion of the sacrum down to and through the center of the external sphincter. The parasagittal fibers of the external sphincter are separated, deepening the incision down to the levator ani and muscle complex. The rectum is separated from the urethra in order to avoid injury to the prostate, seminal vesicles, and vas deferens. The urethral fistula is then closed. Because the rectum is usually ectatic and distended, tailoring is often required to permit it to lie within the muscle structures. The levator ani muscle must be constructed behind the rectum with the distal bowel located within the confines of the muscle complex and external sphincter. The anterior extent of the muscle complex and external sphincter are reapproximated. An anoplasty is performed, as previously described, and the skin is closed. A urethral catheter is usually left in place for between 5 and 7 days.

### Rectovesical Fistula

Rectovesical fistulas represent the extreme in the spectrum of male anorectal defects. The rectum usually opens at the level of the bladder neck. Frequently, the muscle complex and levator ani are only rudimentary structures, and the space available between the urethra and the muscles is usually very narrow. This malformation is often associated with varying degrees of sacral dysgenesis.

Because the rectum cannot be reached through a posterior sagittal approach, these children require a laparotomy as well as a PSARP. The operation commences with a posterior sagittal incision, opening all layers down to the urethra. At this point, a rubber tube is placed immediately behind the urethra and in the presacral space, following the path of the muscle complex. The rubber tube is sutured to the skin, and all muscle structures are reconstructed around the tube. The wound is then closed and the patient placed in the supine position.

The entire body from axilla to foot is prepared, and the abdomen is entered through a long Pfannenstiel incision. The tube is readily found in the retroperitoneum, and the rectum is dissected below the peritoneal reflection to the level of the bladder fistula. The fistula site is closed, the rectum is tapered as appropriate, and then pulled and fixed to the perineum. The operation is completed with an anoplasty, and the abdomen is closed.

### Anorectal Agenesis without Fistula

Surgical treatment for anorectal agenesis without fistula in both males and in females is done in accordance with the same principles.

### Rectal Atresia or Stenosis

Repair of rectal atresia or stenosis in the male is the same as that for the female.

### Secondary Operations for the Treatment of Fecal Incontinence

Infants who were born with an anorectal malformation and who had a conventional procedure done to repair the defect often continue to suffer from fecal incontinence (see Chapter 13). The posterior sagittal approach can be used to repair the muscle injured in prior operations as well as to relocate the rectum properly within the muscle structures.

The ideal candidate for this type of operation is an individual who has at least a favorable potential for continence: relatively normal sacrum and adequate residual muscle as evidenced by a good-looking perineum (e.g., midline raphe and anal dimple). Optimally, the patient should have clinical evidence of an inappropriately located rectum with a well-preserved, intact external sphincter.

The incision is carried out from the middle portion of the sacrum through the center of the external sphincter and around the anus. The repair consists of bringing together both anterior edges of the muscle complex and repairing the perineal body in a manner similar to that previously described.

Because the urethra is not opened, a postoperative urinary catheter is not necessary. Anal dilatation is commenced 2 weeks following the operation.

### Results of Treatment for Anorectal Malformations

It is not unexpected that results will vary, depending on the potential for satisfactory repair that exists with each patient and because of the spectrum of defects being dealt with. Posterior sagittal anorectoplasty permits reconstruction of these defects by placing the rectum in the optimal position to achieve the best functional results. Up to 40% have a "normal" outcome.

Secondary operations for the treatment of fecal incontinence in patients with a normal sacrum reveal some improvement in most.

### *Medical Management of Fecal Incontinence*

Patients who suffer fecal incontinence as a consequence of either poor surgical technique or because of an inadequate sacrum and sphincter muscle can have the condition lessened by a number of medical regimens. This may include laxatives, enemas, or dietary restrictions.

The continued application of such bowel management programs for several months or even years may, through bowel regulation, ultimately permit the medication and enemas to be reduced or even eliminated (see Chapter 13). Some individuals, however, who receive enemas over a long period of time express dissatisfaction with the logistic problem of administration. For this group, consider a continent stoma through which irrigation can be performed, with good results expected.

### NECROTIZING ENTEROCOLITIS

Necrotizing enterocolitis is a serious intestinal disorder that affects predominantly premature infants. As many as 8% of preterm infants with birth weights of 750 to 1,500 g develop the condition, whereas less than 10% are full term. It has also been established that this condition occurs in episodic epidemics, usually after 10 days of life.

## Pathogenesis

The precise pathogenesis of NEC is unknown. However, the well-known predisposing factors include prematurity, hyaline membrane disease, administration of synthetic hyperosmolar formulas, cardiac anomalies, hypovolemia, sepsis, and lack of breast milk. Formula-fed babies suffer NEC six times more frequently than breast-fed newborns. Other less common associated factors are hypothermia, the use of umbilical catheters, and a history of maternal cocaine abuse.

No question remains that bacteria play a prominent role in the pathogenesis of NEC. What remains controversial, however, is the specific sequence of events that eventually produces bowel necrosis, perforation, and generalized sepsis.

Ischemic, necrotic lesions, or both most frequently occur in the terminal ileum, cecum, and ascending colon.

## Clinical Manifestations

Symptoms of NEC most frequently appear in relation to the onset of feeding. This commonly occurs after 10 days of life, generally after the baby has received an artificial formula. Initial, albeit subtle, manifestations include increased gastric residual volumes, abdominal distension, and lethargy. More specific signs are blood-streaked stools and abdominal tenderness. Manifestations of a systemic septic process become evident, including temperature instability, bradycardia, apnea, hypoglycemia, shock, and cyanosis. The platelet and white blood cell counts are persistently low, and severe metabolic acidosis and hypoxia are the rule. The abdominal wall may be noted to be erythematous.

## Radiologic Studies

Radiologic evaluation provides variable images, depending on the stage of the disease. Initial plain and decubitus films may show signs of a nonspecific ileus. Rapid changes in the radiologic images are not uncommonly observed as the disease evolves. Signs of bowel edema and increased peritoneal fluid, as evidenced by a separation of loops of bowel, frequently appear concomitant with the administration of intravenous fluids for resuscitative purposes. Free intraperitoneal gas is obviously a sign of bowel perforation.

## Treatment

Basically, medical management is used to treat NEC, including decompression of the gastrointestinal tract with a nasogastric tube, reliable venous access, aggressive fluid resuscitation, and adequate oxygenation. Broad-spectrum antibiotics are initially started and change in antibiotic therapy is guided by subsequent specific bacteriologic findings. However, intervention by the surgeon is required if medical treatment fails. Ideally, surgical treatment should be initiated when the patient suffers a full-thickness bowel necrosis but which has not yet perforated.

## Operative Treatment

The objectives of surgery are to resect obvious necrotic or perforated bowel and to preserve as much intestine as possible, including questionably necrotic areas with stoma formation. Stomal closure can be performed several weeks later, provided the patient is stable and is growing.

Survival in newborns suffering from NEC has improved during recent years, with reports as high as 72.5% to 80%.

# 19

# Cutaneous Conditions

This chapter describes the skin conditions that affect the perianal area, with emphasis on the differential diagnosis, indications for biopsy, and treatment of the more important diseases. Those conditions that can be found in the anal area that are only incidental to the systemic cutaneous process are mentioned *en passant* if recognition of the disease in the area is felt to be unique or of particular interest.

## CLASSIFICATION

Dermatologic diseases can be categorized in a number of ways: (a) on the basis lesion type (e.g., flat, elevated, depressed); (b) according to whether they are primary or secondary; (c) histopathologically; or (d) by the commonly used classifications of inflammation, infection, and neoplasm. A modification using this last method is illustrated as follows:

### Dermatologic Anal Conditions

#### *Inflammatory Diseases*

Pruritus ani
Psoriasis
Lichen planus
Lichen sclerosus et atrophicus
Atrophoderma
Contact (i.e., allergic) dermatitis
Seborrheic dermatitis
Atopic dermatitis
Radiodermatitis
Behçet's syndrome
Lupus erythematosus
Dermatomyositis
Scleroderma

Erythema multiforme
Familial benign chronic pemphigus (i.e., Hailey-Hailey)
Pemphigus vulgaris
Cicatricial pemphigoid

### *Infectious Diseases*

Nonvenereal
  Pilonidal sinus
  Suppurative hidradenitis
  Fistula-in-ano
  Crohn's disease
  Tuberculosis
  Actinomycosis
  Herpes zoster
  Vaccinia
  Fournier's gangrene
  Tinea cruris
  Candidiasis (i.e., moniliasis)
  "Deep" mycoses
  Amebiasis cutis
  Trichomoniasis
  Schistosomiasis cutis
  Bilharziasis
  Oxyuriasis (e.g., pinworm, enterobiasis)
  Creeping eruption (i.e., larva migrans)
  Larva currens
  Cimicosis (i.e., bedbug bites)
  Pediculosis
  Scabies
Venereal
  Gonorrhea
  Syphilis
  Chancroid
  Granuloma inguinale
  Lymphogranuloma venereum (*Chlamydia* infection)
  Molluscum contagiosum
  Herpes genitalis
  Condylomata acuminata

### *Premalignant and Malignant Diseases*

Acanthosis nigricans
Leukoplakia

Mycosis fungoides
Leukemia cutis
Basal cell carcinoma
Squamous cell carcinoma
Malignant melanoma
Bowen's disease
Extramammary Paget's disease

In addition, a glossary of dermatologic terms to aid in interpreting the description of the lesions is found below.

## INFLAMMATORY CONDITIONS

### Pruritus Ani

Pruritus ani, a frequently heard complaint, is a symptom that was well recognized in antiquity. In the earliest manuscript exclusively devoted to anorectal disorders, the Chester Beatty Medical Papyrus, 10 of its 41 remedies were devoted to the management of anal itching and irritation. By far the most common anorectal symptom presenting to the dermatologist is pruritus ani. The rich nerve supply to the perianal area is thought to be the primary reason for its sensitivity to potential irritants.

### *Symptoms*

Itching is usually noted in the anal or, occasionally, in the genital areas, but the condition is not generalized. Although the anus is frequently the site for auto-eroticism, most individuals do not appear to fall into this category. The condition tends to be worse at night, awakening the patient from sleep. This leads to scratching, which exacerbates the complaint even further. Pruritus ani is more common in men than in women.

### *Differential Diagnosis*

Although the symptoms can be caused by a specific condition (e.g., hemorrhoids, anal fissure, scarring from prior anal surgery) or an associated problem (e.g., constipation or diarrhea), most patients are not found to have significant anorectal pathology, except for the obvious skin changes. Besides anorectal pathology, allergic (i.e., contact) dermatitis, mycoses, seborrhea, diabetes, and oxyuriasis (i.e., pinworm) have all been implicated as causative factors. Other dermatologic problems, such as psoriasis (see later), should be considered. In addition, the possibility of a systemic disease (e.g., diabetes) might necessitate further studies. Anal neurodermatitis can cause violent itching, which can lead to tearing of the perianal area. With chronicity, the skin can become atrophic or hypertrophic, with nodularity and scarring.

## Special Studies

Physiologic studies have demonstrated that in patients with idiopathic pruritus ani, the anal sphincter relaxes in response to rectal distension more readily than in those with no anal disease. It has also been observed that patients with idiopathic pruritus ani have an abnormal rectoanal inhibitory reflex and a lower threshold for internal sphincter relaxation during such studies as the saline continence test. It, therefore, is postulated that pruritus and soiling in some patients occur as a result of a defect in anal sphincter function.

## Glossary of Dermatologic Terms

The following glossary is adapted from Domonkos AN, Arnold HL Jr, Odom RB. Cutaneous symptoms, signs and diagnosis. In: *Andrew's diseases of the skin*, 7th ed. Philadelphia: WB Saunders, 1982:15; Fitzpatrick TB. Fundamentals of dermatologic diagnosis. In: Fitzpatrick TB, Eisen AZ, Wolff K, et al, eds. *Dermatology in general medicine*, 2nd ed. St. Louis: McGraw-Hill, 1979:10; and Rook A, Wilkinson DS. The principles of diagnosis. In: Rook A, Wilkinson DS, Ebling FJG, eds. *Textbook of dermatology*, 3rd ed. Oxford: Blackwell Scientific, 1979:57.

Elevated Lesions
  Abscess
  Bulla (Bullae): bleb; blisters containing serous or seropurulent fluid
  Crusts: dried masses of serum, pus, or blood, with epithelial and bacterial
    debris
  Cyst: sac containing liquid or semisolid material
  Desquamation: scales; results from abnormal keratinization and exfoliation of
    cornified epithelial cells
  Exfoliation: scales; laminated masses of keratin; desquamated epidermis
  Exudate: crusts; dried blood or pus
  Furuncle: necrotizing form of folliculitis; may coalesce to form a carbuncle
  Hyperkeratosis: increased thickening of the stratum corneum
  Keratosis (keratotic): horny growth
  Lichenification (lichenoid): thickened, leathery; exaggerated skin markings
    resembling a mosaic
  Nodule (nodular): larger papule
  Papule (papular, papilloma, papillomatosis): circumscribed solid elevations
    with no fluid
  Plaque: minimal height, relatively large surface area
  Pustule: "pimple"; elevation of the skin containing pus
  Urticaria: wheals
  Vegetation (vegetative): luxuriant, funguslike growth
  Vesicle: blister; circumscribed epidermal elevation
  Wheal: evanescent, edematous, variably sized flat elevation

Flat Lesions
  Infarct: coagulation necrosis resulting from ischemia
  Macule (macular): circumscribed change in skin color
  Sclerosis (sclerotic): induration or hardening
  Telangiectasia: caused by dilatation of capillary vessels and minute arteries
Depressed Lesions
  Atrophy (atrophic): thin, almost transparent epidermis
  Erosion
  Excoriation: mechanical abrasion
  Gangrene
  Scar: cicatrix secondary to injury or disease
  Sinus: tract from a suppurative cavity to skin surface
  Ulcer: excavation of variable depth involving loss of both dermis and epidermis

### Evaluation

Physical examination should include anoscopy and proctosigmoidoscopy to look for a local cause of the symptoms. Usually, however, the procedures are unrewarding. Examination with a magnifying lens may be helpful. Evaluation with a Wood's lamp may reveal fluorescence, but this equipment is usually not readily available in the office practice of most physicians and surgeons. Skin scrapings of the perianal area should be examined using a potassium hydroxide slide preparation and should be cultured on Sabouraud's medium for yeast and fungi if suspicion warrants (see *Fungal Infections*). However, because no good evidence suggests that abnormal fecal flora contributes to the symptomatology, neither qualitative nor quantitative assessmet of the stool is considered appropriate.

### Treatment

Pruritus ani has traditionally been considered a condition that eludes all attempts at cure. Numerous potions, nostrums, and lotions have been used with variable success, as well as more aggressive treatment (e.g., injection of local anesthetics, phenol, methylene blue, and alcohol). Excision and skin grafting have also been suggested.

Psychological factors have been thought to play a role in contributing to the symptoms. However, no objective evidence has ever demonstrated a statistically significant deviation from a normal personality. It is reasonable to assume that severe perianal itching, 24 hours a day, every day, is likely to make an individual rather irascible.

Recently, attention has been drawn to the role of diet in the cause of the condition; therefore, an accurately obtained history will often dictate the appropriate treatment. Items that have been implicated include the following:

• Coffee
• Tea
• Carbonated beverages, especially caffeinated colas

- Milk products
- Alcohol, particularly wine and beer
- Tomatoes and tomato products (e.g., ketchup)
- Cheese
- Chocolate
- Nuts
- Cigarette smoking

Cigarette smoking is another factor. It is postulated that all these products induce mucous discharge, probably through a systemic route, or possibly in some instances by changing the pH of the stool.

A patient may have been told that the problem is psychoneurotic, so reassurance and sympathy are beneficial factors that contribute to a satisfactory resolution. Removing or changing the dietary factor may cause the symptoms to disappear. Additionally, promoting complete evacuation with increased fluids and bulking agents (e.g., bran, psyllium) may help avoid the irritation. Rectal irrigation and a bowel management program also may be necessary for those individuals who experience incontinence or leakage of stool (see Chapter 13).

Despite the validity of the aforementioned suggestions, the most important advice that can be given is usually directed toward the management of anal hygiene. Many individuals perceive their problem to be one of lack of cleanliness; the opposite is more likely. Vigorous scrubbing of the area with soap and water will cause the skin to be defatted, and a contact dermatitis may supervene.

Advise the patient not to use soap in the area! The perineum should be cleansed with plain water, particularly when bathing or showering, and ideally even following defecation. Irrigating the rectum with warm water through a bulb syringe is often ameliorating. Some individuals are actually allergic to toilet paper, so that in stubborn cases a moist cloth should be used for cleansing. Even in a public toilet, a moistened paper towel is preferable to the irritative effects of continued rubbing with toilet paper. For those with copious discharge, a cotton ball placed at the anal verge, changed as necessary, may be helpful.

Many topical creams and ointments, obtained over-the-counter and by prescription, are available for the pruritus ani sufferer. Use of anesthetic ointments and creams (e.g., Nupercainal, Tronolane, Americaine) is not advised. Symptoms are only temporarily masked, the underlying problem is not addressed, and allergic dermatitis can develop. Soothing creams are generally preferred to ointments; many are quite satisfactory (e.g., Balneol, Tucks). For more severe skin cracking, bath treatment with Aveeno colloidal oatmeal may be helpful. However, when the proprietary preparation fails, consider the use of a topical steroid; this almost inevitably will bring immediate relief. It should be discontinued, however, as soon as symptoms resolve, to avoid skin atrophy (see *Atrophoderma*).

In the rare intractable case, sedatives and tranquilizers must be considered. In addition, biofeedback and self-hypnosis have been of demonstrable benefit for some patients. Consultation with a professional familiar with these techniques may be advisable.

## Psoriasis

Psoriasis is a common, chronic inflammatory disease of the skin, character-ized by rounded, circumscribed, erythematous, dry, scaling patches covered by grayish white or silvery white scales. The lesions have a predilection for the scalp and nails; the extensor surfaces of the limbs, elbows, knees; and the sacral region. When the condition occurs in the anal area, it can cause severe pruritic symptoms. Perianal psoriasis is usually sharply marginated, with a characteristic butterfly distribution extending over the coccyx and sacrum (Fig. 19.1). Psoriatic lesions are often present at other sites on the body.

Histologically, characteristic features include epidermal thickening (i.e., acan-thosis), regular elongation of the rete ridges with broadening of the deeper aspect, and elongation with edema of the dermal papillae. Increased mitotic activity may be seen in the epidermis. Cells of the stratum corneum usually have retained nuclei (i.e., parakeratosis). Focal collections of neutrophils in the sub-corneum are known as "Munro microabscesses."

Treatment usually consists of topical corticosteroids, tars, anthralin, or a com-bination of these. In addition, the use of ultraviolet (UV) light has been found to be beneficial. More recently, the so-called "PUV-A treatment" has been advocated. This consists of a combined systemic-external therapy, using a potent photoactive

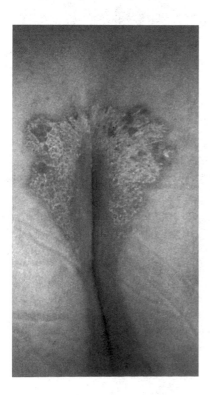

**FIG. 19.1.** Well-marginated erythematosquamous plaque with characteristic silvery scales indicates psoriasis. (Courtesy of Arnold Medved, M.D.)

agent (i.e., psoralen) followed by administration of a special light system emitting long-wave UV-A. Cancer chemotherapeutic drugs (e.g., methotrexate) have also been used.

## Lichen Planus

Lichen planus is a skin condition that consists of an eruption of small, flat-topped papules with a distinct violaceous color and polypoid configuration. The lesion is characteristically found on the flexor surfaces, mucous membranes, genitalia, and occasionally, the perianal area.

Histologically, the papule shows focal thickening of the granular layer, degeneration of the basement membrane and basal cells, and a bandlike lymphocytic infiltrate in the upper dermis. Biopsy of the skin establishes the diagnosis.

Treatment often has less than satisfactory results, corticosteroids appearing to be the most useful therapy for this condition. Topical preparations with occlusive dressings are helpful; systemic administration and intralesional injection have also been used. In mild cases, antipruritic lotions and antihistamines are used. Rest is also helpful.

## Lichen Sclerosus et Atrophicus

Lichen sclerosus et atrophicus (LSA) is an unusual condition of unknown cause. It occurs much more frequently in women than in men. The genital area appears to be the most commonly involved site.

Physical examination may reveal the characteristic "inverted keyhole" distribution. In this situation, the disease extends beyond the mucocutaneous border to involve the skin of the vulva, perineum, and perianal area. In the vulva, the condition affects the labia, vestibule, and introitus (Fig. 19.2). Discomfort, pruritus, dysuria, and dyspareunia are common.

The characteristic histologic change in lichen sclerosus et atrophicus is edema and homogenization of the collagen below the epidermis (Fig. 19.3). The epidermis also shows variable hyperkeratosis and follicular plugging. Lichen sclerosus et atrophicus may be associated with squamous cell carcinoma of the vulva. An association between the condition and squamous cell carcinoma of the perianal region has also been noted.

Treatment is primarily directed at relieving the pruritic complaints in the hope of lessening the risk for leukoplakia and carcinoma. A mild topical steroid sufficient to control the symptoms is advocated. Secondary infection should be treated with appropriate antibiotics.

## Atrophoderma or Atrophy of the Skin

Atrophy of the skin is a reaction to the repeated and prolonged application of topical corticosteroids; it can also follow local injection of these products.

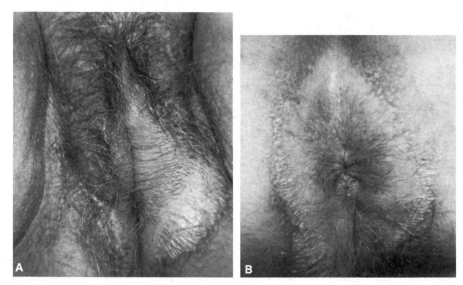

**FIG. 19.2.** Characteristic of lichen sclerosus et atrophicus is a sharply defined dermatosis in the (**A**) vulvar area and (**B**) perianal area with hypopigmentation centrally and hyperpigmentation peripherally. Note the lichenoid papules about the periphery. (Courtesy of John A. Clark, M.D.)

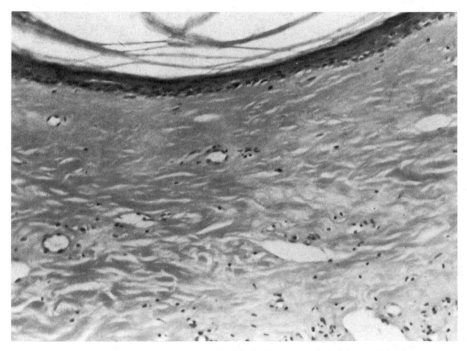

**FIG. 19.3.** Atrophy of the epidermis and hyalinization of the dermis in lichen sclerosis et atrophicus. (Original magnification ×120; courtesy of Rudolf Garret, M.D.)

Telangiectasia occurs, indicating loss of dermal collagen, and the patient who initially complained of pruritus subsequently reports discomfort and burning. The friction of walking rubs the already atrophic and thinned epidermis.

Patients usually report a history of self-application of topical corticosteroids for many years. Attempting to remove the medication is frequently unsuccessful. Biopsy may reveal atrophy and hyperkeratosis. Because of the risk for development of this condition, it is important to discontinue cortisone treatment as soon as possible.

### Contact or Allergic Dermatitis

Substances coming into contact with the skin cause two types of dermatitis:

1. Irritant dermatitis is a nonallergic reaction following exposure to an irritating substance.
2. Allergic (i.e., contact) dermatitis is caused by allergic sensitization to a number of agents.

Irritants include alkalis, acids, metal salts, dusts, gases, and hydrocarbons.

Allergic contact dermatitis results from a delayed type hypersensitivity, also known as cell-mediated hypersensitivity or immunity. A person may be exposed to an allergen for many years before hypersensitivity develops. The allergens, which are numerous and varied, include dyes, oils, resins; chemicals used for fabrics, cosmetics, and insecticides; and products or the substances of bacteria, fungi, and parasites

The most common causes of contact dermatitis are, in order of frequency:

1. Poison ivy, oak, and sumac
2. Paraphenylenediamine
3. Nickel
4. Common rubber compounds
5. Neomycin
6. Dichromates

The patch test is used to detect hypersensitivity to a substance that is in contact with the skin. A nonirritating concentration of agents suspected to be the cause of the contact dermatitis is applied. The patches remain in place for 48 hours, fewer hours if burning or itching occurs. A positive reaction will produce severe pruritus and erythema or vesicles. It is wise to defer this test, however, until the rash has cleared, to limit the likelihood of a severe exacerbation.

Therapy is directed toward removing the underlying cause of the skin problem or the allergen. Iodine and adhesive tape are common dermatitis-inducing products in patients who undergo anal surgery. Soothing compresses such as Aveeno colloidal oatmeal, in addition to corticosteroids, and possibly antipruritics, may be advisable.

## Seborrheic Dermatitis

Seborrheic dermatitis is a chronic, superficial, inflammatory disease of the skin, with a predilection for the scalp, eyebrows, nasolabial crease, ears, axillae, submammary folds, umbilicus, groin, and gluteal crease. The disease is characterized by dry, moist, or greasy scales, and by crusted, pink-yellow patches of diverse size and shape. The condition, believed to result from hypersecretion of sebum, is apparently exacerbated by increased perspiration and emotional stress. A high fat intake is frequently noted.

Histologically, the picture is similar to that of psoriasis, but Munro abscesses are not seen. According to one school of thought, the two conditions are so similar that some justification is seen for thinking their cause must be the same. The application of corticosteroids is the primary therapy. Recent evidence favors a role for yeast organisms in the cause of the condition, with therapy being directed accordingly.

## Atopic Dermatitis or Atopic Eczema

The term *atopy* is derived from the Greek word meaning "out of place" or "strange." It is defined as the tendency for allergies to various substances to develop, manifested by systemic symptoms such as asthma, hay fever, and eczema. The condition is believed to be either a form of immunologic deficiency or possibly a blockade of β-adrenergic receptors in the skin.

Atopic dermatitis can occur as localized, erythematous, scaly, papular, or vesicular patches, or in the form of pruritic, lichenified lesions. The condition is often paroxysmal; emotional upset can initiate an attack. Other factors exacerbating the problem include clothing, certain foods, and dryness of the skin. Superimposed infections (e.g., intertrigo and dermatophytosis) can produce further recurrences.

Histologically, hyperkeratosis and parakeratosis with acanthosis are noted (Fig. 19.4). When lichenification is present, the acanthosis is increased and papillomatosis, with long papillary bodies, reaches to the stratum corneum. These changes somewhat resemble those seen in psoriasis.

Treatment consists of avoiding, if possible, emotional stress; avoiding extremes of cold and heat; limiting the use of stimulant beverages; and using oral antihistamines and topical corticosteroids. Prednisone (30 to 40 mg orally for 4 to 6 weeks or possibly longer) is usually recommended. Alternatively, a parenteral preparation can be substituted.

## Radiodermatitis

Radiodermatitis is a particular problem in the anal area, because current therapy for carcinoma of the rectum, anus, and prostate often involves ionizing radiation. In some individuals, unfortunately, the cancer treatment may actually be worse than the original disease.

Many changes are found in the cell as the result of radiation therapy. Mitoses are temporarily arrested, chromosomal abnormalities occur, and at least a temporary

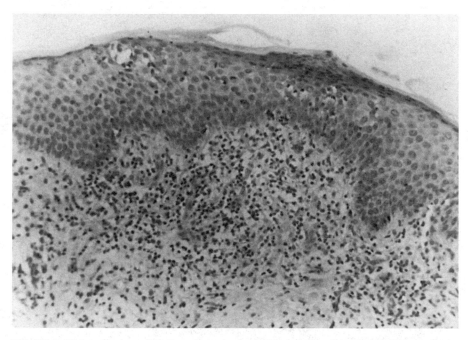

**FIG. 19.4.** Histologic characteristics of atopic dermatitis include mild acanthosis, spongiosis, focal parakeratosis, and dermal mononuclear cell infiltrate. (Original magnification ×180; courtesy of Rudolf Garret, M.D.)

halt occurs in the normal cell cycle. The amount of skin change resulting from radiotherapy depends on the dose. Changes can be manifested as erythema, edema, and ulceration; symptoms can include burning, itching, or severe pain. After a period of time, telangiectasia, atrophy, and freckling may appear. The skin becomes dry, thin, smooth, and shiny (Fig. 19.5). Radiation injury can result in the subsequent development of malignancy, in most cases following a rather prolonged latent period. The incidence of this complication increases with the passage of time.

Results of treatment are often less than satisfactory. If no evidence is seen of malignant change, little or no specific therapy is advisable. Cleansing the area with a mild soap and water, in addition to the use of an emollient, a corticosteroid preparation, or both, may be of help. Biopsy specimens should be taken from any suspicious lesions.

## Behçet's Syndrome

Behçet's syndrome is characterized by four main symptoms: recurrent aphthous ulcers in the mouth, skin lesions, eye lesions, and genital ulcerations. Genital ulcerations can be found in persons of both sexes on the genitocrural fold, on the anus, on the perineum, or in the rectum. Although the cause of the condition is unknown,

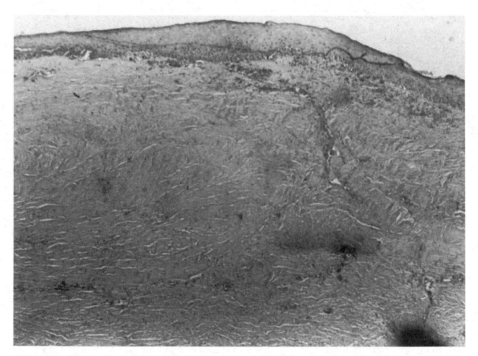

**FIG. 19.5.** Histologic findings of radiodermatitis include fibrosis of the dermis with sclerosis, atrophy of the epidermis, and absence of skin appendages. (Original magnification ×120; courtesy of Rudolf Garret, M.D.)

some evidence suggests that Behçet's syndrome has a viral etiology, or is possibly an autoimmune disease. Histologically, the lesions usually show a vasculitis.

The anal condition can be misdiagnosed as hemorrhoids, fissure, Crohn's disease, condylomata, or venereal disease. Surgery is contraindicated. Corticosteroid treatment, systemically or topically, is the treatment of choice.

## Lupus Erythematosus

Lupus erythematosus, as with other connective tissue diseases, occurs only rarely in the anal area, and still more rarely as an isolated finding in this location. The cutaneous manifestation is called "discoid lupus erythematosus" (DLE). It can begin with single or multiple lesions involving entire regions of the body, especially the head and neck, sternum, vulva, and perineum. The typical plaque is approximately 1 cm or more in diameter, with characteristic scales. Removal of the scales reveals patulous, follicular orifices with dry, horny keratinous plugs. Occasionally, a basal cell or squamous cell carcinoma develops in long-standing DLE lesions.

In laboratory investigation, the LE cell test usually yields a negative result in DLE. Results of the direct immunofluorescence test are usually positive, however, as are antinuclear antibody test results.

Treatment consists of avoidance of strong sunlight, extremes in temperature, and localized trauma. Corticosteroid creams and ointments are particularly beneficial, with intralesional steroid therapy often helpful. Systemic therapy with antimalarials also has been advised.

## Dermatomyositis

Dermatomyositis (i.e., polymyositis) is an inflammatory condition that produces angiopathy in the skin, subcutaneous tissue, and muscles. The disease usually starts in the face and eyelids, and can spread to other areas. It is associated with a number of other disturbances, including Raynaud's phenomenon, alopecia, urticaria, and erythema multiforme. Of particular interest to the surgeon is that in patients above 40 years of age, a visceral cancer is frequently associated with the condition. Histologic changes are similar to those of lupus erythematosus.

Treatment consists of rest, salicylates, steroids, methotrexate, and azathioprine.

## Scleroderma or Progressive Systemic Sclerosis

Scleroderma is characterized by the appearance of circumscribed or diffuse, smooth, hard, ivory-colored areas that are immobile and give the skin the appearance of being "hidebound." The skin becomes smooth, yellowish, and firm, and it shrinks, so that the underlying structures are bound down. Although the condition frequently involves the face and hands, leading to an expressionless facial appearance and a clawlike appearance of the hands, it can progress to involve most of the internal organs. Involvement of the small intestine can cause constipation, diarrhea, and abdominal distension. Although the colon is only rarely affected, it can produce the signs and symptoms of Ogilvie's syndrome. Treatment consists of general supportive measures, baths, a high-protein diet, corticosteroids, and a number of other medications, including immunosuppressives.

## Erythema Multiforme

Erythema multiforme is a clinically and histologically distinctive condition precipitated by the following conditions, among others:

- Viral infections
- Bacterial infections
- Radiotherapy
- Carcinomatosis
- Pregnancy
- Connective tissue diseases
- Drug reactions

The mechanism causing the reaction resulting in erythema multiforme reaction is unknown. The lesions present as flat, dull red maculopapules that can be rather small or can increase to 1 or 2 cm in 48 hours. The periphery may remain red, whereas the center is purpuric. The lesions look almost like targets. They commonly appear in the oral mucous membrane, but genital lesions are also frequent.

Histologically, the abnormality is confined to the upper dermis and lower epidermis. In more severe cases, the whole epidermis is necrotic. Bullae usually are subepidermal.

Treatment consists of symptomatic relief in mild cases. In severe cases, the use of corticosteroids has been suggested. Antibiotics are advised if secondary infection occurs.

### Familial Benign Chronic Pemphigus or Hailey-Hailey

Familial benign chronic pemphigus is a hereditary disease characterized by a recurrent bullous and vesicular dermatitis of the neck, axillae, flexors, and epithelial surfaces that appose. The condition has been found localized to the perianal area and may pose confusion in differential diagnosis. The disease is transmitted as an autosomal dominant trait. The histologic pattern is unique, with prominent intraepidermal vesicles and bullae (Fig. 19.6).

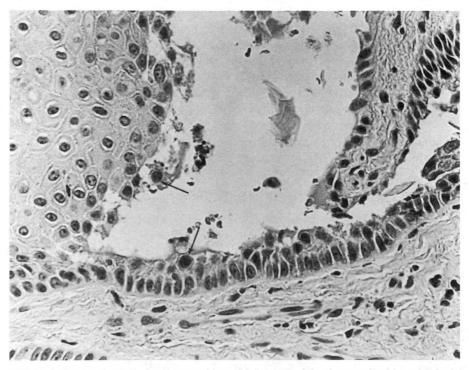

FIG. 19.6. Benign familial chronic pemphigus (Hailey-Hailey) is characterized by suprabasal bullae, such as the one shown here, containing detached prickle cells and good preservation of acantholytic cells. Note the moderate inflammatory reaction in the underlying dermis. (Original magnification ×180; courtesy of Rudolf Garret, M.D.)

Treatment consists of local or systemic antibiotics and the use of topical corticosteroids. Additionally, low-dose radiation treatment has been recommended. Excision and skin grafting have been used to treat localized areas.

## Pemphigus Vulgaris

Pemphigus vulgaris is characterized by bullae appearing on apparently normal skin and mucous membranes. The lesions usually begin first in the mouth, then in the groin, scalp, face, neck, axillae, and genitals. An autoimmune mechanism appears to be the cause. The condition occurs equally in both sexes, usually in adults in their fifth and sixth decades. Circulating intercellular antibodies may be demonstrated in these individuals.

The pathologic changes arc acantholysis, cleft and blister formation in the intraepidermal areas just above the basal cell layer, and the formation of acantholytic cells (Fig. 19.7). Characteristic of the separation of keratinocytes is the presence of the Tzanck cell lining the bulla, as well as lying free in the cavity.

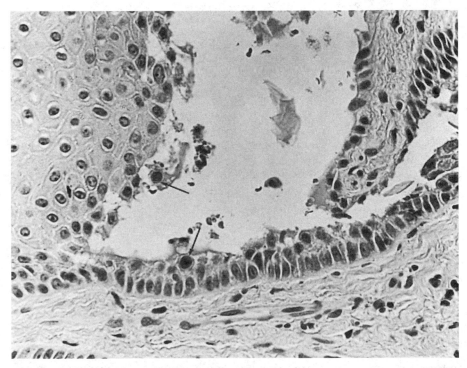

**FIG. 19.7.** Intraepithelial vesicles such as this one are characteristic of pemphigus vulgaris. The *arrows* indicate cells with large hyperchromatic nuclei (Tzanck cells). No inflammatory reaction is seen in the dermis. (Original magnification ×600.)

Because of the pain associated with advanced cases, prolonged daily baths with permanganate solution are advised. Silvadene cream, which is effective in the treatment of burns, is also useful in this condition. High-dose corticosteroids (prednisone, 160 mg daily) remain the primary therapy. Cancer chemotherapeutic agents have also been advised.

### Cicatricial Pemphigoid or Benign Mucosal Pemphigoid

Cicatricial pemphigoid is characterized by the presence of transient vesicles that heal by scarring of mucous membranes. The condition most commonly occurs in the mouth and conjunctivae. Other areas of involvement include the pharynx, esophagus, genitalia, and anus. In rare cases, the lesion has been confined to the genital and anal areas. Direct immunofluorescence of the lesion reveals the presence of antibodies at the basement membrane. The absence of acantholysis differentiates the condition from pemphigus vulgaris.

No effective medication is currently available for cicatricial pemphigoid. Obstructing areas in the larynx and esophagus may require tracheostomy or gastrostomy.

## INFECTIOUS CONDITIONS

For the purposes of discussion, the infectious processes are classified as non-venereal and as those usually attributable to venereal causes.

### Nonvenereal Infections

#### Pilonidal Sinus

Pilonidal sinus is a common infective process occurring in the natal cleft and sacrococcygeal region. It primarily affects young adults and teenagers. There is a 3:1 male predominance. The term literally means "nest of hair"; this is because the epithelium-lined sinus usually is found to contain hair.

When the sinus becomes infected, commonly after puberty, it drains from an opening or openings overlying the coccyx and sacrum. The infected abscess can extend to the perianal area in a presentation that can be mistaken for anal fistula. The disease can also be confused with suppurative hidradenitis. Although the condition is by no means life-threatening, it does cause considerable disability for many individuals.

#### Etiology

The cause of pilonidal sinus has been the subject of some controversy. One possible theory that has been espoused is the failure of fusion in the embryo, with resultant entrapment of hair follicles in the sacrococcygeal region. Proponents of this theory are quick to point out the frequent incidence of eyebrow hair meeting in the midline in such patients. Another theory attributes the problem to the result of trauma, with the introduction of hair shafts into the subdermal area.

## Symptoms and Findings

The patient usually presents with pain, swelling, and purulent drainage at and around the site of the pilonidal opening. Evident, may be the typical appearance of an abscess that can be found anywhere in the skin and subcutaneous tissue. Fever and leukocytosis can also accompany the symptoms.

Some individuals merely observe periodic discharge or intermittent swelling and discomfort. The process can resolve spontaneously or progress to more obvious drainage, swelling, and pain.

## Treatment

Antibiotics have little place in the therapy, except possibly to augment the surgical procedure. For acute pilonidal abscess, incision and drainage will relieve the patient's symptoms. Regardless of the size of the septic process, incision and drainage can usually be done in the physician's office, or in an ambulatory care facility. Whenever possible, it is advisable to drain the abscess and curette or excise the infected sinus simultaneously. The Standards Task Force of the American Society of Colon and Rectal Surgeons has established the following practice parameters for the performance of ambulatory surgery.

> Localized pilonidal abscesses, either primary or recurrent, can usually be incised and drained under local anesthesia in an outpatient setting. For uncomplicated pilonidal sinuses, definitive surgical treatment, including but not limited to excision, curettage, and unroofing, can be accomplished as an outpatient procedure. More complicated surgical procedures, including but not limited to wide excision, creation of skin flaps, and grafting, may require inpatient stay for concern over skin viability or bleeding. Extensive cellulitis in association with pilonidal disease may require inpatient intravenous antibiotic therapy.

Definitive elective treatment of pilonidal disease includes excision and primary closure, excision and grafting, excision leaving the wound open to close secondarily, incision and curettage, follicle excision, and cryosurgical destruction.

Interestingly, almost irrespective of the method of treatment applied, very few patients are troubled with symptoms of persistent pilonidal sinus disease beyond the age of 40 years. Perhaps they simply outgrow the condition. It is important, therefore, to understand that ultimate cure is an almost inevitable result when comparing the value of the various surgical alternatives. Another problem with analyzing the data is that very few so-called prospective, randomized, controlled studies can survive critical review.

*Drainage with or without Excision.* Incision or excision with drainage is simple to do; it requires minimal hospital stay and, in fact, usually can be done with a local anesthetic in the office. A probe is passed from opening to opening and the sinus is unroofed. Alternatively, the multiple openings can be excised *en bloc*, and any further extensions or side tracts curetted out. If the procedure is done on an ambulatory basis, the patient is instructed to remove the packing the following morning, usually while taking a bath.

With this approach, an expeditious surgical procedure and a shortened or eliminated hospital stay, in essence, are exchanged for a prolonged postoperative convalescence, especially in patients with extensive or deep tissue involvement. All too often, these difficult wounds require frequent treatments, necessitating cauterization, shaving, cleansing, and packing. An approach to dealing with this problem is taping the buttocks apart to flatten the intergluteal cleft during the healing process.

Healing per primam can be expected in 60% of cases within 10 weeks. The recurrence rate following initial primary healing is 20%. Those with fewer pits and lateral tracts have a significantly better chance of healing primarily. It is not uncommon for pilonidal sinus wounds that extend toward the anal verge to take 6 months or longer to heal. Delayed healing can persist to the point where re-excision is advised; multiple operative procedures are frequent sequelae under these circumstances. It is for this reason that I am reluctant to advise this particular approach, except for small sinuses. Agreement found in all current writings indicates that wide excision of all tissue down to the sacrum, leaving the wound to heal by granulation, cannot be justified.

*Marsupialization.* Excision with marsupialization is a compromise between a completely open wound and a completely closed one. This operation permits a somewhat smaller opening than does the technique in which the wound is left totally open. If the catgut or long-term absorbable suture succeeds in holding the edges together, more rapid healing should occur. Unfortunately, the sutures frequently pull out, and the individual is left with as wide a wound as would have resulted had excision and packing been done. Even without this complication, the wound still requires careful attention, including packing, shaving, and cleansing.

Marsupialization remains one of the most commonly used options for the treatment of pilonidal sinus. The average healing time is 4 weeks, with some individuals requiring up to 20 weeks for closure. The recurrence rate is approximately 6%, all ultimately healing following remarsupialization.

*Excision with Primary Closure.* Excision with primary closure can be performed in an ambulatory surgical facility if the sinus is relatively small. However, for more extensive lesions, inpatient therapy is recommended. This approach has the disadvantage of a relatively prolonged hospital stay, but it provides the potential benefit of a healed wound within perhaps 10 to 14 days. For large, complex pilonidal sinus problems, particularly when multiple procedures have been performed, the excision and primary closure technique may be effective.

The pilonidal sinus is excised to the gluteal fascia. The fascia is incised, and a periosteal elevator is used to lift the fascia off the sacrum. This maneuver permits the placement of heavy retention sutures through all layers. These are laid into position, and the fascia is reapproximated with absorbable suture material.

The wound is copiously irrigated, and the skin is closed. The retention sutures are secured over a stent dressing, and the dressing is left in place for approximately 10 days.

A technique for limiting the likelihood of recurrence following excision of pilonidal sinus by means of a variation of excision with primary closure has been described. By this technique, each sinus is completely excised through a vertical, eccentric, elliptical incision. By undermining the medial edge and advancing it across the midline, a thick flap is created and the entire suture line is lateralized to reduce the risk for recurrence.

In almost all cases, primary healing should be obtained. Recurrence rates are approximately 20%. As expected, healing is much quicker after primary suture than after excisional therapy alone (median, 14 vs. 64 days).

*Excision with Grafting.* With considerable skin loss, as can occur following multiple operations, it is sometimes useful to rotate skin flaps to cover the defect. This can be done by one of the techniques—advancement or rotation flaps—or even, as has been suggested, by means of a gluteus maximus myocutaneous flap. To eliminate the deep natal cleft with the standard vertical wound, which tends to pull apart, a number of authors have recommended the use of a Z-plasty. Others suggest excision in a rhombic fashion, with coverage affected by means of a so-called "Limberg fasciocutaneous buttock flap." Another modification of the rhombic flap design is the so-called "Dufourmentel technique." In the Z-plasty, the depth of the intergluteal fold with the associated pilonidal sinus disease is excised; skin flaps are then mobilized, rotated, and interdigitated (Fig. 19.8).

Reports of the success of excision and grafting are somewhat difficult to interpret in light of the lack of a control in these studies. The recurrence rate most commonly ranges from 1.7% to 4%, and the failure rate from 3% to 4%. When skin is lost as a consequence of pilonidal sinus disease, particularly in the recurrent situation, mobilizing skin to cover the defect more reliably leads to a satisfactory result.

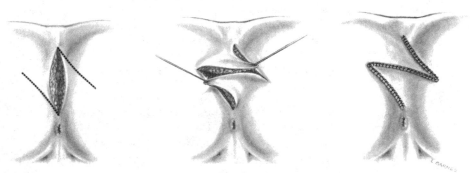

A,B          C

**FIG. 19.8.** Treatment of pilonidal sinus by Z-plasty. **A.** Incisions outlined. **B.** Skin flaps rotated. **C.** Primary closure obliterates natal cleft defect.

*Sinus Extraction.* Other operations have been advocated that require excision of less tissue. The Lord or Bascom modification consists of lateral drainage of the abscess, removal of the hair, and excision of the hair follicle, if present. Minimal excision of a sinus tract can be performed. The cavity is cleansed through incisions adjacent to but not inside the pilonidal sinus. The cavity walls are not excised but are permitted to collapse. The procedure can be carried out in the office or at an ambulatory surgical facility. An alternative approach is to drain the acute abscess and allow the infection to subside before follicle removal is attempted.

This technique is analogous to that of the management of a "horseshoe" fistula, in which the aim is to remove the crypt-bearing area and establish adequate drainage. Certainly, if this can be done satisfactorily, in all probability, healing will result. The same "less is more" approach appears equally valid for selected instances of pilonidal sinus.

The mean disability is 1 day, and the mean wound-healing time is about 3 to 4 weeks. Recurrences appear in approximately 8% to 10%.

*Sclerosing Injection.* Some authors have recommended injection of phenol (80%) into the sinus tract, and have reported recurrence rates as low as 6.3%.

*Cryosurgery.* The use of cryosurgical destruction has also been advocated. The technique consists of surgery (opening of the tracts and side branches), curettage, and electrocoagulation of bleeding points. The open wound is then sprayed with liquid nitrogen for approximately 5 minutes.

*Nonoperative Management.* The role of conservative, nonoperative treatment of pilonidal sinus disease should not be overlooked. Complete healing can be accomplished through meticulous hair control by natal cleft shaving, improved perineal hygiene, and limited lateral incision and drainage for abscess.

*Comment: It is now generally agreed that minimal surgery should be applied to the treatment of pilonidal disease, whenever possible. The concept of removing the hair follicles and the hairs themselves without extensive excision and debridement is an excellent one. Every attempt should be made to keep the patient out of the hospital and to limit the morbidity of the procedure. However, some individuals will benefit from a more generous excision, particularly those who have had multiple procedures or have extensive disease. Under these circumstances, inpatient hospital treatment with excision and primary closure with or without grafting may reduce morbidity, and offer shortened convalescence and more rapid healing.*

### Pilonidal Sinus and Squamous Cell Carcinoma

Squamous cell carcinoma has been reported to arise in pilonidal sinus tracts, almost all inevitably involving long-standing active inflammation. As of 1996, 44 cases were reported. Treatment consists of wide excision and grafting. This is similar to the management of squamous cell carcinoma of the skin anywhere in the body, which can lend itself to this approach. More recently, it has been suggested that because of the high recurrence rate of the malignancy, consideration should be given to adjuvant chemotherapy and radiation.

## Suppurative Hidradenitis or Hidradenitis Suppurativa

Suppurative hidradenitis is an uncommon, chronic, recurrent, indolent infection involving the skin and subcutaneous tissue that arises in the apocrine glands (i.e., axillary, inguinal, genital, perineal, and mammary). The most frequent area of involvement is the axillae, but the perianal area can also be affected. The incidence is increased in women, with most cases occurring between the ages of 16 and 40. Although the cause is unknown, acne appears to be a predisposing factor; poor skin hygiene, hyperhidrosis, and chemical depilatories may play a role. An androgen-based endocrine disorder has also been postulated. No increased association with diabetes mellitus has been documented, but impaired glucose tolerance has been observed. A genetic predisposition based on an increased familial incidence may exist.

The condition can commence with obstruction of the apocrine gland duct, with resultant inspissated secretions. The gland may then rupture, which can lead to extension of the process into the dermis, with consequent secondary involvement of other glands and ducts. In rare instances, the process can extend through the fascia into the underlying muscle.

Suppurative hidradenitis can be confused with anal fistula, Crohn's disease, tuberculosis, pilonidal sinus, infected sebaceous cyst, furunculosis, and other infections in the anal area. In cases in which the disease is long-standing, squamous cell carcinoma has been reported to have developed.

### Physical Examination

Examination reveals tender, erythematous, purulent lesions, which can be associated with adenopathy and systemic signs (e.g., fever, malaise, leukocytosis). The condition frequently produces burrowing sinuses that can extend for many inches around the anus, into the scrotum, buttocks, labia, medial thighs, and sacrum. Although the tracts are usually relatively superficial, they can invade deeply and extend to involve the area around the femoral vessels.

### Histopathology

Microscopically, the earliest inflammatory changes are seen within and around the apocrine glands, the ducts of which can be distended with leukocytes. In the chronic stage, multiple abscesses, intercommunicating sinus tracts, and irregular hypertrophied scars form. The scars, ulceration, and infection extend within the subcutaneous tissue to the fascia.

### Treatment

Antibiotic therapy early in the course of the disease is of value. A number of bacteria have been isolated, including staphylococci, streptococci, *Escherichia coli*, and *Proteus* species. Local and systemic broad-spectrum antibiotics are advised; these include penicillin, erythromycin, and tetracycline in those cases when acne is noted in other areas. The antibiotics should be used until resolution of the process is complete; some patients require treatment for months or even years. Isotretinoin (Accutane) has been shown to benefit some patients. Unfortunately, some individuals do not respond to any medical regimen, and disability is such that surgical intervention is required to treat the extensive sinus tracts and abscesses.

With minimal involvement and inadequate palliation by medical means, incision and drainage of an abscess may result in cure. When the condition progresses to extensive sinus formation, excision is the only means by which the condition can be effectively ameliorated.

The four methods of surgical treatment are as follows:

1. Excision with primary closure
2. Excision with grafting
3. Excision with marsupialization
4. Excision with packing

All four methods can be applied usefully, even in the same patient. Primary closure usually requires a relatively narrow wound; often, however, by elevating the full thickness of skin on either side of the excision site, the wound can be approximated without tension. Wide excision, leaving the wound open to heal by second intention, is probably the most common method of surgical treatment.

Methods to close the wound include the application of a split-thickness graft or some form of plastic procedure (e.g., Z-plasty). Occasionally, it is necessary to perform a diverting colostomy when extensive surgery and grafting are required in the perianal area. Fortunately, the anal canal itself is usually spared. Involvement of the sphincter muscle is so unusual that this observation should prompt consideration of another diagnosis for the problem. In those who have both anterior and posterior disease in the perineal area, it may be wise from the perspective of patient discomfort and disability to perform surgery on one side only and to treat the opposite side after healing has taken place.

### Fistula-in-Ano or Anal Fistula

Anal fistula is another perianal infective process that can be confused with pilonidal sinus and suppurative hidradenitis. Chapter 11 is dedicated to the diagnosis and management of this condition.

### Crohn's Disease

Anal and perianal Crohn's disease present a difficult management problem. This condition is discussed in Chapter 11, and the diagnosis and management of Crohn's disease is presented in Chapter 30.

## Tuberculosis

Tuberculosis distal to the ileocecal valve is uncommon, and it is seldom even considered in the differential diagnosis when the disease process is located in the large intestine. When it affects the perianal area, it can be confused with Crohn's disease, actinomycosis, anal fistula, and other skin conditions. Most reported cases occur in developing countries. The disease, which is seen most commonly in men, is usually but not always, associated with pulmonary tuberculosis. Primary inoculation of the mycobacteria may result from trauma to the skin or mucosa.

The lesion may appear as a brownish red papule that can progress into an ulcerating plaque; this is known as a tuberculous chancre. Regional lymphadenopathy is common. A high index of suspicion is necessary to establish the diagnosis early and to initiate appropriate therapy. An anal fissure in an unusual location that is slow to heal should be pathologically confirmed with appropriate staining and cultures to rule out the presence of the bacterium.

The ulcers are usually painful and indolent, with blue irregular edges. Diagnosis can be established by (a) the determination of acid-fast bacilli in the biopsy specimen; (b) positive guinea pig culture; and (c) the presence of caseating granulomas in the histologic examination of skin lesions.

Antituberculous drugs are the treatment of choice. Therapy with isoniazid, rifampin, and ethambutol will usually resolve the anal condition in a matter of 2 or 3 weeks. However, treatment should be continued for many months following resolution of the local or systemic manifestations.

## Actinomycosis

Actinomycosis is a chronic infectious disease involving the cervicofacial area, thorax, or abdomen. It is caused by an anaerobic, gram-positive bacterium, *Actinomyces israelii*. It produces a suppurative, fibrosing inflammation that forms sinus tracts, discharging granules. In the abdominal form, a mass is usually present, and a psoas abscess occasionally occurs.

Diagnosis is established by identifying the microorganism in cultures of tissue or the exudate of the lesion; the finding of sulfur granules leaves no doubt to the diagnosis. In the anal area, sinus tracts and fistulas can resemble those of Crohn's disease, anal fistula, suppurative hidradenitis, and tuberculosis. The presence of the disease elsewhere, particularly in the abdomen, is helpful in alerting the surgeon to the nature of the problem. The possibility of perianal actinomycosis should be entertained in any individual who has extensive fistula tracts and in whom recurrence develops after what are considered adequate attempts at surgical treatment.

Treatment consists of surgical excision and drainage of the abscess as well as antibiotics—usually penicillin. A 4-week period of treatment is recommended.

## Viral Infections

Virtually any viral infection that affects the skin can involve the perianal area as part of a generalized cutaneous process or by autoinoculation from another site. When lesions are seen in an intertriginous zone, they may not resemble the typical appearance seen elsewhere. A misdiagnosis of condition as secondary syphilis may result. Two common viral infections that are presumed to be non-venereal in origin are mentioned briefly.

### Herpes Zoster

Herpes zoster, caused by reactivation of varicella, can involve the anal area. The condition, also known as "shingles," affects both sexes equally and may be particularly troublesome in patients who have been immunosuppressed by treatment for malignancy. The lesion is characterized by groups of vesicles on an erythematous base along the distribution of a spinal nerve leading to a posterior ganglion. Itching, tenderness, and pain are characteristically located along the region supplied by the nerve.

Diagnosis can be established by means of tissue culture and by demonstration of antibodies in the serum by immunofluorescent techniques. Histologically, vesicles are seen to be intraepidermal; within these vesicles are found large, swollen cells called "balloon cells" (Fig. 19.9).

Treatment consists of medical measures, including rest and the application of heat. Analgesics are advisable for acute neuralgia. Acyclovir (Zovirax; 800 mg) orally four to five times per day for 7 to 10 days) is helpful if initiated early in the course of the disease. For older patients with severe pain, systemic corticosteroid therapy may be considered.

### Vaccinia

Vaccinia virus is an attenuated cowpox virus that has been propagated in laboratories for immunization against smallpox. Perianal vaccinia is a rare complication of vaccination, and usually occurs in young children. It has also been reported as a complication of diarrhea, with probable transmission to the excoriated area by the fingers. In adults, the condition can be confused with syphilis or with herpes simplex infection. The history is helpful if the patient was recently vaccinated or was exposed to someone who had been vaccinated.

Treatment is generally supportive, because complete recovery usually occurs spontaneously. However, vaccinia immune globulin has been recommended in severe cases or to expedite resolution of the process.

### Bacterial Infections

Infective processes associated with bacterial organisms (e.g., pilonidal sinus and suppurative hidradenitis) have already been discussed. However, Fournier's gangrene, a unique infective condition in the perianal area is worthy of discussion.

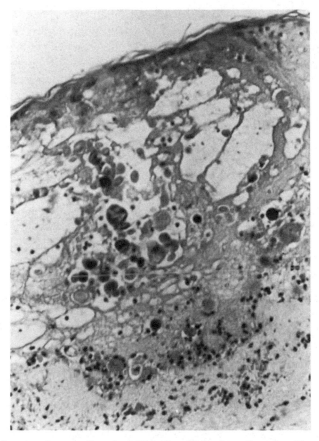

**FIG. 19.9.** Ballooning degeneration of prickle cells with the formation of multilocular vesicles in herpes zoster. Note cells with large inclusion bodies. (Original magnification ×240; courtesy of Rudolf Garret, M.D.)

### *Fournier's Gangrene or Necrotizing Perineal Infection*

In 1883, Fournier described a necrotizing soft-tissue infection of the perineum, groin, and genitalia that almost invariably ended fatally. Because of the prevalence of two or more species of bacteria in the infection, the term *synergistic gangrene* has been employed. *Necrotizing fasciitis* is another expression that has been used to describe the condition. However, it is important to distinguish this entity from clostridial myonecrosis, because the treatment obviously differs.

Why such a fulminant septic process develops in some patients with seemingly trivial septic problems in the rectum, perianal area, or urinary tract is not known. Delay in making the correct diagnosis and initiating appropriate treatment of minor infections probably is the major contributing factor. The high mortality rate associated with these infections may, in part, be attributed to its occurrence in patients with debilitating illnesses, including diabetes. Urinary tract infection, instrumentation, and surgery have all been implicated as contributing factors. Patients having chemotherapy and those with acquired immunodeficiency syndrome (AIDS) are also more susceptible, implying that immunosuppression may play a role. Some have a history of prior anorectal surgery or pelvic surgery for an infective process (e.g., perforated diverticulitis). Rubber ring ligation of hemorrhoids has also been reported to be the precipitating event in a number of cases. Virtually all patients in published series have a demonstrable port of entry for the organism; specifically, perianal infection has become the most common cause. Interestingly, the well-recognized entity in children of perianal cellulitis, caused by hemolytic streptococci, does not seem to predispose to the development of this complication.

The average age is 50 years, with 14% of cases occurring in female patients. The most common etiologic factors were colorectal (33%), idiopathic (26%), and genitourinary (21%). The overall mortality in the series was 22%.

## Symptoms and Findings

The usual presenting complaints are perineal pain and swelling. Frank suppuration or even gangrene of the overlying skin may be apparent in advanced cases. Fever and leukocytosis are invariably present.

A number of organisms have been identified, both aerobic and anaerobic, including *Clostridium welchii*. More commonly, the gangrene is caused by such mixed bacterial flora as the microaerophilic organisms *Streptococcus, Staphylococcus aureus* and *albus, Bacteroides, Klebsiella, Escherichia coli, Enterococcus, Proteus*, and *Citrobacter*. Gram stains and aerobic and anaerobic cultures should be obtained from the margins where infection is advancing.

## Treatment

Broad-spectrum antibiotic therapy is recommended. Because most anaerobic isolates are reported to be sensitive to clindamycin and metronidazole, these are the first-line antibiotics of choice; however, vigorous surgical excision and debridement of all nonviable tissue is imperative. Treatment with hyperbaric oxygen is controversial and may be contraindicated unless the infection is caused by *C. welchii*. A colostomy may be advisable to reduce fecal contamination of the area, but is mandatory if colonic disease is the cause of the perineal sepsis. Debridement must be radical and should be continued until the skin and subcutaneous tissue cannot be readily separated from the fascia. Histologic examination of the margins of excised tissue can be useful in determining the adequacy of debridement. Because of the life-threatening nature of the illness, do not be concerned about the need for subsequent skin coverage or reconstruction. The wounds are left open and packed, and the patient is returned to the operating room if further debridement is deemed advisable. Vigorous irrigation with antiseptic solution (e.g., peroxide, Dakin solution) is recommended. Delayed primary closure, skin grafting, and other reconstructive procedures are often ultimately required.

### Results

Generally, the results of treatment for Fournier' gangrene, applying the principles outlined above, have improved considerably. The mortality rate is reported at 20% to 35%. Anorectal infections are generally more severe and carry a higher mortality rate than those from other causes.

The importance of combined aggressive surgical and medical management, using a team composed of an infectious disease specialist, a surgeon, and, if necessary, a urologist, cannot be overestimated.

## Fungal Infections

Skin is the primary site of involvement of recognized superficial fungal infections. This is presumably because fungi digest and live on keratin. These superficial fungi are called dermatophytes; they include *Microsporum*, *Trichophyton*, and *Epidermophyton*.

### Tinea Cruris; Jock Itch; Crotch Itch

Tinea cruris, also known as ringworm of the groin, is caused by a species of *Trichophyton*. The condition occurs most commonly in the intertriginous areas and is exacerbated by heat and humidity (Fig. 19.10). The differential diagnosis

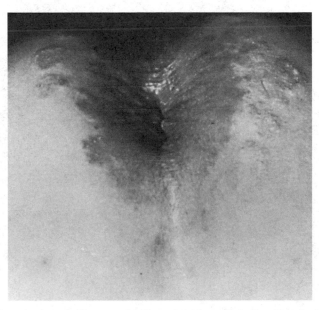

**FIG. 19.10.** Dermatophytosis (tinea cruris). Superficial fungal infection. Note that patches have annular borders with scaling and a tendency toward central clearing. (Courtesy of Samuel L. Moschella, M.D.)

includes moniliasis, erythrasma, seborrheic dermatitis, psoriasis, and vegetative pemphigus. Demonstration of the fungus by potassium hydroxide microscopic examination and culture confirms the diagnosis (Fig. 19.11).

Treatment is aimed at reducing perspiration and enhancing evaporation from the crural area. Loose-fitting clothes are suggested. Griseofulvin has been considered the most effective drug in the treatment of all dermatophytes, but it is rarely needed. Its action is believed to modify keratin so that the fungus will not invade. Treatment for 3 to 4 weeks is advised if topical fungicides such as tolnaftate, clotrimazole, miconazole, econazole, and ciclopirox are not helpful.

### Candidiasis or Moniliasis

Candidiasis is caused by the yeastlike fungus *Candida albicans*. The fungus, a frequent commensal in humans, is present in the alimentary tract and vagina of many healthy people. Intertriginous areas are commonly affected, including the perianal and inguinal folds and the axillae.

The organism is usually found outside the epidermis and behaves primarily as an opportunistic infection, especially in patients who have impaired resistance (e.g., AIDS). The condition may be somewhat difficult to recognize. Pustules

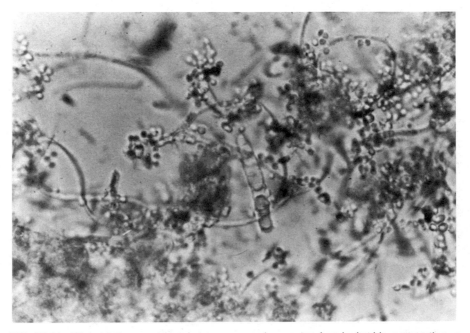

**FIG. 19.11.** *Trichophyton mentagrophytes*, as seen in a potassium hydroxide preparation, a species of *Trichophyton* that can cause tinea cruris (ringworm) of the groin. (Original magnification ×600; courtesy of Rudolf Garret, M.D.)

without surrounding inflammation may leave a "collarette" of scale; satellite lesions can be often seen in adjacent skin. Some eruptions in the inguinal area can resemble tinea cruris, but usually there is less scaling and a greater tendency to fissure. When the condition occurs in children, it is called diaper or napkin dermatitis.

Candidiasis is diagnosed by demonstrating the yeast, spores, or pseudomycelium under the microscope with potassium hydroxide. Culture on Sabouraud's glucose agar shows a growth of creamy, grayish, moist colonies in about 4 days.

Treatment consists of topical nystatin, clotrimazole, or miconazole. For severe cases, usually in patients with immunologic deficiency, oral ketoconazole (Nizoral; 200 mg), or intravenous amphotericin B can be administered.

## Deep Mycoses

Sporotrichosis, coccidioidomycosis, histoplasmosis, North American blastomycosis, chromomycosis, cryptococcosis, nocardiosis, and mycetoma are fungal infections generally known as the "deep" mycoses. They usually come from inhalation of dust contaminated with the fungus, from droppings of animals infected by it, or from contamination from other sources. All have associated skin lesions, which have a good prognosis in the case of primary cutaneous infections. However, when skin involvement is the result of dissemination from a visceral focus, the prognosis is usually much worse. Generally, skin biopsy will reveal the presence of the fungi.

Treatment varies with the type of fungus and with the extent of disease, either localized or systemic. The reader is referred to a textbook of medicine for the clinical features, diagnosis, and management of the conditions.

## Parasitic Diseases

Numerous parasitic diseases have cutaneous manifestations, and many of these also affect the alimentary tract. Included are infections caused by protozoa (i.e., single-cell organisms), nematodes (i.e., roundworms), arthropods, trematodes (i.e., flukes), cestodes (i.e., flatworms), annelids (i.e., leeches), and chordates. A number of these conditions are discussed in some detail in Chapter 33. The discussion that follows is limited to cutaneous manifestations of parasitic diseases.

### Amebiasis Cutis

*Entamoeba histolytica* is an organism that causes disease most commonly in the tropics. Cutaneous amebiasis occurs less frequently than the intestinal condition, except for cutaneous manifestations in the genitalia and perianal area. It is believed that the reason for its presentation in this location is direct extension from the involved bowel. Lesions begin as deep abscesses that rupture and form distinct ulcerations; usually an erythematous halo is seen around the ulcer. Characteristically, skin lesions spread rapidly and may result in death.

Histologically, areas of necrotic ulceration are seen with many lymphocytes, neutrophils, plasma cells, and eosinophils. The organism is frequently demonstrated in the fresh material from the base (see Chapter 33). Although abscesses may require surgical drainage, the cutaneous manifestation will usually respond to either metronidazole or emetine.

### Trichomoniasis

*Trichomonas* vulvovaginitis causes vaginal pruritus, burning, and leukorrhea. The condition is caused by the protozoan *Trichomonas vaginalis*. Because of the discharge and pruritic symptoms, the anal area may be secondarily involved by the irritation. A history of the vaginal discharge should point to the source of the problem. Treatment is metronidazole (Flagyl; 250 mg) for 10 days.

### Schistosomal Dermatitis; Schistosomiasis Cutis; Swimmer's Itch

Schistosomal dermatitis is a severe pruritic, papular dermatitis caused by cercarial species of *Schistosoma*, a genus of trematodes. Exposure to the cercariae (see Fig. 33-17) occurs by swimming or wading in water containing them. They attach by burrowing into the skin. Clinically, severe itching occurs at the time of the exposure secondary to an urticarial reaction. The result is a papular, pruritic lesion that spontaneously regresses after a few days, and disappears by 2 weeks. Antipruritic measures are used for treatment.

Visceral schistosomiasis (i.e., bilharziasis) can produce cutaneous manifestations as a result of deposition of eggs in the dermis. Fistulous tracts can develop in the perineum and buttocks, associated with hard masses, sinus tracts, and seropurulent discharge with a characteristic foul odor. In the severe vegetating form, malignant change in the granulomas has been noted. Treatment consists of trivalent antimony compounds (e.g., tartar emetic, stibophen, triostam, astiban).

### Nematode Infections

#### Oxyuriasis; Pinworm; Threadworm; Enterobiasis

*Enterobius (Oxyuris) vermicularis* is the helminth that most commonly infects humans. Children are more frequently affected than adults, and it is more common in temperate climates than in the tropics. The worm lives in the proximal colon and is often found in the appendix (Fig. 19.12), but the disease is not truly related to the bowel itself. The worms migrate to the rectum at night and emerge on the perianal skin to deposit thousands of ova (Figs. 19.13 and 19.14). The ova are returned to the mouth by the patient through scratching. The larvae then hatch in the duodenum, and migrate to the small and large intestine. Fertilization occurs in the cecum, completing the life cycle.

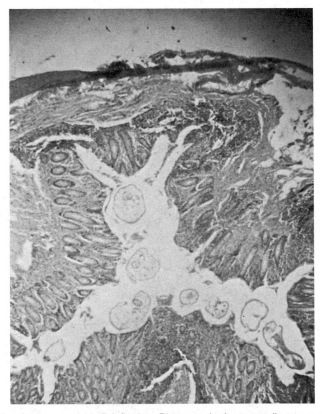

**FIG. 19.12.** *Enterobius vermicularis* infection. Pinworms in the appendix, cross-section. (Original magnification ×80; courtesy of Rudolf Garret, M.D.)

The primary complaint is usually itching, especially interfering with the patient's sleep. Friction and maceration by tight-fitting clothes can lead to superficial or deep folliculitis of the buttocks and perineum. Anal abscess complicating the condition has also been reported.

Diagnosis is usually established by demonstration of the ova in smears taken from the anal area early in the morning. Applying cellophane tape against the perianal region, adding a drop of iodine, and examining the tape under a microscope slide may facilitate detection of the ova. Demonstration of the pinworm in the stool is rarely successful, but occasionally the adult worms can be seen on the perianal skin. Because of the high likelihood of communication, it is appropriate to include members of the patient's family in studies.

Current management of pinworm infestation is mebendazole (Vermox; 100 mg)—a chewable tablet taken once. Other effective medications for the treatment of the condition are piperazine (Antepar) and pyrvinium pamoate (Povan). The former is given in single daily doses of 65 mg/kg (not to exceed 2,500 mg)

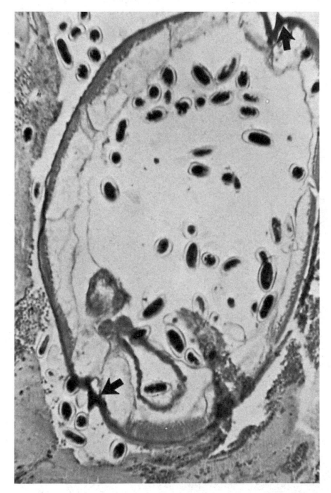

**FIG. 19.13.** Adult pinworm (*Enterobius vermicularis*). Note prominent lateral alae (*arrows*). Numerous ova are seen. (Original magnification ×170; courtesy of Rudolf Garret, M.D.)

1 hour before breakfast for 8 consecutive days; the latter is given in a single dose of 5 mg/kg, and a second dose can be given 1 week after the first treatment. Undergarments, towels, sheets, pajamas, and other clothing should be thoroughly laundered separately from those of other members of the family.

### Creeping Eruption or Larva Migrans

Larva migrans is a cutaneous eruption caused by larvae of several nematodes, most commonly the cat or dog hookworm, *Ancylostoma braziliense* or *Ancylostoma caninum*. The ova of these hookworms are deposited in the soil and

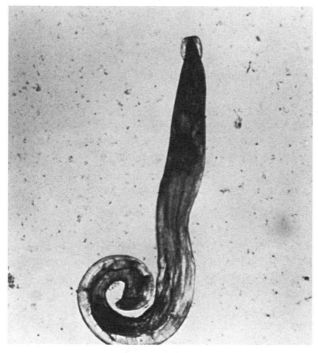

**FIG. 19.14.** *Enterobius vermicularis* the adult pinworm (female). (Courtesy of Rudolf Garret, M.D.)

hatch into infectious larvae that penetrate the skin. People who go barefoot at the beach, children playing in sandboxes, carpenters and plumbers working under houses, and gardeners are the most common victims. Most frequently, the feet, buttocks, hands, and genitals are involved by the process. Raised, pruritic, thin, linear, tunnel-like lesions that contain serous fluid are noted.

The disease is usually self-limited, but freezing of the larvae with ethyl chloride or liquid nitrogen is effective. An alternative internal treatment is thiabendazole (Mintezol).

### Larva Currens

Larva currens is a form of cutaneous larva migrans caused by *Strongyloides stercoralis*. The condition is so called because of the speed of larval migration; in essence, it is caused by an autoinfection, penetration of the perianal skin by larvae excreted in the feces. The eruption, usually associated with intestinal strongyloidiasis, beginning in the skin around the anus, may involve the buttocks, thighs, and back. The itching is quite severe. As the larvae leave the skin to enter the bloodstream and settle in the intestinal mucosa, the rash disappears. The skin demonstrates a papular eruption with edema and urticaria. Treatment consists of thiabendazole (25 to 50 mg/kg) for 2 to 4 days.

## Insect Diseases

### Cimicosis or Bedbug Bites

The bedbug (*Cimex lectularius*) hides in crevices during the daytime and feeds on human blood at night. The bedbug usually produces a linear series of bites on the ankles and buttocks. Because the bites are painless, the patient may not be aware of what has happened until finding the bedclothes stained with blood. Some individuals may react with severe urticaria and pain. Treatment consists of soothing antipruritic lotions. The pests are eliminated by means of fumigation (e.g., with Malathion).

### Pediculosis Pubis or Phthiriasis

Several varieties of *Pediculus* affect humans, but the one of concern in this discussion is *Pediculus pubis* (*Phthirus pubis*), the pubic or crab louse. The condition is usually transmitted by sexual intercourse or acquired from contaminated bedding. The lice are found on the hair or skin, appearing as yellowish brown or gray, glistening specks. The so-called nits are attached to the hair shaft and are best seen under a Wood's light. Symptoms include intense pruritus and the secondary effects of persistent excoriation. The condition frequently coexists with other sexually transmitted diseases. Treatment consists of 1% gamma benzene hexachloride cream or lotion to the pubic area, Kwell, or crotamiton (Eurax). Bed linen and clothing essentially require sterilization.

### Arachnid Infection: Scabies

Scabies is a skin condition resulting from infestation by the mite *Sarcoptes scabiei*. The female burrows into the stratum corneum and there deposits her eggs. Patients complain primarily of itching that is worse at night. Areas commonly involved include the interdigital folds, flexor aspects of the wrist, nipples, navel, genitals, buttocks, and outer aspects of the feet. The lesion appears as a whitish burrow that is tortuous and threadlike. Papules and pustules are frequently seen. The condition is usually contracted by close contact with a person harboring the mite. Diagnosis is made by microscopic examination of scrapings or shave excision of suspected skin for eggs, larvae, adult mites, or feces (Figs. 19.15 and 19.16). Treatment consists of Elimite cream, 10% crotamiton cream (Eurax), or thiabendazole, as well as decontamination of clothing.

## Venereal Diseases

Sexually transmitted diseases are the most common communicable diseases in industrialized countries; one estimate by the World Health Organization indicates that 25 million people are infected annually with gonorrhea and about 3.5 million people with syphilis. Receptive anal intercourse is a particular risk factor, because of the greater fragility of the rectal mucosa in comparison with the squamous mucosa of the vagina. This is certainly a concern in this AIDS era. Sohn and

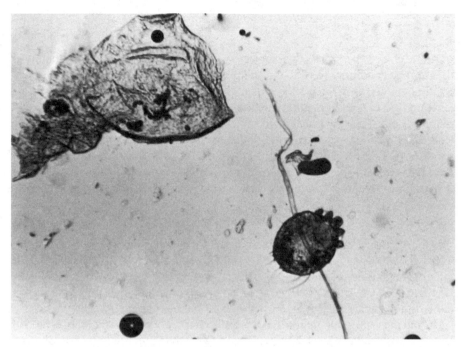

**FIG. 19.15.** Scrapings from a scabies lesion showing the female mite. (Original magnification ×240; courtesy of Rudolf Garret, M.D.)

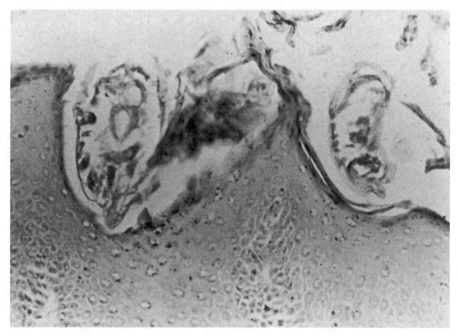

**FIG. 19.16.** A biopsy specimen showing the female mite burrowing into the epidermis. (Original magnification ×280; courtesy of Rudolf Garret, M.D.)

Robilotti coined the phrase "gay bowel syndrome" to indicate a constellation of diseases and conditions to which male homosexuals fall victim. Although the classic venereal diseases, such as syphilis, gonorrhea, chancroid, lymphogranuloma venereum (LGV), and granuloma inguinale, are of interest, they represent only a minority of the sexually transmitted infections in the United States. The epidemic venereal conditions today are condylomata acuminata, anogenital herpes, and, of course, AIDS (see Chapter 20). With the changes in mores and attitudes toward sexual matters, it is incumbent on the surgeon to be knowledgeable about the manifestations, differential diagnosis, and treatment of sexually transmitted disease.

### Gonorrhea

Gonorrhea is a bacterial infection caused by *Neisseria gonorrhoeae*, a gram-negative diplococcus. Humans are the only known reservoir. The disease affects mucous membranes of the urethra, cervix, rectum, and oropharynx. Gonococcal dermatitis is a rare infection that can develop in a wound that has come in contact with the bacterium, including wounds of the genital area.

During the 1980s, the incidence of the disease declined markedly, but the condition is diagnosed at least 10 times more often than syphilis. The incidence in the black population has been reported to be almost 40 times that of whites. The 1995 summary of reported cases by the United States Centers for Disease Control and Prevention (CDC) is 150/100,000 population.

The complication of gonorrheal proctitis is of particular interest to the surgeon. This is usually seen in the gay population as a result of infection from anal intercourse. In women, the condition is frequently caused by spread to the rectum from the genital tract. See Chapter 33 for a discussion of gonococcal proctitis and its treatment.

### Syphilis or Lues

According to the United States Public Health Service, the incidence of primary and secondary syphilis in the United States is about 130,000 cases annually, with 3 cases in men reported for every case in a woman. The disease is caused by the spirochete *Treponema pallidum*. The organism enters the skin or mucous membrane, producing a chancre approximately 3 weeks following the infection. This is the primary stage of the disease. The lesion is usually single and is most commonly found on the penis, but it can also be seen on the lips, tongue, and tonsillar area. In women, it may be inapparent because of its location within the vagina or cervix. In the homosexual population, the chancre is usually situated at the anal margin or in the anal canal. The lesion is usually painless, but sometimes is accompanied by severe discomfort, tenesmus, difficulty with defecation, and discharge. Unless a high index of suspicion exists, the condition can be confused with an anal fissure, but the presence of inguinal adenopathy should alert the examiner to this possibility. The aberrant location of the fissure (e.g., lateral) might arouse some suspicion, but this also could be a finding consistent with anal Crohn's disease.

Most writings on the subject state that the diagnosis is established on the basis of identification of the organism by means of dark-field examination (Fig. 19.17). Because the absence of a positive test result does not exclude the diagnosis, it is probably preferable to treat patients with suspected clinical lesions and await the results of serologic evaluation. It is important to remember, however, that serologic tests for syphilis do not yield positive results until the primary chancre has been present for several weeks.

Although excision of the lesion is not recommended, characteristic histopathologic changes are seen—dense infiltration by round cells, plasma cells, and fibroblasts (Fig. 19.18). Proliferation of endothelial cells results in a progressive arteritis.

### Treatment

Benzathine penicillin (2.4 million units) intramuscularly, repeated 7 days later) is the treatment of choice in nonallergic patients. For those who are allergic to penicillin, tetracycline (500 mg) orally four times daily for 15 days, is recommended. Other tetracyclines can be used as well as erythromycin (500 mg) orally four times daily for 15 days.

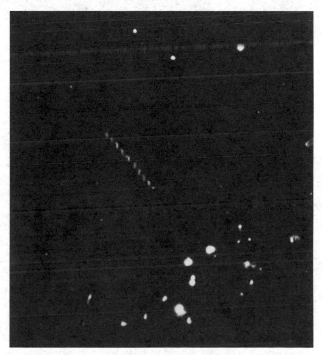

**FIG. 19.17.** *Treponema pallidum*, the causative agent of syphilis, appears as a corkscrew-shaped organism on dark field examination. (Original magnification ×600; courtesy of Rudolf Garret, M.D.)

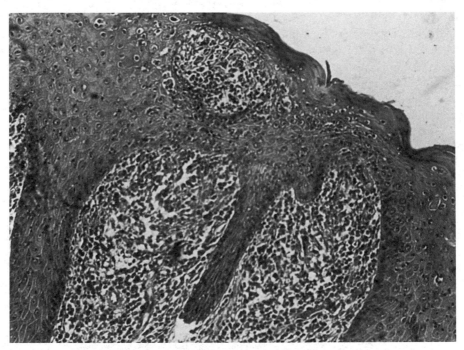

**FIG. 19.18.** Syphilitic chancre demonstrating pseudoepitheliomatous hyperplasia and plasma cell infiltration of the dermis with dilated lymphatics. (Original magnification ×250; courtesy of Rudolf Garret, M.D.)

### Condylomata Lata

The other cutaneous manifestation of lues is the secondary stage of syphilis, condylomata lata. The signs and symptoms of secondary syphilis can develop 2 to 6 months after infection and usually 6 to 8 weeks after the appearance of the primary chancre. Both lesions can exist synchronously. A maculopapular rash develops, which gives rise to a proliferating, weeping mass containing the spirochetes. The lesions may appear rather flat, scaling, red, and indurated. In the anal area particularly, they can become papillomatous and vegetative, with an associated foul odor (Fig. 19.19). Although most literature suggests that the lesions are not pruritic, in some cases this is the primary complaint.

The diagnosis can be established by demonstrating the organism using dark-field microscopic examination, but results of serologic tests are virtually always positive. The histopathology of secondary syphilis varies, depending on the clinical presentation. The lesions of condylomata lata show acanthosis and edema in the epidermis with broadening of the rete ridges (Fig. 19.20). Some lesions demonstrate a nonspecific, chronic inflammatory reaction with a large number of plasma cells.

Treatment with penicillin, erythromycin, or tetracycline is effective. An important part of the management of the patient includes the tracing of all sexual contacts, which, in the case of secondary syphilis, necessitates a 1-year retrospective review.

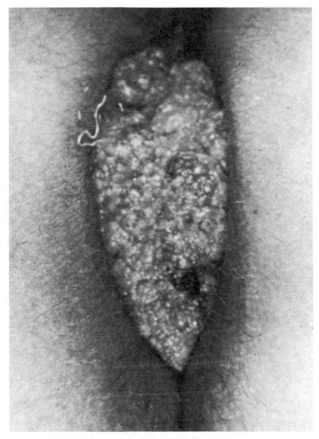

**FIG. 19.19.** Condylomata lata. A large, perianal, mucoid, warty mass composed of smooth-surfaced lobules. (Courtesy of Rudolf Garret, M.D.)

### Chancroid

Chancroid is a rare sexually transmitted disease, but its incidence has increased in the United States in recent years, presumably on the basis of individuals emigrating from the Caribbean, Mexico, and Southeast Asia. The condition is most common in tropical and subtropical areas and in the poorer populations. The disease is caused by the gram-negative bacillus *Haemophilus ducreyi.*

Chancroid begins on the genitals as an inflammatory macule or pustule; the latter ruptures, forming a punched-out ulcer with irregular edges. Within a few days to 2 weeks, inguinal adenitis frequently develops, which can lead to perforation of the lymphatics. The inguinal node is called a "bubo." Characteristic of chancroid is its tendency to autoinoculation. In addition to involvement of the anal area, extragenital lesions may be noted on the hands, eyelids, and elsewhere.

Diagnosis is established by demonstrating the bacterium in smears from the ulcer grown on enhanced chocolate agar vancomycin.

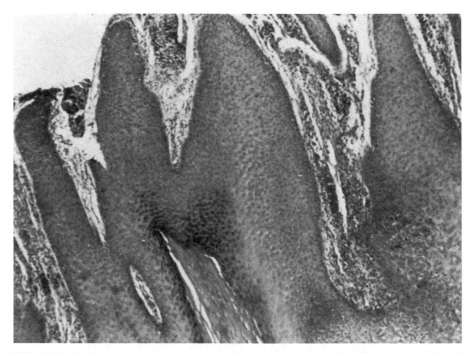

**FIG. 19.20.** Condylomata lata demonstrating dilated lymphatics, proliferation of the prickle cell layer (acanthosis), and an inflammatory exudate. (Original magnification ×250; courtesy of Rudolf Garret, M.D.)

Because many cases are resistant to tetracycline, treatment usually consists of sulfonamides (double-strength trimethoprim-sulfamethoxazole), one tablet orally every 12 hours for 14 days. Third-generation cephalosporins are also effective.

### Granuloma Inguinale, Granuloma Venereum, Donovanosis

Granuloma inguinale is a chronic, granulomatous, ulcerative skin disease caused by *Calymmatobacterium granulomatis*, formerly known as *Donovania granulomatis*. In the United States, fewer than 100 cases are reported annually, almost exclusively in homosexual African-American men. Some question whether it is transmitted nonvenereally as well as venereally. The lesions appear as cauliflowerlike proliferations from which develop pustules and papules (Fig. 19.21). Sinuses and scars are characteristic, with healed areas often devoid of pigment (Fig. 19.22). The lesions can be uncomfortable. Adenopathy is not necessarily present, but secondary infection with abscess of inguinal nodes can occur. Squamous cell carcinoma can develop in long-standing, untreated lesions.

The diagnosis is usually established by the appearance, history, and staining of a punch biopsy specimen. Donovan bodies appear as deeply staining, bipolar, safety pin-shaped rods in the cytoplasm of macrophages (Fig. 19.23). Biopsy usually reveals a massive, predominantly polymorphonuclear inflammatory

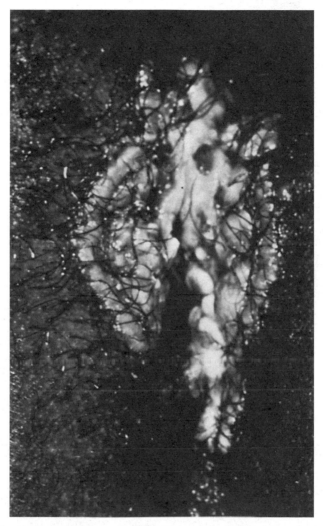

**FIG. 19.21.** Cicatricial granulomatous nodule with a surrounding erythematous border, characteristic of granuloma inguinale. (Courtesy of Rudolf Garret, M.D.)

reaction, thickening of the epidermis at the periphery, and pale-staining macrophages, usually in the upper parts of the granuloma (Fig. 19.24).

A host of antibiotics have been successful in the treatment, a 14-day course of tetracycline being preferred. If irreversible tissue destruction develops, resective surgery may be necessary.

### Chlamydia *Infection, Lymphogranuloma Venereum, Lymphogranuloma Inguinale, Lymphopathia Venereum*

In the United States, health officials consider *Chlamydia* infection the most common sexually transmitted disease, with an estimated 4 million Americans

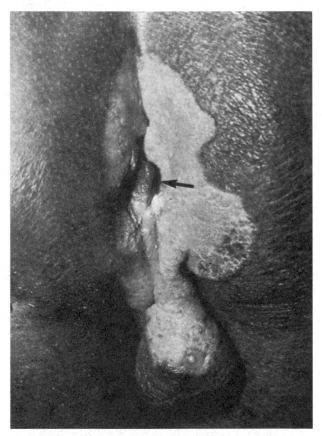

**FIG. 19.22.** Granuloma inguinale. Chronic, irregularly shaped, enlarging ulceration of the perianal area (*arrow*). Note hypertrophic scarring devoid of pigment. (Courtesy of Samuel L. Moschella, M.D.)

affected each year. It is most frequently seen in the homosexual population, with a particularly high incidence among African-Americans. Lymphogranuloma venereum is a suppurative venereal disease caused by *Chlamydia trachomatis*. It has been an uncommon disease in the United States, with fewer than 400 cases noted annually in a 1987 report. The infection is more common in Southeast Asia, Africa, Central and South America, and the Caribbean. However, the incidence is increasing as a complication in patients with AIDS.

Early symptoms are referable to the genitourinary tract, although 25% of men and 50% of women experience no initial symptoms. The lesion initially appears as a herpetiform vesicle on the genitalia or anal area. Complaints, when they occur, include dysuria, pyuria, and mucopurulent discharge. Lower abdominal pain may also be noted, especially in women. The diagnosis can be established by noting the clinical pattern of the genital lesion, followed 1 to 4 weeks later by marked unilateral lymphadenopathy and systemic symptoms. The nodes enlarge, form a large mass, become fluctuant, and drain.

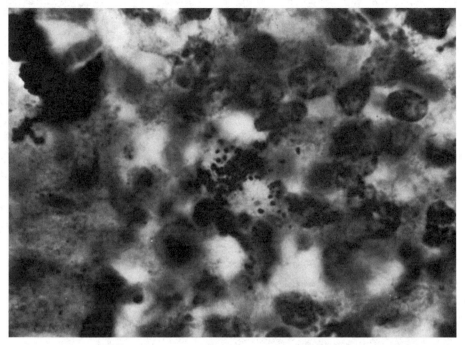

**FIG. 19.23.** Granuloma inguinale. Donovan bodies in macrophages, demonstrated by Leishman's stain. (Original magnification × 600; courtesy of Rudolf Garret, M.D.)

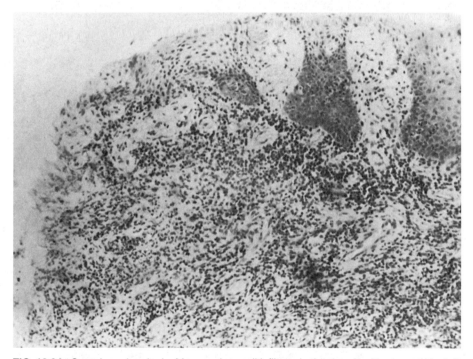

**FIG. 19.24.** Granuloma inguinale. Mononuclear cell infiltrate in the dermis with ulcer on the left. (Original magnification ×120; courtesy of Rudolf Garret, M.D.)

Lymphogranuloma venereum can also start in the rectum as a proctitis. Clinical symptoms under these circumstances are rectal discharge, bleeding, and tenesmus. An associated anal fissure is not uncommon. Perianal and rectovaginal fistulas can develop, and in late cases, progression to severe rectal stricture can occur. Approximately 2 weeks following the appearance of the primary lesion, inguinal lymphadenopathy is evident. Characteristically, in men the nodes fuse together in a large mass. If the primary lesion appears on the cervix or in the rectum, the perirectal and deep iliac nodes will enlarge. Intestinal obstruction and elephantiasis of the genitals are late sequelae.

Histologically, the changes consist of an infectious granuloma with the formation of stellate abscesses (Fig. 19.25). Laboratory studies reveal characteristic abnormalities, such as the frequently observed inversion of the albumin-globulin ratio. The so-called "Frei test" has been classically employed to establish the diagnosis of lymphogranuloma venereum; this is an intradermal test similar to the tuberculin test. However, the procedure has fallen into disrepute and is no longer available in many places. The lymphogranuloma venereum complement fixation test is considered positive at 1:80 or higher, but the microimmunofluorescent test is regarded as being more sensitive. Elevated titers are noted approximately 1 month after the onset of the illness.

Recommended treatments include tetracycline (500 mg) orally four times daily for 21 days; erythromycin (500 mg) orally four times daily for 21 days; and double-strength trimethoprim-sulfamethoxazole every 12 hours for 21 days. Rectal stenosis may require a resective procedure or a diversion.

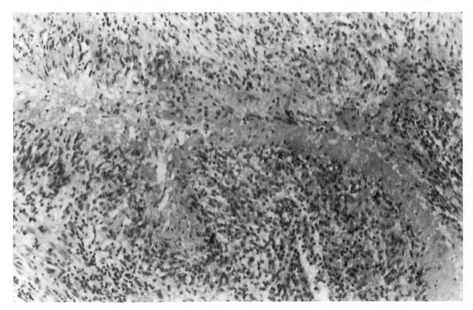

**FIG. 19.25.** Lymphogranuloma venereum. Stellate granuloma in a lymph node. (Original magnification ×280; courtesy of Rudolf Garret, M.D.)

## Molluscum Contagiosum

Molluscum contagiosum is a communicable skin disease caused by a poxvirus. It is seen principally in preschool and elementary school children. In adults, the condition can involve the skin of the abdomen, thighs, groin, genitalia, buttocks, and, in homosexual men, the perianal area. The lesions begin as papules, often develop central umbilication, and can be widely disseminated. They are often asymptomatic but can be pruritic.

Molluscum contagiosum has a characteristic histopathology: a downward proliferation of the rete ridges and envelopment by the connective tissue to form a deep crater. So-called "molluscum bodies" are found in the cytoplasm of the cells of the stratum malpighii (Fig. 19.26).

Treatment may not be required, because the lesions usually heal without scarring unless secondarily infected. Curettage can be done using ethyl chloride spray for freezing. Liquid nitrogen and electrocoagulation also have been effective, as well as 20% podophyllin and saturated solution of trichloroacetic acid.

## Herpes Genitalis; Genital Herpes; Herpes Simplex Infection; Herpes

Herpes simplex is a ubiquitous infection caused by a virus that has been associated with a number of acute, limited, vesicular eruptions near mucocutaneous junc-

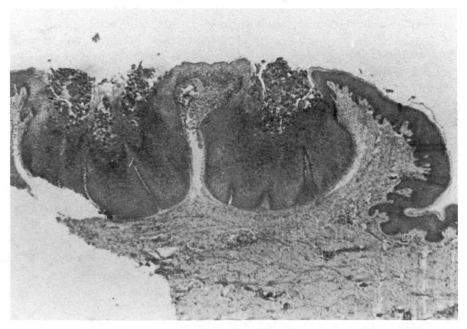

**FIG. 19.26.** Proliferation of squamous cells with formation of pear-shaped lobules and molluscum bodies in the central, craterlike area, which is characteristic of molluscum contagiosum. (Original magnification ×120; courtesy of Rudolf Garret, M.D.)

tions. Synonyms include fever blister, cold sore, herpes febrilis, herpes labialis, and genital herpes. According to the CDC, 300,000 to 500,000 new cases occur annually, with 30 million Americans believed to be harboring the virus. Classically, herpes simplex virus type 1 (HSV-1) commonly appeared above the waistline and was not usually sexually acquired, whereas with the type 2 form (HSV-2), the opposite was often the case. With the increased frequency of oral-genital sex, however, both types can be found in each location. The likelihood of reactivation of herpes simplex infection differs between HSV-1 and HSV-2 infections; the frequency of clinical recurrence with the genital form is six times that of the oral-labial type.

Cutaneous lesions associated with herpes simplex infections are usually characteristic vesicles in small groups. However, patients are often not seen until the vesicles have ulcerated. In the genital area, painful lesions can appear on the prepuce, glans, shaft of the penis, labia, vulva, clitoris, and cervix. The inguinal nodes can be firm and tender. Healing is usually complete by 10 days.

Following infection, the virus travels via an afferent nerve to the associated ganglion (e.g., HSV-2 goes to the sacral ganglion), remaining in the body in a latent state. In the latent stage, no clinical manifestations are seen, but reactivation of the virus can occur, usually two or three times a year, sometimes after a fever, emotional upset trauma, or perhaps menstruation. Prodromal symptoms of exacerbation include itching, tingling, and radiating pain to the pelvis and legs. Recurrent episodes tend to be of shorter duration and intensity. Once infected, the patient is condemned to have herpes for life.

Concerns about herpes infections relate not only to the primary cutaneous process, but also to adverse psychological effects and the risk for transmission from pregnant mothers to newborns. Also an increased frequency of cervical cancer is seen. Untreated neonatal herpes is associated with a 50% mortality rate, but this risk can be reduced by cesarean delivery.

Transmission can result from sexual contact during periods of asymptomatic viral shedding in approximately 70% of individuals. Furthermore, the risk for acquisition of herpes simplex virus is greater in women than in men.

### Diagnosis

A direct fluorescent antibody technique using the fluid from a vesicle is a rapid means to confirm the diagnosis. The Tzanck preparation, in which scrapings are placed on a slide and stained, will reveal intranuclear inclusion bodies and giant cells. The most definitive method for the diagnosis of herpes simplex virus infection is viral culture, but this is a cumbersome, expensive study. The clinical picture of grouped vesicles on an erythematous base anywhere in the body suggests herpes infection, so that laboratory studies serve primarily for confirmation.

### Treatment

Current therapy for the condition is the use of an antiviral preparation, acyclovir (Zovirax), but it does not cure the disease. Acyclovir is a synthetic acyclic purine nucleoside analogue that exhibits *in vitro* inhibitory activity against the virus. Treatment is directed to three areas: management of the initial episode and of the recurrence, and maintenance between attacks. Primary herpes of less than 7 days' duration is treated by oral acyclovir (200 mg) five times daily for 10 days. Intermittent therapy, given at the first sign of recurrence, consists of 200 mg five times daily for 5 days. Chronic suppressive therapy for recurrent disease is 400 mg two times daily for up to 12 months. Patients who present after 1 week but who still have early vesicular lesions or constitutional symptoms may also benefit from therapy. However, acyclovir is not recommended for the management of crusted lesions and for patients who are asymptomatic. Recurrent episodes must be treated within 48 hours if beneficial results are to be expected, but some believe that acyclovir has no measurable effect on the subsequent natural history of the disease. Suppressive therapy is probably most effective in patients subject to frequent exacerbations, but asymptomatic shedding of the virus implies that the individual is still infectious. Continuous or episodic oral acyclovir therapy has been demonstrated to be safe and reasonably effective, with annual rates of recurrence substantially reduced.

### Condylomata Acuminata or Venereal Warts

Condylomata acuminata represent the most common venereal disease seen in the practice of most surgeons. The condition is also among the most troublesome to eliminate. Health officials estimate that genital or anal warts develop in 1 million Americans annually, and two thirds of their sexual partners acquire the condition. The disease is caused by a human papilloma DNA virus, a member of the papovavirus group. Evidence suggests that the virus is antigenically, biochemically, and immunologically distinct from the virus of the common wart, verruca vulgaris. Although the condition can occur in heterosexual men and women, it is most commonly seen in male homosexuals.

#### Symptoms

Patients usually complain of a lump or lumps and often think the problem is caused by hemorrhoids. Other symptoms include discharge, pruritus, difficulty with defecation, anal pain, tenesmus, and rectal bleeding.

#### Examination

The appearance of the lesion usually makes the diagnosis obvious. The warts are usually small, discrete, elevated, pink to gray, vegetative excrescences in the anal canal, perianal skin, and urogenital region (Fig. 19.27). They can be single or multiple, or coalesce to form polypoid masses. Lesions in the anal canal rarely extend into the rectum, but are confined to the squamous epithelium and transitional zones. The wart itself is a hyperplastic epithelial growth with irregular acanthosis and marked hyperkeratosis (Fig. 19.28).

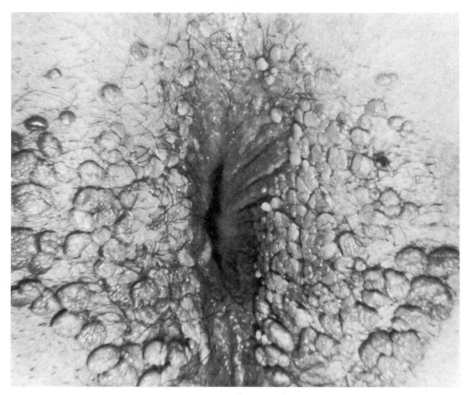

**FIG. 19.27.** Condylomata acuminata. Multiple, closely grouped papillomas creating a cauliflow-erlike appearance. (From Corman ML, Veidenheimer MC, Swinton NW. *Diseases of the anus, rectum and colon.* Part I: Neoplasms. New York: Medcom, 1972.)

## Treatment

The Standards Task Force of the American Society of Colon and Rectal Surgeons has recommended certain practice parameters for ambulatory surgery of anal condylomata.

When condylomata are limited to the perianal skin, treatment with topical medications, local destruction, or harvesting and immunotherapy can be administered in an outpatient setting. Patients with extensive perianal or anal canal condylomata or those patients with associated genital condylomata may require inpatient care. Numerous methods of treating anal condylomata have been proposed, including the following:

- Podophyllin
- Bichloracetic acid and other caustic agents
- Immunotherapy
- Chemotherapy
- Sublesional injection of interferon alpha
- Cryotherapy
- Electrocoagulation
- Laser therapy
- Surgical excision

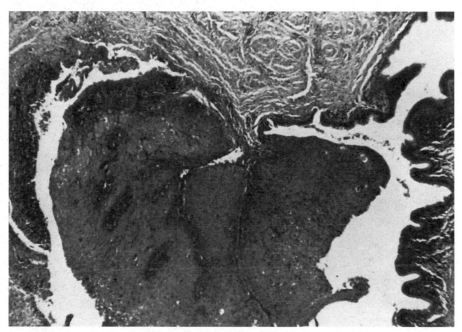

**FIG. 19.28.** Condylomata acuminata in an anal duct. Note the proliferation of squamous cells, vacuolated squamous cells, and hyperchromatic nuclei, and the absence of a cornified layer. Note also the columnar epithelium lining the anal duct. (Original magnification ×120, courtesy of Rudolf Garret, M.D.)

## Podophyllin

Podophyllin is a chemical agent that is cytotoxic for the warts, but it has the disadvantage of being irritating to the skin. It is important, therefore, to apply the liquid with care, and then only to the warts. Podophyllum resin, derived from the plants *Podophyllum emodi* and *Podophyllum peltatum*, contains many biologically active lignin compounds, including podofilox, the most thoroughly characterized and the most active against genital warts. The technique has the advantage of being simple and inexpensive, but its application is limited to external warts. Multiple treatments are often required.

### Bichloracetic Acid or Dichloracetic Acid

Bichloracetic acid, an extremely powerful keratolytic and cauterant, has also been successfully used in the management of condylomata. The chemical rapidly penetrates and cauterizes the skin, keratin, and other tissues. As with podophyllin, it is simple to apply and is inexpensive. Additionally, it has the advantage of being applicable to the anal canal. Multiple office visits are usually required, however, and concern for skin irritation and discomfort exists.

### Immunotherapy

A vaccine is created by excising and washing the condyloma tissue, and a 10% suspension is prepared in Medium 199 supplemented with antibiotics. Following homogenization and freezing, it is then centrifuged, and the supernatant is heated. The inactivated material is then centrifuged again, and the supernatant collected and tested for bacterial sterility. The patient is vaccinated with six consecutive weekly injections (0.5 mL), subcutaneously administered in the deltoid area, with the vaccine frozen between injections.

Although the results of immunotherapy are really good (85% to 95% response), the application of this modality has become a moot issue, because convincing a laboratory to prepare it is virtually impossible. Because of the potential liability hazards and the considerable financial investment needed to perform the clinical and laboratory trials required by the US Food and Drug Administration, no laboratory has been willing to assume the responsibility.

### Topical Cytostatics

Various chemotherapeutic agents have been advocated in the treatment of this condylomata, including 5-fluorouracil, thiotepa and bleomycin. Success rates of 70% have been achieved.

### Interferon

Human leukocyte interferon (Alferon N), because of its antiproliferative and antiviral properties, has been demonstrably effective in the treatment of condylomata acuminata. Interferons are produced and secreted in response to viral infections and to a variety of other synthetic and biologic inducers. Alferon N is manufactured from pooled units of human leukocytes that have been induced by incomplete infection with an avian virus to produce interferon alfa-n3. Randomized, controlled studies have demonstrated a statistically significant reduction in wart area in the treated groups, resulting in early control in 60% to 90% of patients. Long-term studies have yet to be completed.

### Cryotherapy

Cryotherapy is an approach that is also advocated for the treatment of condylomata. Topical application of liquid nitrogen is simple to accomplish and requires little special equipment. Cryotherapy can be performed with a spray or with the use of a cotton-tipped applicator, and can be applied with limited success within the anal canal. As with the aforementioned methods, no pathologic specimen is obtained. Some patients report sufficient discomfort that either a local or regional anesthetic may be required.

### Laser Therapy

Some have recommended laser therapy in the treatment of condylomata, with early success noted in 88% to 95% of cases. Contact lasers are said to produce more predictable, sharply defined areas of thermal necrosis than electrosurgery, although noncontact Nd:YAG as well as carbon dioxide lasers have been successfully used. One of the concerns expressed is the possibility of vaporizing the viral particles, with consequent risk to the surgeon and to the operating room team. Special mask precautions are therefore required. Other disadvantages are the absence of a pathologic specimen and the expensive equipment that is required.

Randomized trials have compared laser therapy with conventional electrocoagulation. No difference was found between the two groups with respect to number of recurrences, postoperative pain, healing time, and rate of scar formation. Furthermore, recurrences are seen more often with the laser. These factors, along with the high cost of the equipment, imply no advantage to this newer form of treatment.

### Electrocoagulation and Surgical Excision

Electrocoagulation with excision of a portion of the specimen to submit for pathologic examination is the "gold standard" for the management of anal condylomata. The technique is limited only by the problem of pain and, of course, the attendant expense of an anesthetic.

The technique of electrocoagulation requires the creation of a first- or at most a second-degree burn. When the needle-tip electrode is used, the wart is virtually exploded, and the residual tissue is wiped away with a dry sponge. If the "burn" is not undertaken too deeply, pain is not severe; it can usually be controlled with a nonnarcotic prescription. Creating a burn deep into the dermis or fat is wrong. Patients will likely complain bitterly of pain, and a risk exists for the subsequent development of an anal stricture if a large area is to be treated.

Close follow-up examination is required to treat recurrent lesions as soon as they are evident. Fewer than one half of patients have resolution of the process after only one treatment. It is important, therefore, for the patient to understand that therapy can be prolonged. Fortunately, once the warts have been removed and the wounds have healed, the condition usually does not recur.

### Giant Condyloma Acuminatum or Buschke—Löwenstein Tumor and Malignant Degeneration

The Buschke-Löwenstein tumor, also known as giant condyloma acuminatum, is a variant of anal condylomata that tends to behave in a locally malignant fashion, burrowing deeply into adjacent structures (Fig. 19.29).

A number of reports have described the development of squamous cell carcinoma in these rare "giant" cases. The hallmark of the disease is the high (66%) recurrence rate and the high (56%) incidence of malignant transformation. Recurrences develop in 50% of those initially treated with radical surgery. Chemoradiation therapy is associated with an improved cure rate in comparison with surgery alone.

However, wide local excision is the recommended initial surgical approach. If the margins are free of tumor, no further treatment is warranted. Occasionally, however, the lesion is so extensive that it is deemed unresectable. Adjuvant ther

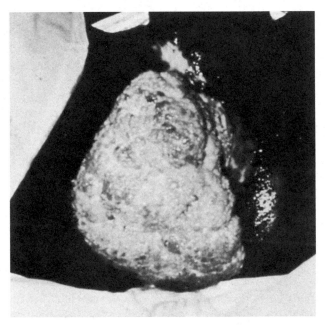

**FIG. 19.29.** Verrucous squamous carcinoma, or tumor of Buschke-Löwenstein. (From Corman ML, Veidenheimer MC, Swinton NW. *Diseases of the anus, rectum and colon.* Part I: Neoplasms. New York: Medcom, 1972.)

apy with lesions of this type should be considered in accordance with the protocol described in Chapter 24.

## PREMALIGNANT AND MALIGNANT DERMATOSES

Malignant neoplasms of the anal margin and perianal skin include basal cell carcinoma, extramammary Paget's disease, Bowen's disease, malignant melanoma, and epidermoid carcinoma. The last two conditions are discussed in Chapter 24. Leukemic and lymphomatous infiltration also can involve the anal area. In addition to these, two other cutaneous lesions may be premalignant or associated with cancer elsewhere: acanthosis nigricans and leukoplakia.

### Acanthosis Nigricans

Acanthosis nigricans is known chiefly to surgeons for its ominous association with abdominal cancer in adults. Regions affected include the face, neck, axillae, external genitalia, groin, inner thighs, umbilicus, and anus. The condition appears usually as a grayish, velvety thickening or roughening of the skin. The pathologic changes are epidermal, with papillomatosis, hyperkeratosis, and hyperpigmentation (Fig. 19.30). Pruritus is the most frequent symptom.

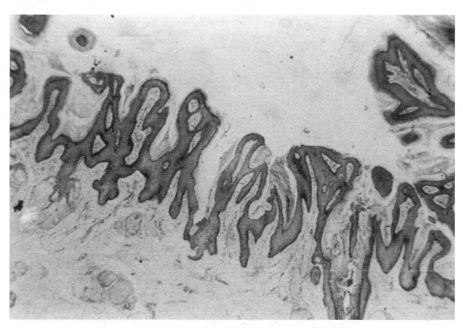

**FIG. 19.30.** Acanthosis nigricans, epithelium in a papillary configuration with pigmented cells in the basal cell layer. (Original magnification ×260; courtesy of Rudolf Garret, M.D.)

The malignant form of acanthosis nigricans may antedate, accompany, or follow the onset of the internal cancer. Most abdominal malignancies are adenocarcinomas, usually of gastric origin (60%). The tumor itself is usually advanced at the time of discovery and has a rapid progression. Treatment is directed to the primary malignant condition.

### Leukoplakia

Leukoplakia is a whitish thickening of the mucous membrane epithelium occurring in patches of diverse size and shape. In the anal canal, it is seen mostly in men and is occasionally associated with delayed wound healing (e.g., following excision of fissure, hemorrhoids, and condylomata). Although the anal condition itself does *not* represent a malignancy, when it occurs in the gingival and buccal mucosa, a high risk exists for the development of epidermoid carcinoma. Bleeding, discharge, and pruritic symptoms are the most common complaints.

Microscopically, hyperkeratosis and squamous metaplasia are seen (Fig. 19.31). Excision of the lesion is generally unsuccessful; the condition simply recurs. However, the likelihood of recurrence can be reduced if an anoplasty is performed, covering the defect with new, full-thickness skin. Because of the problematic potential for malignancy, annual proctosigmoidoscopy (anoscopy) with biopsy of any suspected area is advised.

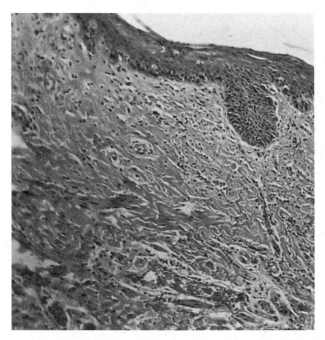

**FIG. 19.31.** Leukoplakia. Parakeratosis with atrophy of the epidermis and fibrosis of the dermis. Note the few cells with hyperchromatic nuclei close to the basal cell layer. (Original magnification ×240; courtesy of Rudolf Garret, M.D.)

## Mycosis Fungoides

Mycosis fungoides is an uncommon, pruritic, usually fatal cutaneous malignant neoplasm of the lymphoreticular system, specifically the thymus-derived lymphocytes (T cells). Subsequent involvement of lymph nodes and internal organs develops as the disease progresses.

The cutaneous lesion can occur anywhere; the overlying skin can have only telangiectasia or be violaceous, often of varied vivid color (Fig. 19.32). As the tumor advances, ulcerations occur (Fig. 19.33), and pain is a predominant symptom. Microscopic changes include epidermal invasion of small groups of abnormal-appearing lymphocytes and perivascular accumulation of lymphocytic cells. As the disease progresses, increased numbers of abnormal, malignant cells are demonstrated (Fig. 19.34).

Treatment is directed toward management of the systemic disease.

## Leukemia Cutis

Infiltration of the perianal area by leukemic cells is uncommon. Occasionally, this can be the first manifestation of the malignancy. Leukemia of the skin can

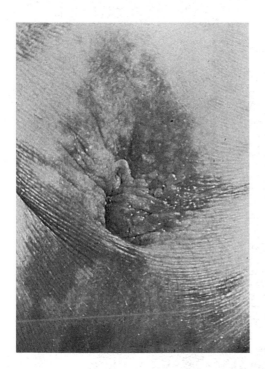

**FIG. 19.32.** A violaceous tumor with adjacent reddish brown, irregularly shaped plaques are indicative of mycosis fungoides. (From Corman ML, Veidenheimer MC, Swinton NW. *Diseases of the anus, rectum and colon.* Part 1: Neoplasms. New York: Medcom, 1972.)

consist of a diffuse infiltration, erythema, and ulceration (Fig. 19.35). Lymphocytic leukemia, characteristically, has a discrete nodular appearance (Fig. 19.36). It can present as a fistula, an abscess, or a tender, erythematous area. Cellulitis can be decidedly marked.

Histologically, masses of cells may be seen in the upper dermis or as nodules in the dermis (Fig. 19.37). The type of cells and immature forms are those of the systemic process; mitoses are infrequently seen in the skin lesions.

Infections in the perianal area are relatively common in patients with myeloproliferative disorders. Because the initial symptoms can be confined to the anal area, biopsy and appropriate hematologic studies may be the only means for establishing an early diagnosis. See Chapter 10 for a discussion of the management of perianal complications of leukemia.

### Basal Cell Carcinoma

Basal cell carcinoma of the anus is an extremely rare tumor, occurring in 1 in 1,500 to 2,000 malignant tumors of the anus and rectum. No gender predominance is seen. Tumors are usually between 1 and 2 cm in size and localized to the anal margin. Symptoms include the sensation of a lump or of an ulcer in two thirds of patients. Bleeding, pain, pruritus, and discharge are other complaints.

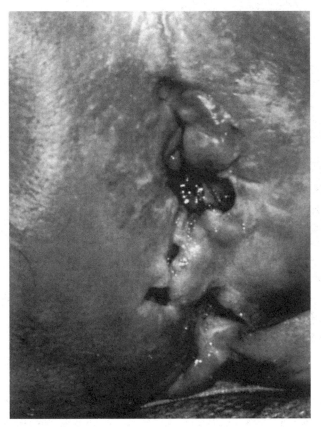

**FIG. 19.33.** Perianal ulceration, nodules, and skin infiltration by biopsy-proved lymphomatous infiltrate. (Courtesy of Daniel Rosenthal, M.D.)

The characteristic appearance of the lesion is that of a chronic, indurated growth with rolled edges (i.e., pearly border) and a central depression or ulceration (Fig. 19.38). Histologically, the tumor arises from the basal cells of the malpighian layer of the skin (Fig. 19.39). Sheets of basophilic-staining cells are seen to contain large, blue-staining nuclei with minimal cytoplasm.

Local excision with adequate margins is the treatment of choice. Radical abdominoperineal resection is performed for neglected, extensive, or infiltrating tumors. The tumor is unlikely to metastasize or cause death.

### Squamous Cell or Epidermoid Carcinoma

Squamous cell carcinoma of the perianal skin is manifested and treated in the same way as lesions occurring elsewhere on the body. The tumor can appear

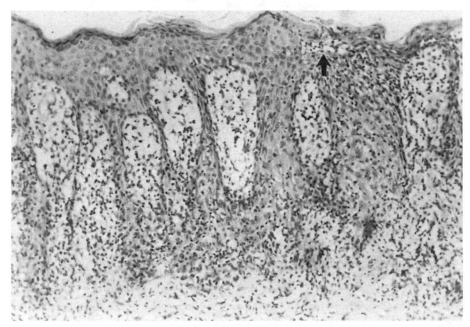

**FIG. 19.34.** Mycosis fungoides, pleomorphic infiltrate of the dermis with characteristic Pautrier's abscess (*arrow*) within the epidermis. (Original magnification ×280; courtesy of Rudolf Garret, M.D.)

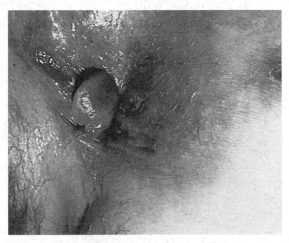

**FIG. 19.35.** An ulcerating, violaceous nodule demonstrated leukemic cells on biopsy, indicating leukemia cutis. (From Corman ML, Veidenheimer MC, Swinton NW. *Diseases of the anus, rectum and colon.* Part 1: Neoplasms. New York: Medcom, 1972.)

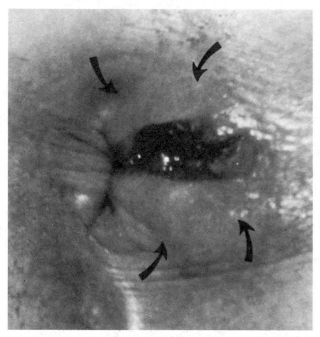

**FIG. 19.36.** Leukemia cutis (lymphocytic leukemia). Diffuse swelling and infiltration (*arrows*) with ulceration. (Courtesy of Daniel Rosenthal, M.D.)

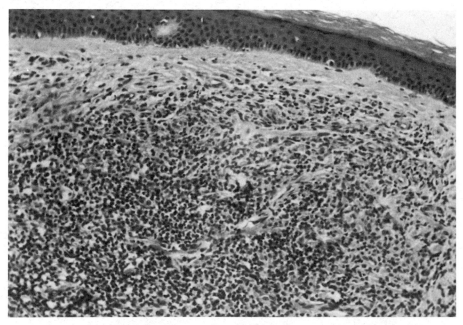

**FIG. 19.37.** Leukemia cutis. Infiltration of the dermis by leukemic cells. Note the collagen bundle separating the mass of tumor cells from the underlying epidermis. (Original magnification ×240; courtesy of Rudolf Garret, M.D.)

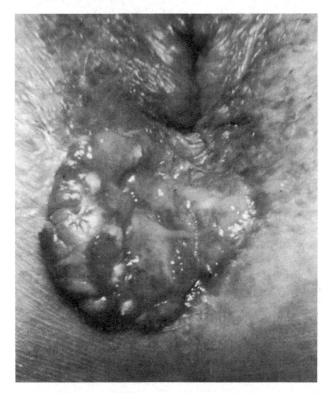

**FIG. 19.38.** Basal cell carcinoma (rodent ulcer). Ulcerating tumor with a pearly border. (From Rosenthal D. Basal cell carcinoma of the anus: report of two cases. *Dis Colon Rectum* 1967;10:397.)

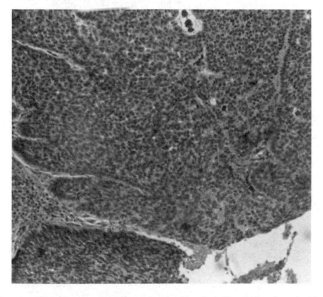

**FIG. 19.39.** Basal cell carcinoma. Proliferating basal cells infiltrate the dermis. Note the peripheral palisading. (Original magnification ×240; courtesy of Rudolf Garret, M.D.)

superficial, discrete, and hard. With progression, it can ulcerate (Fig. 19.40) or become papillomatous or cauliflowerlike (Fig. 19.41). Although this tumor is relatively slow-growing, metastases to regional lymph nodes can occur. Wide local excision is the treatment of choice for most lesions. If a question arises about the site of origin (i.e., anal vs. perianal), treatment is in accordance with the protocol described in Chapter 24.

### Malignant Melanoma

Malignant melanoma is described in Chapter 24.

### Bowen's Disease

Bowen's disease is an intraepidermal squamous cell carcinoma that tends to spread intraepidermally, but it can also invade. It is more commonly seen on the trunk, but more than 100 cases involving the anus have been reported.

### *Symptoms*

The disease usually presents with itching and burning, although pain and bleeding may be noted. Sixty percent present with symptoms, but up to 40% may be found to harbor the condition upon pathologic evaluation of hemorrhoidectomy specimens.

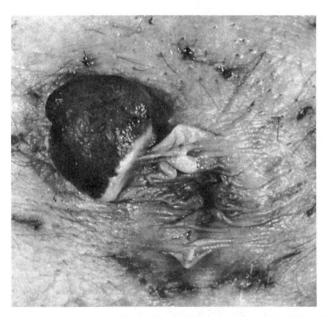

**FIG. 19.40.** Squamous cell carcinoma. Ulcerating, friable tumor. (Courtesy of Rudolf Garret, M.D.)

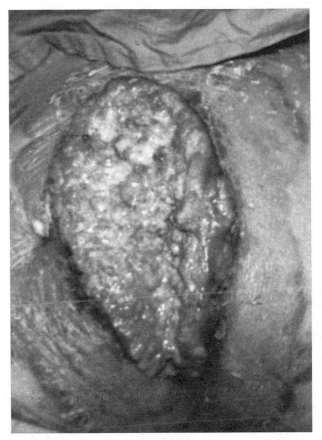

**FIG. 19.41.** Squamous cell carcinoma. Fungating, cauliflowerlike mass. (Courtesy of Daniel Rosenthal, M.D.)

### Appearance

The lesion appears as an erythematous, slightly crusted, plaquelike area with well-defined margins (Fig. 19.42). The condition can be confused with psoriasis and with Paget's disease. Topical staining with toluidine blue has been successfully used as a screening technique for intraepithelial carcinoma of the cervix and vulva. This approach may prove to have value in the diagnosis of Bowen's disease. Microscopically, the epidermis is thickened by hyperkeratosis, and parakeratosis and acanthosis may be seen (Fig. 19.43). In contrast to what is noted in Paget's disease, a bowenoid cell does not pick up aldehyde-fuchsin stain (Fig. 19.44).

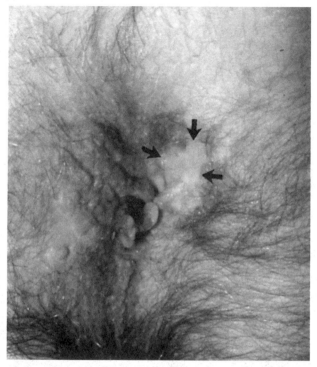

**FIG. 19.42.** Bowen's disease. Indurated erythematosquamous patch involving the perianal area (*arrows*).

## Treatment

Treatment requires wide local excision with frozen-section examination to ensure adequate margins, although radical surgical extirpation has been used when this procedure fails. The condition has also been reported to respond to topical dinitrochlorobenzene and 5-fluorouracil.

## Results

Rarely, is recurrence or metastasis when adequate excision with or without grafting is done. Although recent evidence suggests that a comprehensive search for malignancy in other organs is unwarranted, close follow-up evaluation for recurrence or invasive carcinoma is recommended.

### Bowenoid Papulosis

Bowenoid papulosis is a dermatosis affecting the genitalia, a condition that is similar to Bowen's disease. The condition is often associated with anal condylo-

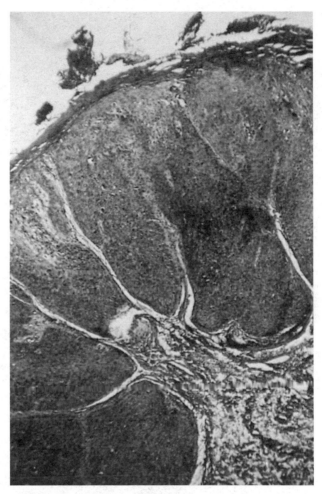

**FIG. 19.43.** Bowen's disease. Disturbance of architecture of the squamous epithelium. (Original magnification ×250; courtesy of Rudolf Garret, M.D.)

mata or genital herpes. Human papillomavirus is believed to be the causative agent. The possibility exists that immunocompromised individuals, especially those with AIDS, are at greater risk for development of cancer on the basis of bowenoid papulosis.

The lesions are described as multiple reddish brown or violaceous papules. Most individuals are asymptomatic or have pruritic complaints. Because the microscopic picture is essentially identical to that of Bowen's disease, the differential diagnosis between the two conditions is made on the basis of age (i.e., patients with bowenoid papulosis tend to be younger) and the fact that bowenoid lesions are small, papular, and multiple. Local excision is the treatment of choice.

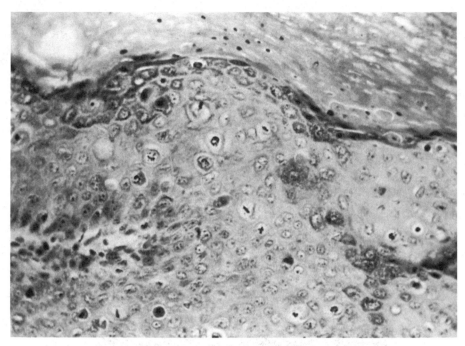

**FIG. 19.44.** Bowen's disease. Note cells with hyperchromatic nuclei (bowenoid cells) scattered throughout the epithelium. Many mitotic figures are seen. (Original magnification ×600; from Corman ML, Veidenheimer MC, Swinton NW. *Diseases of the anus, rectum and colon*. Part I: Neoplasms. New York: Medcom, 1972.)

## Extramammary Paget's Disease

In 1884, Sir James Paget described a cutaneous lesion of the breast that histologically demonstrated the presence of large, round, clear-staining cells with large nuclei. Darier and Couillaud subsequently described the condition in the perineal area, the lesions of extramammary Paget's disease being not unlike those seen in the breast. This is a relatively rare condition, with only about 100 cases reported in the literature. The mean age of onset has been reported to be from 59 to 65 years.

Most patients complain of ulceration, discharge, pruritus, and, occasionally, bleeding and pain. They may be asymptomatic or have a florid type of eczema.

The dermatosis usually appears erythematous to whitish gray, elevated, crusty, scaly, eczematoid, and occasionally papillary (Fig. 19.45). Microscopically, hyperkeratosis, parakeratosis, acanthosis, and pale vacuolated cells are seen within the epidermis (Fig. 19.46). Sialomucin may be identified by periodic acid-Schiff stain. Bowen's disease does not show this positive staining.

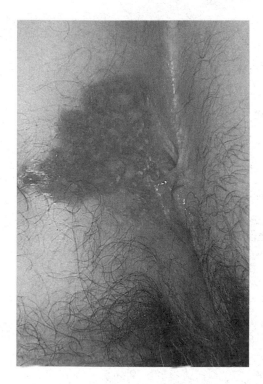

**FIG. 19.45.** Extramammary Paget's disease has caused an irregular but well-marginated erythematous erosive patch with slightly indurated edges in this patient. (Courtesy of Arnold Medved, M.D.)

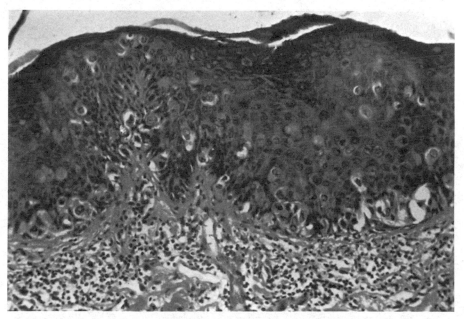

**FIG. 19.46.** Extramammary Paget's disease. Note the large, pagetoid cells within the epithelium. These were mucicarmine-positive, thus ruling out Bowen's disease. (Original magnification ×240; courtesy of Rudolf Garret, M.D.)

### Association with Malignancy

Carcinoma in adjacent areas, especially the anal canal and rectum, is found in a high percentage of patients. In addition, a familial occurrence has been described. A special staining technique is used to assist in the distinction between Paget's disease and so-called "pagetoid spread" as a consequence of an anorectal malignancy.

### Treatment

Treatment depends on the presence or absence of an underlying invasive carcinoma. The use of an oral retinoid, etretinate, may be beneficial in the treatment of the chronic or recurrent form in patients with no concomitant invasive carcinoma. Wide local excision with or without grafting should be adequate for noninvasive disease. A management classification based on the depth of invasion, has been described:

Stage I. Localized perianal disease without carcinoma. Wide local excision
Stage IIA. Localized disease with underlying malignancy. Wide local excision
Stage IIB. Localized disease with associated anorectal carcinoma. Abdominoperineal resection
Stage III. Associated carcinomatous spread to regional lymph nodes. Abdominoperineal resection plus chemoradiation therapy; possible radical inguinal node dissection
Stage IV. Distant metastases. Standard palliative cancer management

### Results

The 5- and 10-year crude survival rates of 54% and 45%, respectively, are significantly lower than what would be anticipated in the normal population. Careful follow-up is considered essential, with recurrence probably dictating a wider excision, provided, of course, no evidence is seen of malignancy. Those managed by local excision should undergo frequent biopsy of any pruritic areas or skin lesions.

# 20

# Colorectal Manifestations of Acquired Immunodeficiency Syndrome (HIV Infection)

## ACQUIRED IMMUNODEFICIENCY SYNDROME

Acquired immunodeficiency syndrome (AIDS) is caused by a retrovirus, an RNA virus that infects cells and causes a DNA template of its RNA to be made and used to reproduce new RNA virus. The International Committee for the Taxonomy of Viruses proposed the name human immunodeficiency virus (HIV). HIV often causes a brief, flulike illness at the time of infection, but the virus can be harbored for many years without producing clinical manifestations. The pandemic of AIDS is of particular concern because it can result in life-threatening opportunistic infections and rare malignant tumors.

Initially, AIDS was confined to the homosexual population, intravenous drug users, and recipients of contaminated blood, but more recently a noticeable increase is noted in the incidence within the heterosexual population. Of cases, 90% occur in individuals between 20 and 50 years of age. AIDS is not a specific disease entity; it is a viral illness that alters immune function, which can lead to many manifestations. The definition of AIDS, therefore, is in the patient who is HIV positive suffering an opportunistic infection.

### Mechanism of Viral Replication

The human immunodeficiency virus survives by invading white blood cells, which in turn provide the resource for replication.

Initially, the virus attaches to receptors on a host cell, releasing its genetic material as RNA. Next, the enzyme reverse transcriptase (RT) converts the viral RNA into DNA. Then, the enzyme integrase splices the viral DNA into the host cell's chromosomes. The infected cell produces new viral RNA, which generates proteins and other viral constituents. The enzyme protease sections the viral proteins into shorter pieces, which then encapsulate to form new HIV. These then bud off to infect other cells.

### Anorectal Immunology and Pathophysiology

The anorectum is composed of both squamous and mucosal elements and is protected by two independent immune systems.

The mucosal layer on the surface of the gut acts as a barrier, supported by IgA as a non–complement-binding antibody that captures pathogens before they can invade the mucosal surface. An antigen that succeeds in penetrating this defense is processed by specialized epithelial cells on the mucosal surface (M cells) and is presented to immunologically competent cells in the lymphoid aggregates. Resident T-cell populations live in the lamina propria and intraepithelial segments of the gut. These T-cell populations have a myriad of functions, including coordinating "memory" cell-mediated immunity, sending messages to other cellular immune elements, and helping to produce immunoglobulin. T cells are named after the receptor protein on their surfaces. The CD4 receptor on T4 cells, (also known as helper T cells) may also be responsible for the demise of these cells, because HIV has a particular affinity for this molecule. HIV will continually destroy resident T cells at a fairly constant rate and, after initial infection, stabilize the rate of viral replication (called the "set point") in an individual. This continues until the capacity of the immune system to restore itself is exhausted. Therefore, measurement of plasma HIV-1 RNA now appears to be a better prognostic indicator of disease activity than the CD4 count.

It has been suggested that HIV-laden sperm have a special affinity for rectal mucosal cells. It has also been postulated that a difference for the increase in heterosexual transmission rates in underdeveloped nations is the presence of a unique subtype (E) that has increased affinity for vaginal epithelium.

In the gastrointestinal tract, the depletion of T4 cells adversely affects immunoglobulin production and mucosal integrity, thereby promoting translocation of bacteria and subsequent bacterial invasion. In addition, some evidence suggests the enterocyte itself is damaged by HIV, causing an effect on absorptive and secretory function.

The skin around the anus allows for a different barrier mechanism. Keratinocytes are cells that are protected from invasion by HIV, because they lack CD4 receptors. The disruption of the skin by sexual trauma or coincident inflammation or ulceration, however, allows penetration and subsequent infection by HIV.

### Colonic Manifestations of HIV Infection

A variety of disease processes, which can affect the colon in an individual who harbors HIV, can present in a number of ways. These include colitides that are frequently aggravated by immunosuppression; a number of malignancies that can cause bleeding, obstruction, or intussusception; and lymphadenopathy itself which can cause severe abdominal pain and compression of viscera, primarily through a *Mycobacterium avium* complex (MAC) infection.

Generally, the goal in management of the acute abdomen in a patient with HIV is to *try to avoid surgery* because of the high morbidity and mortality rates with operations in these patients.

### Cytomegalovirus Infection

Cytomegalovirus (CMV) is a double-stranded DNA virus from the herpesvirus family. Infection with CMV is extremely common in patients with AIDS. The condition can cause ulceration of the gut anywhere from the mouth to the anus, but the major colorectal manifestation is ileocolitis. In addition, up to 10% may experience sight-threatening infections resulting from chorioretinitis.

#### Symptoms and Findings

A mild case of CMV infection usually presents with diarrhea, although up to 30% of patients complain of fever and weight loss *without* diarrhea. As the virally induced vasculitis progresses, frank ulceration, toxic megacolon, hemorrhage, and perforation can occur. Cytomegalovirus enterocolitis was the single most common reason for abdominal surgery in the AIDS population; however, effective antiviral therapy has reduced the incidence of this intervention.

#### Diagnosis

Diagnosis is made by endoscopic identification of the mucosal ulcerations. However, in 25% of patients with CMV colitis, the mucosa appears endoscopically normal.

#### Pathology

Biopsy usually reveals an inflammatory infiltrate, including lymphocytes and plasma cells with polymorphonuclear leukocytes and histiocytes in some areas. The most characteristic histologic feature is the presence of intranuclear inclusions in the colonic mucosal cells. The retrieval of CMV inclusions appears to depend on the number of biopsy specimens, the skill of the pathologist, and whether the material was taken from an endoscopically abnormal colon. Cultures for CMV have been inconsistent in predicting the presence of active infection. Immunoperoxidase staining for CMV antigen and *in situ* DNA hybridization have also been used, but with conflicting results. Polymerase chain reaction amplification of cytomegalovirus DNA offers the best method for both diagnosis and monitoring of the efficacy of therapy.

Radiologic investigation, specifically computed tomography, usually reveals nonspecific changes, but the colonic wall can be thickened and is often associated with mural ulceration.

## Management

Medical management includes ganciclovir and foscarnet. Relapse, however, is common; therefore, maintenance therapy should always be considered.

Surgical intervention is reserved for perforation, massive bleeding, and toxic megacolon. However, a patient with mild peritoneal signs, without free air, and with the presumptive diagnosis of CMV colitis can be treated with both ganciclovir and appropriate antibiotics for aerobic and anaerobic organisms and observed cautiously. Most individuals will respond without the need for surgical intervention. However, when emergency surgery is required, resection of the involved segment of colon is necessary; no anastomosis should be performed under these circumstances.

## Results of Surgery

Approximately two thirds of patients with AIDS who had emergency bowel resection by Wexner and colleagues had CMV ileocolitis. The postoperative mortality was 28% at 1 day, 71% at 1 month, and 86% at 6 months. Death often is a consequence of sepsis and pneumonia caused by *Pneumocystis carinii*.

## Mycobacterium avium *Complex Infection*

*Mycobacterium avium* complex (MAC) affects about 5% of severely immunocompromised patients with HIV and is diagnosed in 50% of those with AIDS. It is an environmental bacterium that enters through both the gastrointestinal and respiratory tracts. In addition to severe diarrhea, intraabdominal lymphadenopathy can lead to severe abdominal pain. This is readily diagnosed by computed tomography and needle aspiration. Blood cultures are more helpful than either stool or respiratory specimens for establishing the diagnosis with certainty.

Treatment consists of medical management and includes rifabutin, clarithromycin, and ethambutol. Surgery is rarely indicated.

## Extranodal Lymphoma

Aggressive non-Hodgkin's lymphoma has been increasingly described in the AIDS population. It tends to occur in advanced disease in those individuals with a CD4-cell count of less than $50/mm^3$. The Epstein-Barr virus and a human herpesvirus-8 DNA sequence have both been implicated in promoting non-Hodgkin's lymphoma.

The biology of these lymphomas varies in relationship to morphologic type, anatomic site, and overall state of immunodeficiency. Approximately 25% of the time, the gastrointestinal tract is the only site of disease.

Chemotherapy is effective treatment, with surgical therapy reserved for bleeding, perforation, or obstruction. Surgical resection should be reserved for localized disease only after an extensive search has been made for a disseminated process.

Median survivals of up to 42 months have been reported.

## Kaposi's Sarcoma

Kaposi's sarcoma is usually an indolent cutaneous disorder in older men of central European origin, but the neoplasm is more aggressive in immunocompromised patients and resembles a disorder seen in young blacks from central Africa. Kaposi's sarcoma is at least 20,000 times more common than would be expected from its incidence rates in the United States before the beginning of the AIDS epidemic. A herpeslike virus has been identified as the etiologic agent.

### Clinical Presentation

Kaposi's sarcoma lesions vary in their clinical presentation and affect predominantly the skin, oral mucosa, and visceral organs. They range in color from light pink to dark purple. The gastrointestinal tract appears to be uniquely susceptible to dissemination by this tumor, and occasionally, gastrointestinal lesions antedate skin manifestations. Lesions can be well localized or multifocal in presentation.

### Symptoms

Symptoms include diarrhea, mucous discharge, bleeding, rectal pain, and incontinence. The presence of characteristic raised, purple, nontender skin lesions, especially on the feet, should alert the physician to the diagnosis.

### Endoscopy

The lesions appear submucosal, purple, spongy, and irregularly shaped. When viewed endoscopically, they vary in size from a few millimeters up to 2 cm. Biopsy specimens can be taken if clinical management may be altered by the results. A deep biopsy is usually needed because of the location of the lesions. Because of the tendency to hemorrhage following rectal biopsy, rubber band ligation of the site has been recommended and then sampling the more superficial portion. Because the patient usually has other obvious lesions on the skin, this is the preferred site for making the diagnosis.

### Histopathology

On histology, spindlelike cells with hemorrhage are frequently demonstrated. Kaposi's sarcoma cells, which are thought to arise from the mesenchymal cells, are characterized by intense neovascularization with spindle cells. Three features make up the histologic appearance of Kaposi's sarcoma: proliferation of vascular spaces, a background of spindle cells, and extravasation of red cells. Kaposi's sarcoma cells have been shown to have features of vascular channel and endothelial cell lineage.

### Radiologic Studies

Contrast study may reveal changes in the stomach and duodenum suggestive of diffuse nodularity, multiple polypoid lesions, or the presence of an infiltrative mass. In the small bowel, thickening and irregularity of the folds may be noted. In the colon, all of the above findings have been reported.

### Treatment

Treatment is generally supportive as most of these patients die of opportunistic infections within 2 years. Surgical excision, cryotherapy, intralesional injections of chemotherapeutic agents, or electrosurgery can be used to remove localized lesions. "Aggressive" attempts at surgical management are not indicated, except for the rare case of bleeding or obstruction. Medical treatment is rapidly changing but includes the Vinca alkaloids, bleomycin, paclitaxel, and doxorubicin. Cutaneous lesions have been irradiated successfully.

### Clostridium difficile *Infection*

Many patients who are infected with HIV receive a variety of antimicrobial agents, either for prophylaxis or for treatment of bacterial diseases, which increases the risk of *Clostridium difficile* infection, which can progress to acute megacolon, as well as to life-threatening diarrhea. The colitis may lack characteristic pseudomembranes in the patient with AIDS and can also involve a secondary pathogen (e.g., CMV). See Chapter 33 for a more comprehensive discussion of antibiotic-associated colitis.

### *Diarrheal Conditions*

The cause of diarrhea in the patient who is HIV-positive is multifactorial. Noninfective problems can be caused by the HIV virus. This includes minor alterations in the architecture of the villi, leading to mild malabsorption of carbohydrates, increased permeability resulting from cytokine activation by foreign antigens, and amino acid sequences of the HIV virus similar to those of vasoactive intestinal peptide (VIP) which can induce diarrhea by upregulation of VIP receptors.

Infective causes of diarrhea include the protozoa *Cryptosporidia* and the organisms *Microsporidia*, *Giardia, M. avium*, and *Isospora*.

With a comprehensive investigation, involving three stool samples, colonoscopy with biopsy and, occasionally, upper gastrointestinal endoscopy a causative agent can be found in 90% of patients. See Chapter 33 for a comprehensive overview of a number of infectious and noninfectious colitides.

## Anorectal Disease in the Patient Infected with HIV

A host of coexisting factors make evaluation of the anorectum in patients infected with HIV perplexing.

### Examination and Diagnosis: General Principles

Much can be ascertained by clinical examination of the patient who is HIV positive. Visual inspection of the perineum may reveal condylomata, the blisters of herpes simplex, the linear lesions of a sacral root herpes zoster, the erythema of an ischiorectal abscess, or the excoriated anus of a patient with intractable diarrhea and a lax sphincter. Before performing a digital examination, it is important to manipulate the perianal tissue, looking for the discharge of pus or air bubbles that would suggest a deep infection. Spreading the buttocks gently can help in identifying an anal fissure. Palpation of the anus and low rectum may demonstrate a mass or an ulcer. Rigid sigmoidoscopy will assess the rectal mucosa for evidence of colitis. In any patient in whom evaluation is too painful, it is wise to proceed to an examination under anesthesia (EUA).

A few caveats are helpful as well as cost-effective. Any exudate associated with a fistula or ulcer should be sent for acid-fast stain and culture. Rarely is useful information obtained from routine aerobic and anaerobic culture. Any exudate found in the anus or distal rectum without a demonstrable fistula should be cultured and stained for *Neisseria gonorrhoeae, Chlamydia*, amebae, and herpes simplex virus. For inflammation extending proximal to 15 cm from the anal verge, request cultures for all enteric pathogens, ova and parasites, and *C. difficile* and perform colonoscopy if preliminary results are nondiagnostic. Tissue from all ulcerative lesions that are shallow and not suggestive of an idiopathic AIDS-related ulcer should be sent for CMV and herpes simplex virus culture as well as for histopathology. A noncutting seton should be placed in all identified fistula tracts. Biopsy should be performed on any mass.

## Nonsexually Transmitted Anal Disease in the Patient Who is HIV-Positive

The anus of the patient infected with HIV can be affected by a number of conditions not necessarily related to HIV.

### Anal Fissure

The differentiation diagnosis of an anal fissure from an idiopathic AIDS-related ulcer is critical to proper management. If concern exists about the possibility of impairment for bowel control, anorectal manometry can be performed to assess the anal canal pressure preoperatively and to determine whether the procedure can be done with minimal morbidity.

### Perianal Suppuration

Perianal abscess in the patient with HIV is analogous to the problem observed in an individual with Crohn's disease. No place is seen for nonoperative management in the presence of perianal suppuration.

A generous incision should be made, but the wound should not be packed. If a fistula is found, a noncutting seton should be placed. Any purulent material should be sent for acid-fast stain and for culture. Untreated perianal sepsis can progress to necrotizing gangrene (see Chapter 19) or lead to disseminated abscesses.

### Fistula-in-Ano

Generally, any anal fistula should be treated conservatively, without performing a definitive operation because many of these patients have attenuated sphincters. A fistulotomy can be considered only when the tract is superficial.

### Hemorrhoids

External thrombosed hemorrhoids can be safely excised. It is safe to offer surgical hemorrhoidectomy to the patient with symptomatic grade III hemorrhoids if the HIV disease is early in its course. However, it is extremely difficult to treat grades III and IV hemorrhoids in patients with advanced AIDS.

### Pruritus Ani

Severe pruritus, which occurs secondary to leakage of pus, fecal incontinence, and fungal overgrowth, is readily treated by antifungal powders and the avoidance of sensitizing over-the-counter preparations (see Chapter 19). If possible, the source of the excessive moisture should be eliminated. Persistence of pruritus despite therapy should lead to the consideration of biopsy to rule out Bowen's disease and other specific perianal conditions.

### Sexually Transmitted Disease in the HIV-Infected Population

#### Gonorrhea

The anus of the practicing homosexual can be infected with a variety of pathogens, one of the most common of which is *Neisseria gonorrhoeae*.

The classic clinical presentation is that of a thick, yellow mucopurulent discharge with or without proctitis, occurring 5 days after inoculation. Diagnosis is confirmed by the presence of gram-negative intracellular diplococci. At the time of diagnosis, patients should also be screened for syphilis. If untreated, gonorrhea can progress to fulminant perihepatitis, meningitis, endocarditis, pericarditis, and arthritis. See Chapters 19 and 33 for a more comprehensive discussion of this infection.

### Chlamydia Infection and Lymphogranuloma Venereum

*Chlamydia trachomatis* is the most common sexually transmitted infectious pathogen in the United States. Depending on the serotype, the infection can present as a mild proctitis or progress to lymphogranuloma venereum. Ten days after inoculation, non-lymphogranuloma venereum proctitis presents with pain, tenesmus, fever, and nonulcerative proctitis. When lymphogranuloma venereum develops, ulceration and stenosis mimicking Crohn's disease occur. However, whereas lymphadenopathy is present in lymphogranuloma venereum, it is absent with Crohn's disease. Once a stricture develops, fecal diversion is the preferred option. Further details concerning epidemiology, symptoms, and treatment are found in Chapter 19.

### Syphilis

Anal syphilis is caused by *Treponema pallidum*, developing 2 to 6 weeks following inoculation. The disease progresses in approximately one third of patients, and in one third it remains latent. When it progresses, the second stage usually is recognized 2 months following resolution of the chancre. The presentation is that of a verrucous, flat lesion (condyloma latum). This is associated with a maculopapular rash on the soles of the feet and the palms of the hand. A high incidence is seen of neurosyphilis with a lack of a predictable serologic response to treatment in the HIV-positive population. This translates into either doing a spinal tap on diagnosis or empirically treating all patients for neurosyphilis. See Chapter 19 for an additional discussion.

### Herpes Simplex

Herpes simplex virus infection is important, not only because of its high incidence, but also because the associated break in the epithelial integrity of the skin probably facilitates the transmission of HIV. After primary infection, the virus remains latent in the sacral root ganglia. On reactivation, it can cause root symptoms along the affected dermatomes, leading to dysuria, leg pain, and constipation. Blistering is often followed by ulceration.

Both tissue culture and biopsy specimens for histopathology are recommended.

Empiric treatment, which should be undertaken before biopsy results are obtained, consists of acyclovir. Those who are acyclovir-resistant usually respond well to foscarnet (Foscavir). Herpes genitalis is discussed also in Chapter 20 and herpes simplex proctitis in Chapter 33.

### Cytomegalovirus Infection

Because CMV is ubiquitous in the AIDS population, it may actually be a nonpathogenic bystander or secondary pathogen rather than the primary cause of disease.

### Anal Condylomata Acuminata

*Etiology and Pathogenesis.* Condylomata are caused by human papillomavirus, a sexually transmitted virus ubiquitous in the homosexual population. Human papillomavirus has multiple subtypes, with subtypes 6 and 11 responsible for most anal condylomata acuminata. Certain subtypes, notably 16, 18, and perhaps 31, 33, and 35, have been associated with malignant transformation. The mechanism is believed to be the transcriptional integration of the E6 and E7 genes into the host genome and binding to the p53 and Rb proteins, respectively. Loss of these tumor suppressor genes is thought to be responsible for malignant transformation. HIV may be a cofactor in E6 and E7 gene expression.

Human papillomavirus typically causes infection by direct inoculation, invading the basal layer of the skin, but anoreceptive intercourse is not required for anal infection. As the virus propagates upward through the layers of the epithelium, a characteristic lesion is seen. The lesions occur typically after a 6-week inoculation time. Visible warts are infectious to others, but the stimulus for propagation is unknown.

*Anal Intraepithelial Neoplasia.* In men infected with HIV, it appears that human papillomavirus infection occurs with clinically normal but histologically abnormal epithelium. Progression to anal intraepithelial neoplasia appears to be directly related to the level of immunosuppression rather than to the specific subtype of human papillomavirus retrieved.

No longitudinal study has identified the expected outbreak of squamous cell carcinoma in patients with precursor lesions.

*Principles of Management.* Anal warts should be destroyed, with follow-up every 2 months. Our preferred method is cytodestruction (electrocautery). Some suggest interferon alfa-2b injected into the operative bed significantly reduces frequency and severity of recurrence. Larger flat lesions should be excised. Noninvasive flat lesions that are determined to be carcinoma *in situ* with negative margins do not need any additional therapy. Ablative prophylactic therapy for anal intraepithelial neoplasia is not indicated. These patients should be observed at 3-month intervals; biopsy specimens can safely be taken from any suspicious lesions, which can be treated as they become apparent. Although a variety of methods have been described in treating anal condyloma acuminatum, high recurrence rates remain a problem (see also Chapter 19).

## Aids-Specific Disease

Idiopathic AIDS-related ulcers occur in advanced disease, usually when T4-cell counts fall below 200/μL. Their characteristic appearance is one of an extremely caustic and ulcerative process that occurs more proximally than do benign anal fissures, undermining what appears to be normal mucosa and traversing normal tissue planes. Symptoms include a sensation of pressure caused by pocketing of stool, pus, and vegetable matter, and severe pain that is worse on defecation.

Treatment consists of operative debridement to eliminate the pocketing effect and injection of a depot steroid preparation into the base and sides of the ulcers. Another agent, thalidomide, has been used anecdotally in both anal and oral aphthous ulceration. Its presumed mechanism of action is also downregulation of cytokine production.

## Anorectal Malignancy

The anorectum can be the initiating site for non-Hodgkin's lymphoma, which can present as either a mass or a fissure; biopsy is diagnostic. Kaposi's sarcoma is usually an incidental finding and rarely causes significant anorectal symptoms.

The greatest controversy in the patient infected with AIDS concerns the management of squamous cell carcinoma. Classic treatment for squamous cell carcinoma of the anus begins with a chemotherapy-radiation protocol (see Chapter 24). However, several small series have documented the inability of patients to complete the protocol without intolerable morbidity. Some have recommended resection for those with advanced disease or severe diarrhea and reserve chemoradiation only for individuals with early HIV disease. It is hoped that new antiviral agents will improve the management of these difficult cases.

## Wound Healing and AIDS

Although impairment of healing is indeed seen, no consistently predictive factor has been implicated. Overall performance status of the patient, rather than T4 count alone, seems to predict the rate of wound healing. Despite unpredictable healing, most operations still produce symptomatic relief.

## Protection of the Surgeon

Seroconversion to an HIV-positive state following percutaneous exposure with a hypodermic needle (0.3%) and mucous membrane exposure (0.1%) has been documented. However, seroconversions after being stuck with a suture needle have been reported. Furthermore, no seroconversions occurred following exposure if the skin remained intact. Although universal precautions should be routinely instituted, certain special efforts should be made when operating on an identified or suspected HIV-infected individual. The following recommendations should be enforced:

- Eyeglasses should be worn, in addition to water-resistant foot covering.
- Double gloves with a disposable sleeve insert should be used to prevent blood from reaching the wrists of the surgeon.
- Scalpels should be disposed of once skin incisions have been made.
- When suturing, the senior surgeon should dictate a choregraphed procedure.
- If a serious exposure occurs, triple therapy is recommended.

### Antiviral Therapy

The goal of all current antiviral therapies appears to be achieved by early intervention with low-dose zidovudine (Retrovir): to suppress the replication of the virus and to slow the clinical progression of the disease. This, along with management of the other sequelae, forms the basis for treatment.

### CONCLUSIONS

Advances in combination medical therapy and a better understanding of the pathophysiology of HIV may be transforming HIV infection from a terminal into a chronic disease. New drugs are available, which, when combined with zidovudine (AZT), seem to have an improved effect on progression of disease. Most investigators suggest aggressive therapy early in the course of the illness, while the body's HIV population is homogeneous and has not mutated. It is important, therefore, that individuals treating this condition keep abreast of the literature, because changes will obviously affect the management of the myriad problems encountered in this population.

# 21

# Polypoid Diseases

This chapter discusses a number of benign polypoid conditions that are commonly observed in the practice of general and colon and rectal surgeons. A polyp is a well-circumscribed projection above the surface epithelium. It can be pedunculated or sessile. It can vary in size from 1 or 2 mm to more than 10 cm. It is not a histologic diagnosis, however; polyp is merely a descriptive term. Three types of polyps are discussed in this chapter: hyperplastic (metaplastic), hamartomatous, and adenomatous.

## HYPERPLASTIC OR METAPLASTIC POLYP

### Clinical Appearance

Hyperplastic polyps are usually found in the rectum and sigmoid, often at the summit of mucosal folds and on the apex of the valves of Houston (Fig. 21.1). They are nearly always multiple and can present in such large numbers that on both endoscopic examination and barium enema they can simulate familial (multiple) polyposis. Their usual size is from 2 to 5 mm. They appear approximately the same color as the rectal mucosa, or slightly paler; often, they are overlooked.

### Histology

Microscopically, crypts are seen to be lined by a hyperplastic epithelium that gives the crypt lumen a scalloped appearance (Fig. 21.2). The structure is different from that of an adenomatous polyp. The lining epithelium loses its regular columnar and goblet cell pattern and appears serrated because of flattening of the cells (Fig. 21.3). Goblet cells are diminished and the lamina propria may demonstrate increased inflammatory reaction: plasma cells and lymphocytes.

### Management

Because it has been generally accepted that hyperplastic polyps are not neoplasms and do not connote increased risk for the development of tumors, either

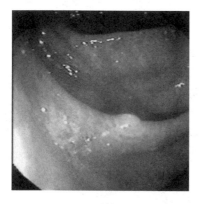

**FIG. 21.1.** A hyperplastic polyp can be seen on the surface of one of the valves of Houston. Note the coexisting melanosis coli, which serves to demarcate clearly the nonpigmented lesion.

benign or malignant, the question of how to treat them demands a decision. The fact that a patient harbors hyperplastic polyps would seem of no clinical significance; hence, therapy is unnecessary. The problem arises, however, in establishing with certainty the nature of the tumor. This can be accomplished only by submitting the lesion for pathologic confirmation. This is an important consideration, because if it is discovered that the tumor is a neoplasm (e.g., a polypoid adenoma), the need for total colonic evaluation and follow-up is different.

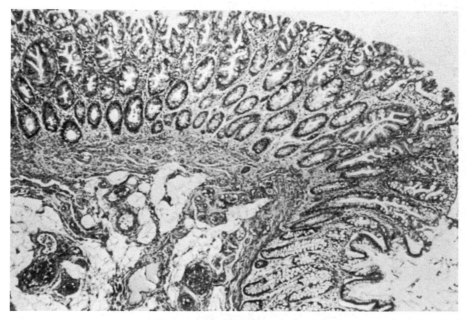

**FIG. 21.2.** Hyperplastic (metaplastic) polyp. Note the hyperplastic changes in the mucosa, and the serrated glands near the surface with papillary projections. (Original magnification ×240.) (Reproduced with permission from Corman ML, Veidenheimer MC, Swinton NW. *Diseases of the anus, rectum, and colon.* Part I: Neoplasms. New York: Medcom, 1972.)

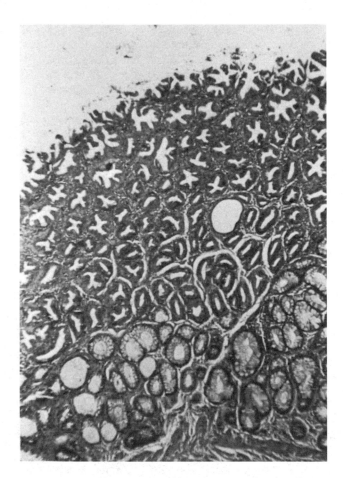

**FIG. 21.3.** Hyperplastic (metaplastic) polyp. A lesion has serrated glands, some of which are cystically dilated. (Original magnification ×280; courtesy of Rudolf Garret, M.D.)

Small colonic polyps are usually neoplastic, but even if hyperplastic, are associated with adenomas elsewhere in 33% to 75% of cases. Small rectal polyps are usually hyperplastic but are associated with neoplasms elsewhere in 63%. Total colonoscopy is probably appropriate for even proved hyperplastic polyps. Many authors have concluded that small adenomatous and hyperplastic polyps cannot reliably be distinguished by their endoscopic appearance.

### Hyperplastic Polyposis

Hyperplastic polyps can show spatial clustering with neoplastic polyps, suggesting that regions with prior polyps merit close surveillance. A number of cases of so-called "hyperplastic polyposis" have appeared in the literature. This particular entity seems to have an increased association with colorectal cancer. Interestingly, disappearance of the hyperplastic polyps has been reported following resection.

*Comment*: My own philosophy is to effect a compromise between an aggressive "search and destroy" attitude with every identifiable mucosal excrescence and a *laissez-faire* approach. I recommend the following protocol.

Excise the lesion initially to confirm the diagnosis. No follow-up other than the routine colorectal cancer screening appropriate for any patient free of a prior history of neoplasm is suggested, if the polyp is nonneoplastic. If an individual is found on subsequent routine endoscopic examination to harbor additional lesions, no treatment is advised, except possibly fulguration or cold biopsy of the relatively larger ones. I have four reasons why I suggest ignoring them. First, they tend to disappear spontaneously and recur elsewhere; some patients simply are hyperplastic polyp creators. Second, I am reluctant to create further anxiety by reinforcing the phobia most people have about cancer. Third, complications are associated with excision of lesions; bleeding and perforation are encountered more frequently when small lesions are removed than when large tumors are biopsied. This occurs because sometimes normal bowel must be injured to completely extirpate the growth. If the surgeon performs procedures through the endoscope frequently enough, inevitably a complication will result. Finally, it adds considerably to the cost of medical care.

## HAMARTOMAS

A hamartoma is defined as a nonneoplastic growth composed of an abnormal mixture of normal tissue. In the colon, this includes juvenile and Peutz–Jeghers polyps.

### Juvenile Polyps

The juvenile polyp (congenital polyp, retention polyp, juvenile adenoma) is usually found in children under 10 years of age, but it is also seen in older children and in adults at any age. It is an uncommon condition, occurring in approximately 1% of asymptomatic children. The age distribution has been reported to have a bimodal pattern, with the childhood group having a modal age of 4 years, whereas the adult group is found to have a modal age of 18 years. The incidence is twice as frequent in boys, and a 13:1 ratio of men to women is seen in adults.

Although juvenile polyps are the most common colorectal tumors in children, benign and malignant neoplasms can present at virtually any age. Solitary adenomas account for 7% to 8% of all polyps found in patients under 20 years of age.

#### Symptoms and Signs

The most common presenting complaint is rectal bleeding, followed by prolapse or protrusion of the mass, passing of tissue, and abdominal pain. Autoamputation is noted in up to 10% of patients. Diarrhea, mucus, proctalgia, tenesmus, and rectal prolapse are also identifiable complaints.

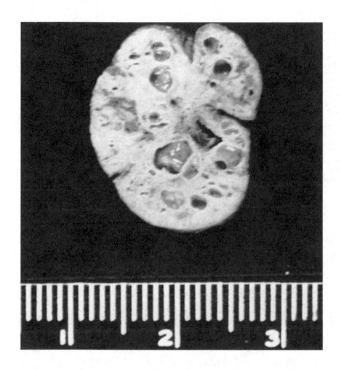

**FIG. 21.4.** Juvenile polyp. Note the characteristic cystic spaces in cross section. (Courtesy of Rudolf Garret, M.D.)

### *Distribution*

Of the polyps, 60% are located within 10 cm of the anal verge; only 10% are located farther away than 20 cm, but these are scattered throughout the colon. Approximately three fourths are more than 1 cm in diameter.

### *Appearance*

Macroscopically, the lesions are usually round or oval, with a smooth, continuous surface, in contrast to the papillary surface that characterizes the adenomatous polyp. They usually have a short stalk. The cut surface demonstrates numerous cystic spaces filled with mucus (Fig. 21.4).

### *Histology*

Microscopic examination reveals that juvenile polyps are composed of an epithelial and a connective tissue element, with the latter contributing the bulk of the tumor mass (Fig. 21.5). Acute and chronic inflammatory cells are frequently seen.

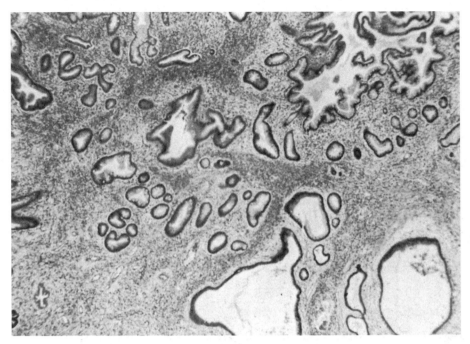

**FIG. 21.5.** Juvenile polyp. Note the cystically dilated glands lined by normal-appearing epithelium. (Original magnification ×170; courtesy of Rudolf Garret, M.D.)

### Etiology

A frequent microscopic finding is infiltration by eosinophils. It has been postulated that because eosinophils usually connote an allergic response, the polyps are the result of allergy. In support of this theory is the observation that a statistically significant increased incidence of allergy is seen in children with polyps and in the families of those children.

Despite the suggestion by some that juvenile polyps may be neoplastic, most pathologists today agree that the lesion is a hamartoma. This is based on the observation that an abnormality of the mucosal connective tissue or lamina propria is present and that this connective tissue stroma bears a resemblance to primitive mesenchyme. This lends support to the contention that the lesion is a malformation rather than a neoplasm. One theory holds that the polyp is a form of retention cyst that takes on a polypoid form from traction caused by peristalsis. Juvenile polyps also have been reported at the site of a ureterosigmoidoscopy.

### Diagnosis and Management

The diagnosis is usually confirmed by means of proctosigmoidoscopy, and the lesion is removed transanally. In many centers, colonoscopy is the initial means used to investigate children with undiagnosed rectal bleeding.

Despite the likelihood that a lesion proximal to a juvenile polyp in the rectum is most probably another juvenile polyp, an aggressive attitude should be taken to confirm its true histologic nature. It is, however, generally agreed that a juvenile polyp, itself, is neither a neoplasm nor a premalignant condition. Once the polyp is removed, no further follow-up is required.

## Juvenile Polyposis

Juvenile polyposis is an uncommon condition characterized by the development of multiple juvenile polyps, primarily in the colon, but also in the remainder of the intestinal tract. A family history is found in 20% to 50% of patients with an apparent autosomal dominant hereditary pattern. The gene has not yet been identified. The condition should be distinguished from multiple juvenile polyposis. Many of these individuals have a family history of adenomatous polyposis and of carcinoma of the colon. As suggested, in addition to the colon, the polyps occasionally are found in the small intestine and stomach. The recurrence rate for solitary juvenile polyps is less than 20%, whereas the rate approaches 90% in familial cases.

Patients with juvenile polyposis have a much different clinical course when compared with those who have solitary juvenile polyps. Hematochezia, iron deficiency anemia, hypoproteinemia, hypokalemia, anergy, finger clubbing, and a failure to thrive are much more likely to occur in the former condition. Other extracolonic congenital and acquired manifestations in this condition include macrocephaly, alopecia, bony swellings, cleft lip, cleft palate, abnormalities of the vitellointestinal duct, double renal pelvis and ureter, acute glomerulonephritis, undescended testicle, and bifid uterus and vagina. Of course, some of the associations may be purely coincidental. The rare and often fatal form, juvenile polyposis of infancy, is associated with profuse diarrhea, protein-losing enteropathy, bleeding, and rectal prolapse.

A strong association exists with benign and malignant neoplasms of the colon as well as gastroduodenal polyps. The condition usually presents in childhood, with only 15% being identified in the adult population.

### *Management*

Because juvenile polyposis should be considered a potentially premalignant condition, an aggressive approach to management is indicated. Unless truly satisfied that the colon has been "cleared" (usually by means of colonoscopy and polypectomies), total colectomy is the recommended procedure. Consideration should be given to ileoanal anastomosis with intervening pouch if the rectum is densely involved. Neoplasms within the ileal reservoir following this operation have been reported. Periodic endoscopic surveillance of the ileal pouch as well as upper gastrointestinal endoscopy should be considered following restorative proctocolectomy. Proctocolectomy and ileostomy are required in some cases. Finally, family members should have colorectal evaluation.

## Cronkhite–Canada Syndrome

In 1955, Cronkhite and Canada described a syndrome of gastrointestinal polyposis, hyperpigmentation, alopecia, and nail dystrophy. The syndrome is felt to be a variant of juvenile polyposis with ectodermal changes and without evidence of genetic transmission. Some have suggested that the disease is caused by an abnormality of ectodermal and endodermal proliferation. The polyps can be seen in association with neoplasms of the colon, which is considered by some authors to represent a premalignant condition.

### *Symptoms and Signs*

Diarrhea and malabsorption produce severe vitamin deficiency, hypoproteinemia, and fluid and electrolyte abnormalities. Anemia and rectal bleeding are commonly reported. Other symptoms include weight loss, abdominal pain, weakness, nausea and vomiting, hypogeusia (loss of taste), and a variety of neurologic complaints. Hair loss and nail and skin changes may be evident before the gastrointestinal symptoms become manifested.

Polyps involve the stomach and large bowel in virtually every case, but the small intestine probably frequently contains the tumors; it is simply that the small bowel is more difficult to evaluate. As with juvenile polyposis, pathologic study confirms their hamartomatous nature. The observation of dysplasia in a biopsy specimen should encourage the endoscopist to pursue an aggressive surveillance program.

### *Management*

Most patients have been treated symptomatically by means of nutritional support, including home parenteral nutrition. Resection is indicated when massive involvement is limited to a segment amenable to excision, whether it be stomach, small bowel or colon. The cause of death is attributable to the disease and its complications.

## Peutz–Jeghers Polyps

In 1921, Peutz reported a familial syndrome of polyps of the gastrointestinal tract with pigmentation of the mouth and other parts of the body. Later, Jeghers and his colleagues established the syndrome by describing a number of cases. The disease appears to be transmitted in an autosomal dominant fashion, but *de novo* cases have been reported without any suggestive family history.

The polyps are found most frequently in the small bowel, particularly the jejunum, but they also can occur in the stomach, colon, and rectum.

### *Signs, Symptoms, and Diagnosis*

Cutaneous pigmentation usually is noted at birth or in infancy; the skin changes may actually disappear after puberty. They consist of clusters of black or dark brown frecklelike spots, 1 to 2 mm in diameter, on and around the lips and buccal mucosa, fingers, and toes. The most common symptom and the one most difficult to manage is abdominal pain, often caused by intestinal obstruction. The obstruction is usually the result of a polyp or of an intussusception. The other frequent complaint is rectal bleeding. Additional signs and symptoms include prolapse of the polyp, passage of the polyp, hematemesis, and anemia. Diagnosis of the syndrome usually can be made on the basis of family history, skin pigmentation, and gastrointestinal symptoms. Contrast studies in addition to endoscopy confirm the extent of the polypoid disease.

### *Pathology*

Macroscopically, the polyps vary in size. They can be as large as several centimeters in diameter and, with increasing size, tend to become pedunculated. Visually, they look much like adenomatous polyps.

Microscopically, the polyps seem to originate from intestinal glandular epithelium along with a muscular branching framework that arises from the muscularis mucosa (Fig. 21.6). The tubules of epithelium rest on the branching bands of smooth muscle in a relationship similar to that which the glandular

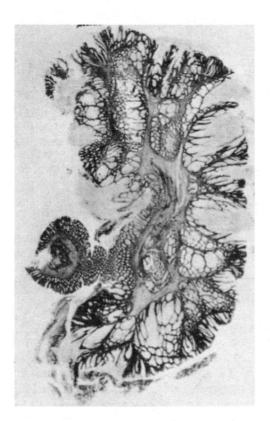

**FIG. 21.6.** Peutz–Jeghers polyp of the large intestine. Note the treelike muscular framework. (Reproduced with permission from Morson BC. Some peculiarities in the histology of intestinal polyps. *Dis Colon Rectum* 1962;5:337.)

epithelium has to the muscularis mucosa of the normal bowel. Because no evidence is seen of hyperplasia, cytologic variation, or loss of differentiation, the lesion probably represents a hamartomatous process or malformation, rather than a neoplasm.

### Treatment

The major problem with this condition lies with the treatment, particularly for the most frequent manifestation—small bowel involvement. Many of these young individuals have multiple abdominal operations because of small bowel obstruction and bleeding. Under these circumstances, multiple polyps can be removed by enterotomy and invagination, not resection, or by endoscopic polypectomies via enterotomy. Alternatively, an orally introduced endoscope has been successfully used at the time of laparotomy by telescoping the small bowel over the instrument. Another approach is to perform operative endoscopy by means of an enterotomy. Massive small bowel resection should rarely be necessary, thus avoiding the consequences of a short bowel syndrome. Evidence suggests that an aggressive approach is justified because the frequency of recurrent tumors decreases as the patient becomes older.

### Relationship to Cancer

Another concern that has been expressed is the suggestion of an association between Peutz–Jeghers syndrome and the development of gastrointestinal benign and malignant tumors. As many as 50% may develop malignancy, a rate 18 times greater than would be expected. The increased frequency is noted for cancers of both gastrointestinal and nongastrointestinal origin. Neoplastic transformation—not a rare event—suggests a hamartoma-adenoma-carcinoma sequence in Peutz–Jeghers polyposis.

As of this writing, the question of surveillance for malignancy is an unresolved issue. With the probability of an increased incidence of breast, ovarian, and pancreatic cancers, annual mammography and ultrasound may be useful.

Of course, it is of paramount importance to distinguish and identify those lesions that represent true (adenomatous) polyps from the hamartomatous tumors. The malignant potential of the former is not a subject for debate.

## ADENOMAS

Whereas a hyperplastic polyp is the most common "tumor" of the colon and rectum, an adenoma is by far the most frequently observed neoplasm. Adenomas are classified into three categories: polypoid, villous, and mixed. The lesions are by definition benign, but their relationship to the subsequent development of cancer is important (see *Polyp-Cancer Sequence*).

## Polypoid Adenoma, Adenomatous Polyp, and Tubular Adenoma

Approximately 75% of the benign tumors in the colon are classified as adenomatous polyps and 10% as villous adenomas. The lesions can be as small as 1 mm or larger than 5 cm. They can be pedunculated or sessile, with a relatively smooth surface broken by clefts into multiple nodules. The smaller tumors are more likely to have a regular outline and the larger adenomas a lobulated pattern.

### *Histology*

Microscopically, polypoid adenomas consist of closely packed epithelial tubules separated by normal lamina propria, which grow and branch horizontally to the muscularis mucosae. However, no consistent appearance of the tubules is seen; they can be regular or irregular, with or without inflammatory reaction (Fig. 21.7). The epithelial cells can become distorted, the nuclei can be hyperchromic (stain more deeply) with increased number, and mucus is reduced. Mitoses can be observed frequently, but not invasion of the muscularis mucosae. Whereas some authors describe certain changes as representative of *in situ* carcinoma, others may call the same phenomenon "atypia" or "dysplasia."

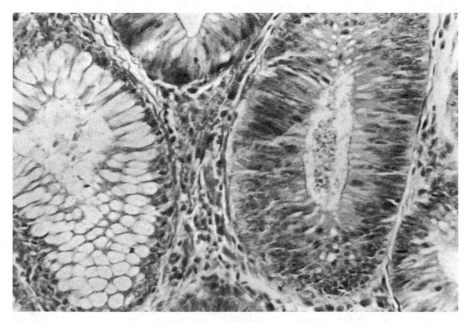

**FIG. 21.7.** This section from the edge of a polypoid adenoma illustrates a neoplastic and a normal gland, side by side. Note the crowding of cells, piling up of nuclei, and the loss of ability to produce mucus in the neoplastic gland on the right. (Reproduced with permission from Corman ML, Veidenheimer MC, Swinton NW. *Diseases of the anus, rectum, and colon.* Part I: Neoplasms. New York: Medcom, 1972.)

Of the adenomas, 20% were found to contain aneuploid cells compared with 63% of adenocarcinomas, which correlates with increasing degrees of dysplasia. A positive correlation was seen between the size of the diploid adenomas and proliferative activity.

### Rate of Growth

Normal surface epithelial cells of the colonic mucosa are replaced every 4 to 8 days. Cell division and migration balance exfoliation of the cells. Epithelial surfaces are increased up to 226 times in adenomatous polyps when compared with the normal mucosa. Furthermore, the number of cells is increased up to 370 times. The increased number is not primarily dependent on mitotic activity but on amitotic nuclear fragmentation.

### Pseudocarcinomatous Invasion

Benign-appearing glandular tissue has been described deep to the muscularis mucosae; this condition has been termed "pseudocarcinomatous invasion." It is believed to be associated with larger tumors, those with a long pedicle, and lesions of the sigmoid colon. The histologic appearance may be caused by trauma, possibly secondary to repeated twisting of the stalk.

Histologic examination reveals glandlike or cystlike structures in the submucosa that show a cytologic appearance similar to that of the overlying benign tumor.

Differentiation of pseudocarcinomatous invasion from invasive cancer is important, in that no patient develops a recurrence or metastasis following excision.

### Villous Adenoma or Villous Papilloma

The villous adenoma generally appears larger than a polypoid adenoma and is more frequently sessile. The margins are usually less well defined than with adenomatous polyps. Despite its size, however, its velvety soft texture can cause it to be missed on digital examination of the rectum. One third are asymptomatic; 7% are less than 1 cm, and 61% are less than 3 cm. However, sigmoidoscopy will readily demonstrate the presence of a lesion. Large tumors can prolapse through the anal canal. The median age at diagnosis is 64 years (range, 36 to 82 years).

### Symptoms

Although rectal bleeding is the most frequent presenting complaint for both adenomatous conditions, change in bowel habits and mucous discharge are much more frequent concerns in a patient with a large villous adenoma. In fact, a unique symptom complex is associated with villous adenoma that today has become rare: hypokalemia and dehydration. The syndrome is attributed to the loss of copious fluid and electrolytes from the mucus-secreting tumor. Sodium loss is as frequently seen and may be the dominant feature of this syndrome in some cases.

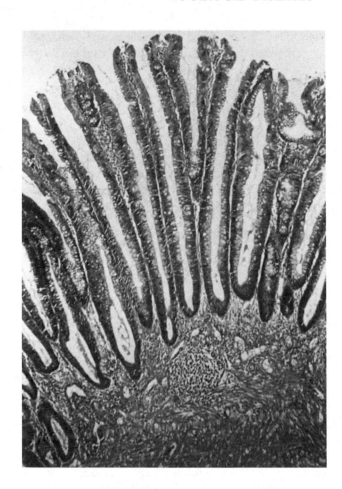

**FIG. 21.8.** Villous adenoma. Papillary fronds extend from the mucosa. (Original magnification ×280.) (Reproduced with permission from Corman ML, Veidenheimer MC, Swinton NW. *Diseases of the anus, rectum, and colon.* Part I: Neoplasms. New York: Medcom, 1972.)

## Histology

Microscopically, the villous adenoma consists of fingerlike processes, each made up of a core of lamina propria covered by epithelial cells growing vertically toward the bowel lumen (Fig. 21.8). The epithelium sits on the muscularis mucosae and, in the benign lesion, no evidence is seen of invasion. Whereas mucus is decreased in polypoid adenomas, some villous adenomas actually demonstrate an increase. Atypia or dysplasia is commonly observed.

### Tubulovillous Adenoma, Villoglandular Adenoma, Papillary Adenoma, Villoglandular Polyp, Mixed Adenoma, and Polypoid-Villous Adenoma

The combination of polypoid and villous elements is frequently seen with benign neoplasms of the colon and rectum. Histologically, the changes are intermediate between a villous and a polypoid adenoma. The distinction, however, between this presentation and that of a "pure" polypoid adenoma is academic. The patient's symptoms, the methods of diagnosis, and the therapy for the benign lesion are identical.

### Evaluation and Diagnosis

Adenomas are commonly observed in countries wherein a high incidence of colorectal cancer is found; their frequency increases with the age of the patient. Benign neoplasms of the colon and rectum have been observed in from 12% to 60%. The three methods for diagnosing polypoid disease are proctosigmoidoscopy, barium enema, and fiberoptic colonoscopy. The relative merits of these approaches and the techniques, themselves, are discussed in Chapters 4 and 5.

### Sigmoidoscopy

Benign lesions are found in approximately 9% of asymptomatic individuals.

### Radiologic Evaluation

Depending on the barium enema technique used, polyps of the colon can be identified in from 1% to 13% of patients; the double-contrast (air-contrast) approach gives a higher yield. The air-contrast enema is considered the preferred option by many radiologists for evaluating the colon, especially when the patient has a prior history of polyps or carcinoma; lesions as small as 2 or 3 mm are identifiable by this technique.

The radiologist cannot ascertain the histologic nature of a polyp, although certain characteristic features can be identified. Of particular importance, note the presence or absence of a pedicle or stalk. Although a pedicle does not connote benignity, it implies that at least an attempt should be made to remove the lesion by means of the colonoscope, and that an adequate margin will probably be obtained. Sessile lesions are more likely to be malignant and are more difficult to remove by colonoscopy.

Villous adenomas have a characteristic radiologic appearance. They have an irregular surface because of the frondlike growths; barium in the interstices of the tumor surface produces striated or lacelike radiographic features.

### Colonoscopy

Colonoscopy and colonoscopy-polypectomy are the diagnostic and therapeutic modalities that have been responsible for the quantum advance in our knowledge of polypoid disease over the past 25 years. The comparative overall inaccuracy rate for air-contrast barium enema (false-positive and false-negative findings) is 30%. The major morbidity is the "lost polyp." In a comparison of the two techniques, a demonstrated 90% accuracy of air-contrast enema and 91% accuracy of colonoscopy has been shown.

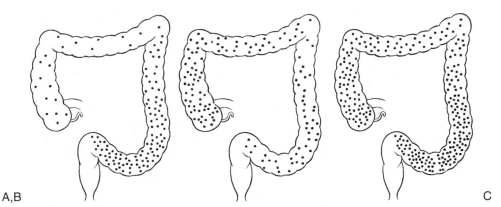

A,B                                                                                              C

**FIG. 21.9.** Distribution of colonic polyps. **A.** Radiologically suspected. **B.** Unsuspected. **C.** Total distribution. (Illustration by Steckel, FE; based on data from Coller JA, Corman ML, Veidenheimer MC. Colonic polypoid disease: need for total colonoscopy. *Am J Surg* 1976;131:490.)

With increasing polyp size, a greater tendency is seen to villous involvement; this is associated with a higher incidence of malignant change. Invasive cancer can be found in polyps less than 1 cm in diameter.

Despite generalizations concerning size, color, and presence or absence of a pedicle, the only definitive means for establishing the diagnosis is histologic confirmation. Five criteria suggestive of malignant change include friability, ulceration, firmness, lobulation, and asymmetry. Also the "dunce cap" appearance (a broad base tapering to a narrow tip) can be indicative of invasive carcinoma.

Total colonoscopy is a requisite for patients found to harbor a neoplasm of the colon. Two thirds of the unsuspected neoplasms were found proximal to the splenic flexure, resulting in a more uniform distribution of neoplastic colonic polypoid disease (Fig. 21.9).

What about a screening colonoscopy in the asymptomatic patient? Currently, the procedure should certainly be performed on individuals at an increased risk for the development of neoplasms, but some have suggested that it may be reasonable to consider this evaluation every 5 to 7 years for all asymptomatic adults.

## Polyp-Cancer Sequence

The significance of neoplastic polyps would be of academic interest only, were it not for the relationship between these lesions and the subsequent development of carcinoma.

### Synchronous Cancer

Many authors have demonstrated that from 13% to 50% of resected specimens for colon and rectal cancer harbor one or more adenomas. Numerous colonoscopy studies have confirmed this frequent association.

## Metachronous Cancer

Marked reductions have been demonstrated in the incidence of large bowel cancers by a program of follow-up proctosigmoidoscopy after polypectomy. Only 15% of the statistically anticipated carcinomas develop, and each of these is an early lesion.

It has been known that patients who have undergone colon resection for carcinoma are at an increased risk for the subsequent development of a malignancy. The metachronous cancer rate is approximately 4%. The average time interval is about 10 years, implying that the polyp-cancer development period, specifically, is that length of time. The frequency of identifying benign neoplasms in such patients is also high.

Patients who have previously undergone polypectomy are more likely than the general population to develop more polyps. The rate can be 15 to 16 times that expected in a population of similar age and gender during the first year. Furthermore, in those who develop a recurrent polyp, one third develop another recurrence.

## Geographic Distribution

Carcinoma of the colon and rectum is a disease of Western civilization. Adenomatous polyps parallel the geographic distribution, with a high incidence in Europe and in the United States, in other high meat-consuming countries, and in urban populations. The epidemiology of carcinoma is discussed in Chapter 22.

## Anatomic Distribution

The distribution of benign tumors of the colon is similar to that of cancers: more frequent in the distal bowel, with a relatively high incidence in the cecum. Additional studies have demonstrated a more uniform distribution for adenomas than for carcinomas; this observation may be anticipating a further trend to more proximal cancers. A left-to-right shift was apparent in the decade from 1971 to 1980 in comparison with the prior 10-year period.

## Age

It should be expected that adenomatous polyps antedate cancer by several years, but until recently this could not be well documented. The probable reason for this is that cancer patients are usually symptomatic, and the date of onset can be accurately reported. Polyps, especially when small, can be asymptomatic for a considerable period of time. The evolution of the polyp-cancer sequence is estimated to be approximately 7 to 10 years. The mean age of patients who have colonoscopy-polypectomy is 55 years compared with patients with colorectal cancer (mean age 62 years).

## Gender

Men and women have an approximately equal frequency of colorectal cancer; the same observation is true for adenomas. Women have a slightly greater number of right-sided lesions (both benign and malignant).

## Miscellaneous Factors

The high incidence of polyps parallels that of colorectal cancer in every population-based study. Whether this is diet-related or caused by other environmental factors, the validity of the observation cannot be denied. Cigarette smoking, beer consumption, cirrhosis, and alcoholism are independent risk factors for the development of colonic adenomas. Immunodeficiency has also been suggested to play a possible role in the pathogenesis.

## Family History

The adenoma-carcinoma sequence suggests an increased risk of colorectal cancer in the families of patients who harbor adenomatous polyps. Siblings and parents of patients with adenomatous polyps are at an increased risk for the development of colorectal cancer, particularly if the adenoma is diagnosed before the age of 60, or in the case of siblings, when a parent has had a colorectal cancer.

## Evolution

Three situations are seen in which the life history of the adenoma-carcinoma sequence can be demonstrated: first, in the unusual opportunity in which a patient with a benign polyp refuses removal of the lesion and subsequently develops a carcinoma at the same site; second, in familial polyposis, a condition that always results in a bowel cancer if the colon is not resected (see later); and third, in hereditary nonpolyposis colorectal cancer (see Chapter 22; *Lynch Syndromes*). Because the histologic nature of the polyps in the familial polyposis condition does not differ from that seen in the common, solitary adenoma, a cause and effect relationship is inferred. The huge number of polyps present in the bowel implies that the risk is multiplied many times.

Actuarial analysis of patients with polyps larger than 1 cm in size, who have elected observation, reveal that the cumulative risk of diagnosis of cancer at the polyp site at 5, 10, and 20 years is 2.5%, 8%, and 24%, respectively.

## Histologic Change

The most direct evidence for the polyp–cancer sequence is the demonstration of all stages in the development of malignancy within the same specimen: normal epithelium, adenomatous tissue, atypia, and frank invasion. In large series of colonoscopy-polypectomies, 4% to 5% of polyps demonstrated some element of invasive carcinoma. Generally, the larger the lesion, the greater the likelihood of malignant degeneration. Polypoid adenomas smaller than 1 cm have been shown to have a 1% incidence of malignant change; those from 1 to 2 cm have a 10% incidence, and those over 2 cm, a 35% incidence. In patients with villous adenomas, the incidence has been reported as follows: less than 1 cm, 10%; 1 to 2 cm, 10%; and more than 2 cm, 53%.

### De Novo *Carcinoma Versus the Polyp-Cancer Sequence*

If carcinomas of the large bowel arose *de novo* from normal mucosa, without passing through the stage of benignity, it would not be uncommon to observe a cancer of 0.5 cm in diameter. Because this is not the case, most colorectal cancers are assumed to arise from benign polyps. It has been said that, if one seeks vigorously enough and performs sufficient serial sections of the pathologic specimen, an element of benign polyp can virtually always be found in a cancer, particularly if the tumor is relatively small. However, compelling evidence indicates that some malignant tumors of the rectum and colon arise from the mucosa without passing through a benign stage. The implications of this observation are applied to the follow-up evaluation of individuals with long-standing ulcerative colitis (see Chapter 29; *Relationship to Malignancy*).

### *Genetics*

This section on genetics has been contributed by Dr. Anthony A. Goodman.

Carcinogenesis has been well established as a multistep process involving the accumulation of mutations in the genome of somatic cells. In the case of colorectal cancers, the progression from normal cells to benign adenomas and finally to carcinomas has been among the best studied. It is now well established that virtually all colorectal carcinomas derive from preexisting benign adenomas.

#### Cancer and Natural Selection

It has become increasingly clear that the development of all forms of cancer is based on the accumulation of mutations in the cellular DNA and the subsequent natural selection of these mutated clones of cells. In the case of normal colon epithelium, the cells arise from several lines of stem cells, and thus are polyclonal. The adenomas (and ultimately, the carcinomas) arise from a single mutated cell line and, therefore, are monoclonal. The mutations that give rise to the single abnormal cell provide a significant growth advantage to that cell, and its progeny, therefore, will predominate; this results in the neoplasm. This can be viewed as a microevolutionary process in which the rules of survival of the fittest cell (or the fittest DNA) will dominate.

## Multistep Carcinogenesis

The process of carcinogenesis can be seen to occur in four basic phases. Each step or phase of the multistep process is driven by genetic damage primarily to somatic cells. The somatic DNA is exposed to some form of carcinogen (chemical, viral, physical), which permanently alters the structure of the DNA. This confers a selective growth advantage on the cell by increasing the cell's responsiveness to intra- and intercellular growth signals. In the case of colorectal cancers, the mucosal cells are exposed to many carcinogens residing in the fecal mass. Because of the rapid turnover rate of the mutated clonal cells, these changes will lead to selective clonal expansion and natural selection, which ultimately increases the turnover rate and leads to more DNA damage. The speeding up of cell replication interferes with the processes that allow for discovery and repair of DNA errors. Then, epigenetic changes occur, which can alter the expression of the genetic damage without necessarily further altering the genome. Finally, after accumulation of enough mutations, the cell expresses the malignant phenotype and emerges as a clinical cancer.

*Initiation.* Initiation involves the modification of cellular DNA by the carcinogen in the form of irreversible genetic damage to the DNA. At the molecular level, what usually takes place during initiation is the activation of an oncogene, (or, actually the conversion of a proto-oncogene to an oncogene), or the inactivation of a tumor suppressor gene. The resulting oncogenes can cause growth abnormalities by one or more of several mechanisms:

Overexpression of a gene product, which leads to an increased concentration of an active protein (dosage hypothesis)
Expression of a gene at an inappropriate time in the cell cycle, bypassing resting phases and increasing rate of replication (unscheduled gene expression)
Expression of a gene product in an inappropriate cell type
Some structural alteration of a gene protein or product to make the same amount of product more potent

The proto-oncogenes are the "wild-type" or normal form of the oncogene. In general, oncogenes behave as if they were dominant genes, as described by Mendelian inheritance. Another form of gene, the tumor suppressor gene, generally behaves as if it were a recessive Mendelian gene. However, in the case of colorectal cancers, as with some other cancers, exceptions are found to these rules of dominant and recessive genes, which are discussed below. Finally, the mutations that occur here ultimately confer on the mutated cell, growth and survival advantage, in addition to the ability to later invade and to further mutate. In general, because mutations are random events, it is the accumulation of the mutations and not the order of their occurrence in the stages of tumorigenesis that is important in the development of cancers of all kinds. However, in the case of colorectal cancer, it appears that the order as well as the accumulation of mutations also has some importance.

*Promotion.* During the promotion phase, the predominant events involve expansion of the initiated clone of cells. It is here that more errors are made, because the rate of accumulation of mutations is proportional to the rate of cell division. This explains why most human cancers are carcinomas, because the most rapidly proliferating cells, in general, are epithelial. The immediate effect of environmental promoters (chemical, viral and physical) is to stimulate division in cells that would not ordinarily be dividing. Tumor promoters are not generally mutagenic after initiation is complete. Although initiators and promoters tend to be separate classes of carcinogens, some chemicals can both initiate and promote. These are called "complete carcinogens," and include such substances as benzo-α-biphenyl and 4-aminobiphenyl. Common promoters include dioxin, saccharin, cigarette smoke condensates, ultraviolet-B light, cyclamates, estrogens, chronic inflammation, and aflatoxins produced by *Aspergillus flavus*. The promoters can act by either directly promoting genetic damage (tobacco smoke, aflatoxin) or by enlarging the tumor cell populations. These can then undergo further genetic damage through more mutations. The promoters can also induce tumor formation in conjunction with doses of initiators that would have been too low for carcinogenesis.

Cells that have undergone initiation and promotion, although containing permanent genetic damage, are still in a reversible stage. Until these cells express malignant behavior (i.e., express the malignant phenotype), the process can generally be reversed. After the next step (malignant conversion), the process becomes irreversible, and clinical cancer is present, although not necessarily diagnosable.

*Malignant Conversion.* The change from the stages of promotion to malignant conversion requires that more genetic alterations occur in the DNA. The important steps here include multiple, frequent doses of tumor promoters over time, rather than a single large dose. If that critical point (conversion) does not occur, the process can be reversed, for example, in smokers whose risk returns to that of a nonsmoker after about 10 to 15 years following the discontinuation of tobacco use. Malignant conversion is often mediated by the activation of more oncogenes and the loss of more tumor suppressor genes.

*Tumor Progression.* The final stage in multistep carcinogenesis is called "tumor progression." This stage represents the clinical expression of the malignant phenotype. It is here that the surgeon deals with the clinical aspects of invasion and metastases in the individual with clinical cancer. The process of natural selection continues with the most aggressive and resistant tumor cell clones dominating the clinical picture.

### *Molecular Mechanisms of Carcinogenesis*

General release of growth constraints derives mainly from mutations that result in either (a) activation of proto-oncogenes to oncogenes or (b) inactivation of tumor suppressor genes. The role of the oncogene as it relates to the stimulation of inappropriate growth of cells has been discussed. Many authors have likened this to the car with its accelerator stuck on the floor. Tumor suppressor genes could be thought of as failure of the brakes.

Oncogenes function as *dominant* genes, in that a mutation in only one of the alleles is necessary to initiate tumorigenesis. Actually, the abnormal proteins made by the mutant allele are sufficient for carcinogenesis. The tumor suppressor gene, on the other hand, behaves in most instances as if it were a *recessive* gene, and requires both alleles to be mutated or inactivated before it plays its role in the processes of carcinogenesis. This is because the single "wild-type" tumor suppressor gene can still function as the cell's *brake*, even when the other allele is inactivated or absent. An important exception is seen to this last concept: the *dominant negative*. It seems that in certain situations the protein of the mutated tumor suppressor gene can overwhelm the wild-type protein in a number of ways, and still destroy the "brake" function of the remaining allele. Such may be the case with p53 colorectal cancers.

A gene whose function it is to detect errors in the replication of DNA, is p53. Its protein checks for errors in DNA, and it can then halt the cell cycle while repairs are made. However, if the damage is too serious to repair, p53 can trigger apoptosis—programmed cell death. More recent information suggests that p53 works by activating another nearby gene—WAF1 (identical to p21). WAF1, a powerful suppressor of tumor growth, acts by inhibiting cell cycle-controlling kinase systems. The mutated form of p53 not only fails to do its job as a brake on replication, but in the worst case mutations, it can actually stimulate even faster replication, even in the face of major DNA errors. Furthermore, loss of p53 can confer resistance on the tumor cell to therapies such as radiation and chemotherapy. Parenthetically, radiation does not "fry" cells as was once thought, but instead does sufficient damage to the DNA that p53 then can take over and trigger apoptosis. A similar event occurs in some forms of chemotherapy. If the p53 is inactivated, then the damage done by the radiation or chemotherapy will not trigger apoptosis, and cell death may not occur.

Finally, a group of genes functions neither as oncogenes nor tumor suppressor genes. These are what have been called "mutator genes." This recently discovered class of genes does not control the intrinsic pathways for regulation of growth and replication, but rather controls the rate at which other genes can mutate. Because these mutations will also occur in proto-oncogenes and tumor suppressor genes, aberrant mutator genes will increase the probability of tumorigenesis.

### Molecular Changes Leading to Colorectal Cancers

At least five alterations are common to the cellular biology of most colorectal cancers. These occur in both the sporadic and the hereditary forms of the disease. As has been discussed, virtually all colorectal cancers arise from preexisting benign adenomas. The sequential steps from the first changes in these adenomas appear to be consistent as they progress from small adenomas to large adenomas, and then through stages of hyperplasia, dysplasia, and finally to invasive cancer.

Several features should be kept in mind as the steps in colorectal carcinogenesis are analyzed. First, both activation of proto-oncogenes to oncogenes and the inactivation of tumor suppressor genes are vital to the early initiation and promotion of these tumors. Second, it is now generally agreed that the total accumulation of the genetic changes is a critical factor in tumorigenesis, as well as the actual temporal sequence of the changes. Finally, even though the general paradigm suggests that tumor suppressor genes act in a "dominant" fashion, instances are seen in carcinogenesis in which even the heterozygous expression of the mutant tumor suppressor gene can dominate the cellular phenotype. Mutant p53 expression is just such an example.

### Specific Genetic Alterations in the Development of Colorectal Cancers

One of the most commonly mutated genes in the evolution of colon polyps and cancers is the adenomatous polyposis coli (APC). It is located at 5q21 (on the "q" or long arm of chromosome 5). This is a tumor suppressor gene, and the loss of heterozygosity at this location is found in more than 70% of colorectal cancers and small adenomatous polyps. This gene is altered in the germline of families with familial adenomatous polyposis (FAP) as well as in sporadic polyps and cancers. The "wild-type" APC gene appears to function in cell-to-cell adhesion and intercellular communication. Mutations or inactivation of the APC gene produce a pattern of hyperplasia often without dysplastic changes. The resulting cell pattern is seen in early adenomas. Also located on chromosome 5q is a tumor suppressor gene named "mutated in colon carcinoma" (MCC). This gene, which is present in invasive colon carcinomas, is often classified as a tumor initiator. Another epigenetic event that appears to occur early in the genesis of colon cancer is the hypomethylation of DNA. This loss of methyl groups has been postulated to inhibit the condensation of chromosome material and lead to nondisjunction. The affected chromosomes would then be at risk for possible allelic losses.

Of the several genes involved in the evolution of colorectal cancers, perhaps the most important is the *ras* oncogene. This is located on chromosome 12p (chromosome 12, on the small "p" or "petite" arm). This gene is found mutated in approximately 50% of adenomas more than 1 cm in diameter and fewer than 10% of adenomas less than 1 cm. The "wild-type" K*ras* gene (other family members include H*ras* and N*ras*) produces a protein whose function in normal cells is to stimulate cell division and differentiation when signaled to do so by extracellular growth factors. It is involved, therefore, in what is called "intracellular signal transduction," as a mitogenic signaling pathway from cell surface receptors. The mutated version (*ras* oncogene) continues to promote cell division even in the absence of any signals to do so. The result is continued replication in an inappropriate setting, as well as failure to enter terminal differentiation. This mutation tends to enter the carcinogenesis progression in the conversion from an early small adenoma to the larger and more dysplastic intermediate adenoma. Cells affected by K*ras* mutations, which show abnormal histologic patterns of differentiation, are seen in dysplastic polyps.

The next important mutation or allelic loss involves a tumor suppressor gene that is rare in polyps but very common in colon carcinomas (70%) and in late adenomas (50%). This gene is called "deleted in colon carcinoma" (DCC) and is located on chromosome 18q21. The gene product of the "wild-type" is a 190-kd protein, which appears to function in cell-cell and cell-extracellular matrix adhesion processes. It also appears to function in cell differentiation. The degree of mutation of this gene has been found to correlate with prognosis in Dukes' B colorectal cancers. Patients with allelic loss of DCC behave more like patients with Dukes' C, whereas those with intact DCC behave more like patients with Dukes' A.

However, DCC is not found in hereditary nonpolyposis colon cancer syndromes (see Chapter 22). A locus on chromosome 2p22-21 has been found in hereditary nonpolyposis colorectal cancer (HNPCC) or Lynch syndrome, called "MSH2" (the human homologue of the bacterial gene, *mut*S). The gene at this location has been shown to be responsible for mismatch repairs. These were found in both somatic and germline cells in patients with this disease. Other genes that are commonly mutated in HNPCC include MLH1, PMS1, and PMS2. Each (MSH2, MLH1, PMS1, PMS2) encodes substances that are involved in the detection and correction of mismatch repairs of DNA. As would be expected, patients with HNPCC tend to have large numbers of cells with errors in their DNA replication. Carcinogenesis and the natural selection that take place among the aberrant cells seem to be the consequence of these accumulated errors.

The clinical differences between the familial cancer syndromes (FAP and HNPCC) can be correlated with differences in the molecular biology of the two diseases. In FAP, patients develop thousands of benign polyps, which have a relatively low rate of further mutation to cancer. So only one or a few will go on to develop a carcinoma. In HNPCC are seen only a small number of benign tumors, but with a high propensity for conversion to the malignant phenotype. Both diseases become clinically evident decades before sporadic colon cancers. So, in looking at the general theory of carcinogenesis, FAP seems to be a defect in tumor initiation (APC gene leading to multiple benign adenomata), whereas HNPCC is a disease characterized by the changes that take place in tumor promotion and conversion.

The latest event in the chronology and accumulation of genetic mutations or losses in colon cancer involves p53. This tumor suppressor gene is mutated in more than 50% of all cancers worldwide, and in most colon cancers. Its mutated form is uncommon in adenomas. The "wild-type" p53 protein functions as the last brake on cell replication in the face of DNA errors. It checks the DNA for errors. If errors are found, it will generally halt the cell cycle until repairs can be made. If the damage is too extensive, it will initiate cellular apoptosis. The mutated form of p53 is doubly dangerous in the genesis of cancers. In many cases, it will not only fail to stop the cell cycle and fail to trigger apoptosis, but it can actually increase the rate of replication of the abnormal cells. Another important facet of the activity of p53 that should be reemphasized is that, although it is a tumor suppressor gene, it can act in a dominant fashion. Thus, it can function in carcinogenesis even when only one of the alleles has mutated. This can result from the abnormal p53 protein, which can tie up and render useless the normal p53 protein produced by the remaining "wild-type" p53 allele. This kind of interaction is referred to as a "dominant negative." P53 can also act in the pathway of tumor angiogenesis. P53, in its "wild-type," acts to stimulate the release of thrombospondin-1, a potent angiogenesis inhibitor. The mutated form of p53 loses this function, and, therefore, the suppression of angiogenesis is lost as well. Tumor angiogenesis is critical to the development of tumors from microscopic to larger masses, as well as for permitting and encouraging blood-borne metastases.

The loss of p53 in the final stages of colon carcinogenesis not only allows the cells to divide at an unrestrained rate, but this rapid replication further promotes the development of even more cellular genetic mutations because the cell cycle is not interrupted when errors are detected.

The complex sequences of oncogene activation and tumor suppressor gene inactivation or loss fits well into the classic concepts of tumorigenesis (Fig. 21.10). However, it should be remembered that APC, *ras,* and p53 mutations or deletions do not occur in all colorectal cancers. The remainder of the colon cancers has other aberrations in their genome, aberrations that can develop from another different set of errors. However, the action of promoters to enhance rapid replication and perpetuate genetic errors will not occur if the initiating event has not taken place. For example, mutant p53 may not have as ominous an effect in a normally replicating cell if its rate has not been stepped up by the loss of an APC "brake."

Other genes have been identified in the genesis of colorectal cancers and other malignancies. A metastasis suppressor gene, nm23-h1, has been implicated with high tumor metastasis potential and poor prognosis in colon and breast cancers. This gene appears to be involved in signal transduction through transforming growth factor-β. Its mutated expression has been used as a predictor for staging colorectal cancers. Decrease in motility and responsiveness to motility signals may account for the mode of action of normal nm23. Similarly, a protective effect by normal nm23 has also been noted in the outcome of colorectal cancers.

## Treatment and Results

With the advent of colonoscopy, the presence of a polypoid lesion virtually dictates endoscopic evaluation and, in most cases, polypectomy. There is no justification for observation to determine the lesion's change in appearance or size with the passage of time except in the rare situation when the risk of endoscopy is too great.

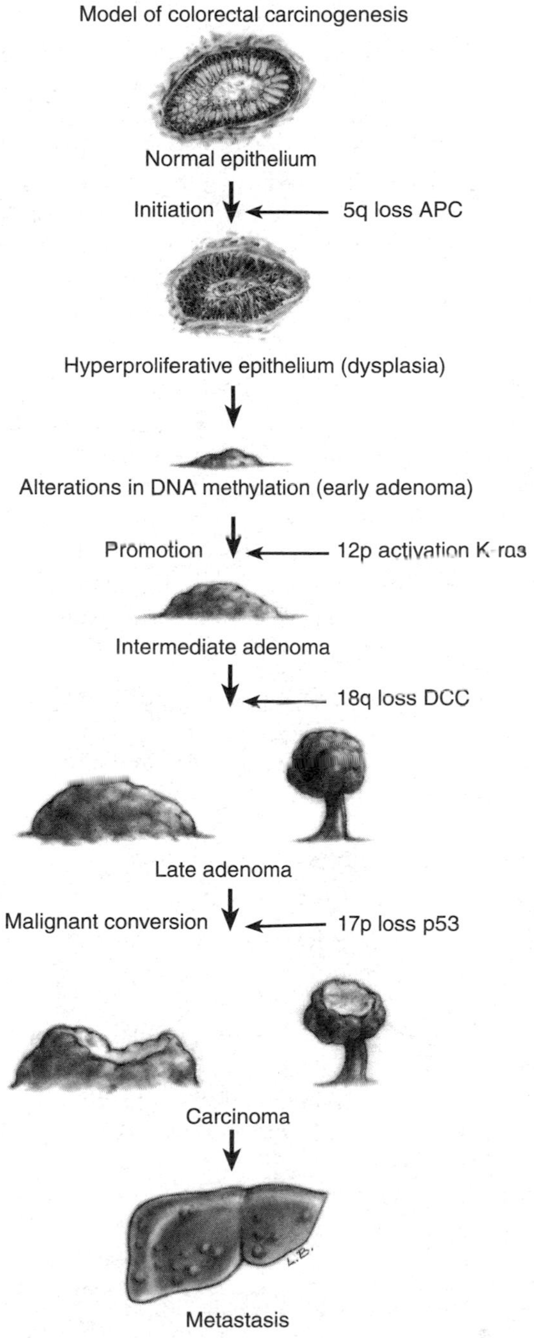

Model of colorectal carcinogenesis

Normal epithelium

Initiation ↓ ← 5q loss APC

Hyperproliferative epithelium (dysplasia)

↓

Alterations in DNA methylation (early adenoma)

Promotion ↓ ← 12p activation K-ras

Intermediate adenoma

↓ ← 18q loss DCC

Late adenoma

Malignant conversion ↓ ← 17p loss p53

Carcinoma

↓

Metastasis

**FIG. 21.10.** Model of colorectal carcinogenesis. (From Fearon ER, Vogelstein B. A genetic model of colorectal cancer tumorigenesis. *Cell* 1990;61:759.)

### Colonoscopy–Polypectomy

The technique of colonoscopy–polypectomy is discussed in Chapter 5, and the protocol for follow-up evaluation is presented in the following section. Pedunculated polyps can usually be snare-excised as can small sessile lesions.

The problem of the management of the sessile lesion has been the subject of debate. Most examiners today, however, depending on the "aggressiveness" and experience of the endoscopist, would recommend at least an attempt at colonoscopic removal of a benign-appearing lesion. For those patients at high risk for an anesthetic and for laparotomy, the endoscopist should attempt removal of even very large tumors.

### Management of Malignant Polyp

The most controversial management issue is the problem of what to do if invasive carcinoma is found in the polypectomy specimen. Some selectively advise resection (e.g., in individuals with poorly differentiated lesions, or simply in young patients). Others recommend resection if the cancer is close to the plane of resection, if tumor is in the lymphatics, or if the lesion is poorly differentiated.

Haggitt et al. determined the prognostic significance of invasion at different levels in colorectal carcinomas arising in adenomas. The level of invasion was defined according to the following criteria:

Level 1: carcinoma invading through the muscularis mucosae into the submucosa, but limited to the head of the polyp
Level 2: carcinoma invading to the level of the junction between adenoma and stalk
Level 3: carcinoma invading any part of the stalk
Level 4: carcinoma invading into the submucosa of the bowel wall but above the muscularis propria (Fig. 21.11)

Level 0 lesions are not defined as carcinomas because the muscularis mucosa is not breached. Level 4 invasion and rectal location were the only statistically significant adverse prognostic factors.

In patients having bowel resection after removal of sessile polyps containing invasive carcinoma, the incidence of lymph node metastasis is as much as 10%. Of these, 80% may result in lymphovascular invasion. For pedunculated polyps, the incidence of lymph node metastasis is 6%, but as little as zero if the depth of invasion is limited to levels 1, 2, or 3 (see above).

Many authors affirm that the patient can be treated for pedunculated lesions by endoscopic polypectomy alone if the following criteria are applied

Visual confidence of complete excision
Proper preparation and examination of the removed malignant polyp
Absence of a poorly differentiated tumor
Absence of lymphatic or vascular invasion
Absence of invasion at the margin

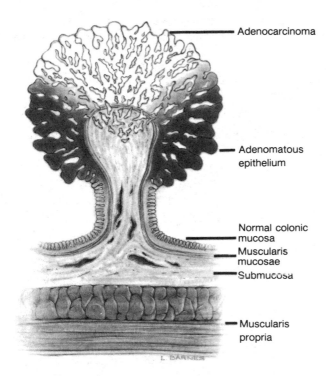

Adenocarcinoma

Adenomatous epithelium

Normal colonic mucosa

Muscularis mucosae

Submucosa

Muscularis propria

L. BARNES

**FIG. 21.11.** A pedunculated adenoma has various structures that determine the significance of invasion at different levels. (Adapted from Haggitt RC, Glotzbach RE, Soffer EE, Wruble LD Prognostic factors in colorectal carcinomas arising in adenomas: implications for lesions removed by endoscopic polypectomy. *Gastroenterology* 1985;89:328.)

Preparation of the specimen by using an elastic tissue (van Gieson) stain is helpful for identifying venous invasion.

The key to proper management, therefore, is competent interpretation of the microscopic findings. This is particularly difficult when many terms are used by different pathologists: severe dysplasia, adenoma with atypia, carcinoma *in situ*, superficial carcinoma, focal carcinoma, and intramucosal carcinoma. Be well advised to look at the slides yourself, so that with the pathologist you can make a reasoned judgment about the validity of pursuing a more aggressive approach.

*Comment*: With respect to pedunculated tumors, if the cancer invades the pedicle it is theoretically possible for it to metastasize. The likelihood, however, is extremely remote if the margin is free. In this situation, I prefer to inform the patient that in all probability cure has been achieved, but a remote possibility (perhaps 1% or 2%) remains that residual tumor may still be present. The determination for or against resection is left to the individual on that basis. This is usually a highly personal decision, based on age, risk of surgery, anxiety level, and a host of subjective concerns. However, if the margin is not clear, resection is strongly encouraged. Parenthetically, if laparotomy is performed, it is important for the surgeon to know exactly where the lesion originally was located. If the specimen is opened, it is usually possible to recognize the site of the polypectomy, even up to 5 weeks later. One alternative to facilitate identification of the polypectomy site and to avoid blind colon resection is to preoperatively tattoo the area endoscopically with a dye, such as India ink, indocyanine green or methylene blue. The color can be easily perceived on the serosal aspect. Another option is to perform intraoperative colonoscopy (see later).

### Colotomy and Polypectomy

Colotomy and polypectomy for pedunculated lesions is a procedure that has been relegated almost completely to the realm of historic interest. If the technique of colonoscopy is unavailable, if the lesion is felt to be beyond the limit of the endoscopist's ability, if the instrument cannot be passed to the level of the lesion, or if adequate control cannot be obtained during an attempt at polypectomy, abdominal operation may be justified. But even with one of these criteria fulfilled, a second opinion from another endoscopist would be the prudent alternative.

The major concerns for laparotomy as the method for removing the lesion are, of course, the operative morbidity and mortality, hospital costs, and time lost from work. Before the advent of colonoscopy, the generally quoted operative mortality was from 1% to 2%. Some rationale may be seen for deferring surgery in the patient at high risk who harbors a relatively small lesion, because of the slight risk of cancer (<1% for a tumor of <1 cm). Unfortunately, this information is not particularly helpful in management, because lesions of this diameter can usually be removed by means of the colonoscope. Those that cannot are larger, and hence the likelihood of the presence of a cancer is that much greater. Whether the new approach of laparoscopic colon surgery will reestablish the validity of colotomy and polypectomy is a matter of conjecture at this time.

When laparotomy is required for pedunculated polyps, a colotomy and polypectomy is, indeed, an adequate operation. However, the preferred treatment of sessile lesions for which laparotomy is required is resection. Frozen section examination should be performed when sessile tumors are removed (if resection is not performed) and for pedunculated tumors with a short pedicle or in which is seen some indication of possible cancerous change.

### Operative Colonoscopy

An alternative to colotomy and polypectomy when colonoscopy has been unsuccessful is operative colonoscopy: laparotomy and transanal polypectomy. The patient is placed in the perineolithotomy position as if for combined abdominoperineal resection. Following laparotomy, the colonoscope is inserted into the rectum; a noncrushing clamp is placed proximal to the tumor to avoid air insufflation beyond the area for polyp excision. With the guidance of the abdominal surgeon, the endoscope is expeditiously passed and the polyp is removed by the endoscopist.

Others have been pleased with the technique in the infrequent circumstance when it has been advised. In addition to cases of unsuccessful colonoscopy, the procedure can be usefully performed in combination with laparotomy for other conditions (e.g., cholelithiasis), in order to avoid opening the colon, and for localization of nonpalpable known colonic lesions. Although the advantages of the approach are limited, consideration should be given to its application in the occasional difficult polypectomy problem.

## Management of Benign Rectal Tumors

Large, benign neoplasms of the rectum that do not lend themselves readily to endoscopic excision, are tumor management problems. Villous adenomas, in particular, have an increased likelihood of malignant degeneration when compared with polypoid adenomas.

Biopsy results of any grossly benign polyp are notoriously inaccurate, but with villous adenoma this dictum is especially true. The tumor should be inspected carefully, and pale or white areas suggestive of malignant change should be noted. These are the areas that should be biopsied. Palpation is often helpful in identifying firm or hard sites for biopsy. Certainly, the presence of ulcer implies cancerous change. The most important criterion for determining the type of operative approach is the clinical impression gained by palpation and inspection.

### Techniques

Basically five methods are used to remove rectal tumors: transanal excision, transcoccygeal excision (Kraske), transsphincteric excision (Mason), transperineal excision, and rectal resection with or without restoration of intestinal continuity. These methods are discussed in Chapter 23, but transanal excision, and the transcoccygeal and transperineal approaches are worth reviewing here.

*Transanal Excision.* Transanal excision is the preferred operation, especially if resection precludes restoration of continuity. The procedure can be performed by snare electrocoagulation, laser therapy, conventional excision with some type of retractor, or by means of transanal endoscopic microsurgery (TEM). Generally, I prefer to use the first approach for larger lesions and transanal excision for the smaller ones. The reason for this apparent contradiction is that it is helpful to have the specimen removed intact and submitted for pathologic evaluation. With a small lesion, this can usually be achieved by excision; however, excision of large or circumferential tumors requires a tedious, often bloody dissection. A compromise is suggested, wherein a wire-loop snare is used to remove the bulk of the mass, and the base is electrocoagulated.

*Snare/Electrocoagulation.* With snare/electrocoagulation of a large tumor, inpatient management may be necessary. A bowel preparation, as if for colectomy, is advisable, as are perioperative antibiotics. However, only a small volume enema is given for relatively small tumors; this type of problem can usually be dealt with on an outpatient basis. The patient is placed in the prone jackknife position if the lesion is situated anteriorly, and in the lithotomy position if the tumor is primarily posterior. A moderate sphincter stretch is undertaken and, depending on the level of the lesion, an operating anoscope or anal retractors is inserted. The tumor is pared down with the wire loop until only a minimal residual remains or has been completely extirpated. The base is coagulated along with any residual tumor, making certain that an adequate margin has been created. It may be helpful to inject saline solution submucosally to facilitate excision and to minimize bleeding.

*Excision.* A complete excision of the tumor can be done by electrocautery without paring down the tumor. The lesion is outlined by the electrocautery, in order to be certain that the excision margins will be adequate, and then the tumor is completely excised.

Another option is "cold" knife or scissors dissection. The tumor is visualized, and an anchoring suture is placed distally. Infiltration of the submucosa with saline solution or, possibly, dilute adrenaline may facilitate dissection and limit blood loss. If necessary, the full thickness of the bowel can be excised to obtain an adequate margin around the tumor. The rectum can be reapproximated as the dissection proceeds. Each suture is held for traction. An error is made when attempting to place the suture proximally and then carry the dissection in a distal manner. Traction can also be effected by elevating a mucosal flap somewhat distal to the tumor. These techniques have the advantage of obtaining a complete, undistorted pathologic specimen.

Another approach has been described in which a pseudostalk composed of normal mucosa and submucosa is created by traction on the tumor with Allis or Babcock forceps, and a stapling device is applied across the base. Another option is to use a laparoscopic stapler to excise the lesion and to maintain hemostasis. The tumor is then removed. Even if the muscularis is incorporated by the staple line, bowel closure should still be secure. Another option is to use an endoscopic clipping apparatus as the polyp is excised to maintain hemostasis. The concept of rectal mucosectomy, as adapted from restorative proctocolectomy, has been used to manage large, benign tumors of the rectum. This approach is recommended for large or circumferential, benign lesions and is illustrated in Figure 21.12.

*Photoablation.* With respect to photoablation, the laser is an effective tool for vaporizing and destroying rectal tumors with minimal risk of bleeding. A number of investigators have successfully used either the noncontact Nd-YAG laser or the contact endoprobe with coaxial water to destroy both benign and malignant lesions. The major problem, however, is that because the target site is destroyed, it is not available for complete histologic study. The equipment is expensive, the technique is time-consuming, and operating room safety is always a concern.

*Transanal endoscopic microsurgery (TEM).* TEM is an endoluminal, minimally invasive technique that permits transanal excision of rectal lesions up to about 20 cm without the requirement for major abdominal operation. The pro-

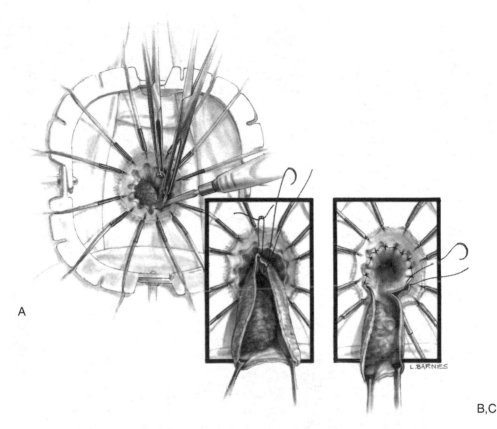

A

B,C

**FIG. 21.12.** Excision of large rectal tumor. **A.** Lone Star self-retaining retractor provides exposure of the anal canal and lower rectum. A circumferential incision is made distal to the tumor, just above the dentate line. **B.** Following dissection and freeing of the rectal mucosa circumferentially, including the tumor, the rectal mucosal sleeve is incised. Sutures are placed between the proximal rectal mucosa and the dentate line to prevent retraction. **C.** The rectal mucosa above the tumor is progressively divided, and the anastomosis is completed with interrupted sutures as the tumor is being excised. (From Keck JO, Schoetz DJ Jr, Roberts PL, et al. Rectal mucosectomy in the treatment of giant rectal villous tumors. *Dis Colon Rectum* 1995;38:233.)

cedure has been recommended primarily for benign tumors at a higher level than has been mentioned, especially for those who would require an abdominal operation to extirpate.

The instrument is a modified operating rectoscope, 4 cm in diameter. It holds a stereoscopic optical visual attachment with four gas-tight ports to allow simultaneous use of four instruments. Carbon dioxide is constantly infused, and a variety of instruments (e.g., tissue graspers, a high-frequency knife, suction, and needle holders) are inserted through the face piece. Adenomas that are even circumferential as well as selected carcinomas can be removed with TEM instrumentation.

The two major disadvantages are: a limited space within the lumen to undertake suturing, and the equipment is expensive, especially because it cannot be readily applied to other uses.

*Transcoccygeal Excision/Resection.* Transcoccygeal excision is a satisfactory alternative approach to the removal of benign midrectal lesions that do not permit resection and reestablishment of intestinal continuity by a more conventional means. It can also be used for excision of a more distal lesion when the surgeon wishes to accomplish a partial rectal resection rather than simply a tumor excision. However, the operation should not be performed for malignant lesions because of no removal of the associated lymph-bearing area. The so-called "Kraske approach" is discussed in a number of areas within this text as applied to several conditions (e.g., rectal prolapse, rectourethral fistula, rectal cancer, and rectal stricture).

*Technique.* A complete bowel preparation is recommended. The patient is placed in the prone jackknife position with the buttocks taped apart. Through a midline incision from just outside the anal verge to just above the coccyx, the coccyx is exposed (Fig. 21.13). The dissection can be facilitated by removal of

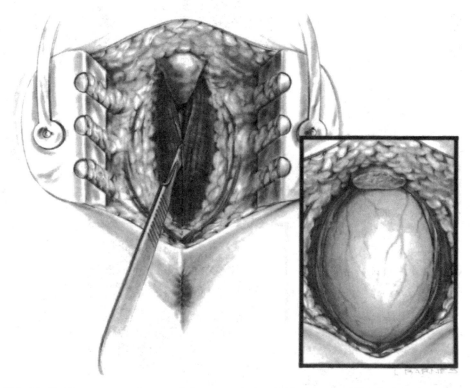

**FIG. 21.13.** Transcoccygeal approach to removal of rectal tumors. A midline incision is made and the levator ani muscle divided. The coccyx is excised and the posterior wall of the rectum exposed (*inset*).

the coccyx and even the lower sacral segments, if necessary. The levatores are incised, in addition to the deep portion of the external sphincter. The entire sphincter can be divided and repaired if this is required for complete excision of the tumor. The posterior wall of the rectum is then exposed (Fig. 21.13, inset). Allis forceps is placed on the posterior rectal wall and a transverse proctotomy is performed. A partial wall excision is then performed (Fig. 21.14). The rectal incisions can then be closed individually (Fig. 21.14A), and the sphincter repair accomplished (Fig. 21.14B).

If it is necessary to resect the bowel or to perform an excision of a tumor on the posterior wall, it is especially important to make the proctotomy incision at the correct level (not through the tumor!). Partial wall excision or proctectomy can be performed and an anastomosis effected by either a hand-sewn or stapling technique (Fig. 21.15; see Fig. 23.51). Only 5 or 6 cm can usually be safely resected without opening the peritoneal cavity to obtain sufficient bowel for performing an anastomosis. If necessary, this can be accomplished by opening the anterior peritoneum and delivering the sigmoid colon through the pelvic pouch of Douglas.

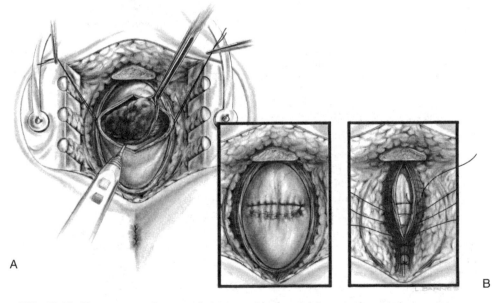

A

B

**FIG. 21.14.** Transcoccygeal approach to removal of rectal tumors. A posterior proctotomy reveals a tumor on the anterior wall. This is excised by means of electrocautery. Tumor excision alone or full-thickness excision of the bowel wall can be accomplished. **A.** The enterotomy wounds can be closed separately. **B.** Repair of the sphincter muscles is accomplished in a layered fashion.

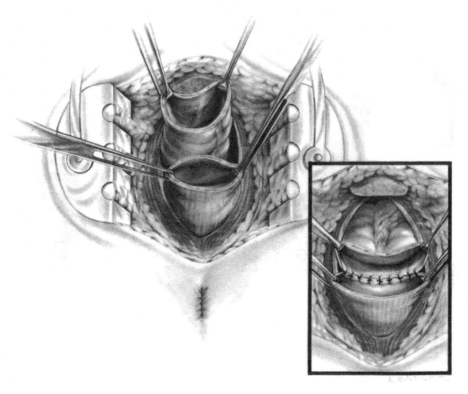

**FIG. 21.15.** Transcoccygeal approach to removal of rectal tumors. Sleeve resection can be performed, if necessary, but additional length may be required through the floor of the pelvis. Anastomosis is shown by means of an interrupted suture technique (*inset*).

*Intersphincteric Excision.* Selvaggi et al. suggest an unusual approach for the treatment of benign tumors of the rectum: anterior intersphincteric access. This apparently offers a good view of the posterior rectal wall, enabling the surgeon to perform excision of the neoplasm. The operation, in essence, is the reverse of transcoccygeal excision.

A transverse, curvilinear, transperineal, anterior incision is made outside the anal verge. Through the intersphincteric plane, the supralevator area is exposed. An anterior proctotomy is created, and the tumor on the posterior rectal wall directly visualized and excised. Repair follows the general principles of standard layered closure.

*Transsphincteric Excision.* See Chapter 23.

## Medical Treatment

As has been mentioned and as is discussed in Chapter 22, a diet high in vegetables and fruits is associated with a lower risk of cancer of the colon. Particular interest has been seen in supplementary antioxidant vitamins to prevent colorectal cancer, because these are present in these food groups.

## Polyp Follow-Up

How to follow patients who have undergone colonoscopy-polypectomy is a subject of some controversy. As mentioned, if the patient has had only a polypectomy, the entire colon should have complete endoscopic evaluation as soon as possible. Unfortunately, however, little objective evidence is found that recommends the correct intervals for follow-up examination.

A reasonable recommendation would be a colonoscopy every 2 years if more than one adenoma was removed and every 3 years in patients with only one index lesion. Most recent reports seem to agree that the presence of multiple polyps on initial examination is a significant consideration in predicting the likelihood of the subsequent development of tumors.

Epidemiologic studies have demonstrated that relatives of patients with colorectal cancer are at an increased risk for the development of malignancy. This has also been confirmed, not only in families of cancer patients, but also in families where relatives harbored adenomatous polyps (excluding the polyposis syndromes). Therefore, these individuals also should be subjected to a screening and follow-up protocol (see Chapter 22).

*Comment*: The assumption is the risk of the presence of a synchronous adenoma in a patient with a known neoplasm is at least 25%. Therefore, no debate occurs about the merit of "clearing the colon." Even after such a procedure, published studies of colonoscopic examinations performed 1 year later usually find that 25% or more of the patients have additional neoplasms. How important are these benign tumors? Because they are invariably small, the fact that they are merely present is not a threat to survival. Therefore, if a vigorous, effective, polyp-cancer surveillance program is to be carried out for an individual who has had prior polypectomy for neoplastic disease (benign or malignant), I advocate no radiologic investigation and limit the procedure to colonoscopy every 3 years. To help ensure maximal patient commitment to follow-up, a flexible sigmoidoscopy is advised at a yearly visit.

Exceptions to this regimen include individuals felt to be at an increased risk: Those who have had multiple adenomas removed, who initially harbored a large neoplasm, who had a sessile tumor, or who had evidence of invasive carcinoma. These people may require more frequent examinations.

With respect to villous adenomas, local recurrence is not uncommon, especially when large, sessile lesions of the rectum are removed by snare electrocoagulation or by local excision. Although the incidence of malignant degeneration is high, when it occurs, the tumors are usually well differentiated and relatively slow growing. Frequent follow-up examination is mandatory. Every 3 months is recommended until recurrence is no longer observed. Usually, if the patient is free of recurrence after 1 year, I am willing to pursue an annual follow-up program. Even confronted with tumor at each visit, I am willing to continue to perform local treatment, as long as the biopsies results are benign if the alternative is an abdominoperineal resection.

## Familial Adenomatous Polyposis

Occurring in 1 of every 7,000 to 10,000 births FAP is an inheritable (autosomally dominant) disease in which the colon is involved with innumerable adenomatous polyps. Despite the well-recognized inheritance pattern, approximately 20% of patients have no family history. Presumably, these cases represent spontaneous genetic mutations.

Distinction should be made between FAP and the condition of multiple adenomas. In the former, colon polyps number as many as several thousand, whereas in the latter it is usually fewer than 100. The number, 100, is generally used as the cut-off point to distinguish between the two conditions. FAP becomes apparent during youth and, if colectomy is not performed, it is associated with a high incidence of colorectal cancer, usually by the age of 40.

### Gene Identification

Recent studies have suggested that a gene on chromosome 5q21 (APC) is responsible for the inheritance of FAP and, therefore, is important for the development of colorectal carcinoma. Additionally, two genes tightly linked to FAP have been found to be somatically altered in tumors from patients with sporadic colorectal cancer. Identification of these genes should permit a better understanding of the pathogenesis of colorectal neoplasms and, therefore, aid in counseling individuals with a possible predisposition to these tumors. The identification and characterization of the FAP gene has been accomplished by demonstrating mutations which, essentially, were base substitutions or deletions.

Familial polyposis DNA testing for patients and family members, and for prenatal investigation (amniocentesis) is now commercially available. More than 80% of family members tested will have clinical features of FAP or be at risk for the disease.

As mentioned, gene therapy of somatic cells may in the future provide a nonsurgical means for dealing with this condition. In the prenatal situation, if somatic gene therapy can be successfully applied to fetuses with FAP, it might obviate the need to terminate pregnancies. This issue raises important ethical and legal questions concerning altering the human gene pool, with its unknown effect on future generations.

### Signs, Symptoms, and Manifestations

Polyps can be present for a number of years before the onset of symptoms. That is why family members of known patients with polyposis should be routinely screened for their presence. The mean age of the appearance of polyps is 22. The polyps probably exist for at least a decade before causing symptoms of sufficient import to stimulate the patient to seek medical attention. With the formation of polyposis registries, a significant decrease has occurred in the percentage of patients having cancer at the time of colon resection.

Bleeding is the most common complaint (80%), followed by diarrhea (70%), abdominal pain, and mucous discharge. Weight loss, anemia, and intestinal obstruction are ominous signs, implying the presence of a cancer. Approximately one quarter will have colorectal cancer at the time of presentation. In addition to the complaints and findings indicative of intestinal polypoid disease, patients can develop symptoms from extracolonic manifestations.

### Gardner's Syndrome

Gardner's syndrome is characterized by the presence of multiple osteomata (usually skull and mandible), cysts, and soft-tissue tumors. Other conditions associated with the syndrome include desmoid tumors of the abdominal wall, mesentery, and retroperitoneum; dental abnormalities; thyroid carcinoma; periampullary carcinoma; and gastrointestinal adenomatosis and carcinoma. With careful scrutiny of individuals with FAP, the presence of extracolonic manifestations probably represents the rule rather than the exception.

*Osteomas.* Osteomata were originally described in the skull and mandible but more recently have been shown to involve other areas; they may be the only extracolonic manifestations. The bony tumors can be present for many years before the onset of intestinal symptoms. Because of the potential for use as a marker for Gardner's syndrome, some have suggested screening x-ray studies of the skull and mandible.

*Epidermoid Cysts (Oldfield's syndrome).* The association of epidermoid (sebaceous) cysts with familial polyposis has been termed, "Oldfield's syndrome." Because of the common occurrence in the general population of these cutaneous lesions, however, little thought is usually given to the possibility of its being associated with the condition. But because they are uncommon prior to the age of puberty, epidermoid cysts in this age group should alert the physician to pursue colorectal investigation.

*Desmoid Tumors.* Desmoid tumors are usually benign fibromata that tend to infiltrate locally into adjacent tissue. They are reported to arise in from 3.5% to 5.7% of patients who have Gardner's syndrome. Although the lesion appears occasionally to emulate fibrosarcoma, metastasis does not occur. Local recurrence is the rule rather than the exception. The mass tends to develop in abdominal incisions, in the abdominal cavity (particularly the small bowel mesentery), and the retroperitoneum. The condition can antedate the appearance of the polyposis by developing in an abdominal incision performed for another purpose (e.g., appendectomy). Usually, however, desmoid tumors become manifest from 1 to 3 years following surgery for polyposis. Studies have shown that the absolute risk of desmoids in patients with FAP is 2.56/1,000 person years, with the comparative risk 852 times that of the general population. Desmoids can, however, occur in the absence of Gardner's syndrome. Intraabdominal desmoids behave unpredictably but are an important source of mortality in those with FAP.

*Dental Anomalies.* Dental abnormalities have been recognized as part of the syndrome complex, including impacted supernumerary teeth, unerupted teeth, early cavities, edentulousness, dentigerous cysts, and abnormal mandibular bone structure.

*Thyroid Disease.* Thyroid carcinoma has been reported to be associated with Gardner's syndrome. Unique to observation is the fact that the proliferative abnormalities of the syndrome as listed above are of mesenchymal origin, whereas thyroid tumors are not; this suggests a broader potential for the genetic defect. Young women (<35 years) are at a particular risk for developing thyroid cancer, mainly of the papillary type. This group especially warrants periodic thyroid evaluation. A recent association with thyroiditis has also been observed.

*Periampullary Tumors.* Periampullary carcinoma is a well-recognized disease that is associated with Gardner's syndrome. Up to 12% of patients who survive for 5 years after colectomy may develop a carcinoma of the duodenum, ampulla of Vater, or pancreas. The mean age is 45 years.

*Upper Gastrointestinal Tumors.* Gastrointestinal polyps and cancer have been frequently reported with Gardner's syndrome. Invasive upper gastrointestinal adenocarcinoma is found in 4.5% of patients with FAP. The most frequent sites were the duodenum, pancreatic ampulla, and then, stomach. Japanese studies reveal the incidence of gastric polyps to be as high as 70% with Gardner's syndrome, whereas the incidence of duodenal polyps approaches 100%.

Numerous case reports indicate the association of gastroduodenal polyps (including villous adenoma) as well as an association with small bowel carcinoma. Periodic upper gastrointestinal radiologic investigation (optimally with double-contrast technique), or preferably endoscopy at intervals in all patients found to have FAP is recommended to diagnose and treat lesions at an earlier stage, before invasive carcinoma supervenes. Their kindred should also be studied.

*Pancreatitis.* Acute pancreatitis has been reported to be associated with familial polyposis. The pancreatitis can be secondary to the duodenal tumor or, possibly, result from trauma when a biopsy of the lesion is attempted. However, some suggestion is found that pancreatitis develops before the periampullary tumor is recognized.

*Hepatoblastoma.* Hepatoblastoma is a rare childhood tumor affecting approximately 1 in 100,000 children under the age of 15 years. The condition may precede the development of FAP by many years.

*Congenital Hypertrophy of the Retinal Pigment Epithelium.* Pigmented ocular fundus lesions (e.g., congenital hypertrophy of the retinal pigment epithelium [CHRPE]) have been noted in patients with Gardner's syndrome and in some family members. When such lesions are identified in both retinas, they suggest inheritance of the gene for polyposis. Absence of this ophthalmologic finding, however, does not guarantee that an individual is protected.

*Miscellaneous Associations.* Other conditions believed to represent manifestations of this syndrome include carcinoid of the small bowel, adrenal cancer, adrenal adenoma, skin pigmentation, and lymphoid polyposis. However, the possibility exists that the observations may merely be coincidental. By considering Gardner's syndrome in terms of a family unit rather than for a specific, affected individual, signals the increased risk for the development of colorectal tumors as well as the possibility of extracolonic manifestations.

## Turcot's Syndrome

Turcot's syndrome is the eponym given to familial polyposis in association with malignant tumors of the central nervous system (i.e., tumors of neuroepithelial origin). The condition was originally described by Turcot et al. in 1959.

Turcot's syndrome is thought to be distinct from Gardner's syndrome because of the pattern of inheritance; a generation is frequently missed. Some have attributed this observation to variable gene penetrance. Others suggest that the disease is transmitted as an autosomal recessive trait.

## Evaluation

Historically, proctosigmoidoscopy has been the procedure used to identify familial polyposis in relatives of a family member known to harbor the condition. The rectum, however, can be relatively or even totally spared, and patients may be given false reassurance.

In addition to considering the means of evaluation, the age at which screening should begin must be addressed. Because barium enema was not always diagnostic of polyps, some authors recommend colonoscopy and biopsy in children at risk.

## Treatment and Results

### Colon

The four bowel operations that can be used to treat familial polyposis are:

- Proctocolectomy and ileostomy
- Total colectomy with ileorectal anastomosis (periodically fulgurating residual or recurrent rectal polyps)
- Total proctocolectomy and ileoanal anastomosis
- Proctocolectomy with reservoir-anal anastomosis

The technical aspects of total colectomy and ileorectal anastomosis are discussed in Chapter 22; the other procedures are detailed in Chapter 29. Total colectomy with ileorectal anastomosis for this condition has also been undertaken laparoscopically.

Many surgeons recommend total colectomy and ileorectal anastomosis for this condition, especially if the rectum is relatively spared. Early surgical intervention (before age 20), with anastomosis at approximately 12 cm from the dentate line, and close follow-up (every 6 months) is felt to be critical. Colectomy and ileorectal anastomosis is a relatively safe operation that results in minimal disturbance of bowel function. It is certainly agreed that the choice of operation should be based on the perceived risk of cancer developing in the residual rectum.

Some authors now recommend ileal pouch anal anastomosis for most patients with polyposis, except for those who do not wish to risk impairment of sexual function. Parenthetically, others have also observed pouchitis to develop following reservoir construction for FAP. Obviously, this complication, therefore, is not limited to those who have the procedure for inflammatory bowel disease. Furthermore, pouch polyposis following this procedure has also been observed. In fact, procto-colectomy and ileo-pouch—anal anastomosis does not truly cure FAP. Be aware of the possibility that polyps can develop in the reservoir itself. The greater morbidity of ileo-pouch—anal anastomosis may limit its application to those at higher risk for developing rectal cancer, those who refuse or cannot have close follow-up, those with large or confluent rectal polyps, and those with curable colon cancer at the initial operation. Irrespective of the method of pouch construction, reports from every series indicate that patients with polyposis have better bowel control and fewer evacuations than those who have the operation for ulcerative colitis.

With respect to life expectancy and comparing age- and sex-matched controls, the relative risk of dying for FAP is calculated to be 3.35 times as great as the normal population. The three main causes of death are upper gastrointestinal malignancy, desmoid disease, and perioperative complications.

*Regression of Rectal Polyps.* A number of authors have pointed out that polyps can spontaneously regress following total colectomy. A lowered pH of the stool has been stated to be a possible factor. Antioxidant vitamins and lactulose use have also been felt to increase the tendency to regression. Although the regression may be only temporary, the avoidance of an esoteric operation or an ileostomy in an individual who is likely to comply with the follow-up regimen makes colectomy and ileorectal anastomosis an appealing surgical option for many patients. Certainly, when the rectum is relatively free of polyps, total colectomy with ileorectal anastomosis is the preferred alternative. It is important to reemphasize that initial polyp regression does not prevent the subsequent development of rectal cancer.

The drug, sulindac, a nonsteroidal anti-inflammatory agent (a long-acting analogue of indomethacin), (150 or 200 mg twice a day [in adults]), has been demonstrated to produce regression of rectal polyps following total colectomy. It has been applied orally and even rectally. A low-dose rectal sulindac maintenance therapy achieved complete adenoma remission without relapse in 87% of patients after a 33-month follow-up. Long-term treatment is, of course, mandated. Great recent interest has been expressed with the newer COX-2 inhibitors. Randomized, controlled trials are awaited.

Oral calcium has been shown to inhibit rectal epithelial proliferation in patients with FAP. The mechanism of action is believed to be its ability to reduce colorectal cell turnover.

*Development of Colorectal Cancer.* As mentioned, all patients with FAP will develop colorectal carcinoma if untreated. For many years, total colectomy and ileorectal anastomosis had been the procedure of choice for many surgeons. The cumulative risk of the development of cancer in the retained rectum has been computed at 3.6%. Most groups now recommend 6-month proctoscopic examinations when polyps are seen and removed, and yearly reevaluation when the rectum is free of neoplasms.

*Ileal Tumors.* In addition to the concern for neoplasms to develop in the rectal remnant of patients with FAP, ileal adenomas have been observed following colectomy. Endoscopic examination of the terminal ileum is necessary as well, not merely rectal evaluation. Carcinoma of an ileostomy in an individual who has had proctocolectomy many years previously has also been described.

*Extracolonic Manifestations. Desmoid tumors.* A desmoid tumor is by far the most troublesome, indeed disabling, consequence of Gardner's syndrome. Complete extirpation in some patients may not be possible, but this certainly represents the best possibility for cure. Involvement of retroperitoneal structures can cause urinary obstruction which, in turn, may require a diversionary procedure. Because of the variation in the way they present, no one specific method of management exists. Even after aggressive surgical excision, recurrence is likely.

When the tumor is incorporated within the small bowel mesentery, if excision is performed, meticulous dissection of the mesenteric vessels must be done to assure that when the resection is completed the proximal and distal bowel will have an intact blood supply. A bypass procedure is often the wiser alternative. Abdominal wall tumors can usually be treated by wide excision, with abdominal wall reconstruction if necessary.

For unresectable lesions, radiotherapy and chemotherapy have been used with limited success. In the experience of many, however, intraabdominal desmoids do not respond to radiation therapy.

Inhibition of prostaglandin synthesis has been attempted to enhance the immune response. If the tumor is not resectable, the nonsteroidal anti-inflammatory drug, sulindac (Clinoril; 100 mg), twice daily, has been reported to diminish the size of the tumor. Another possible alternative, the antiestrogen and prostaglandin inhibitor, tamoxifen (Nolvadex), has also been suggested.

A combined chemotherapy program with vincristine, azathioprine, cyclophosphamide, and prednisone has also been suggested. Others avow that chemotherapy should be reserved for those individuals who do not respond to a trial of noncytotoxic drug therapy. Although many pharmacologic approaches have been advocated, it is difficult to evaluate the results, because the experience is often anecdotal.

*Gastroduodenal tumors.* Tumors of the stomach and duodenum can be treated by endoscopic removal. Gastric resection is necessary for malignant lesions, and pancreaticoduodenectomy (Whipple operation) is required for periampullary carcinomas. Villous tumors of the duodenum present a particular management problem, because even when biopsies are available, malignant change is often missed. Complete excision, either by endoscopy or duodenotomy, is necessary to advise the patient accurately. As mentioned, a number of reports have demonstrated regression or disappearance of colonic polyps with sulindac therapy. Interestingly, a case of such disappearance with duodenal polyps has been reported. Others now feel it is useful to consider this drug as an adjunct following duodenal clearance.

*Comment*: Conventional proctocolectomy and ileostomy achieve complete extirpation of the polyp-bearing intestine, but at the loss of intestinal continuity. The fear of having a permanent stoma can dissuade some patients from having needed surgery or members of families with polyposis from having screening evaluation. But if one is to consider retaining the rectum, a considerable burden of responsibility falls on the surgeon and the patient. The confidence of being relatively asymptomatic lulls patients into a false sense of security; rationalization and denial are frequently employed defense mechanisms. Under such circumstances, when rectal bleeding or a change in bowel habits develops, the cancer is often far advanced. The patient must be informed of the risk and be willing to have sigmoidoscopy every 6 months for an indefinite period. It is easier to justify this position if the rectum is relatively spared. If rectal polyposis cannot be adequately treated by a local procedure, a sphincter-saving operation should be considered.

Although the ileo-pouch—anal anastomosis is preferred to conventional ileostomy, the procedure has a relatively high morbidity, and the functional results are certainly less than perfect. The individual should not be "convinced" by the surgeon to have this operation; rather, considerable motivation to avoid an ileostomy must exist.

# 22

# Carcinoma of the Colon

Excluding cancer of the skin, colorectal carcinoma is the most common malignancy found in most Western countries. In women, lung and breast cancers are more common, whereas in men, lung and prostate cancers are more frequently observed. The American Cancer Society's estimates for the year 2000 were 93,800 new cases of colorectal carcinoma would be diagnosed in the United States, and 47,700 deaths would occur. The chance of colorectal carcinoma developing during the life of an infant born in the United States today is 5%.

The incidence and death rates of colorectal cancer now appear to be decreasing. The American Cancer Society's estimate for 2000 was approximately 41,000 fewer cases than in 1997. This suggests that the fall in colorectal cancer incidence, especially among whites, may be attributable to more effective preventative measures. The trends in cancer incidence, mortality, and patient survival in the United States are derived from the SEER Program (Survey of Epidemiology and End Results) of the National Cancer Institute.

## ETIOLOGY AND EPIDEMIOLOGY

### Distribution and Nationality

The incidence of colorectal cancer varies from one population to another, but is particularly high in the United States and Western European countries. In addition, a difference in the incidence of cancer has been observed from country to country when urban populations are compared with rural populations. With respect to immigrants, colorectal cancer is less common among Japanese-Americans than American whites. However, the rates for Japanese-Americans are higher than those for Japanese living in Japan. The children of these immigrants have an incidence approximating native American whites. A similar phenomenon has been seen in other populations.

## Race

The risk for large-bowel cancer in American Indians is less than one half that of whites. However, little difference is seen between African-Americans and whites within each community and region of the country.

## Religion

Jews have a higher incidence than people of other religions. Members of the Church of Jesus Christ of Latter-Day Saints (Mormons) have a low incidence. Their religion prohibits the use of tobacco, alcohol, tea, and coffee. Seventh-Day Adventists have a significantly lower rate of colorectal cancer; their church proscribes tobacco and alcohol.

## Alcohol and Tobacco

A prospective study of Japanese men in Hawaii revealed an association between the consumption of alcohol and rectal cancer, attributable to a monthly consumption of 500 oz (15 L) or more of beer. No causative relationship seems to exist between smoking and malignancy of the colon and rectum.

## Diet

Diet is the epidemiologic area that has received the most attention during the past 20 years. Studies have demonstrated correlations between colorectal cancer and additional dietary factors. The addition of fiber has been shown to inhibit the cancer that can be induced by carcinogens. The mechanism by which this protects the individual from the development of large-bowel cancer remains speculative. Some investigators have observed that fiber associated with high butyrate concentrations in the distal large bowel is protective against large-bowel cancer, whereas soluble fibers that do not raise distal butyrate concentrations are not protective.

## Fecal Bile Acids

Fecal bile acid concentration is increased by dietary fat and decreased by dietary cereal fiber. Some have shown an unambiguous connection between the fecal bile acid level and the incidence of dimethylhydrazine-induced colon cancer. The feces of people in Western countries exhibit a high concentration of bile acids when compared with the feces of residents of African and eastern countries.

## Cholesterol

Some investigators have demonstrated a strong correlation between colorectal cancer and a high intake of animal fat and protein. Others opine that the consumption of red meat, or total or saturated fat, has only a weak association with the development of colorectal cancer. Populations with a high consumption of beef generally have the highest incidence of bowel cancer.

## Bacteria

Bacteria are thought to play a role in the causation of colorectal cancer; presumably, their action on ingested fat or metabolites is a critical factor. It has been demonstrated that people in the United States and Great Britain have a higher colony count of anaerobic flora and a lower count of aerobic bacteria. A similarity is seen between the chemical structure of bile salts and the carcinogen, methylcholanthrene. It is not unreasonable to hypothesize that the action of bacteria on bile salts might produce a substance capable of inducing malignant degeneration.

## Cholecystectomy

Clinical evidence indicates an increased quantity of secondary bile acids in the feces of patients with bowel cancer. Experimental studies have demonstrated that secondary bile acids promote chemical carcinogenesis. Consequently, cholecystectomy has been implicated as a possible precipitating factor, although the evidence is not compelling.

## Ulcer Surgery

An association has been reported between colorectal cancer and prior peptic ulcer surgery, specifically truncal vagotomy. It is thought that abnormalities in bile acid metabolism as a consequence of vagotomy might explain the increased risk for the development of colorectal cancer.

## Aspirin

Considerable evidence now suggests that regular use of aspirin and other nonsteroidal anti-inflammatory agents reduces the risk for the development of colorectal cancer, particularly after 10 years of use.

## Inflammatory Bowel Disease

Patients with inflammatory bowel disease, especially ulcerative colitis, are at increased risk for the development of a malignancy; this risk is as high as 60% with 30 years of active, total-bowel disease (see Chapter 29). With respect to Crohn's disease, a number of reports have been published implicating an association between regional enteritis and small-bowel carcinoma. The relationship between granulomatous colitis and large-bowel cancer is less well documented but appears to be real (see Chapter 30).

## Radiation

Considerable differences of opinion are found about the risk for development of colorectal cancer following pelvic irradiation. Most believe the risk is not increased.

## Appendectomy

Most studies have failed to substantiate a relationship between appendectomy and an increased incidence of colorectal cancer. However, a prior history of appendectomy has been found to be an independent risk factor for decreased survival, worsening the prognosis for those in whom carcinoma of the cecum subsequently developed.

## Ureterosigmoidostomy

A number of authors have recognized the relationship between ureterosigmoidostomy and carcinoma of the colon at the site of the ureteral implant into the colon. The frequency of this complication may be several hundred times greater than that expected in the general population. The cause of this complication is not clearly understood; it might be related to urine bathing the colonic mucosa, the presence of a carcinogen in the urine, or the effects of the ureter itself implanted into the colon. It is suggested that this type of diversion of the urinary tract be abandoned, especially in young patients with benign disease.

## Extracolonic Tumors

An association between sebaceous gland tumors and internal malignancies has been called the "Muir-Torre syndrome." The incidence of colorectal malignancies is estimated to be almost 50%. It is important to screen all individuals with sebaceous gland tumors for underlying gastrointestinal as well as genitourinary and breast malignancies. Others have identified an increased risk of colorectal malignancy after the diagnosis of breast cancer.

## Genetic Predisposition

Genetic influences have been known for some time to be an independent risk factor for the development of colorectal cancer. The relative risk of cancer in persons with affected first-degree relatives, compared with persons without a family history, was 1.72 for one relative and 2.75 for two or more. This increased risk for disease was especially evident among younger individuals (5.37).

Rapid advances in the identification of genetic events that are important in colonic carcinogenesis have been made in the past few years. Both acquired and genetic anomalies (*ras* gene point mutations; *c-myc* gene amplification; allelic deletion at specific sites on chromosomes 5, 17, and 18) seem to be capable of mediating steps in the progression from normal to malignant colonic mucosa (Fig. 22.1).

### *Hereditary Nonpolyposis Colorectal Cancer (HNPCC)*

Excluding the polyposis syndromes (see Chapter 21), carcinoma of the colon has been reported in cancer families, the so-called "cancer family syndrome" or

Model of colorectal carcinogenesis

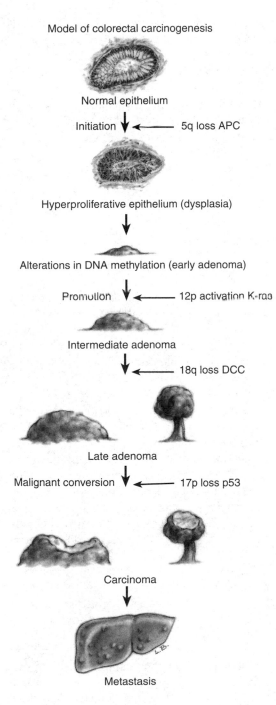

Normal epithelium

Initiation ↓ ←——— 5q loss APC

Hyperproliferative epithelium (dysplasia)

↓

Alterations in DNA methylation (early adenoma)

Promotion ↓ ←——— 12p activation K-ras

Intermediate adenoma

↓ ←——— 18q loss DCC

Late adenoma

Malignant conversion ↓ ←——— 17p loss p53

Carcinoma

↓

Metastasis

**FIG. 22.1.** Model of colorectal carcinogenesis. (From Fearon ER, Vogelstein B. A genetic model of colorectal cancer tumorigenesis. *Cell* 1990;61:759.)

"hereditary nonpolyposis colorectal cancer." This hereditary predisposition has been reported to account for up to 5% of all cases of colorectal cancer. Lynch et al. estimate that the risk for development of colorectal cancer is three times greater than that of the general population for individuals with a first-degree relative with this condition. They also described two variants of HNPCC. These were initially known as Lynch family syndrome (I), where the tumors were localized to the colon and rectum, and Lynch family syndrome (II), associated with extracolonic tumors. Recently, however, the distinctions have been eliminated. They have been grouped together simply as HNPCC.

Diagnosis of this syndrome is by the so-called "Amsterdam criteria":

• At least three relatives with histologically verified colorectal cancer, one of them a first-degree relative of the other two
• At least two successive generations affected
• In one of the relatives, colorectal cancer should be diagnosed under the age of 50 years
• Familial adenomatous polyposis (FAP) is excluded

The Amsterdam criteria, however, do not take into account the presence of extracolonic tumors. Furthermore, it may be difficult to satisfy the criteria if the family is small.

Extracolonic tumors have been found in many organs, especially stomach, uterus (endometrium), ovary, breast, and upper urinary tract. Some investigators have noted that the risk for breast cancer is increased fivefold. The lifetime risk is estimated at 1 in 3.7 for first-degree relatives of persons with HNPCC.

Specific findings of the patients identified by Lynch et al. were (a) mean age at the initial colon cancer diagnosis was 44.6 years; (b) of first colon cancers, 72.3% were located in the right side of the colon and only 25% were in the sigmoid and rectum; and (c) 18.1% of the patients had synchronous colon cancer, with a risk for metachronous lesions at 10 years of 40%. Studies have shown the existence of a genetic defect that is transmitted in a Mendelian, dominant mode. These defects affect DNA repair mechanisms, which results in microsatellite instability. This is thought to increase the risk of malignancy by causing abnormalities of the tumor suppressor genes. The identified abnormal repair genes are seen in Table 22.1.

Evidence suggests that microsatellite instability is uncommon in sporadic colorectal cancer but is present in more than 90% of those with HNPCC. Researchers have identified a panel of molecular markers to identify a patient at risk for microsatellite instability. However, the expensive germline mutation analysis is reserved for those individuals who demonstrate a positive test to the molecular markers. Consensus is lacking to which of the microsatellite markers is the most appropriate, but most investigators agree that an abnormality of two or a minimum of four microsatellites should be regarded as diagnostic, and, therefore, requires more detailed genetic testing. Once the diagnosis has been established, genetic counseling is strongly advised.

**TABLE 22.1.** *Abnormal repair genes*

| DNA mismatch gene | HNPCC populationwith defect (%) |
| --- | --- |
| hMSH2 | 50–60 |
| hMLH1 | 20–30 |
| hPMS1 | Rare |
| hPMS2 | Rare |
| hMSH3 | Rare |
| hMSH6 | Rare |

With respect to screening, colonoscopy every 1 to 3 years is generally felt to be the preferred evaluation in these individuals. Because of the increased risk for harboring benign and malignant tumors, colonoscopy is recommended for screening asymptomatic individuals with first-degree relatives having colon cancer, even in the absence of one of the Lynch syndromes.

With respect to extracolonic manifestations of tumors, annual pelvic examinations are recommended beginning at age 25, including endometrial aspiration biopsy and ovarian ultrasonography. Prophylactic hysterectomy with bilateral salpingo-oophorectomy should be considered in postmenopausal women and in those who have completed childbearing.

Lynch et al. pleaded for the establishment of computerized registries, such as have been developed for familial adenomatous polyposis, to transmit information about the diagnosis, surveillance, and management of hereditary colon cancer syndromes. Recognizing families and individuals at high risk who would benefit from surveillance should help reduce the incidence of this common malignancy.

Some people, however, do not require genetic screening for HNPCC. They are:

- A person under the age of 18 years
- A person with a known diagnosis of ulcerative colitis for 7 or more years, familial adenomatous polyposis or Gardner's syndrome, hereditary flat adenoma syndrome, Peutz–Jeghers syndrome, familial juvenile polyposis syndrome, or hereditary discrete polyp-carcinoma syndrome
- A cognitively impaired person or one unable to provide informed consent
- Someone who has a psychological condition precluding testing

## AGE AND GENDER

The incidence of carcinoma of the colon and rectum increases with age, but the progression also varies by anatomic site, population, and gender.

In women, colorectal cancer ranks third in the United States in number of cancer deaths, 11%. Lung (25%) and breast (15%) are first and second, respectively. The 2000 estimated cancer incidence is third, after breast and lung (30%, 12%, and 11%, respectively).

In men, colorectal cancer (10%) ranks third, after lung (31%) and prostate (11%), for deaths. Prostate cancer is now the single most common cancer (29%); lung is second (14%), and colorectal, third (10%).

## SYMPTOMS AND SIGNS

### Change in Bowel Habits

Change in bowel habits is the most frequent complaint of patients with colorectal cancer. Generally, a more distal lesion creates more obvious symptoms than a proximal one. The reasons for this are threefold: first, it is more difficult for formed stool in the distal colon to pass through an area of narrowing than for the relatively liquid stool present in the proximal bowel; second, the lumen of the bowel itself is larger proximally than distally; and third, because of the presence of other symptoms (bleeding, pain, discharge), the patient is more likely to pay attention when a distal tumor produces a change in bowel habits.

### Bleeding

Bleeding is the second most common symptom of colorectal cancer. It can be overt or occult. The blood can be bright red, purple, mahogany, black, or inapparent. The more distal the location of the lesion, the less altered the blood will be, and the redder it will appear.

### Mucus

Mucus, either as a discharge (implying a distal lesion) or mixed with the stool, often accompanies bleeding. The presence of mucus and bleeding should be considered a highly suggestive combination that necessitates bowel investigation.

### Pain

Rectal pain is a less common presenting symptom of cancer. When rectal cancer produces pain, the lesion usually is very distal or very large. Pain can result from infiltration of the sensitive anal canal or from sphincteric invasion.

Abdominal pain resulting from tumor implies an obstructing or partially obstructing lesion. This pain is usually colicky in nature and can be associated with abdominal distension, nausea, or vomiting. Back pain from retroperitoneal extension of a tumor of the ascending or descending colon is an unusual and late sign.

### Mass

A palpable or visible abdominal mass in the absence of other signs and symptoms is more common with right-sided cancers. This presentation implies a slow-growing, infiltrative process that may be much more amenable to surgical extirpation than might otherwise be anticipated.

## Weight Loss

Weight loss, in the absence of other symptoms, is a poor prognostic sign. Inanition and loss of strength and appetite suggest metastatic disease, most commonly to the liver, and is the presentation in approximately 5% of patients with colorectal cancer. Hepatomegaly is a frequent observation, but pulmonary, cerebral, lymph node, and osseous metastases as isolated findings may reveal an occult colorectal primary on investigation.

## Peritonitis

Perforation with peritonitis is an unusual presentation. Differentiating carcinoma from perforated diverticulitis, particularly with a sigmoid lesion, can be extremely difficult (see *Surgical Treatment*).

## "Appendicitis"

A carcinoma of the cecum can obstruct the lumen of the appendix and cause signs and symptoms suggestive of acute appendicitis. More common is perforation of the appendix from an obstructing carcinoma of the more distal bowel. Although such presentations are unusual, any individual over the age of 50 years with a presentation of acute appendicitis should be evaluated carefully at the time of surgery for an underlying carcinoma.

## Septicemia

Septicemia from *Streptococcus bovis* is associated with gastrointestinal neoplasms, especially colonic neoplasms. Secondary infections of hepatic metastases in an individual with a known primary tumor of the colon are well recognized. Also, colonic cancer can be an underlying cause of pyogenic liver abscesses in the absence of metastases. In these uncommon situations, after the usual causes have been excluded, an asymptomatic colon cancer should be considered in the differential diagnosis, especially if a coliform organism is discovered on culture.

## Cutaneous Manifestations

A number of conditions have been associated with gastrointestinal malignancy, including acanthosis nigricans, dermatomyositis, pemphigoid, and others. Such manifestations are rare, but any disseminated skin condition that is unresponsive to conventional therapy should prompt the consideration of gastrointestinal investigation.

Cutaneous metastases from colorectal carcinoma are extremely unusual except, of course, in the incision, at port site (see later), or at the site of a stoma.

## Intussusception

Intussusception in the adult is always a condition that requires surgical treatment. This is in contradistinction to children, for whom medical management (e.g., reduction by barium or air-contrast enema) may result in cure. Patients usually present with signs and symptoms of intestinal obstruction.

The most common causes of intussusception in adults include malignant neoplasm, benign tumor, metastatic lesion, and Meckel's diverticulum. Two thirds of the colonic intussusceptions are associated with primary carcinoma of the colon, whereas only one third of the intussusceptions of the small intestine are associated with an underlying cancer; most of those malignancies are metastatic.

## Duration of Symptoms

Those with a short history of symptoms do not have a better prognosis than patients who present with symptoms of greater than 6 months' duration. Individuals with symptoms of less than 5 months' duration have a higher incidence of resection for cure, but the actual long-term survival has not been shown to be improved.

## EVALUATION

### Practice Parameters for the Detection of Colorectal Neoplasms

Colorectal cancer screening is relatively inexpensive compared with screening for breast and cervical cancer, with cost estimates suggesting that the amount necessary to prevent one cancer is essentially equivalent to that required to treat a symptomatic patient. Although the most cost-effective approach has yet to be identified, screening can decrease mortality by making possible the identification of tumors at an earlier stage and the removal of benign lesions before they become malignant, thus preventing the subsequent development of cancer.

In 1992, the American Society of Colon and Rectal Surgeons published guidelines for the detection of colorectal neoplasms. These guidelines are reproduced in Table 22.2.

### Determination of Occult Blood

The stool guaiac or orthotoluidine test has been the subject of a number of reports (see Chapter 4).

Evaluation of a patient with a positive guaiac determination can be expensive, but other pathologic entities that can be significant are worth identifying.

**TABLE 22.2.** *Screening guidelines*

| Risk | Procedure | Onset | Frequency |
|---|---|---|---|
| Asymptomatic low risk | Digital and fecal occult blood | Age 40 | Yearly |
| | Sigmoidoscopy | Age 50 | 3–5 yr |
| Asymptomatic high risk | Fecal occult blood | Age 35 | Yearly |
| | Colonoscopy or barium enema and sigmoidoscopy | Age 40 | 3–5 yr |
| Familial adenomatous polyposis | Sigmoidoscopy | Age 10 | Yearly until age 40; then follow asymptomatic high-risk guidelines |
| Ulcerative colitis (pancolitis) | Colonoscopy | Disease years 7 and 8 | Every 2 yr until 20 yr of disease; then annually |
| Ulcerative left-sided colitis (or Crohn's colitis) | Colonoscopy | Disease year 15 | Every 2 yr |
| Symptomatic patient | Barium enema or colonoscopy (preferred if bleeding, occult blood, or melena) | — | — |
| Polyp surveillance (adenoma) | Colonoscopy | — | Yearly until colon cleared; then every 3–5 yr |
| Hyperplasia | Colonoscopy | — | Repeat colonoscopy in 1 yr; then revert to asymptomatic, low-risk guidelines if colon cleared |
| Colon cancer surveillance after resection | | | |
| If colonoscopy or barium enema cleared colon preoperatively | Colonoscopy or barium enema | — | 1 yr postoperatively; then every 3 yr until colon is cleared |
| If colon is not cleared preoperatively by barium enema or colonoscopy | Colonoscopy or barium enema | — | Within 6 mo; then every 3 yr if colon is cleared |

From Practice parameters for the detection of colorectal neoplasms—supporting documentation. *Dis Colon Rectum* 1992;35:391–393, with permission.

Although the cost versus the benefit of a massive screening program is debatable, no doubts exist to the value of early diagnosis, especially before a malignancy supervenes. The problem is the variable efficacy of the tests. A false-positive finding can be caused by diet and a false–negative finding is possible if the tumor is not bleeding at the time of the investigation. Despite these issues, the American Cancer Society recommends yearly fecal occult blood testing together with flexible sigmoidoscopy to screen for colorectal malignancy.

## Digital Rectal Examination

Only 10% of colorectal cancers are potentially within reach of the examiner's finger. Even when the cancer is palpable, sufficient cautious and diligence are required to permit discovery of a lesion. The risks of the examination, however, are nonexistent, and no one can argue the cost versus the benefit.

Digital examination will identify the location of the tumor, anterior or posterior, and whether it occupies part or the whole of the circumference. The tumor can be fixed or movable, ulcerated or scirrhous, exophytic or invasive. Careful palpation of the presacral space may reveal hard lymph nodes suggestive of tumor metastases, which may be a valuable prognostic sign. The fact that the tumor is palpable will often suggest the type of operation possible or whether the lesion is indeed resectable. Fixity may indicate a need for supplemental treatment (e.g., radiotherapy). Therefore, despite the numerous, often esoteric studies available to evaluate today's patient, digital examination of the rectum is still an important adjunct.

## Proctosigmoidoscopy

Examination with the rigid sigmoidoscope may reveal mucosal excrescences, polyps, polypoid lesions, cancer, inflammatory changes, strictures, vascular malformation, and anatomic distortion from extraluminal masses. It can also detect numerous anal conditions (e.g., fistulas, hemorrhoids, fissures, and abscesses). When a rectal or distal rectal tumor is identified, a rigid sigmoidoscopy is mandatory for accurate assessment of the level of the tumor, noting the distance from the anal verge to the lower level of the lesion. Also, the size, macroscopic appearance (ulcerated or polypoid), and location should be recorded.

It is also generally superior for evaluating the state of the anastomosis as part of a follow-up protocol or when the patient experiences symptoms following resective surgery.

When a tumor is identified, a biopsy of the lesion should be performed. For polypoid, exophytic lesions, appreciable bleeding is rarely a concern after a biopsy. If electrocoagulation equipment is not readily available and bleeding is encountered, pressure with a long, cotton-tip applicator soaked in a topical solution of adrenaline will usually suffice.

The sample for biopsy should be taken from the edge of the lesion at the junction of the tumor and the normal-appearing bowel, and placed in a fixative solution.

The flexible sigmoidoscope has virtually replaced the rigid instrument for screening purposes (see later and Chapter 5), because more of the colon can be visualized. (See Chapter 4 for additional information.)

### Flexible Fiberoptic Sigmoidoscopy, Video-Endoscopy, and Colonoscopy

See Chapter 5 for information on indications, preparation, and technique.

*Comment*: Complete visualization of the colon must be accomplished within a reasonable time following identification of a bowel neoplasm. Optimally, this should be performed preoperatively, because it can alter the type of operation. If total colonoscopy is not possible before surgery (usually because of an obstructing cancer), it should be carried out by the sixth postoperative week.

## Cytology

Establishing the diagnosis of carcinoma of the colon by cytologic evaluation, washing out the colon with saline solution has been advocated by some authors (see Chapter 4). They believe that brush cytology improves the yield of tissue diagnosis when combined with biopsy, but lavage cytology alone does not seem to be as useful.

Although we have had only limited experience with this technique, the addition of brushing or lavage appears relatively academic. If the nature of the lesion can be identified with an accuracy rate of only 90%, exploratory laparotomy and segmental resection are advisable. We believe this technique should be relegated to that of a historical curiosity.

## Barium Enema and Air-Contrast Enema Examination

No studies have evaluated whether screening double-contrast (air-contrast) barium enema alone reduces the incidence or mortality of colorectal cancer in individuals who are at average risk for development of the disease.

The barium enema has traditionally been the most commonly employed investigative study for the evaluation of carcinoma of the large bowel, but for screening and preoperative assessment it has essentially been replaced by colonoscopy. Most believe that, despite meticulous double-contrast technique, the examination cannot be performed with the accuracy of colonoscopy (see Chapter 4). Also, the absence of any therapeutic potential relegates this examination to a second choice for most physicians.

Differentiating between diverticulitis and carcinoma of the sigmoid colon is often difficult. It is sometimes said that the presence of diverticula excludes the diagnosis of carcinoma. This is certainly not true. The most important radiologic distinction is that the mucosal pattern usually is maintained in diverticular disease, whereas in carcinoma the mucosa is destroyed or the pattern is lost. In some patients, however, it is impossible to distinguish between the two conditions, and a resection must be performed.

It is important to remember that not all tumors of the colon originate within the bowel. Metastasis of cancers from an ovary, breast, or other sites, as well as direct extension from adjacent organs, can produce a radiologic picture virtually identical with that of an intrinsic lesion. This is another area in which colonoscopy with biopsy has a particular advantage.

## Urologic Evaluation

For many surgeons in the past, an integral part of the preoperative evaluation of a patient about to undergo bowel surgery was intravenous pyelography (IVP).

However, with the ubiquitous application of computed tomography (CT) in the preoperative assessment of individuals with colorectal cancer, IVP seems unnecessary. The urinary tract is generally well visualized by means of computed tomography.

## Other Imaging Studies

### *Computed Tomography*

Sophisticated radiologic studies may be worthwhile if they can help in therapeutic decision making before the operation. Computed tomography can diagnose metastatic disease, but whether this investigation causes the surgery to be altered is problematic. Preoperative CT changes the planned intervention uncommonly.

Computed tomography has also been used to assess the stage of the primary tumor, but studies have failed to demonstrate that the technique is sufficiently accurate. The place of CT and ultrasonographic evaluation of an individual with known or suspected metastatic disease is discussed later in this chapter.

### *Ultrasonography*

Ultrasonographic examination is useful to screen the liver as an alternative to CT in patients with colorectal carcinoma. In England, liver ultrasound has become mandatory as part of the workup, before performing colorectal resectional surgery for adenocarcinoma.

Transcolorectal endosonography has been suggested to offer an important advantage. The application of this modality for assessing rectal cancers is well established and is discussed in Chapters 4, 6, and 23. The accuracy of staging rectal and colonic carcinomas is 81% and 93%, respectively. Although the potential for benefit in managing patients with rectal cancer is genuine (there may be other surgical options besides resection), the alternatives to colon resection constitute a less valid proposition.

## Carcinoembryonic Antigen

Carcinoembryonic antigen (CEA) is a glycoprotein absent from normal adult intestinal mucosa but present in primitive endoderm. In cancer localized to the mucosa and submucosa, without invasion into the muscularis propria, the percentage of patients with an elevated test result is between 30% and 40%.

Levels of CEA can be applied usefully in assessing the prognosis of individuals with colorectal cancer. If the tumor has been completely excised, any elevated level preoperatively should return to normal within a few days. A limited fall to an intermediate, albeit elevated, level is indicative of incomplete excision. Subsequent elevation after return to normal implies recurrence of tumor (see later).

The CEA is of limited value in the search for a primary site if metastatic carcinoma is noted. The antigen is detected in about 50% of tumors of the breast, stomach, and lung, and in other solid tumors. Levels above normal have also been found in heavy smokers and in persons with cirrhosis, pancreatitis, uremia, peptic ulcer, intestinal metaplasia of the stomach, and ulcerative colitis.

## Nuclear Medicine Studies

### *Liver Scan*

The liver scan has been virtually abandoned for the evaluation of this organ in patients with colorectal cancer, either preoperatively or postoperatively. The study has been supplanted CT.

### *Pelvic Lymphoscintigraphy*

Pelvic lymphoscintigraphy has been used to try to discriminate between normal and diseased large bowel and to determine the extent of nodal uptake, but it has no demonstrable value in the diagnosis or staging of colorectal cancer. Angiography of the mesenteric arteries likewise has not been proved useful in the preoperative evaluation of colon carcinoma.

### *Radiolabeled Antibody Imaging*

#### *Anticarcinoembryonic Antigen*

Anticarcinoembryonic antigen is a CEA assay that involves the use of radiolabeled antibodies to the antigen followed by an external photoscan. The main role of this investigation is for evaluation of those with recurrent cancer that produces CEA, and in whom accurate staging may influence surgical management. However, this test has been largely replaced by the positron emission test (PET) scan as the preferred investigation for staging recurrent colorectal cancer.

#### *Gastrointestinal Cancer Antigen*

Gastrointestinal cancer antigen (CA 19-9) is a monoclonal antibody produced against human colorectal carcinoma cell line SW1116. However, this antigen is not specific for cancer and has been found in certain normal tissues, most notably pancreas, gallbladder, and gastric mucosa. This antigen is more commonly elevated in those with foregut cancer (e.g., stomach and pancreas).

#### *Other Antibody Imaging Options*

Researchers have addressed the concept of the application of monoclonal antibodies that react with epithelial membrane antigen. Those examined include

[111]In-M8, [111]In-77-1, NCC-ST 439, anti-p53, CA 242, and CA M43. They are all only research tools at the present time.

### Vasoactive Intestinal Peptide Receptor Imaging

Vasoactive intestinal peptide (VIP) is a major regulator of water and electrolyte secretion in the gut. Various endocrine tumors, as well as intestinal adenocarcinomas, express large numbers of high-affinity receptors for VIP. Some authors have investigated colorectal cancer with radiolabeled VIP in an attempt to visualize intestinal tumors and metastases. To date, this is not part of the routine workup of colorectal carcinoma.

*Comment*: The reader is referred to the discussion on the postoperative application of these techniques in the section on *Follow-up Evaluation*.

### Leukocyte Adherence Inhibition

The leukocyte adherence inhibition (LAI) assay is an *in vitro* test based on the observation that, following incubation with tumor extracts from the same organ, leukocytes from cancer patients lose their ability to adhere to glass surfaces. However, the lack of specificity for localization of the growth and inconsistencies in the performance of the technique relegate the procedure at this time to the status of a research tool.

## PATHOLOGY

By far the most common malignant lesion affecting the colon and rectum is adenocarcinoma. The tumor arises from the glandular epithelium, and it can invade microscopic blood vessels as well as metastasize to distant organs, most commonly the liver. It can spread by way of the lymphatics to regional lymph nodes and ultimately pass into the systemic circulation. The tumor can also extend locally into adjacent organs (e.g., posterior vaginal wall, uterus, bladder, small bowel, stomach, and retroperitoneal structures).

### Microscopic Appearance

Histologically, the cancer may appear well differentiated, moderately differentiated, or poorly differentiated. The tumor can produce so much mucin that the nucleus is pushed to one side of the cell, creating a signet ring appearance. Some debate whether the presence of this cell type is an indication of a poor prognosis, but most believe that mucin production and signet ring formation are ominous prognostic variables.

### Macroscopic Appearance

In addition to degree of differentiation, tumor morphology—whether polypoid, infiltrative, or ulcerated—has been found to be an important prognostic variable. Generally, the more poorly differentiated tumors are more invasive at the time of diagnosis, and the more invasive the tumor, the poorer the prognosis.

## Factors Affecting Rates of Growth and Spread of Tumor

Carcinomas of the colon and rectum are relatively slow-growing tumors. Symptoms usually appear early in the development of the disease, and metastases occur relatively late. Tumor growth and spread display considerable variation, depending partly on histologic grade (based on cellular arrangement and differentiation); increased ameboid action of some cancer cells; enzymes, such as hyaluronidase; decreased adhesiveness of the tumor cells; lesion size at the primary site; and length of time the tumor has been present. Additional variables include location of the tumor, indeterminate host factors, manipulation at surgery, and the age and sex of the patient.

Ideally, as more information is developed about prognostic factors, more meaningful recommendations with respect to supplementary therapy will be made.

Tumor doubling time has been calculated to be between 130 and 636 days. The longer time is probably more accurate and thought to be caused by desquamation from the surface of the tumor.

In comparison, doubling time of pulmonary metastases from colon and rectal carcinomas has been calculated radiographically and found to be from 109 to 155 days. It is theorized that the absence of desquamation in the metastatic site accounts for this observed difference.

## Staging and Prognosis

### *Classifications*

The importance of tumor invasion and its prognostic implications were initially postulated by Dukes for rectal cancer. This staging was later expanded to include liver metastases and colon carcinoma.

Others have introduced their own classifications, subdividing Dukes' system and broadening it to include colon cancer and disseminated metastases, degree of differentiation, tumor morphology, and histogram pattern, among others. Jass et al. suggested a classification based on prognosis:

I. Excellent prognosis
II. Good
III. Fair
IV. Poor

Most observers, however, believe that the Dukes' classification is of greater prognostic value and more reproducible than that of Jass.

Figure 22.2 illustrates the more popular staging systems. The more "substages" used, the greater the refinement potential to predict tumor behavior, and therefore to gain more information about the possible outcome. The tumor-node-

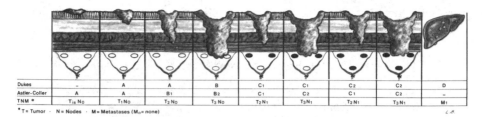

| Dukes | – | A | A | B | C₁ | C₁ | C₂ | C₂ | D |
|---|---|---|---|---|---|---|---|---|---|
| Astler-Coller | A | A | B₁ | B₂ | C₁ | C₂ | C₁ | C₂ | – |
| TNM * | T$_{is}$ N0 | T₁ N0 | T₂ N0 | T₃ N0 | T₂ N₁ | T₃ N₁ | T₂ N₁ | T₃ N₁ | M₁ |

* T = Tumor · N = Nodes · M = Metastases (M₀= none)

**FIG. 22.2.** Comparison of staging classifications for colorectal carcinoma.

metastasis (TNM) staging system is now the most widely accepted system for colorectal carcinoma.

Recently, researchers have attempted to identify indicators, particularly in patients with stage 3 disease, to ascertain those with a poorer prognosis, and therefore, those who may benefit from adjuvant therapy. These include: blood vessel invasion, neural invasion, DNA content or DNA ploidy, oncogene analysis, nuclear organizer regions, nuclear morphology, proliferating cell nuclear antigen expression, tumor budding, and other immunologic markers.

Debate occurs whether lymphatic invasion is an independent prognostic marker, but certainly, lymph node involvement with tumor, as shown by Dukes, influences survival.

### Blood Vessel and Neural Invasion

The prognostic implication of blood vessel invasion and neural invasion has been well established as indicators of a poorer prognosis.

### DNA Content or DNA Ploidy

A number of studies have suggested that tumor DNA content, as determined by flow cytometry, provides valuable information about the biologic behavior of neoplastic cells and, therefore, is an important prognostic factor in determining survival. Aneuploid (nondiploid) tumors contain a population of cells that exhibit a DNA content distinctly different from the DNA noted in "normal" (diploid) malignant cells. It should be remembered, however, that, although tumor cell DNA content is perhaps an independent prognostic factor, most believe Dukes' stage, patient age, and tumor differentiation are the variables most closely related to survival, and that conventional histologic variables remain the best predictors of prognosis for this condition.

### Oncogene Analysis

Oncogenes exist in the normal human genome as proto-oncogenes but can be activated by various means in tumors, including overexpression and mutation (see Chapter 21). Some authors have observed that the combination of ploidy status and oncogene expression predicts survival better than ploidy alone.

### Nucleolar Organizer Regions

Nucleolar organizer regions are loops of ribosomal DNA in nuclei that direct ribosome and protein formation. Researchers have concluded that nucleolar organizer regions are the most important individual variables for predicting survival, whereas ploidy values are equivalent to histologic differentiation.

### Nuclear Morphology

Nuclear shape factor is defined as the degree of circularity of the nucleus, with a perfect circle recorded as 1.0. A shape value greater than 0.84 is associated with a poor outcome, and indeed, according to some, is the most significant predictor of survival even when corrections are made for sex, age, histologic grade, and Dukes' classification.

### Doppler Perfusion Index

Leen et al. assessed the relative value of Dukes' staging and the Doppler perfusion index (DPI) as prognostic indices in individuals who had apparently curative surgery for colorectal surgery. This index, the ratio of hepatic arterial to total liver blood flow, was measured before resection by means of duplex or color Doppler sonography. The authors observed that the DPI identified two groups of individuals—78% of those with an abnormally elevated DPI value had recurrent disease or died, whereas 97% of those with a normal DPI value survived. The implications concerning the suitability for adjuvant therapy following apparent curative resection are clear.

### Proliferating Cell Nuclear Antigen Expression

Cellular proliferative activity has been shown to be a useful indicator of biologic aggressiveness in colorectal carcinoma. Investigators using immunohistochemical methods involving a monoclonal antibody to proliferating cell nuclear antigen, determined that this antigen found at the invasive tumor margin was a valuable predictor for determining those individuals with a higher potential for metastasis or recurrence.

### Tumor Budding

Tumor "budding" refers to microscopic clusters of undifferentiated cancer cells ahead of the invasive front of the lesion. Severe budding is associated with a poorer prognosis and paralleled a poorer Dukes' classification.

## Immunologic Markers

Investigators have evaluated many different markers, including antigens CD44v6, CD30, HLA-DR, and antibodies against cardiolipin. The CD44v6 antigen is associated with lymph node metastases and a poorer prognosis. Those with HLA-DR expression have a much improved 5-year survival (50% vs. 19%). The anticardiolipin antibody titer correlates with an improved disease-free survival. The CD30 is only found in those with advanced colorectal cancer. How these markers will affect the management of colorectal cancer has yet to be determined.

*Comment*: It is useful to obtain flow cytometry, cell differentiation studies, or both to make decisions, especially with respect to whether a local procedure should be considered (see Chapter 23).

# SURGICAL TREATMENT

## Preoperative Preparation

For elective colonic resection, patients are usually admitted to the hospital 1 day before the operation. A more prolonged hospitalization to prepare the bowel or to perform preoperative testing is generally not felt to be necessary and, in the era of cost containment in the United States, can rarely be justified to insurance carriers, even when the indications are reasonable. Further pressures to decrease the cost of medical care have mandated outpatient bowel preparation, required by many insurance carriers and health maintenance organizations.

Certainly, if the preoperative preparation cannot be performed with safety because of medical conditions (cardiac, renal, hepatic) or because of logistic concerns, the procedure should be done in a hospital setting.

## Mechanical Preparation

The bowel preparation regimen consists of appropriate dietary restriction, mechanical cleansing, and nonabsorbable antibiotics. The patient is placed on a clear liquid diet 24 hours before surgery. The mechanical preparation begins in the afternoon, the day before surgery. A vigorous cathartic is administered at this time so that its effect will have dissipated in time for the patient to have a reasonable night of sleep. The choice of laxative is a matter of the surgeon's personal experience or prejudice, because when adjusted for dosage, most laxatives have a comparable effect. Choices include castor oil (2 oz), magnesium citrate (10 oz), X-Prep liquid (2.5 oz), and oral Fleet PHOSPHO-SODA (60 to 90 mL) to produce the desired result. In the morning of surgery, we advise two Fleet enemas to ensure that the large bowel is adequately cleansed.

## Antibiotics

The use of a broad-spectrum systemic antibiotic immediately preoperatively, intraoperatively, and for one or two doses postoperatively has been suggested in numerous experimental regimens to reduce the incidence of infection following elective colon resection. In addition, nonabsorbable oral antibiotic regimen, taken the day before surgery, may reduce the incidence of infections.

*Comment*: In the case of a poorly prepared bowel; in the presence of obstruction, perforation, abscess, or fecal contamination; with a prolonged operative time; and with considerable blood loss, I believe that antibiotics should be continued beyond the first postoperative day. Any patient with valvular heart disease also requires systemic antibiotic prophylaxis (see Chapter 4).

### Urinary Catheter

An indwelling urinary catheter should be placed for all bowel operations. For an abdominoperineal resection or low pelvic operation, the urinary catheter should remain in place for 5 to 7 days to minimize the likelihood of subsequent urinary retention. With colonic surgery, the removal time is at the discretion of the surgeon and quite variable.

### Ureteral Catheters

Ureteral catheters are not harmless; severe oliguria and anuria are recognized rare but with serious potential consequences. Generally, these catheters are more useful in reoperative pelvic surgery as an aid in identifying the ureters.

### Hydration

Overnight intravenous hydration before surgery is advisable for any patient who might be susceptible to adverse cardiac or renal consequences of excessive fluid loss.

### Hyperalimentation

Hyperalimentation has been advocated before surgery for the nutritionally depleted patient to prepare for the assault on the patient's metabolic processes. However, with the exception of weight loss, laboratory abnormalities can usually be corrected by 2 or 3 days of appropriate therapy. Delaying surgical intervention for a week or more to administer hyperalimentation is an expensive, time-consuming extravagance that has in itself an associated morbidity. Balance the benefits and risks when considering hyperalimentation.

### Nasogastric Intubation

The routine use of a nasogastric tube is discouraged for colon resections. It does not protect the anastomosis and merely causes patient discomfort. Prospective studies comparing the preoperative use of a long intestinal tube (Cantor), a nasogastric tube, and no tube, have shown no significant differences in the lengths of hospital stay, duration of postoperative ileus, adequacy of intraoperative intestinal decompression, gastric dilatation, and postoperative complications. Obviously, however, on a therapeutic basis (intestinal obstruction, postoperative vomiting), gastric drainage is usually required.

### Thrombophlebitis Prophylaxis

Antiembolism stockings and subcutaneous heparin have proven valuable in preventing postoperative thrombophlebitis and pulmonary embolism. I prefer to use PASR Pulsatile Anti-Embolism Stockings (Baxter Healthcare Corp., Valencia, California), worn the evening before surgery, and until the patient is fully ambulating. Routine use of anticoagulants on a prophylactic basis is not suggested, unless the person is at an increased risk for the development of thrombophlebitis.

## OPERATIVE TECHNIQUE

### General Principles

With the occasional exception, most surgeons prefer to perform colon operations through a midline incision. This permits ready access to both sides of the abdomen and allows rapid entry into the peritoneal cavity. Furthermore, it leaves both sides of the abdomen free should a colostomy or ileostomy be required. Some surgeons use a right-sided oblique or a transverse incision for right colon resections. These wounds heal well and are perhaps associated with less discomfort, but exposure may be compromised. A Pfannenstiel incision can also be used if concerned with a cosmetic effect. The abdominal contents are examined carefully for the presence of metastatic disease and any other incidental lesion. The cancer itself is examined last. It is important to determine whether (a) the tumor is freely movable or fixed; (b) sepsis or perforation is present; (c) the mesentery is invaded by tumor; and (d) seeding of the peritoneal cavity has occurred. It is often difficult to determine by inspection alone whether lymph nodes contain tumor or are uninvolved. Large, firm nodes may prove to be inflamed when examined under the microscope.

As with all operations for malignancy, surgery for carcinoma of the colon is aimed at (a) removing the growth with an adequate margin by a wide excision of the tumor-bearing area and associated lymphatics, with attention to the blood supply to that segment (Fig. 22.3), and (b) creating an anastomosis without tension. The use of topical tumoricidal agents has been suggested to minimize the risk for implantation metastases, especially with respect to resection of the rectum (see Chapter 23). In the absence of pus, no drains are employed.

For wound closure, the use of a nonabsorbable monofilament suture, a nonabsorbable multifilament suture, or a long-term absorbable suture has been demonstrated to be associated with no statistically significant difference in the incidence of wound infection, wound dehiscence, and incisional hernia.

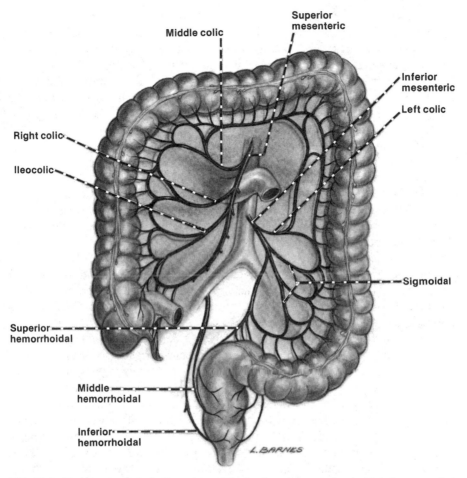

Middle colic

Superior mesenteric

Inferior mesenteric

Left colic

Right colic

Ileocolic

Sigmoidal

Superior hemorrhoidal

Middle hemorrhoidal

Inferior hemorrhoidal

*L. BARNES*

**FIG. 22.3.** The blood supply to the colon originates from the superior and inferior mesenteric arteries.

The operations generally done for cancer above the rectum include right colectomy, transverse colectomy, left colectomy, sigmoid colectomy, high anterior resection, subtotal colectomy, and total colectomy. Other, more limited resections are occasionally performed for palliation, but these generally should be condemned because of the problems of inadequate blood supply, insufficient mesenteric removal, and tension on the anastomosis.

## Right Hemicolectomy

Lesions of the cecum, ascending colon, and hepatic flexure usually are treated by right hemicolectomy, as the blood supply to this area comes from the ileocolic and right colic arteries. After incision, resectability of the tumor is evaluated with a minimum of manipulation. The small bowel is retracted into the left half of the abdominal cavity, and the root of the mesentery and the base of the transverse mesocolon are exposed. Some surgeons ligate the ileocolic, and right and middle colic vessels as the first maneuver. However, most mobilize the bowel before vessel ligation. The terminal ileum and right colon are elevated from the retroperitoneal structures by dividing the peritoneum along the lateral gutter. Included in the resected specimen is any lateral peritoneum involved by serosal tumor. Care must be taken to avoid injury to the ureter, spermatic or ovarian vessels, and inferior vena cava. The duodenum is identified and is displaced carefully as the colon is freed from its retroperitoneal attachments. The developmental adhesions from the gallbladder and liver to the hepatic flexure are incised. When the head of the pancreas is in view, the duodenum is sufficiently clear from the dissection so that clamping of the blood supply can be accomplished with safety.

It is often advisable to enter the lesser sac, dividing the gastrocolic omentum as far to the left as possible. This maneuver expedites entrance into the sac and permits the posterior wall of the stomach to be retracted out of harm's way. The remainder of the gastrocolic omentum is then divided until the hepatic flexure is no longer tethered. The omentum is incised to the point where the anastomosis will be performed. With all the blood supply divided to the segment, the bowel is resected, leaving open the ends that are to be anastomosed.

Not uncommonly, a discrepancy exists between the luminal sizes of the ileum and the transverse colon, the latter being considerably larger. Under such circumstances, it is usually advisable to make a Cheatle cut into the antimesenteric portion of the ileum when performing a hand-sewn anastomosis. This anastomosis can be performed by (a) an interrupted, full thickness, one-layer technique; (b) two continuous layers; (c) one continuous layer; or (d) a one-layer, interrupted seromuscular closure. The suture material can be absorbable monofilament (PDS, Maxon), nonabsorbable monofilament (Prolene, nylon), absorbable braided (Vicryl), or nonabsorbable braided (silk).

After a satisfactory anastomosis has been secured, the mesenteric defect is closed with either an interrupted or continuous technique. This prevents herniation of small bowel through the defect in the mesentery. It can also be useful to place omentum around all colonic anastomoses to protect further against the possibility of leakage.

## Surgery for Carcinoma of the Transverse Colon

Carcinoma of the transverse colon often presents a challenge in the choice of operative procedure. The blood supply to this area is derived from the middle colic artery as well as from the right and left colic vessels. Anastomosis in the region of the splenic flexure poses some risk for compromise of the blood supply to the bowel, because with the middle colic artery divided, the blood supply must come from the inferior mesenteric artery. In the region of the hepatic flexure, however, blood supply is not usually a problem, because of the contribution from the ileocolic and right colic vessels.

In addition to the concerns about blood supply with anastomoses in the transverse colon, another problem is the lymph-bearing area. A carcinoma in this location can spread to regional lymphatics through the middle colic, right colic, and left colic branches. Generally, for proximal lesions, right hemicolectomy is advised; for distal lesions, left partial or hemicolectomy (Fig. 22.4) with anastomosis of the transverse colon to the sigmoid colon (Fig. 22.5); and for lesions of the midtransverse colon, limited transverse colectomy may be considered. However, if tension or technical difficulty prevents a safe anastomosis between the proximal and distal transverse colon (Fig. 22.6), subtotal or total colectomy and ileosigmoid or ileorectal anastomosis are suggested. Mobilization of the splenic flexure is facilitated, first, by division of the gastrocolic omentum to within a few

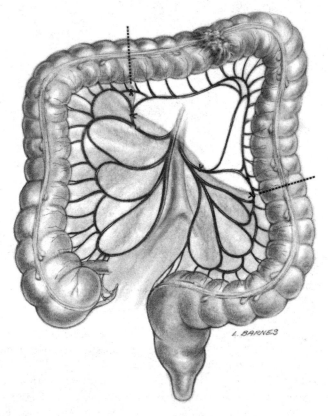

**FIG. 22.4.** Left partial colectomy. With tumors of the left portion of the transverse colon, resection of the descending colon is required to obtain a safe anastomosis while removing lymphatic drainage areas.

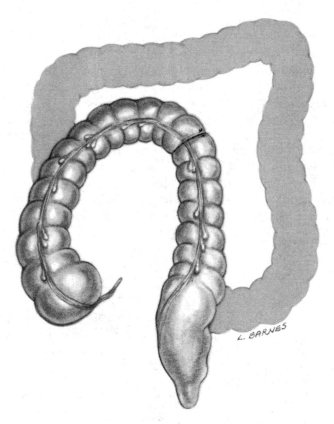

**FIG. 22.5.** Left partial colectomy. Anastomosis between the midtransverse colon and the upper sigmoid is usually possible without difficulty, except in obese patients.

centimeters of the flexure and, second, by incision of the lateral peritoneal attachments along the descending and sigmoid colon. As the splenic flexure is approached, the spleen is seen and the lienocolic and phrenicocolic ligaments are divided, the splenic flexure is delivered into the wound. The technique of anastomosis does not differ from that already described.

## Splenectomy

Locally invasive tumors of the splenic flexure usually are not amenable to wide excision unless the spleen and tail of the pancreas are also removed. Removal of the spleen, whether intentional or inadvertent in conjunction with a colonic resection, is associated with a high morbidity and an increased mortality rate. With splenic injury, topical hemostatic agents (e.g., Avitene, Surgicel, Helistat, and Gelfoam) have been recommended as well as primary suture repair and even partial splenectomy. If conservation of the spleen is not possible, appropriate coun-

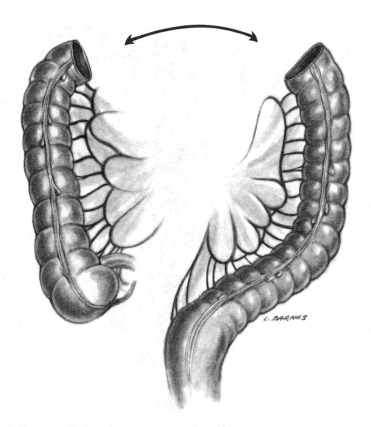

**FIG. 22.6.** Transverse colon resection. Anastomosis may not be feasible because of tension.

seling concerning the implications is advised, and the administration of polyvalent pneumococcal vaccine (Pneumovax) is strongly encouraged.

## Left Partial Colectomy or Hemicolectomy

Left partial colectomy is the operation of choice for tumors involving the distal transverse colon, splenic flexure, and descending colon. The right branch of the middle colic artery should be kept intact proximally, and the left colic artery is ligated, care being taken to preserve the inferior mesenteric artery (Fig. 22.7). The anastomosis is effected between the midtransverse colon and the upper sigmoid. In most instances, sufficient redundancy of the sigmoid colon is present to permit an anastomosis without tension. Occasionally, with an obese patient or with someone who has undergone a prior resection, such an anastomosis is not possible. Under these circumstances, total or subtotal colectomy is recommended. Usually, the colonic mesenteric defect is left unrepaired.

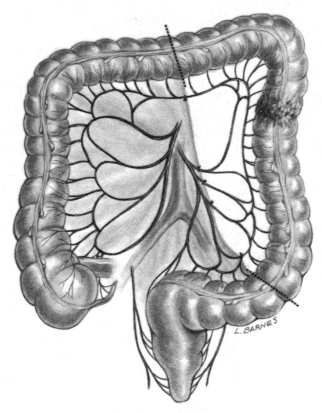

**FIG. 22.7.** Left partial colectomy. Area of resection for lesion of descending colon, with preservation of sigmoid and rectal vessels.

### Sigmoid Colectomy and High Anterior Resection
### (Anastomosis into the Upper Rectum)

Removal of the sigmoid colon for carcinoma is the standard operation for tumors in this location. Dividing only the sigmoid branches has not been associated with a poorer prognosis when compared with ligation of the inferior mesenteric artery at its origin.

In mobilization of the sigmoid colon, a major concern is to avoid traumatizing the left ureter. Most injuries to this structure take place at the level of the iliac vessels. The left ureter should be retracted laterally and displaced from the area of resection. Then, the left hand is passed beneath the inferior mesenteric vessels, and the peritoneum is incised on the right side. The inferior mesenteric vessels are then cross-clamped, divided, and ligated, and the arcade vessels to the upper sigmoid are divided. Anastomosis is optimally performed into the upper rectum. For distal sigmoid lesions, it may be necessary to mobilize the rectum slightly and preserve a portion of proximal sigmoid to effect a safe anastomosis without tension. Conversely, for proximal sigmoid lesions, I prefer to preserve the distal sigmoid and perform an anastomosis between the lower descending colon and the distal sigmoid colon rather than to mobilize the splenic flexure to obtain an adequate length without tension. This is different from the principle of resection described for sigmoid diverticulitis (see Chapter 26).

## Left Hemicolectomy

Left hemicolectomy should rarely be performed for left colon or sigmoid lesions. Despite the potential advantage of radical removal of the lymphatics, the additional dissection required, the prolongation of the operative time, the possibility of injury to the spleen, and the technical difficulty associated with a transverse colon–rectal anastomosis all militate against this approach. This procedure involves bringing the proximal ascending colon or transverse colon stump through the distal ileal mesenteric defect to reach the rectum in a tensionless fashion.

## Use of Drains

The application of intraabdominal drains following elective colon resection has traditionally been a stimulating subject for debate at surgical meetings. Absolutely no difference was seen in outcome in studies comparing those with and those without the use of drains.

## Subtotal or Total Colectomy

Removal of all or most of the colon and anastomosing the bowel to the upper rectum or sigmoid colon is a more extensive operation but permits a technically simple anastomosis. The procedure is indicated when (a) tumors are found synchronously on the left and on the right side of the colon; (b) multiple tumors (benign, malignant, or both) are present; (c) a resection has been performed previously; (d) the distal colon is obstructed (see *Management of Obstruction*); or (e) technical factors preclude a limited bowel resection. Although it has been shown that more than one intestinal anastomosis can be safely performed without a diversionary procedure if the bowel preparation has been satisfactory, with minimal fecal soilage and lack of tension on the suture lines, it is not recommended and should be applied selectively.

## No-Touch Technique

Although the theoretic value of early ligation of the vascular pedicle seems reasonable, it is difficult to understand how the excellent cure rates reported by the Cleveland Clinic group are achieved solely by this maneuver. One possible explanation for Turnbull's results is that a somewhat different classification was used for staging cancers of the colon. Others have concluded that no statistically significant advantage is seen for the no-touch technique. I believe the value of the no-touch technique has been greatly overstated.

### Radical Lymphadenectomy

As mentioned, the concepts of high ligation of the inferior mesenteric artery and of radical lymphadenectomy have failed to show any survival benefit. Certainly, with respect to radical lymphadenectomy, the complications far outweigh the theoretic advantages.

### Colonoscopy

The importance of complete evaluation of the colon before performing a colectomy for cancer cannot be overestimated. However, instances are found when such an evaluation may not be feasible, such as when an obstructing lesion prohibits passage of the instrument. Under such circumstances, careful palpation of the colon is mandatory, and a colonoscopy performed by 6 weeks is essential.

### Stapling Techniques

Stapling instruments have replaced conventional suture techniques for many surgeons today. Except for avoidance of the risk for needle injury and some slight savings in time, however, stapling devices offer no great advantages over conventional suture technique for standard colon anastomoses in other than low pelvic procedures (see Chapter 23).

### Other Anastomotic Devices

#### Biofragmentable Ring (Valtrac)

In 1985, Hardy et al. described a biofragmentable ring for sutureless intestinal anastomosis. The ring is composed of two segments containing polyglycolic acid (Dexon) and 12% barium sulfate. The major advantage, when compared with the classic Murphy button, is that it does not produce necrosis but fragments during the third week following implantation.

Since the original publication of the experimental reports, hundreds of patients have undergone resection and anastomosis by this method. In randomized, multicenter, prospective, clinical trials that compared the biofragmentable ring with suture technique and with stapling, no significant difference was found in morbidity, mortality, or clinical course of the patients.

#### Circular Compression Device

A mechanical device for creating a circular anastomosis through compression has been described. This is much more like the Murphy button, in that both innovations effect an anastomosis by means of compression. The apparatus consists of three molded polypropylene rings carried by a gun that introduces them into the bowel. For a colorectal anastomosis, transanal insertion is done in the same way as with the conventional circular stapling instruments (see Chapter 23). Firing of the gun causes simultaneous assemblage of the rings, expulsion of the entire anastomotic apparatus, and disengagement of the gun, with the creation of two tissue rings. The rings are evacuated between the 9th and 13th postoperative days. In contrast to the circular stapler, it leaves no staples or foreign material within the bowel. We have not yet had any experience with this device.

### Magnetic Ring Anastomosis

A modification of the Murphy button has been described. An anastomotic apparatus consisting of two magnetic rings embedded in polyester progressively compresses and causes necrosis in the intervening bowel through increasing magnetic force while healing takes place. We have had no experience with this method. No recent contributions have appeared in the literature on this subject.

## Specific Management Situations

### *Obstruction*

### Proximal Colon Obstruction

Carcinoma that obstructs the proximal colon usually can be treated by resection and primary anastomosis, without a diversionary procedure. Technically, the resection can be relatively easily performed and an anastomosis effected between the ileum and the distal bowel.

When the ileocecal valve is intact, the distal ileum is usually of normal caliber. Even when the small bowel is dilated, an anastomosis can and should be accomplished. Whenever carcinoma of the right and transverse colon presents with obstruction, the resected bowel proximal to the lesion should always include the colon to the level of the distal ileum. If diversion of a proximal colonic obstruction is believed necessary at the first stage, or if a protective stoma after ileocolonic anastomosis is indicated, loop ileostomy is the diversionary procedure of choice.

### Left Colon Obstruction

When carcinoma precipitates a left-sided obstruction, a more difficult decision must be addressed. Should primary resection be undertaken? Should an anastomosis be performed? Should a diversion be created? It is difficult to answer these questions dogmatically, because nuances in the presentation or in the findings might lead to an alternative course of action.

Temporary or permanent diversion in patients with malignant colonic obstruction can be created by the use of a Wallstent enteral endoprosthesis. This is a metal self-expanding stent with an internal diameter of 20 mm and a column length of 80 mm that can be placed endoscopically under fluoroscopic guidance to palliate colonic obstruction. An elective, segmental resection of the involved bowel can be then done. Alternatively, if the patient is not sufficiently fit for surgery, the stent itself can provide adequate palliation.

If the dilatation is minimal or moderate and the resection can be accomplished without an extensive dissection (as for a sigmoid lesion), resection is advisable. After removing the tumor adequately, an anastomosis can then be considered. If this is done, however, a proximal colostomy, or ileostomy should be performed. Not to do so in a situation in which the bowel is unprepared and the colon is dilated invites disaster, with a clinical leakage rate of up to 18%.

Alternatively, the anastomosis can be deferred in favor of, for example, a sigmoid colostomy and mucous fistula—a safe, acceptable alternative. Remember, however, that a dilated stoma (especially sigmoid colostomy) tends to retract. An extra length should be delivered to avoid this complication. When left-sided obstruction produces so much dilatation that resection is contraindicated, or when considerable dissection is required for removal (as with lesions of the splenic flexure, upper descending colon, or distal transverse colon), a loop or divided transverse colostomy may be considered. Ten days to 2 weeks later, elective resection can be done. The diversionary stoma may or may not be closed or resected at the same time, as the rate of wound infection for the combined procedures is high.

Several other options, however, permit resection and re-establishment of intestinal continuity in the first instance for malignant left-sided colonic obstruction.

*On-Table Lavage.* On-table lavage is particularly applicable to obstructing rectal cancers, but it has been recommended as an alternative for left-sided colon lesions as well. The irrigation can be accomplished in an antegrade or retrograde fashion, either before or after the tumor has been removed, through the open bowel, a cecotomy, or an appendicostomy. Some authors report relatively good results (a clinical anastomotic leak rate of 5% to 7%), but others note a clinical and radiologic leak rate of 10% to 14% and a mortality rate of up to 17%.

*Intracolonic or Intraluminal Bypass.* The procedure, which involves only a limited resection, is applicable to obstruction and to perforation. The technique and results are described in Chapter 26.

*Subtotal or Total Colectomy.* The optimal way of dealing with an obstructed colon is to perform subtotal or total colectomy and ileosigmoid or ileorectal anastomosis. This operation has the additional merit of removing any synchronous lesions, especially if unsuspected. The procedure is obviously technically more difficult and requires experience, but results indicate that the morbidity and mortality rates do not exceed, and in most series are considerably better than those of staged operations. This procedure is also preferred for the management of perforation, in which situation it is of paramount importance to remove the bowel in the first instance (see later). The functional results are reviewed in Chapter 16.

## Proximal Colon Obstruction

Enteroenterostomy is a reasonably safe alternative for patients with obstructing tumors and for those unresectable cancers that are likely to obstruct. To effect a safe bypass, the enterostomy, ideally, should be at least 20 cm from the lesion proximally and distally, and the anastomosis should be free of areas of tumor implantation if this is possible. A colocolostomy is preferred to decrease the likelihood of diarrhea. For right-sided lesions, an ileotransverse colostomy is usually performed, but if the entire colon is in jeopardy for recurrent tumor, ileorectal or ileosigmoid bypass is suggested.

Colostomy or ileostomy obviously bypasses the lesion, but efforts should be made to avoid a stoma for palliation unless an internal shunt is not possible. When a stoma is employed for obstruction, it should be either a loop or divided with the distal end exteriorized. If the distal end is closed, subsequent obstruction can lead to perforation of the oversewn bowel. If the stoma is to be permanent, a loop ileostomy is preferred to transverse colostomy, because the appliance is easier to manage, the patient has the alternative of a reusable or a disposable appliance, and odor is less a source of concern. I do not recommend the use of a cecostomy, because it is difficult to manage and diverts inadequately (see Chapter 31).

## Perforation

Carcinoma of the colon with perforation is a challenging surgical problem. All too often, the pathologic diagnosis is not clearly established preoperatively or even intraoperatively. The patient may present with a rigid abdomen, generalized peritonitis, and a pneumoperitoneum. Surgery often is required without benefit of gastrointestinal investigation or even a meaningful history from the patient.

Although extravasation is demonstrated on a limited water-soluble enema, the differential diagnosis (especially for a sigmoid lesion) always includes diverticulitis. Failure to demonstrate a carcinoma by means of colonoscopy at or near the site of a known perforation does not exclude cancer.

Diagnosis can usually be confirmed with certainty only by an exploratory laparotomy and resection of the involved segment of bowel. It should be emphasized repeatedly to all surgical trainees that limited exploration and blind diversionary procedures for suspected colonic perforation are to be condemned. In all patients suspected of having a bowel perforation, the lesion should be clearly demonstrable before definitive treatment is undertaken. Parenthetically, it is important to evaluate the rectum before an incision is made. It is impossible to evaluate the extraperitoneal rectum through an exploratory laparotomy. By simply passing a rigid sigmoidoscope with the patient on the operating table, the surgeon should be able to confirm adequately that the rectum is spared of disease.

The surgical options in the treatment of perforation are somewhat more limited than those for obstruction. The goal should be to remove the diseased segment.

Surgical alternatives for removal of a perforated bowel include resection of the disease-bearing segment; anastomosis, if convenient; always a protective colostomy or ileostomy; and drainage of the area of contamination. With a right-sided perforation, the surgeon can perform either an end-ileostomy and mucous fistula of the colon, ileocolic anastomosis with protective loop ileostomy, or end-ileostomy with closure of the colonic stump. With more distal lesions, attempt an anastomosis with protective loop colostomy or loop ileostomy, end-stoma with mucous fistula, or end-stoma with closure of the distal stump.

Subtotal or total colectomy with ileosigmoid or ileorectal anastomosis is another alternative for the treatment of perforation. It fulfills the criterion of removing the disease, and it permits a relatively safe anastomosis for left-sided perforations. Even with a technically secure anastomosis, loop ileostomy should be considered when contamination has occurred.

When a primary resection is contemplated, blunt dissection should be used as often as possible. Unless invasion by the tumor has caused fixation of the bowel, sharp dissection invites injury to the ureter and other retroperitoneal structures. In addition, because of the poor prognosis of perforating carcinomas of the colon and the high risk for local recurrence, clips should be applied to serve as markers for subsequent radiotherapy. Adjuvant postoperative radiotherapy should be initiated for the perforated tumor (see later). Metallic clips (e.g., stainless steel), although readily visible on plane radiographs, often distort and interfere with the interpretation of computed tomograms. Plastic clips cannot be seen on the plane film, but because they produce much less artifact than steel, titanium clips are preferred.

Finally, vigorous irrigation of the peritoneal cavity should be performed with many liters of saline solution. Continuous postoperative lavage may also be helpful for up to 72 hours.

### Preventing Adhesions

Recent years have seen renewed concern and therapeutic effort regarding the prevention of intestinal adhesions. The magnitude of the problem is not insignificant. Some authors have noted that approximately 1% of adult general surgical admissions to the hospital is for intestinal obstruction, and 3.3% of laparotomies are for this complication.

Considerable research has been done on products to reduce adhesion formation. One such product, Seprafilm, is composed of a sodium salt of hyaluronic acid, sodium hyaluronate, combined with another polyanionic polysaccharide, carboxymethyl cellulose. In both clinical and animal studies, it has been shown to decrease adhesion formation and has been recommended as an adjuvant for preventing postoperative anterior abdominal wall adhesions. A randomized, controlled, blinded, prospective multicenter study is currently being conducted to ascertain whether this treatment can actually reduce the incidence of intestinal obstruction.

## Liver Metastases

### Intraoperative Ultrasonography

Accurate staging before liver resection is essential. It is the optimal investigation for identifying liver metastases, but requires either a laparotomy or laparoscopy to accomplish.

### General Principles

If a small focus of disease is present on the margin of the liver and no other lesion can be palpated or identified by operative ultrasonography, it is reasonable to remove it at the same time as resecting the primary tumor. For any other situation, resection is not advised. The location and size of the residual tumor or tumors are determined, and the patient is re-evaluated following the operation. A computed tomogram is obtained during the postoperative convalescence. If multiple or bilobar tumors are confirmed, no attempt is made to resect them. If solitary or unilobar disease is seen on the first scan, then repeat investigation should occur using spiral CT during venous and arterial phases after contrast injection. If only localized disease persists, exploratory laparotomy or laparoscopy with intraoperative ultrasound is performed at about 12 weeks postresection of the primary tumor. Resection is recommended in accordance with the protocol discussed in *Treatment of Recurrence: Liver Metastases.*

## Resection of Other Organs

### Excision in Continuity

Resection of adjacent small or large intestine, bladder wall, uterus, tubes and ovaries, stomach, spleen, tail of pancreas, duodenum, kidney, and portions of the abdominal wall can be done for cure or to offer better palliation. Because of the differences in the biologic nature of neoplasms, occasionally a tumor will invade locally and not metastasize until late in the course of the disease. If this locally invasive tumor is not removed, the patient can experience many months or years of pain, or intestinal obstruction or a visible protrusion of the tumor can develop—all situations that may be preventable by a more aggressive attempt at extirpation at the time of the initial operation. However, major resection of the abdominal wall, alloplasty, hemicorporectomy, and total pelvic exenteration, in the hope of improving the likelihood of cure for colorectal cancer, should be discouraged. The morbidity and mortality rates associated with these operations are so high that they almost preclude the possibility of a meaningful lifestyle.

## Oophorectomy

The incidence of metastatic tumor to the ovaries (6%) is approximately five times that of a primary ovarian malignant neoplasm. This is usually found in younger, premenopausal women, often concomitantly with diffuse intraabdominal metastases. Removal of the involved ovaries is the appropriate treatment. The question of the role of prophylactic oophorectomy has been a matter of some controversy. The additional procedure adds minimal risk and increases operative time only slightly. However, in the premenopausal patient, replacement estrogen therapy is required, and the operation will obviously precipitate an early menopause. To date, no objective, compelling data support prophylactic oophorectomy in the premenopausal woman.

## Cholecystectomy

The morbidity and mortality rates of cholecystectomy for cholelithiasis when performed concomitantly with colectomy are not higher than for colectomy alone. Consequently, our policy always is to perform a cholecystectomy during elective colon resection when cholelithiasis is present, unless the operative time would be inappropriately prolonged or the incision would need to be extended for an unreasonable length.

## Appendectomy

It had been advocated that appendectomy should be performed concomitantly with cholecystectomy, gynecologic procedures, and bowel resections. On the basis of a number of actuarial studies, appendectomy as a preventive measure is not cost-effective in individuals above the age of 40. Furthermore, although the morbidity associated with the appendectomy itself is extremely low, the differential diagnostic concerns may be increased when an intraabdominal septic problem develops in a patient following colectomy. Therefore, I do not recommend appendectomy and do not perform it.

## Meckel's Diverticulectomy

Meckel's diverticulum is the most common congenital abnormality of the small intestine (see Chapter 28). Most agree that a Meckel's diverticulum in the older patient should probably be left alone. In younger patients, the issue is still a subject for debate. Still, if the diverticulum is "wide-mouthed," then it should be left alone.

## Incidental Abdominal Aortic Aneurysmectomy

The incidence of colonic cancer coexisting with an aneurysm of the abdominal aorta is approximately 2%. Concerning management, the opinions of 46 professors of general and vascular surgery have been polled in one article. Whenever the preoperative diagnosis was clearly established, approximately one third favored excision of the carcinoma first, one third stated that priority should be given to the aneurysm, and the remaining one third stated that they would make a decision at the time of the laparotomy. Only two felt that simultaneous operations should be attempted. Because of risk for sepsis in the graft and the potentially catastrophic consequences of such a complication, I believe that this last position is without justification.

## POSTOPERATIVE CARE

The relative merits of postoperative antibiotics and the use of an indwelling urinary catheter were discussed above. The lack of benefit of a nasogastric tube has also been addressed. Adequate control of postoperative pain must be achieved (see Chapter 7).

## COMPLICATIONS

The complications of colon and rectal surgery, especially as applied to cancer, are discussed in Chapter 23.

## MORTALITY AND RECURRENCE FOLLOWING RESECTION

Considerable difficulty is encountered in analyzing the survival results after resection for colorectal carcinoma at various institutions. Many reports use actuarial methods, correcting the data for the age of the patient, thereby theoretically giving more accurate survival statistics. Another method commonly used to analyze results divides patients who have undergone surgery into two categories: (a) those who have had resection and in whom the surgeon believes the disease is potentially curable; and (b) those whose disease is considered incurable and for whom the operation is palliative.

A third method of analysis is to determine the "crude" survival rate. This is calculated on the basis of the number of patients alive 5 years after treatment. Obviously, this may not be a true estimate of the number of deaths from cancer, because the patient may have died of another cause during the interim.

The prognostic implication of Dukes' classification has been well established. Recently, many modifications have been proposed to stage the tumor more accurately and to predict survival better.

Survival rates also correlate with the extent of lymph node involvement. The number of positive nodes in the specimen appears to be as important as the level of nodes involved by tumor. Apical lymph node involvement anticipates a poor survival. Five-year survival rates of 45% and 17% have been reported for patients without and with apical lymph node involvement, respectively, and 44% and 6% with four or fewer nodes involved versus more than four involved, respectively.

Other variables include histologic grade, level of direct spread, presence of venous invasion, age and sex of the patient, tumor ploidy, mucin production, and the presence of obstruction.

### Significance of Blood Transfusion

Perioperative blood transfusion, possibly because of the potential for immunosuppression, can be associated with an increased risk for the development of recurrence, according to some studies, even when this variable is controlled for age, sex, Dukes' stage, and histologic differentiation. However, others have found no relationship between transfusion status and tumor recurrence, tumor behavior, or patient survival. The association between blood transfusions and prognosis in colorectal cancer is probably a result of circumstances that necessitate the transfusions in the first place. The association may be greater with the development of local recurrence than with distant metastases.

### Obstructing and Perforating Carcinoma

Patients who present with obstruction or perforation have a poorer prognosis than other individuals with colorectal carcinoma. Often, they have evidence of metastatic disease at the time of presentation. The operative morbidity and mortality are also much higher.

### Carcinoma in Younger Patients

Colorectal carcinoma has been felt to be associated with a poor prognosis when it develops in young patients. Only a small percentage of these individuals will have a predisposing factor (e.g., familial adenomatous polyposis). Although the incidence is much lower in the younger group, it is imperative, at least, to consider investigating anyone who presents with symptoms suggestive of a bowel tumor (e.g., vague abdominal pain, nausea and vomiting, weight loss, rectal bleeding, or change in bowel habits).

Because of the symptoms at presentation and the difficulty in interpreting their significance, delay in diagnosis and treatment is one of the major factors responsible for the poor survival rates. Even for the same stage of lesion, however, younger persons have been felt to do less well when compared with older individuals. The overall 5-year survival rate has been reported to be 39%. Patients with Dukes' C lesions, in the same series, had a 5-year survival rate of 21%.

Carcinoma of the colon is extremely uncommon in children. In contrast to the presentation in adults, the most frequent symptom is abdominal pain, often with vomiting. Basically, three factors contribute to the increased mortality in these individuals: delay in diagnosis, advanced stage of disease, and poorly differentiated histology.

## Carcinoma in the Elderly

Simply stated, no justification is found for avoiding needed surgery simply on the basis of a patient's age. Generally, no differences are seen with respect to presentation, location, Dukes' classification, and prognosis in comparison with younger individuals. All studies confirm no statistically significant differences exist in age-corrected survival curves. However, emergency operations are associated with a high morbidity and mortality in this age group.

## Carcinoma in Pregnancy

Colorectal carcinoma in pregnancy is extremely unusual. As with carcinoma in young patients, and for essentially the same reasons, prognosis is poor. Management is determined by the gestational age of the fetus at the time of diagnosis, as well as religious and ethical considerations. The question of oophorectomy is problematic, especially during the first trimester, because of the risk for spontaneous abortion.

## Palliative Resection

Because carcinoma of the colon is a relatively slow-growing tumor, a palliative resection should be performed whenever possible, subject to a few relative contraindications. Even with extensive metastatic disease, patients can live a relatively long time and be free of the often miserable sequelae associated with an untreated primary lesion.

Contraindications to performing palliative resection include the presence of ascites, massive peritoneal seeding, jaundice, or severe debilitation. Obviously, the decision to carry out such a procedure is a matter of surgical judgment.

## FOLLOW-UP EVALUATION

How to follow patients who have undergone resection for carcinoma of the colon is a subject worthy of some discussion. Methods of evaluation include physical examination, fecal occult blood testing, proctosigmoidoscopy, colonoscopy, barium enema examination, chest radiography, determination of CEA levels, liver function studies, liver scan, ultrasonographic evaluation, CT, and exploratory laparotomy at an interval after operation.

The frequency with which evaluation should be undertaken is also the subject of some debate. One school of thought postulates that the patient should be discharged after recovery from surgery and report only if symptoms develop. So nihilistic is the attitude of many physicians and surgeons that earlier diagnosis and treatment of recurrent disease fail to result in a sufficiently improved survival rate to justify the cost and the effort. Others have found that an intensive follow-up program, at best, is associated with only a minimally increased survival rate, but for those individuals fortunate enough to have recurrent tumors that are amenable to curative re-resection, it would seem important.

## Physical Examination

Physical examination is often unrewarding for identifying an early recurrence. By the time palpation of the abdomen reveals a tumor in the liver or a recurrent lesion in the peritoneal cavity, the cancer is usually unresectable. Palpation of the abdomen, pelvic examination, and evaluation of supraclavicular and inguinal nodes serve primarily to reassure the patient and the physician. The primary value of such examinations and findings is to follow the response to supplementary treatment once an obvious tumor has been identified.

## Occult Blood Determination

The importance of examination of the stool for occult blood has been emphasized earlier in this chapter and in Chapter 4. As with the early identification of a primary tumor, the main purpose of performing this test is to look for a second (metachronous) lesion. However, with the recommended colonoscopic follow-up regimen, this investigation has little place in the management of the postoperative patient.

## Proctosigmoidoscopy and Flexible Fiberoptic Sigmoidoscopy

On an annual basis, or even more frequently, proctosigmoidoscopy is of particular value if the anastomosis can be seen with the instrument. Recurrence at the suture line, which most often results from inward growth of the tumor from the pelvis and not from residual cancer within the bowel wall or mucosa, can be identified, so that re-resection for possible cure can be done. Flexible sigmoidoscopy serves the same purpose if the anastomosis can be seen within range of this instrument. If the anastomosis is above this level, the only purpose of either examination is to identify a metachronous lesion within the limitations of the instrument.

## Colonoscopy

Colonoscopy should be used to evaluate the residual colon following resection if the procedure was not performed preoperatively or if visualization of the entire bowel was not accomplished. Many studies have demonstrated the high incidence of benign and malignant lesions harbored in the residual colon, presumably missed at the time of resection.

The procedure is also of value in identifying recurrent disease at the anastomosis. Some advise colonoscopy every 3 years once the bowel has been demonstrated to be completely free of neoplasm. The combined findings of anastomotic recurrences, metachronous colon cancers, and polyps represented an interval yield of 3% to 5% annually. Others believe that an annual evaluation with this instrument for the first 4 years after curative resection is preferable. It must be remembered that endoscopy is a poor tool for evaluating extramucosal, locally recurrent disease. Any follow-up program must, therefore, address this concern through additional studies.

## Barium Enema Examination

The barium enema examination is of limited benefit in the follow-up evaluation of the patient with colorectal cancer. A possible exception to this dictum, however, is that extrinsic compression might be perceived more readily with a barium enema study than by a colonoscopy. As suggested, in the follow-up evaluation of the bowel of patients who have had resection for colorectal cancer, colonoscopy appears to be the preferred technique.

## Chest Radiography

Chest radiography should be done annually to identify patients with pulmonary metastases; some of these individuals may still be operated on for cure (see *Treatment of Recurrence: Pulmonary Metastases*).

## Liver Function Studies

Traditionally, liver function studies have been considered useful in the follow-up evaluation of patients with colorectal cancer. However, this is an insensitive test and plays no role in current colorectal cancer follow-up.

## Liver Scan

Computed tomography has virtually replaced this study in the evaluation of colorectal cancer patients.

## Computed Tomography

Computed tomography offers a simple, noninvasive method for the evaluation of metastatic colon tumor by enabling visualization of the liver, pelvis, retroperitoneum, and adrenal glands. In addition, the CT-guided aspiration technique is useful for obtaining cytologic confirmation of malignancy. However, routine CT scanning as part of the follow-up has not been shown to improve prognosis.

## Magnetic Resonance Imaging

Magnetic resonance imaging is a promising new modality that has certain advantages in comparison with CT, even replacing it as the diagnostic study of choice for lesions of the central nervous system. However, this advantage does not translate as well to the evaluation of tumor in other organs. CT is still the preferred alternative for the detection and follow-up of metastatic liver tumors.

## Tumor Markers

The primary role of tumor markers today is in the postoperative surveillance of individuals who, theoretically, had surgery for cure and, therefore, are at risk for recurrence. The most frequently used such marker is the serum CEA. In addition, monoclonal antibodies labeled with radioisotopes are being used to identify possible sites of recurrent disease.

### *Carcinoembryonic Antigen*

Some believe that CEA has a lack of specificity and question whether it is a sufficiently early diagnostic marker of recurrent disease to make cure possible. However, most researchers generally agree that increasing levels are found with more advanced disease, that a failure of elevated levels of CEA to return to normal after resection is associated with a poor prognosis, and that elevated levels usually appear before any clinical evidence of recurrence.

### *Radiolabeled Imaging*

The advent of monoclonal antibody technology has permitted the development of radiolabeled tumor reactive probes, which can be used in conjunction with gamma camera imaging equipment to identify the presence of a malignancy within a patient. A number of studies have been published concerning the value of radioimmunolocalization with radiolabeled antibody to CEA in individuals with no physical signs of local recurrence but with elevated CEA levels. Generally, these tests can distinguish between localized disseminated disease and often are more accurate than conventional radiologic studies, including CT.

A number of other monoclonal antibodies have also been developed, including monoclonal antibody B72.3. This is a murine monoclonal antibody of the IgG1 subclass; it detects a glycoprotein, TAG-72, associated with high-molecular-weight tumors. This glycoprotein is expressed on certain human colon and breast carcinoma cell lines. To serve as a useful diagnostic agent, however, it must be coupled or conjugated to a radionuclide for imaging purposes. The monoclonal antibody conjugate, termed CYT-103, is labeled with indium 111 ($^{111}$In) for diagnostic imaging. It has been used in a study in those cases in which standard diagnostic modalities did not provide sufficient information for patient management decisions. The antibody imaging study detected occult (inapparent) disease in 70%, a finding responsible for altering or canceling the planned procedure. A total of 83% of the patients was found to have benefited from the study.

### Gamma-Guided Surgery; Radioimmunoguided Surgery

The application of this radiolabeled monoclonal antibody technique is discussed in the section on *Second-Look Operation.*

## *Other Markers*

Other markers used in an attempt to increase the sensitivity of monitoring for tumor recurrence include several acute-phase reactive proteins (APRP), serum protein hexose, transferrin, and ceruloplasmin. As mentioned, other tumor-associated antigens, such as carbohydrate antigen 19-9 (CA 19-9), have also been used. More work must be done, however, before the true value of all these newer techniques can be accurately assessed.

### Positron Emission Tomography

Positron emission tomography may be of benefit in localizing tumor recurrence following resection of colorectal cancer. This is a whole-body imaging technique utilizing $^{18}$F-fluorodeoxyglucose. It has been reported that whole-body PET affects management in a significant number of patients studied. The main disadvantages are the cost and the limited availability. As with radiolabeled imaging, the indications for the use of this modality are limited: an equivocal evaluation or a presumed isolated recurrence. PET may be of particular benefit in evaluating the resectability of a presacral mass of equivocal nature on CT or magnetic resonance imaging.

*Comment*: The various radiolabeled imaging techniques that have been applied to the follow-up management of patients who have had resection for colorectal cancer certainly have added much to our knowledge of the pathologic processes. The question remains: Is there a tangible survival benefit? For the present, these modalities are of value in only two scenarios: that of an individual who will have re-exploratory surgery for a presumed isolated recurrence, and that of someone with a rising CEA in whom other evaluations fail to identify the site of recurrence. Before embarking on a second-look procedure (see later), newer imaging modalities should be applied. In some instances, the tumor will be localized; in others, cancer beyond the limits of surgical cure may be identified. In both instances, the operative procedure would be changed. As the technology improves, it is hoped that the sensitivity and specificity will be high enough so that the surgeon can make a strong recommendation to the patient concerning the appropriateness of re-exploration.

## *Second-Look Operation*

When recurrence of tumor is discovered, surgical resection offers the best possible chance for cure in those patients who have localized disease. Some surgeons have proposed second-look procedures in an attempt to improve the cure of colorectal cancer. Sugarbaker found improved survival with re-exploration of the abdomen in those with a raised CEA level. However, with the advent of newer investigative modalities, this approach is less likely to be considered.

*Comment*: Having stated that after investigations fail to reveal a source of a rising CEA determination, provided that the patient is at a reasonable risk to undergo the procedure, and there has been appropriate informed consent, an offer is made to re-explore the abdomen. Whether the morbidity, mortality, and cost of a second-look procedure are justified remains unanswered.

## Gamma-Guided Surgery; Radioimmunoguided Surgery

It is axiomatic that accurate assessment of the extent and location of tumor within the abdomen is necessary for the performance of a truly useful exercise by reoperation. Standard methods of visual examination and palpation and the time of surgery, of course, are supplemented by the information gleaned through the preoperative methods discussed. It has been suggested that radioimmunolocalization using labeled monoclonal antibodies potentially may complement the traditional approaches.

### *Technique*

One of the monoclonal antibody tumor markers previously discussed (e.g., as anti-CEA labeled with $^{111}$In-MoAb) is injected preoperatively. At the time of laparotomy, a hand-held gamma-detecting probe is used to locate foci of malignancy (e.g., Neoprobe Corp., Dublin, Ohio) (Fig. 22.8). Depending on the location of the tumor or tumors, an *en bloc* excision or "tumorectomy" is carried out.

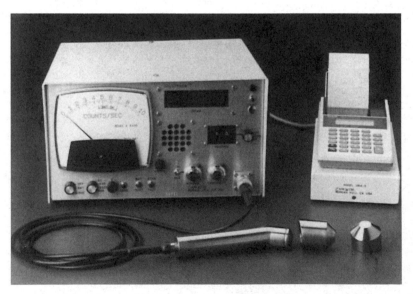

**FIG. 22.8.** A C-Trak system with probe for gamma detection of recurrent tumor at the time of laparotomy. (Courtesy of Care Wise Medical Products Corp.)

If dealing with lymph nodes that are producing the uptake seen on the imager, the operation may become little more than "cherry picking."

*Comment*: The problem with radioimmunoguided surgery, is that therapeutic efforts to remove lymph nodes by identification through radiolocalization are not consistent with the concepts of cancer operative technique. In other words, "cherry picking" of highlighted lymph nodes adds nothing to the survival benefit for an individual with metastatic disease at that focus. This has been discussed previously with respect to apical nodes in the resected specimen. Still, the technique has value, particularly with respect to upstaging. The pathologist can identify tumor only within the specimens submitted for examination. The surgeon, on the other hand, may be able to identify tumor beyond the reach of surgical excision. This obviously would have an influence on subsequent management decisions (e.g., adjuvant therapy). Weigh the theoretic benefit of changing the classification of the patient's tumor against the additional cost, both in terms of equipment and increased operative time.

## TREATMENT OF RECURRENCE

### Anastomotic Recurrence

Anastomotic recurrence following resection for colon carcinoma is much less commonly seen than after resection for rectal cancer. It is usually much more feasible to perform an adequate, wide excision of the cancer-bearing segment than when limitations are imposed by the confines of the pelvis. Symptoms of recurrence include abdominal pain, anorexia, nausea, vomiting, weight loss, change in bowel habits, and rectal bleeding. If a tumor is identified in the bowel, an aggressive surgical attitude should be adopted because the so-called recurrence may, in reality, be a missed synchronous lesion. Excluding this possibility, in contrast to recurrence following rectal resection, in which an inadequate lateral or distal margin is often the precipitating factor, anastomotic recurrence that develops after a more proximal bowel resection is usually a result of initial retroperitoneal fixation by that tumor.

The specific problems of anastomotic recurrence and local recurrence following rectal excision are discussed in Chapter 23.

### Pulmonary Metastases

Solitary lung metastases from colorectal cancer have been resected for cure more often than metastases to all other sites combined. It still should be remembered, however, that primary lung cancer is the second most common visceral malignancy in men and that an isolated pulmonary metastasis should not contraindicate radical surgical removal of the bowel tumor. Also, in resection of a solitary lung lesion that has metastasized from a primary colonic carcinoma, the chance of a cure is better than when the lesion is a primary bronchogenic carcinoma.

Investigators from Memorial Sloan-Kettering Cancer Center reported 10- and 5-year survival rates after resection for pulmonary metastases as 40% and 30%, respectively. Several studies have attempted to identify prognostic factors. The only factor that appears to be significant is the disease-free interval; the longer the interval, the better the survival rate.

## Ovarian Metastases

The ovary may be the only site of macroscopic spread of disease; it is the site of metastases in 3% to 5% of patients. Bilateral oophorectomy has been recommended on a prophylactic basis in all postmenopausal women who have colorectal cancer because of the risk for harboring a metastatic focus as well as for the prevention of primary ovarian carcinoma (see earlier discussion). No question remains to the advisability of therapeutic oophorectomy when macroscopic tumor is evident in the adnexa. The likelihood of cure in such circumstances, however, is virtually nil.

## Liver Metastases

The overall mean survival of patients with untreated metastatic colorectal cancer to the liver is approximately 23 months. Studies analyzing unresectable hepatic metastases from colon and rectal cancer identified six independent determinants of survival in the following order: percentage of liver volume replaced by tumor, grade of malignancy of the primary tumor, presence of extrahepatic disease, mesenteric lymph node involvement, serum CEA determination, and age. The investigators felt able to provide a prognostic tree that displayed median survival times for a number of subgroups of these variables.

The poor prognosis has stimulated a number of resective approaches that have yielded successful results. It has been estimated that 15% to 25% of individuals with metastatic disease are candidates for these procedures. Before embarking on such an effort, however, it is imperative to determine the extent of disease and the surgical anatomy. This can be accomplished by several preoperative and intraoperative methods.

### *Computed Tomography with Arterial Portography*

Although CT is important in the preliminary assessment of an individual who is being evaluated for a rising CEA, particularly with respect to identifying liver metastases, it is not as sensitive as would be wished. It is now well established that CT examination during arterial portography (CTAP) is the most sensitive preoperative imaging technique for the detection of hepatic metastases from colorectal cancer. Knowledge of the extent of the metastases is important, not only in intraoperative decision making, but also in determining which patients are not candidates for a resective approach.

### Hepatic Angiography

Liver angiography has been considered a useful guide in the preoperative assessment of known hepatic metastatic tumor, as well as in the evaluation of vascular anatomy, particularly if a major hepatic resection is contemplated. However, this has been generally replaced by CTAP in the workup of those considered for hepatic resection.

### Hepatic Resection

The precise steps in the performance of the various hepatic resection maneuvers are not within the purview of this text. Options include right hepatic lobectomy, right trisegmentectomy, left hepatectomy, left lateral segmentectomy, wedge resection, extended left hepatectomy (left trisegmentectomy), and segmental resections.

### Results

Many studies confirm that hepatic resection for colorectal metastatic disease can be done in a number of individuals for cure. Factors reported to improve the outcome include resection margins of at least 1 cm and fewer than four metastatic nodules. Generally, it has been concluded that major liver resection can be performed safely, with less than a 5% operative mortality, and a cure rate between 20% and 25%. In those with a solitary metastasis, the cure rate can be as high as 40%. Repeat hepatic resection for isolated metastases can result in long-term survival in selected patients.

### Intraoperative Ultrasonography

The area of occult hepatic metastases has been emphasized earlier with respect to the application of intraoperative ultrasonography. Many centers are recommending its routine use during surgery for colorectal cancer. Some have found that more metastases were diagnosed by intraoperative ultrasonography than by palpation, abdominal ultrasonography, or CT.

Operative ultrasonography has certain advantages of particular importance in hepatic surgery: (a) Because no energy is lost in passage through the abdominal wall, greater resolution is possible and smaller lesions can be detected; (b) landmarks on the liver parenchyma can be easily correlated with the position of the probe; and (c) ultrasonographic guidance can facilitate both biopsy and other hepatobiliary procedures. The technique can be used to confirm the presence of tumor in the liver that was suspected on the basis of preoperative evaluation. It can prevent the surgeon from embarking on an ill-advised resection when cure is unattainable (e.g., when multiple lesions are involved). Finally, it can establish the relationship between tumor and intrahepatic vessels, thus possibly preventing vascular injury and perhaps making radical hepatic resection safer.

### Cryosurgery

Intraoperative ultrasonography has also been used to direct the application of treatment, specifically cryotherapy. The technique is relatively safe and has been used successfully, especially in those individuals with low volume, unresectable metastatic disease. *In situ* destruction of tumors by means of freezing has been applied to the management of skin, rectal, prostatic, gynecologic, and head and neck cancers, so it is not surprising that some centers have begun to use this approach in the treatment of primary and metastatic lesions of the liver. The cryoprobe, which uses circulating liquid nitrogen and produces a spherical ball of ice around each treated metastatic site, is controlled by the imaging technique. A technique has also been described that uses cryosurgery in combination with hepatic resection, in essence excising the ice ball.

Cryodestruction can accomplish a number of things:

- Treat multiple areas of involvement focally
- Preserve a maximal amount of normal liver tissue
- Destroy tumors deep in the liver parenchyma without the need for major resection
- Avoid large vessels or vital structures
- Minimize blood loss
- Is associated with lower morbidity and mortality than resection
- Can be combined with other modalities (e.g., resection of one lobe and cryosurgical destruction in other areas)

### Osseous Metastases

Osseous metastases from colonic and rectal cancer are relatively uncommon, occurring in up to 9% of reported series. Most of these tumors had spread to bone in association with widespread metastases elsewhere. The median survival time from establishment of the diagnosis is only 7 months. Bone scanning is felt to be more sensitive for diagnosing metastases than is radiography. Palliative treatment by means of radiation therapy for the bone pain is usually effective.

### Cerebral Metastases

Metastatic carcinoma to the brain is uncommon and is usually associated with metastatic disease elsewhere, especially in the lung. Rarely, will a metastatic focus be present in the brain with no other evidence of disease. Under these circumstances, craniotomy is indicated to remove the metastatic lesion, with the expectation that, even if cure cannot be attained, good palliation of neurologic signs and symptoms will result.

Occasionally, a patient will present with neurologic signs and symptoms as the initial manifestation of colorectal cancer. Subsequent gastrointestinal investigation can be stimulated by the histologic interpretation after the intracranial tumor has been removed.

## Penile Metastases

Metastatic tumors to the penis are uncommon; more than 80% of them originate in the bladder, prostate, rectum, sigmoid colon, and kidney. Direct invasion, retrograde venous extension, retrograde lymphatic extension, perineural spread, and arterial embolism are proposed mechanisms for the spread. Surgical excision with or without chemoradiation therapy is the primary treatment. Prognosis for long-term survival is poor.

## Chemotherapy

It is self-evident, despite the high rate of resectability and the improvement in the surgical management of patients with colorectal cancer, almost one half die of recurrent disease. It is for this reason that approximately 60% of patients are treated with systemic chemotherapy for metastatic disease, at diagnosis, for disease recurrence, or as adjuvant therapy.

Initially, 5-fluorouracil (5FU) was the primary chemotherapeutic agent. This drug had a response rate of only 20% to 30%. Later, with the addition of levamisole or leucovorin, an increased effect of the 5FU was noted. Moertels, at the Mayo Clinic, showed that adjuvant therapy with these combined agents improved survival by 33% in those with stage 3 disease (TNM). The regimen of 5FU and leucovorin for 6 months, therefore, has become standard adjuvant therapy in the patients with lymph node metastases. More recently, infusional 5FU has been used because of fewer side effects.

Remember, however, that chemotherapy is not innocuous—potential complications are myriad. These include bone marrow depression, alopecia, sepsis, renal and hepatic toxicity, gastrointestinal hemorrhage, mutagenesis, typhlitis, and bowel wall necrosis. Close monitoring, therefore, is essential.

Recently, newer therapeutic agents have been used in an attempt to better deal with metastatic disease and, it is hoped, to reduce the incidence of side effects. Furthermore, analysis of the tumor behavior and its response allows selection of combinations of these agents, which may improve the outcome. This has been greatly enhanced by a better understanding of the pathways of action of these chemotherapeutic agents.

Ethynyluracil is an analogue of uracil that inactivates dihydropyrimidine dehydrogenase (DPD), the enzyme responsible for 5FU degradation. Phase 3 trials are now being conducted.

Ftorafur is an oral pro-drug of 5FU. It is completely absorbed through the gastrointestinal mucosa and metabolized to 5FU. This agent has been combined with oral leucovorin in an attempt to improve activity. A phase 2 trial showed a

42% response rate in those with metastatic colorectal cancer. Worldwide prospective randomized trials are being conducted.

An oral formulation of Ftorafur and its modulators (5-chlorodihydopyrimidine, and Oxonic acid) S-1 is now undergoing trials in North America and Europe.

Capecitabine is another pro-drug of 5FU, but it is absorbed through the gastrointestinal mucosa as an intact molecule. This is used to circumvent the gastrointestinal toxicity associated with this treatment. Phase 3 trials have been completed, and the results are being awaited.

Some colorectal tumors have demonstrated 5FU resistance. 5FU inhibits thymidine synthase (TS) by binding with the TS. TS is essential for production of thymidine monophosphate (TMP), which is anabolized in cells to the triphosphate, essential for DNA synthesis and repair. Consequently, raltitrexed (Tomudex), which is a thymidine synthase inhibitor, was developed. Phase 2 trials revealed a 26% response rate. Phase 3 trials using various regimens have shown similar response and palliation rates when compared with 5FU and leucovorin. However, because of side effects, doubt exists to whether this drug will be approved for use in North America.

Oxaliplatin, a third generation platinum compound, produces inter- and intrastrand DNA links. In those with mismatch repair deficiencies (e.g., HNPCC), this drug may be a good therapeutic choice. It is used in those with colorectal cancer that is refractory to other therapies.

Irinotecan (CPT-11) is a pro-drug that is converted in the liver to an active metabolite, SN-38. Dose-limiting toxicity is diarrhea and neutropenia. This drug has been shown to improve survival when compared with 5FU (10.5 months vs. 8.5 months) and best supportive care (9.2 months vs. 6.5 months) in those individuals with metastatic colorectal cancer. Current studies are being performed using this drug in adjuvant settings.

As one can appreciate, chemotherapy is rapidly evolving.

### Hepatic Artery Infusion, Ligation, Dearterialization; Portal Vein Infusion

Hepatic artery infusion is sometimes recommended; in the opinion of some authors, it produces higher regression rates and slightly longer remissions than other techniques. However, these advantages are at the cost of increased morbidity, time in the hospital, and technical difficulties, which may make this route less than desirable. Also, most believe no improvement in survival occurs, because patients generally succumb to extra-hepatic metastatic disease.

Hepatic artery ligation and hepatic dearterialization also have been used, primarily making subsequent resectional surgery safer rather than by curing the patient as a definitive treatment.

Portal vein infusion with 5-FU has also been done, with mixed results. Some report significant prolongation of survival, as well as a qualitative and quantitative improvement in a host of other variables.

## Immunotherapy

Chemotherapeutic agents, especially 5-FU, have been used in combination with other treatment modalities (e.g., surgery, radiation, and immunotherapy). The value of chemoimmunotherapy has been studied, through the use of 5-FU plus BCG. This has been shown to produce a longer disease-free period with increased survival in some patients. These studies have not yet been confirmed by randomized, controlled trials from other institutions.

Immunotherapy with BCG is most effective when the tumor mass is reduced to a minimum when (a) it is administered directly into or close to the tumor; (b) the patient is able to respond to BCG; and (c) a large enough dose is given. Routes of administration include direct insertion into the tumor; administration can also be intradermal (by skin scarification), intracavitary, or oral.

Another study used adjuvant immunochemotherapy with PSKR, an immuno-modulator composed of a protein-bound polysaccharide extracted from mycelia of *Coriorus versicolor*. The PSKR group received this agent orally over 3 years, in addition to mitomycin C and 5-FU. The median follow-up time was 4 years. When the patients taking PSKR were compared with the control group (chemotherapy alone), a statistically significant improvement was noted in the disease-free survival curve.

Immunotherapy with agents such as interferon-$\alpha_{2a}$, monoclonal antibody 17-1, and autologous tumor vaccines is also under investigation, and preliminary results suggest improved survival. The German Cancer Aid 17-1A study group designed a protocol in which a monoclonal antibody (17-1A) was used to target minimal residual disease (i.e., Dukes' C patients). Patients were randomly assigned to an observation regimen or to postoperative treatment with this antibody, infused each month. Antibody treatment reduced the overall death rate by 30% and decreased the recurrence rate by 27%.

Durrant et al., from England, have experimented with 105AD7, a human anti-idiotype antibody that mimics the CD55 antigen, in an attempt to stimulate CD4 and CD8 response with resultant tumor cell death. They treated 18 patients with advanced colorectal cancer, demonstrating a good response in 14. However, few patients produced a sustained activation. This will obviously need further investigation before being clinically useful.

## Radiotherapy

Radiotherapy has been applied primarily in the treatment of rectal cancer (see Chapter 23). However, conventional external radiation therapy should still be considered when macroscopic tumor remains or when fixity of the lesion precludes complete excision. Usually, 45 to 60 Gy (4,500 to 6,000 rads) is administered over a period of 5 to 6 weeks. Evidence suggests that this reduces the likelihood of local recurrence and improves survival rates.

When 5-FU is combined with radiation therapy, a modest improvement takes place in length of remission and survival compared with survival after radiation therapy alone in patients with local, inoperable, or recurrent disease.

*Comment*:  In reviewing the experience with colorectal carcinoma for the past 40 years, it seems apparent that no significant improvement in operative mortality and cure rate has taken place. It appears, then, that surgery has accomplished all it possibly can for this condition. Any further improvement in survival rates will depend on patients having surgery earlier and on the effectiveness of other modalities of therapy.

# 23

# Carcinoma of the Rectum

Chapter 22 addressed the diagnosis and treatment of cancer of the colon, including presentation, evaluation, management, and results of treatment of cancer of the rectum.

## SIGNS, SYMPTOMS, AND DIAGNOSIS

The signs and symptoms of cancer of the rectum have been discussed in Chapter 22. Bleeding is the most common complaint (35% to 40%), followed by diarrhea, change in bowel habits, and abdominal pain. Rectal pain, as a presenting symptom, is not common.

### Carcinoma of the Prostate

Potential confusion occasionally exists in the differential diagnosis. Be wary of the rectal mass caused by invasion by carcinoma of the prostate; such involvement of the prostate can lead to rectal ulceration. The tumor can become so large that the rectum is completely encircled and obstructive symptoms are produced.

Biopsy may show adenocarcinoma, but if poorly differentiated, special staining may be required to establish the tumor to be of prostatic origin (acid phosphatase [PSA]). Because of the frequency of both conditions, the two tumors can occasionally occur synchronously. If a pyelogram or computed tomography (CT) is performed, a consistent finding is the presence of ureteral dilatation.

## FACTORS INFLUENCING THE CHOICE OF OPERATION

To save or not to save the sphincter is a perennial question. Is there a level below which an anastomosis should not be attempted? Conversely, too often, in a zealous effort to avoid a colostomy and to reestablish intestinal continuity, surgeons compromise on the margins of resection. The consequences are often tragic: recurrent disease, anastomotic obstruction, unremitting pelvic pain, and the requirement for subsequent surgery, including a colostomy.

A number of procedures available, under particular circumstances, can be the preferred approach for a given patient:

- Abdominoperineal resection
- Low anterior resection
- Colostomy or ileostomy
- Hartmann resection
- Abdominoanal pull-through
- Abdominosacral (coccygeal) resection
- Transsacral resection (Kraske)
- Transsphincteric excision
- Transanal (local) excision
- Electrocoagulation
- Laser coagulation
- Cryosurgical destruction
- Radiation (obviously not an operation, but it can be the sole modality of treatment in some instances)

If another resective procedure is contemplated, it should rarely be other than an anterior resection. If embarking on another procedure, be able to justify it as the optimal treatment of the patient under the circumstances.

In recent years, many surgeons have used a more scientific approach to determining the proper surgical alternative. Sophisticated staging techniques have been suggested, including not only standard examination with biopsy and hematologic and radiologic studies, but also tumor DNA content, acute phase reactive proteins, and endoluminal ultrasonography. Factors that are helpful in determining the choice of operation for cancer in the rectum are summarized here:

- Level
- Macroscopic appearance (ulcerated, polypoid)
- Extent of circumferential involvement
- Fixity
- Degree of differentiation (histologic appearance)
- Tumor cell DNA content
- Endorectal ultrasound determination
- Magnetic resonance imaging (MRI) assessment
- Presacral adenopathy
- Body habitus
- Gender
- Age
- Metastatic disease
- Other systemic disease
- Other conditions that might contraindicate colostomy (e.g., blindness, severe arthritis, mental incapacity)

## Lesion Level

The distance of the lower edge of the tumor from the anal verge is probably the single most important variable that aids the surgeon in the choice of operation. This distance should be carefully measured using the rigid proctosigmoidoscope. The flexible sigmoidoscope is not as accurate for this determination.

## Macroscopic Appearance

Generally, the distal margin of resection should be approximately 4 cm below the tumor; for infiltrative carcinomas, however, the risk of anastomotic recurrence may be increased with a margin of less than 7 cm. The length of distal intramural spread of tumor in resected specimens is extremely variable. Ascertaining the appearance of the lesion, whether ulcerated, scirrhous (infiltrative), or polypoid, helps in determining the choice of operation.

## Extent of Circumferential Involvement

Usually, more highly aggressive tumors tend to involve a greater circumference of the bowel wall when they present. Under these circumstances, a greater margin of resection is required.

## Fixity

Fixity of the tumor in the pelvis implies a poor prognosis. A greater likelihood exists of residual tumor following resection, and anastomotic recurrence is a frequent sequela. An abdominoperineal resection probably offers better palliation, because the need for subsequent reoperation is less likely. The presence of a fixed tumor might also prompt the consideration of preoperative radiotherapy (see later).

## Histologic Appearance

A biopsy is mandatory. It is done routinely, usually at the time of initial discovery of the lesion. Ideally, the material obtained should be from the edge of the lesion. Generally, tumors regarded as poorly differentiated have highly irregular glands or no glandular differentiation. The more anaplastic, the more aggressive is the lesion; the more aggressive, the greater is the resection margin that would be required. The chance of local recurrence is much greater with a poorly differentiated cancer than with one that is well differentiated. Therefore, do not overestimate the importance of degree of differentiation (Broder's classification), depth of penetration, and the presence or absence of venous or perineural invasion (PNI) in making the appropriate choice of operation.

A particularly useful microscopic variable to identify is the extent of lymphocytic infiltration at the border of the tumor. Patients who harbor tumors that demonstrate pronounced lymphocytic infiltration have a better prognosis than those who do not. Optimally, view the histologic evidence yourself to make the most reasoned recommendation to the patient.

## Tumor Cell DNA Content

Reports of DNA measurements in human cancers suggest that flow cytometry assays of DNA ploidy have prognostic value. Hence, this may affect the choice of operation. A DNA histogram of normal colonic epithelium reveals that more than 90% of the cells have a single diploid peak. Carcinomas that are nearly diploid have a better prognosis than those that are aneuploid.

## Presacral Adenopathy

By careful palpation of the rectum, the surgeon can occasionally identify a hard lesion, a lymph node with metastasis. Such a finding suggests that the tumor has spread beyond the bowel wall and that recurrence, therefore, is more likely, especially if a local procedure is performed. This is the type of situation in which preoperative radiotherapy may be of benefit.

## Computed Tomography

Computed tomography (CT) is of great value in identifying metastatic disease, especially in the liver and elsewhere within the abdomen. It has no significant value in identifying depth of invasion preoperatively.

## Magnetic Resonance Imaging

Magnetic resonance imaging (MRI) has also been used for preoperative assessment, but it has not been of particular advantage when compared with CT or endoluminal ultrasound.

### *Magnetic Resonance Imaging with Endorectal Coil*

A recent improvement in MRI technique is the use of surface MRI coils to allow a higher definition of image to be obtained with a smaller field of view. In this way, a more local accurate staging might be possible. As with endoluminal ultrasound, the technology is now available for the office evaluation of patients. Although initially promising for local staging of rectal cancer, this modality does not improve the staging accuracy of MRI to a clinically useful level.

## Endorectal or Transrectal Ultrasound Examination

Endorectal ultrasound has developed into an extremely useful tool for the preoperative assessment of patients with rectal cancer. After a small enema is administered, the probe is introduced into the rectum beyond the tumor. A balloon is filled with approximately 50 mL of water, and an acoustic contact is produced between the rotating part of the transducer and the rectal wall.

Each layer of the rectum can be sonographically visualized, with a tumor usually appearing as a hypoechoic disruption of the rectal wall. The procedure can also reveal if underlying lymph nodes are affected. Sensitivity and specificity for bowel wall involvement are above 90%. An additional benefit is that invasive carcinoma can be detected within an otherwise villous lesion with this technique. Lymph node metastases can be predicted with an accuracy of nearly 70% and inflammatory lymph nodes with a specificity of nearly 85%.

Optimal results can only be obtained with consistency in both technique and interpretation. Accuracy improves considerably with increased experience. As experience is acquired with this instrument, patients with limited rectal wall involvement can be offered a less than radical surgical alternative to the treatment of their condition. In addition, the technique offers the opportunity for clear visualization of the full thickness of an anastomotic area in those patients who have had restoration of rectal continuity, especially with respect to the possibility of early detection of recurrent cancer, and for the effect of preoperative radiotherapy. Further information can be obtained by means of ultrasonographically guided biopsies.

A new modality has been recently introduced—three-dimensional endoluminal ultrasound. Although it has many of the limitations associated with conventional transrectal ultrasound examination (TRUS), it seems to provide significantly more information on spatial relationships. This is particularly useful when considering biopsy of extrarectal lymph nodes, for example. Whether this modality will ultimately result in improved staging of rectal cancer awaits further investigations.

### Rectal Endoscopic Lymphoscintigraphy

Rectal endoscopic lymphoscintigraphy involves the endoscopic injection of 0.1 mL of radiocolloid (rhenium sulfur marked with technetium 99m) into the submucosa of the extraperitoneal rectum bilaterally. The diffusion of the tracer along the lymphatics is registered by a computerized gamma camera. Preliminary studies report the technique to have a sensitivity rate of 85%, a specificity rate of 68%, an overall accuracy of 76%, a positive predictive value of 71%, and a negative predictive value of 71%. Its value awaits further study.

### Other Factors

The aforementioned factors concerned the tumor, itself. The following variables that can influence the choice of operation are related to the patient.

## Body Habitus

A rectal resection on an asthenic patient usually permits a technically lower anastomosis than does an operation for the same level of lesion in an obese individual.

## Gender

An anastomotic procedure is more likely to be possible in women than in men. A broad pelvis, furthermore, usually permits a wider resection, whereas a narrow pelvis tends to impede dissection, potentially limiting the adequacy of tumor margins and the use of conventional anastomotic techniques.

## Age

A resection involving an anastomosis is a higher-risk procedure than an abdominoperineal resection; morbidity is greater, and operative mortality is higher. Furthermore, the possible need for a second operation (e.g., closure of a colostomy) increases the risk still further.

## Metastatic Disease

Anastomotic procedures are often mistakenly embarked on in the presence of metastatic disease to avoid colostomy during the terminal phase of the patient's illness. All too often, however, the patient returns to have a colostomy because of complications related to recurrence in the pelvis. Operative mortality, furthermore, is much greater for palliative resections, including abdominoperineal resection. A colostomy or a Hartmann resection can be adequate, or a local procedure may be the best choice if symptoms can be controlled by this means.

## Systemic Disease

Any patient, regardless of age, is at an increased risk if systemic disease (e.g., cardiovascular, pulmonary, renal) is present. Such individuals are more safely treated by a procedure that does not involve an anastomosis. Balance the risks with the advantage of avoiding a colostomy.

## Other Conditions

Avoiding a colostomy in a patient who cannot cope with an appliance or a stoma is an unusual, albeit legitimate, reason for choosing an alternative procedure. This can happen if the individual is blind, has severe impairment in the use of hands (e.g., arthritis), or cannot learn how to use the appliance. Obviously, alternatives exist to support the patient (e.g., care by a family member, a visiting nurse, or a home helper).

## ABDOMINOPERINEAL RESECTION

As originally advocated, abdominoperineal resection involved an abdominal dissection and mobilization of the rectum; the rectum was then buried beneath the reconstituted pelvic floor. It was then excised through the perineal route, classically in the left lateral position. Since the original description, only minor modifications in the surgical technique have been introduced.

The major modification was the introduction of the synchronous combined (two-team) abdominoperineal resection, which originally had been proposed by Mayo as early as 1904. The technique involves two teams of surgeons operating synchronously once the resectability of the tumor has been ascertained. This method permits easier access to the pelvis and allows an attack on the area from two directions. It is particularly helpful when confronted with a bulky or fixed tumor, or in a patient with a narrow pelvis. Blood loss can be reduced and operative time decreased by using a two-team method.

### Indications

When tumors are less than 8 cm from the anal verge, the standard treatment is abdominoperineal resection. Higher lesions generally permit restoration of intestinal continuity, usually by low anterior resection. As a palliative procedure (even in the presence of metastatic disease), if the patient's life expectancy may be several months or more, greater patient comfort can often be achieved with resection than by a diversionary procedure alone. This is particularly true when (a) the tumor invades the sphincter mechanism to produce tenesmus; (b) it extends to the perineum; or (c) bleeding is a major concern. Abdominoperineal resection is the most consistently successful operation for carcinoma, and it is the procedure against which alternative sphincter-saving operations must be compared.

### Preoperative Preparation

Evaluation of the proximal bowel by colonoscopy or barium enema (to look for synchronous lesions) should be done, except when the rectal tumor appears to be virtually obstructing. A CT scan is recommended, not only to ascertain evidence of metastatic disease, but also to evaluate tumor extent and the presence of any compression, dilatation, or deviation of the ureters. The bowel preparation consists of laxatives, enemas, and nonabsorbable antibiotics. Determine the optimal location of a stoma site before surgery.

### Anesthesia

A general, endotracheal anesthetic is advised for this procedure, but a spinal anesthetic can also be used. A Foley catheter with a 30-mL balloon is inserted into the bladder. Use of a nasogastric tube is not necessary. Whether to place ureteral catheters prophylactically in operations involving the rectum is some-what controversial, at least at the initial procedure. However, in reoperative rec-tal surgery or for those in whom radiation had been performed, the prophylactic use of ureteral catheterization is strongly recommended. The risk of ureteral injury as a direct result of catheter insertion is small (1.1%). Although the pres-ence of such catheters does not ensure the prevention of ureteral injuries, imme-diate recognition is usually evident. Complications of this procedure include renal colic, oliguria, and anuria, but these are infrequently observed.

## Technique

The patient is placed in the perineolithotomy position with the legs in stirrups. The knees can be flexed, but the hips should be relatively extended and the thighs abducted to allow simultaneous, unlimited access to both the abdomen and the perineum. Too much hip flexion can interfere with the abdominal operator's maneuverability. A moderate degree of Trendelenburg (head-down) tilt aids in the dissection.

One of the concerns of placing the patient in the perineolithotomy position is its association with the development of a compartment syndrome. This occurs when an elevated pressure in an osteofascial compartment compromises local perfusion. This can result in neurovascular damage and permanent disability, emphasizing the importance of prevention and early diagnosis. Intermittent, sequential compression of the lower limbs is strongly encouraged to prevent venous stasis.

A purse-string suture is placed around the anus using a nonabsorbable reten-tion material. The location of the incision is important, not only for the obvious reason of access to the abdomen, but also to avoid interference with the subse-quent placement of the stoma. A midline hypogastric incision is advised, extend-ing through the umbilicus if necessary. Ideally, the colostomy should be sited over the rectus muscle and brought out through the split thickness of the muscle. Paracolostomy herniation is less likely to occur if the stoma is brought through the muscle rather than a pararectus location. It should never be brought out through the incision; a left paramedian incision, therefore, is relatively con-traindicated. Furthermore, ideally the stoma should be situated below the belt-line at a distance from bony promontories and from the umbilicus (Fig. 23.1). The consequences and management of poorly placed stomas are discussed in Chapters 31 and 32.

After the insertion of a self-retaining (e.g., Balfour, Bookwalter) retractor, the abdomen is explored for evidence of metastatic disease, synchronous colon lesion presence, or other pathology. The small intestine is packed into the upper abdomen using moist pads. Rarely, should it be necessary to exteriorize the bowel. Keeping the viscera warm and moist and within the abdomen reduces the likelihood of postoperative ileus, and a nasogastric tube may be avoided. This can be more easily accomplished if the incision can be kept below the umbilicus.

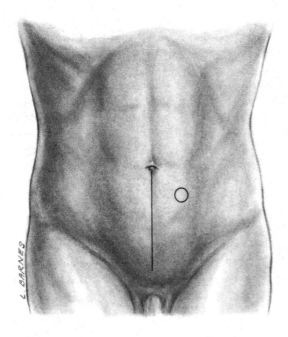

**FIG. 23.1.** The proper position for the sigmoid colostomy site of abdominoperineal resection is away from any bony promontories, the umbilicus, scars, and skin folds, and within the rectus muscle.

Mobilization of the sigmoid colon and rectum commences along the left colic gutter, lysing the developmental adhesions to obtain sufficient mobility to deliver the bowel to the abdominal wall at the level of the proposed colostomy.

The peritoneum on the left lateral aspect is incised, and the left ureter is identified and retracted laterally. Injury to the ureter most commonly occurs during this phase of the procedure, at the level of the iliac artery; it should always be visualized and protected. Incision of the peritoneum is continued anteriorly to the base of the bladder.

The technique of abdominoperineal resection requires identification and control of the inferior mesenteric vessels, the middle hemorrhoidal arteries (which pass adjacent to the lateral ligaments of the rectum), and the inferior hemorrhoidal vessels.

Then the left hand is passed beneath the inferior mesenteric vessels, and a peritoneal incision is performed in a similar fashion on the right side. The mesenteric vascular pedicle is ligated between clamps; always check to be certain that the left ureter has not been incorporated. It is less important to visualize the right ureter because it should not be involved in this aspect of the dissection. Exceptions to this dictum include a congenital anomaly or a history of prior surgery that might have caused medial deviation of this structure. Injury to the right ureter is usually caused at the time of pelvic floor reconstruction by mobilization and suture of the peritoneum on that side.

Ligation of the inferior mesenteric artery at its origin is unnecessary because nodal involvement at that level is found only in patients with incurable cancer, and survival rates are not improved. Ligation distal to the first branch of the inferior mesenteric artery ensures a viable blood supply to the bowel from which the stoma will be created. Pelvic peritoneal incisions are then joined across the base of the bladder (or at the vaginal apex in women).

Attention is then turned to the retrorectal space. Often, surgeons commence blunt dissection at the level of the sacral promontory; when doing so, however, the plane may be improperly entered, the presacral vessels can be torn, and profuse bleeding ensues. Hemorrhage, in fact, is often caused by bleeding from basivertebral veins through the sacral foramina and not from injury to the presacral venous plexus. When such vessels are encountered, attempt at ligation may be unsuccessful, especially if the bleeding emanates directly from bone. Rather than attempt to electrocoagulate and accept additional blood loss, apply direct pressure with a large pad for a few minutes. Failure to achieve hemostasis may necessitate the use of packing, or even the application of a hemorrhage occluder pin (thumbtack) placed into the sacrum. The risk of bleeding can be minimized if the dissection is performed, as much as possible, under direct visualization and by sharp dissection (Fig. 23.2). Gentle anterior traction is placed

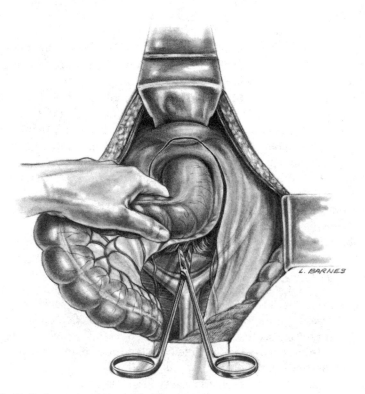

**FIG. 23.2.** Abdominoperineal resection. The presacral space is entered by sharp dissection.

on the rectosigmoid and the scissors inserted anterior to the sacral promontory. The presacral space is relatively avascular and usually readily entered. The loose areolar tissue is identified and incised. The presacral nerves can usually be seen clearly and, therefore, can be displaced out of harm's way.

Once the presacral space has been opened as far as convenient by retraction and under direct visualization, the right hand can be inserted and the dissection carried out bluntly (Fig. 23.3). It is still preferable to perform as much of the dissection under direct visualization, cutting with the scissors as distally as possible. The rectum is freed to the tip of the coccyx in a plane anterior to the sacral fascia, avoiding injury to the presacral veins (Fig. 23.4).

If posterior mobilization of the rectum is impeded by tumor extension, the abdominal operator should wait for the perineal surgeon to develop a plane, rather than to proceed blindly. If a synchronous combined procedure is not being performed or if no plane can be developed from either direction, the surgeon must dissect wherever the plane is presumed to have been, fully recognizing that the possibility for cure may be compromised. If performing a synchronous approach, at this point in the operation the abdominal operator meets the peri-

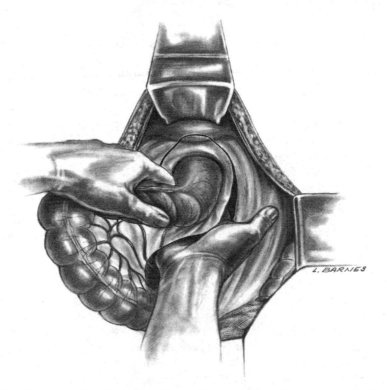

**FIG. 23.3.** Abdominoperineal resection. The rectum is mobilized from the lower pelvic adhesions by blunt dissection; this produces a characteristic "sucking" sound.

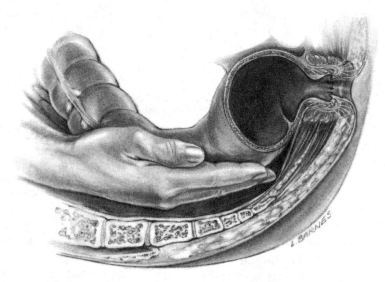

**FIG. 23.4.** Abdominoperineal resection. The lateral view illustrates that, ideally, the sacral fascia is not breached when the rectum is bluntly dissected.

neal surgeon (in the posterior midline) when the rectococcygeus ligament has been divided.

Attention is then turned to the anterior part of the dissection. The posterior wall of the bladder and seminal vesicles (or uterus and posterior vaginal wall in women) ideally are demonstrated visually. This is accomplished by using a 7-inch St. Mark's pattern retractor with turned-back lip (Thackray, Inc., Woburn, MA) and by a combination of sharp and blunt dissection (Fig. 23.5). Denonvilliers' fascia must be incised to separate the rectum completely from the prostate and the seminal vesicles. By means of retraction of the bladder and prostatic area and countertraction on the rectum, the dissection is carried distally until the inferior margin of the prostate and the urethra with its contained catheter can be palpated. In women, the posterior vaginal wall is swept anteriorly to the point where it is to be incised or removed (Fig. 23.6). Dissection is facilitated by placing the left hand as distally as possible and compressing the anterior rectal wall.

Attention is then turned to the lateral ligaments and to the middle hemorrhoidal vessels. A single crushing clamp is used, and the lateral ligament and the middle hemorrhoidal vessel transected medial to the clamp. Back-bleeding from the artery rarely occurs, but can be controlled easily and safely by rotating the rectum and directly visualizing the bleeding point. When the lateral ligament has been divided, the rectum on that side is readily mobilized.

The left lateral ligament is divided in a similar way. On completion of this step, the rectum is completely isolated anteriorly, laterally, and posteriorly. A few fibrous strands may require division, but no important vascular structures need to be controlled to complete the pelvic dissection.

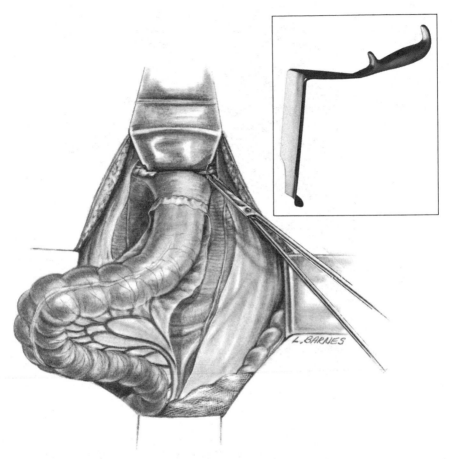

**FIG. 23.5.** Abdominoperineal resection. The anterior peritoneal dissection in the male patient reveals the seminal vesicles and prostate. The mobilization is facilitated by use of the St. Mark's pattern retractor (*inset*).

The sigmoid colon is then held up to the abdominal wound and a point (usually at the apex) is selected for creation of the colostomy. The arcade vessel is then divided.

The site of the colostomy is now prepared by grasping the skin with a Kocher clamp and by excising a disk of skin, the diameter of which should approximate the diameter of the sigmoid colon to be used for the stoma. The subcutaneous, fatty tissue is bluntly retracted (not excised) and the anterior sheath of the rectus muscle is incised in a cruciate fashion (Fig. 23.7A, B). The rectus muscle fibers are then split in a longitudinal direction, and the peritoneal cavity is entered with scissors (Fig. 23.7C). The colostomy aperture in the peritoneum, muscle, and skin should permit the insertion of two fingers. Now, inspect the abdominal wall for possible injury to the inferior epigastric vessels.

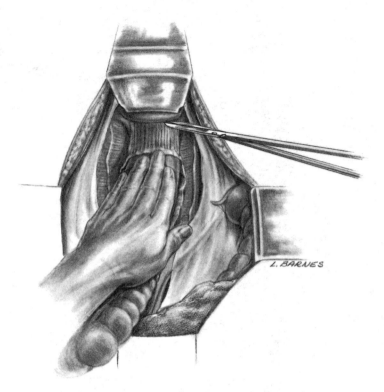

**FIG. 23.6.** Abdominoperineal resection. The posterior vaginal wall is exposed below the retractor. By using the St. Mark's pattern retractor with the turned-back lip, the dissection between the rectum and vagina is facilitated.

A crushing clamp is passed through the colostomy wound into the abdominal cavity to grasp the prepared colon at the site of the proposed stoma. The distal rectosigmoid is also clamped, and the bowel is divided between the two clamps. The proximal bowel is drawn through the abdominal wall to lie without tension on the anterior abdominal surface.

The divided distal bowel is sealed from contamination by grasping it with a doubly gloved hand and tying the removed outer glove over the stump of the rectosigmoid as the clamp is released (Fig. 23.8). The rectum is then delivered through the perineal opening (in a synchronous combined operation) or buried in the pelvic cavity (with the classical Miles approach).

When certain that hemostasis has been established, place Kocher clamps on the cut edge of the peritoneum. By gentle finger dissection and judicious use of the scissors, the peritoneum is mobilized to a degree that permits closure without tension; a continuous absorbable suture is suggested. Closure of the lateral paracolostomy opening (gutter) is not recommended. Too often, a narrow opening results if a suture cuts through or breaks; a large defect is preferred to a narrow one.

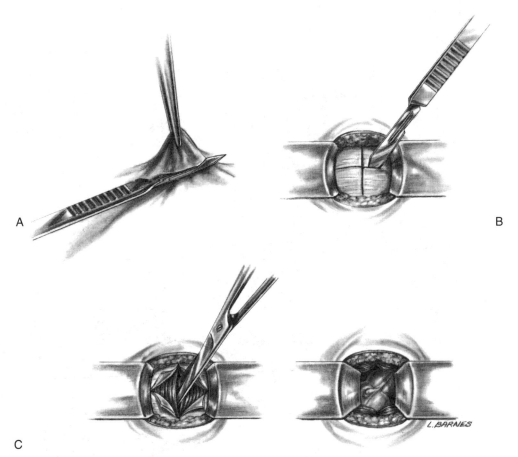

**FIG. 23.7.** Abdominoperineal resection. Creating the abdominal wall opening for the colostomy. **A.** A cruciate incision is made in the anterior rectus fascia. **B.** The rectus muscle is split longitudinally. **C.** The completed abdominal wall opening.

Following abdominal wound closure, the redundant bowel is excised and the colostomy primarily "matured" by using approximately eight sutures of no. 4-0 chromic catgut through the full thickness of the bowel and the skin.

### Perineal Dissection

In the synchronous-combined excision, the perineal dissection is commenced as soon as the abdominal operator determines that the lesion is resectable. If two teams are not available, the perineal portion of the operation is performed after the entire abdominal operation has been completed, and the pelvic peritoneum has been closed above the stump of the rectosigmoid. Under no circumstances should the perineal operation be undertaken initially.

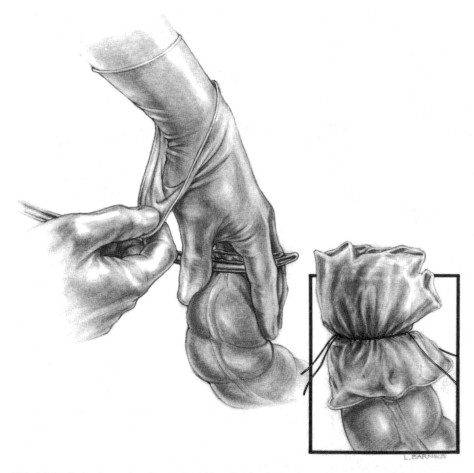

**FIG. 23.8.** Abdominoperineal resection. The distal colonic stump is encompassed by a rubber glove, then everted and secured with heavy ligatures (*inset*).

An elliptical incision is made outside of the sphincter muscle, including a generous margin of perianal skin (Fig. 23.9). The skin edges are grasped with Kocher clamps. The dissection is carried out at least initially with electrocautery, and the assistant clamps any bleeding vessel with a curved hemostat. Usually, two vascular bundles are encountered lying anteriorly and posteriorly on either side in the ischiorectal fat. These are the inferior hemorrhoidal vessels (Fig. 23.10).

Once the ischiorectal fossa has been entered, a self-retaining retractor facilitates the exposure. The anterior dissection proceeds by incising the deep transverse perineal muscle. The presacral space is now entered by dividing the rectococcygeus, commencing at the level of the tip of the coccyx (Fig. 23.11). The coccyx is not removed unless the tumor proves to be so large that it cannot be delivered through the perineal opening. Care should be taken to dissect sufficiently anterior to the

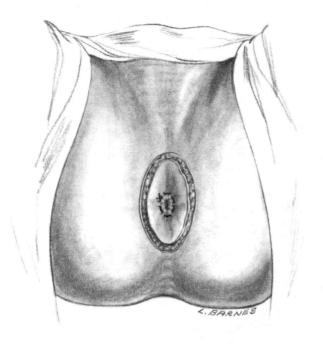

**FIG. 23.9.** Perineal dissection. An elliptical incision is made outside the anus.

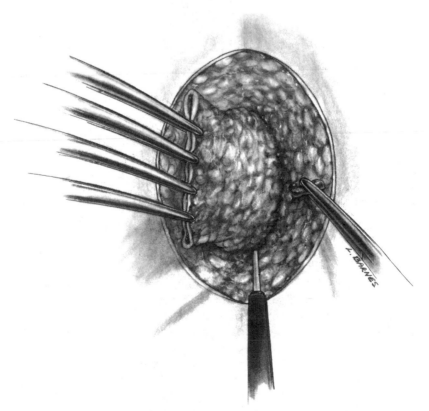

**FIG. 23.10.** Perineal dissection. Serial Kocher clamps are applied to the perianal skin and the incision is deepened. The inferior hemorrhoidal vessels are clamped and divided.

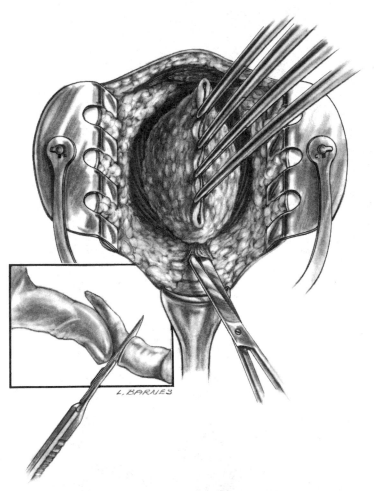

**FIG. 23.11.** Perineal dissection. The presacral space is entered, usually at the level of the tip of the coccyx. If necessary, the coccyx can be disarticulated (*inset*).

sacrum. Conversely, be careful not to dissect too far anteriorly because of the risk of entering the rectum. This is particularly likely to occur if the tumor is relatively fixed posteriorly. With the synchronous combined operation, the abdominal operator can direct the perineal surgeon into the proper plane. The rectum and anus should now be free in the midline posteriorly.

After the presacral space is entered, a finger is swept across the superior aspect of the levator muscles on the left and right sides of the pelvis. The levatores are then divided near the pelvic wall attachments with scissors or electrocautery. This is a relatively avascular dissection (Fig. 23.12).

Sometimes one or both lateral ligaments are divided from below. The perineal operator must take care to avoid injury to the ureters by this maneuver. The peri-

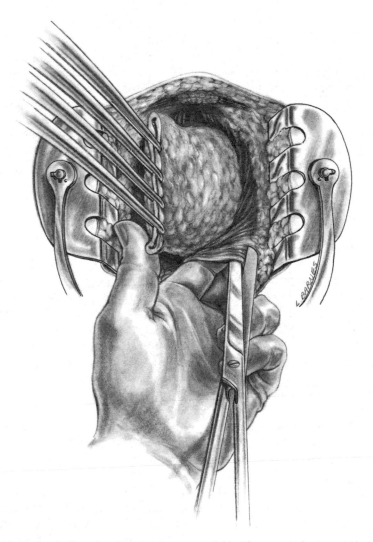

**FIG. 23.12.** Perineal dissection. The levatores are divided from posterior to anterior on each side.

neal operator cuts the distal ureter more frequently during combined abdominoperineal resection than does the abdominal surgeon.

The proximal rectum can now be delivered out of the pelvis. By vigorous traction, the remaining attachments of the rectourethralis muscle and fascia in the region of the urethra are sharply divided. By palpating the catheter, the surgeon should be able to determine the location of the urethra and avoid it.

After the bowel has been removed, the perineal wound is copiously irrigated with saline solution and the skin closed. (I do not advocate continuous irrigation or irrigating with antibiotics, although some have advocated these maneuvers.) No attempt is made to reapproximate the levatores in a cancer operation, a different approach than when proctectomy is performed for inflammatory bowel disease (see Chapter 29). A closed suction drain (e.g., Jackson-Pratt) is placed into the pelvic cavity and brought out, either through the incision, itself, a stab wound in the abdominal wall, or preferably through a stab wound in the buttock. In any case the perineal wound is closed primarily.

As mentioned, diffuse bleeding from pelvic veins can persist because of difficulty encountered because of tumor extension, prior pelvic surgery, or dissection in the improper plane. Under these circumstances, packing the pelvis with gauze usually controls the source of the bleeding. If this is necessary, the packing is left in place for 3 to 4 days and then removed at the bedside with the aid of a narcotic analgesic.

### "Nerve-Preserving" Operation

Urinary and sexual dysfunction are common sequelae of abdominoperineal resection (see later). Impotence is directly related to the extent of lateral pelvic dissection, hence, my reluctance to perform so-called "radical lymphadenectomy" as a routine in the treatment of rectal cancer. Injury to the sacral parasympathetic nerves, especially in relation to the lateral ligaments where their course may be variable, is a clear risk. In recent years, a number of publications have addressed the issue of autonomic nerve-preserving pelvic wall dissections, which theoretically combine the benefits of *en bloc* parietal pelvic dissection with nerve preservation.

The technique involves identification, dissection, and preservation of the hypogastric (sympathetic) nerves from above the aortic bifurcation to a point anteriad to the lateral ligaments of the rectum. Preservation of the sympathetic nerves can be readily achieved because they can be clearly visualized. Identification of the parasympathetic nerves is another matter, and I see no difference with the methods described than that which has previously been presented. Frankly, as will be discussed, the preoperative libido seems to be the most important issue with respect to postoperative potency, not the nature of the dissection, except, of course if an ultraradical operation is performed.

### Perineal Dissection in Women

Unless the tumor is very small and exophytic, or localized only to the posterior wall of the rectum, a posterior vaginectomy should always be performed coincident with an abdominoperineal resection. Remember, the distance between the rectum and vagina, in some areas, is less than 1 mm. For distal lesions, excision of the lower one third or the lower portion of the posterior vaginal wall may be all that is required; for more extensive or more proximal tumors, the vagina should be excised to the level of the posterior cul-de-sac (Fig. 23.13).

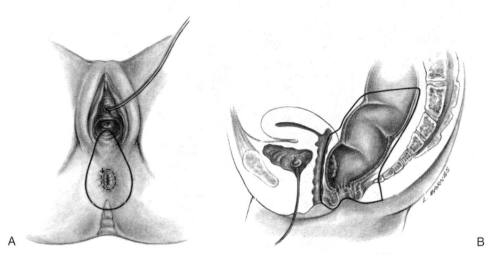

**FIG. 23.13.** Perineal dissection in women. **A.** Outline of the incision for excising the posterior vaginal wall. **B.** Lateral view showing the extent of removal.

Following posterior vaginectomy, the perineal skin closure is carried out until the forchette has been reconstituted. The posterior vaginal defect is left open, but the cut edges are sutured with an absorbable material for hemostasis. A drain is brought out through the defect in the vaginal wall rather than through the perineum. The vagina will eventually heal with minimal or no narrowing, depending on the extent of the vaginectomy. Obviously, if much of the vagina is removed, a stenosis will result.

### Concomitant Hysterectomy

Hysterectomy concomitant with abdominoperineal resection should not be done routinely, unless the presence of the uterus precludes visualization of the area of dissection. However, if the tumor breaches the muscular wall with invasion of the cervix, lower uterine segment, or body of the uterus, an "incontinuity" hysterectomy must be performed to adequately extirpate the tumor.

The incision of the peritoneum in the floor of the pelvis must be wider than that for abdominoperineal resection (Fig. 23.14). Both ureters are in greater danger of injury when this operation is performed. Therefore, they should be clearly identified virtually throughout their lengths. The peritoneum is swept off the uterus, and the bladder is bluntly pushed away from the cervix and vaginal wall. The infundibulopelvic and round ligaments are cross-clamped, divided, and ligated (Fig. 23.15). The broad ligament is dissected away from the pelvic wall, exposing the uterine artery. By retraction of the uterus to the contralateral side, the uterine artery is cross-clamped, divided, and ligated. Division of the cardinal ligament poses the greatest threat to the ureter. If the tumor approaches this area, the cardinal ligament should be clamped close to the pelvic wall; thus, the ureter

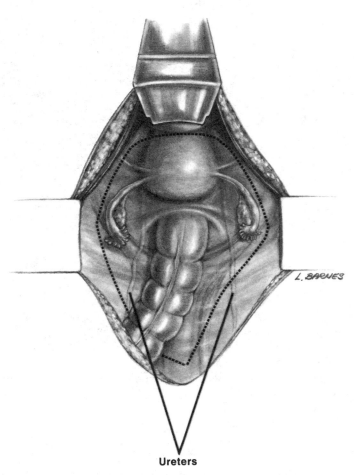

**Ureters**

**FIG. 23.14.** Hysterectomy concomitant with abdominoperineal resection. Peritoneal incision (*dotted line*) must be wide to incorporate the uterus and rectum for removal in continuity.

must be clearly visualized (Fig. 23.16). I prefer to use a single curved Kocher clamp, dividing the tissue on the medial aspect, a maneuver analogous to the technique used to divide the lateral ligaments. The clamp is replaced more distally after each suture ligature is tied.

When the dissection has been completed on both sides, the anterior vaginal wall is incised and the posterior vaginal wall removed with the proctectomy specimen. The vagina can be closed or left open to facilitate drainage, depending on how much of the posterior vaginal wall has been excised.

### Oophorectomy

Metastatic disease apparent at the time of surgery is an indication for therapeutic oophorectomy, but the value of prophylactic oophorectomy has been the

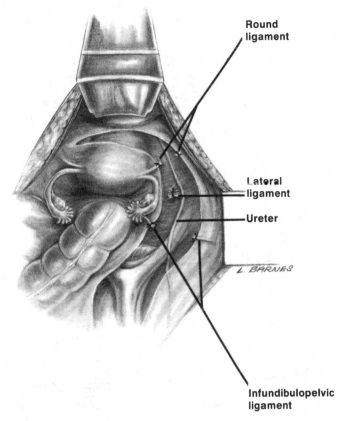

Round ligament

Lateral ligament

Ureter

L. BARNES

Infundibulopelvic ligament

**FIG. 23.15.** Concomitant hysterectomy. The uterus and rectum are mobilized on the right side by dividing the round, infundibulopelvic, and lateral ligaments.

subject of debate. This controversy is discussed in Chapter 22, but it appears that the prevention of primary ovarian cancer is probably the main benefit. With the low incidence of microscopic metastatic involvement, it is difficult to justify prophylactic oophorectomy in the premenopausal age group, but removal of the ovaries in the postmenopausal patient appears a reasonable course. Parenthetically, oophorectomy is as appropriate for cecal carcinoma as it is for a rectal or sigmoid lesion.

### Reconstruction of the Pelvic Floor

One of the concerns expressed in the application of postoperative as well as preoperative radiotherapy is the possibility of injury to the small bowel. The likelihood of such a complication is considerably reduced if doses do not exceed 50 Gy. However, evidence suggests that if higher dosages are applied recurrence rates may diminish. A number of techniques have been suggested to minimize radiation to this relatively vulnerable organ by excluding the small bowel from

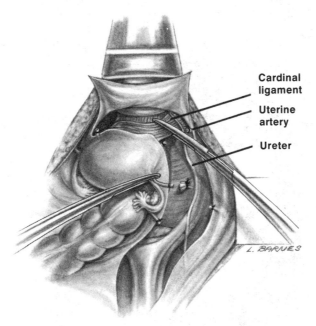

**FIG. 23.16.** Concomitant hysterectomy. The uterine artery has been divided, and the cardinal ligament is clamped. The ureter is extremely vulnerable to injury at this point.

the pelvis. These include suturing the terminal ileum and its mesentery around the linea terminalis, constructing an omental envelope; and using a synthetic absorbable or nonabsorbable mesh sling, a breast prosthesis, and a synthetic polymer mold. The possibility of infection with nonabsorbable material is, of course, a concern, as well as an inconvenience if it must be removed. The concern for failure to maintain the small bowel in the proper position during the course of the treatment must also be considered.

*Technique.* I prefer to use either Dexon or Vicryl mesh for this procedure, a technique which is recommended whenever postoperative radiation, following either abdominoperineal resection or even anterior resection, is being considered. Commencing at the level of the sacral promontory, the mesh is anchored. Using a continuous, locking suture technique, the mesh is anchored laterally on each side to the peritoneum. The mesh is then brought to the anterior abdominal wall and secured in place, creating a halter or sling that keeps the small bowel out of the pelvis.

### Incidental Appendectomy

Incidental appendectomy is not recommended at the time of proctectomy or with any bowel resection. It is sufficiently difficult to evaluate postoperative lower abdominal signs and symptoms, fever, and leukocytosis, without adding an unnecessary variable.

## Sacrectomy and Exenteration

Total pelvic exenteration is defined as the removal of the distal colon and rectum, along with the lower ureters, bladder, internal reproductive organs, perineum, draining lymph nodes, and pelvic peritoneum.

*Comment*: Operative mortality has been reported at 8% to 10%, but it is often difficult to interpret the results of this procedure from the literature because the indications are variable and may include a large percentage of individuals with carcinoma of the uterine cervix. Furthermore, a major problem with most published studies is that, to report more than an anecdotal experience, authors tend to supplement their reports with patients who have limited follow-up. Certainly, it is an option for locally recurrent, invasive disease.

## Postoperative Care

An indwelling catheter should be left in place for 5 to 7 days, longer if the patient has had a history of difficulty in voiding or has prostatic hypertrophy. Generally, women have fewer problems with micturition following abdominoperineal resection than men.

A nasogastric tube is not routinely used. With reasonably expeditious surgery and no intraoperative complications or extenuating circumstances, most patients tolerate the absence of a tube very well. Occasionally, a patient complains of nausea, but antiemetic medication usually suffices. If vomiting ensues, a nasogastric tube should be placed until gas is passed or gastric output is minimal.

A concerted effort is made to institute oral feedings as soon as the patient can tolerate it. Flatus from the stoma may not be necessary before advancement of diet. Generally, a progressive diet is instituted, advancing through full liquids and then to a selected diet, usually over 2 to 3 days.

Early ambulation is advised following abdominoperineal resection. Patients may be asked to sit or stand the evening of surgery and encouraged to walk on the first postoperative day. Fear of evisceration through the perineal wound is not justified. The use of a foam rubber donut will ameliorate the patient's discomfort.

The perineal drain is removed on the third postoperative day, if the drainage is less than 75 mL in 24 hours. Otherwise, it is left in place until the drainage reaches this level. If the wound has been left open, it is vigorously irrigated with saline, three times daily. If the drainage appears foul, one-half strength Dakin's solution or povidone-iodine (Betadine) is used. Sitz baths, which are also useful for comfort, are advised immediately following the irrigation. Sitz baths alone, however, are inadequate for cleansing the perineal cavity. Hematoma, pus, and debris are effectively removed only by irrigation.

If the perineal wound required packing, the pack is removed at 3 or 4 days. This is done at the bedside and usually requires a parenteral narcotic. Rarely, is it necessary to return the patient to the operating room to remove the pack.

## Complications

Complications following abdominoperineal resection are extremely common, with reported incidences in the range of 60%.

### *Intraoperative Complications*

Injury to small bowel usually is easily dealt with by standard reparative techniques, as long as the problem is recognized at the time of surgery. Likewise, slippage of ligatures on vessels or injury to vessels can be readily addressed by conventional hemostatic maneuvers.

By far the greatest fear that confronts the surgeon performing an abdominoperineal resection is that of injury to the ureter. However, the operator can take some solace in the fact that, in most cases, recognition of the injury at that time usually leads to a good functional result through the application of proper principles of repair. The degree of difficulty in effecting a delayed repair is much greater, and the results of such maneuvers are not as successful when compared with early recognition. The same techniques are applicable in the situation when part of the ureter is intentionally excised as a consequence of invasion by tumor.

### *Ureteral Injury*

Despite advances in the surgical treatment of patients, ureteral injuries still occur relatively frequently during pelvic operations, especially hysterectomy, low anterior resection, and abdominoperineal resection. It is because of this risk that it is often helpful to have the benefit of CT or a preoperative intravenous pyelogram, so that the surgeon can embark on repair knowing the status of urinary tract anatomy. It is also useful to know that the patient had two functioning kidneys before the operation. Injury to the ureter usually occurs at one of three points during removal of the rectum.

First, during the ligation of the inferior mesenteric vessels, the left ureter can be incorporated in the ligature or divided when the vessels themselves are divided. Care must be taken to displace the left ureter laterally, away from the vascular pedicle. Also, when dividing the inferior mesenteric vessels, always look a second time to be certain that the left ureter is out of harm's way.

The second area of injury occurs deep in the pelvis and is produced usually coincident with the division of the lateral ligaments. The ureter is particularly exposed to danger if a synchronous hysterectomy is being carried out. Retracting both ureters laterally and visualizing them throughout their lengths reduces the risk of injury. However, this is often cumbersome and unnecessary if the growth is not adherent to the pelvic wall or if no prior surgery has caused displacement. A practical means for avoiding ureteral injury during the course of division of the lateral ligaments is to use only one clamp. Minimal dissection is required, and so there is less likelihood of incorporating the ureter in the laterally placed hemostat. Back-bleeding is rarely evident, but it can be easily controlled by separate applications of a clamp with the rectum freed and the vascular area rotated anteriorly.

Use of ureteral catheters does not necessarily protect the ureter from harm. However, when repeated pelvic surgery is performed or when a difficult dissection is expected, preoperative placement of ureteral catheters can aid the surgeon in identifying the structures. If the ureter and the catheter are divided, the injury is usually self-evident.

Injury to the lower ureter is more likely to occur during synchronous-combined abdominoperineal resection than if the single-team approach is used. If the lateral ligaments are divided from below or blind scissors dissection is employed, the ureter can be unknowingly injured. Great care must be taken by the perineal surgeon when dividing the ligaments or when dissecting in the supralevator area.

The third area of vulnerability is a consequence of mobilization of the peritoneum and the closure of the pelvic peritoneal floor. One or both ureters may be divided as the peritoneum is elevated, or they may be incorporated in the suture during the closure. It is imperative that the ureters be clearly visualized during the reperitonealization maneuver and that they be displaced laterally.

Only 20% to 30% of ureteral injuries are recognized at the time of operation. If concerned about the possibility of ureteral injury during a difficult pelvic dissection, the injury site can be identified by injecting 12.5 g of mannitol intravenously followed by the intravenous administration of 5 mL of indigo carmine dye. The presence of a blue stain in the operative field is diagnostic of injury. If the distal ureter cannot be identified, a cystotomy should be made and a ureteral catheter placed through the ureteral orifice until it presents in the operative field. If ligation without penetration is suspected, a proximal linear ureterotomy permits antegrade insertion of a ureteral catheter to test the patency.

As suggested, most ureteral injuries probably go unrecognized and, indeed, may forever be unrecognized if a single ureter has been ligated. Flank pain, fever, leukocytosis, and tenderness are the most often presenting signs and symptoms of ureteral ligation during the early postoperative period. Urinary fistula can be suspected if copious serous or serosanguineous perineal wound drainage occurs in the early postoperative period. A blue stain appearing on the perineal or abdominal wound dressing after intravenous administration of indigo carmine confirms the diagnosis.

Late urinary fistula can occur because of ureteral necrosis from devascularization injury, from the membranous urethra, or from the base of the bladder.

### Treatment

With crush injury from a hemostat or with partial ligation, removing the ligature and performing a limited repair or tube decompression requires careful patient selection to avoid postoperative difficulties. Occasionally, if the patient's poor general condition precludes prolonging the operation by the performance of a definitive reconstruction, a temporary feeding-tube proximal diversion can be used. Proximal ureteral ligation with the expectation of renal death in the patient at poor risk who has a limited life expectancy is generally to be condemned because of the complications of sepsis and fistula formation. Also exercise concern regarding the function of the contralateral kidney.

*Injury to the lower ureter.* Ureteroneocystotomy is the procedure of choice for injuries of the pelvic ureter. Injuries within 5 cm of the bladder and often at greater distances are suitable for this approach. The procedure achieves an antirefluxing ureteral anastomosis.

A midline cystotomy is made, and 3 mL of saline solution is injected through a 23-gauge needle, raising a small bleb of mucosa. An ellipse of mucosa is excised, and a 3-cm submucosal tunnel is created with a right-angle clamp (Fig. 23.17). The clamp is then rotated to point through the bladder wall, and the detrusor muscle is pierced. The distal ureter is pulled through the tunnel with the aid of traction sutures and spatulated for approximately 1 cm. A no. 6 or no. 8 French catheter is inserted to make certain that the ureter pursues a direct course. The ureter is then sutured to the bladder with interrupted no. 5-0 chromic catgut sutures. Deep bites of detrusor must be included in the two distal sutures at the 5 and 7 o'clock positions to help restore normal ureterovesical function. A no. 5 feeding tube, used as a ureteral stent, is brought out alongside a suprapubic cystotomy catheter. It is removed on the seventh day.

Ureteral reimplantation into the bladder is the best method for restoring continuity following ureteral injury; every effort should be made to accomplish this. If the ureter cannot be brought down without tension, a Boari bladder flap tube technique can be used, or preferably a so-called "psoas bladder hitch maneuver" can be used. These techniques are best accomplished by a urologist who is familiar with the specialized approaches to ureterovesical surgery. It is always wise to take advantage of the availability of urologic consultation when injury to the urinary tract has occurred.

Transureteroureterostomy is another alternative that can be used for the injured ureter. However, because of the possibility of injury to the recipient ureter, it should be used only sparingly and then limited to injuries of the upper pelvic ureter when reimplantation cannot be accomplished. The technique is shown in Figure 23.18. The injured ureter should be resected at a point of certain viability, taking care to preserve the adventitia and blood supply. The recipient ureter should not be mobilized from its bed.

*Injury to the mid- and upper ureter.* Injuries to the proximal ureter are the most difficult and least satisfactory to treat. Fortunately, this is a rare complication of bowel surgery. Because of the distance, reimplantation into the bladder is not possible, and the blood supply is less adequate. Direct repair by end-to-end ureteroureterostomy is the treatment of choice. With loss of ureteral length from excision or necrosis, defects of up to 8 cm can be traversed by this method using a renal-lowering technique. If direct repair is impossible, consider the highly specialized techniques of ileal interposition and autotransplantation. Nephrec-

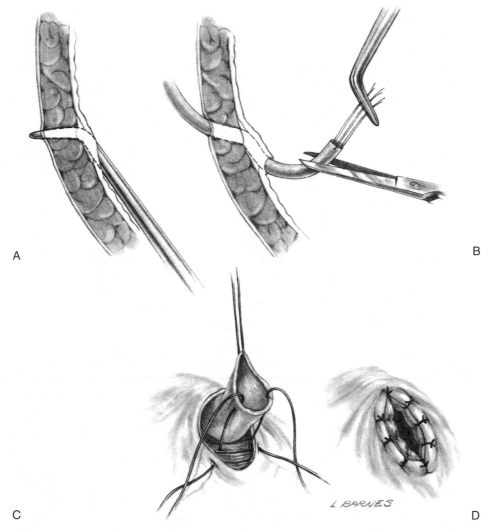

**FIG. 23.17.** Ureteroneocystotomy. **A.** A right-angle clamp pierces the detrusor muscle. **B.** The ureter is pulled through the submucosal tunnel; the distal ureter is cut at a 45° angle, creating a new ureteral meatus. **C.** The ureter is anchored to the bladder detrusor muscle. **D.** Completion of the anastomosis to the bladder mucosa. (Adapted from Libertino JA, Zinman L. Technique for ureteroneocystotomy in renal transplantation and reflux. *Surg Clin North Am* 1973;53:459.)

tomy can be used if the surgeon is satisfied that contralateral kidney function is adequate and calculous disease or other conditions that might affect the kidney are not present.

Whenever a direct repair of a ureteral injury is performed, proximal diversion is advised. The cut edges of the ureter are debrided and spatulated, and the kid-

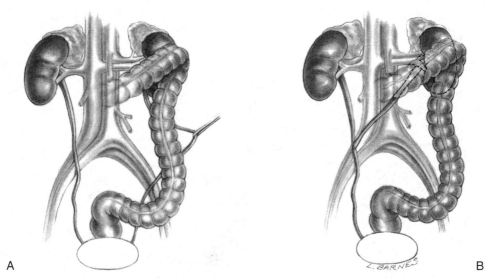

A                                                              B

**FIG. 23.18.** Transureteroureterostomy. **A.** A tunnel is developed by retroperitoneal dissection after exposure of the upper ureter lateral to the colon. **B.** The ureter is brought across the retroperitoneal space and anastomosed. (Adapted from Libertino JA, Zinman L. Technique for ureteroneocystotomy in renal transplantation and reflux. *Surg Clin North Am* 1973;53:459.)

ney, ureter, or both are adequately mobilized. The ureter is spatulated on opposing sides of each end to prevent stricture (Fig. 23.19A). Anastomosis is effected with interrupted no. 5-0 chromic catgut or long-term absorbable sutures placed full thickness, with the knots on the outside, inverting the mucosa (Fig. 23.19B). Noncrushing, vascular forceps can be used to grasp the tissue; the presence of a catheter within the lumen facilitates the procedure. A continuous suture should never be used. The ureter can be wrapped in omentum if the anastomosis is felt to be precarious. A soft rubber drain (Penrose) is placed at the site of the uretero-ureterostomy and brought out through a stab wound. The stent is removed on postoperative day 10, followed by the drain 48 hours later (if no urine drainage is present).

Before discharge, an intravenous pyelogram should be performed for all patients who have ureteral repair, to determine the adequacy of the reconstruction.

### Bladder Injury

Bladder injury that is recognized at the time of surgery can usually be repaired by a layered closure of no. 2-0 chromic catgut or long-term absorbable suture. When injury to the bladder neck or trigone has occurred, great care must be taken to avoid incorporating the distal ureters in the suture. A cystotomy with insertion of small catheters in a retrograde fashion through the ureteral orifices

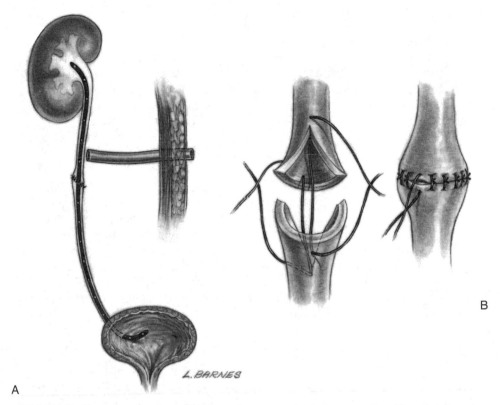

A

B

**FIG. 23.19.** Ureteroureterostomy. **A.** The ureters are spatulated on opposing sides of each end to achieve oblique anastomosis. **B.** The edges are approximated with interrupted fine catgut sutures placed through the full thickness of the ureteral wall, inverting the mucosa. (Adapted from Libertino JA, Zinman L. Technique for ureteroneocystotomy in renal transplantation and reflux. *Surg Clin North Am* 1973;53:459.)

is useful to prevent this complication. Drainage of the area is advised. Suprapubic cystotomy is prudent when the injury is to the bladder neck or trigone.

### Urethral Injury

Injury to the urethra occurs most often as a result of too vigorous electrocoagulation in the prostatic area. Also, tumor can invade the prostate and, in attempting to perform a curative resection, the prostatic urethra may be entered. External trauma can cause a delayed urethral stricture, which may require catheterization or subsequent reconstruction. If injury to this area is recognized at the time of proctectomy, direct repair or urethroplasty may be indicated. A urologist should be consulted if the surgeon is not experienced with reparative approaches.

### Seminal Vesicle Injury

Injury to the seminal vesicles probably occurs much more frequently than is generally suspected. This may be responsible for some problems related to fertility, but should otherwise be of no consequence. However, seminal vesicle–rectal fistulae have been reported. Also, a fistula to the perineum following an abdominoperineal resection has been seen. Treatment in this case included percutaneous drainage of the abscess, antibiotics, and oral administration of finasteride (Proscar).

## Postoperative Complications

### Perineal Hemorrhage

Returning the patient to the operating room is certainly a defeat for the surgeon and a risk to the patient. Fortunately, perineal hemorrhage can usually be controlled by opening the perineal wound and finding the bleeding vessel or by packing. Occasionally, however, laparotomy must be redone. This complication is usually preventable. Perineal wound hemostasis should be adequate before the patient is permitted to leave the operating room. If the bleeding is so diffuse that a specific vessel cannot be identified, packing with or without a supplementary hemostatic agent may be necessary.

### Necrotic Colostomy

By preserving the first branch of the artery, blood supply to the descending colon and residual sigmoid colon is less likely to be impaired. Despite this precaution, division of the inferior mesenteric artery or one of its major branches can result in necrosis or frank gangrene of the bowel. This occurs when the colon receives much or all of its vascular supply from the inferior mesenteric artery. Although the use of Doppler ultrasound or the intravenous injection of 5 mL of fluorescein dye, followed by the use of a long-wave ultraviolet lamp have been advocated, such relatively esoteric studies are unnecessary, because bowel ischemia can usually be assessed adequately by clinical inspection alone.

Despite careful attention to the viability of the intestine, the colostomy at the time of abdominal wound closure may appear ischemic. This is usually noted when the surgeon has difficulty creating the stoma, either because of the patient's obesity or because of tension on the bowel itself. By making certain that sufficient bowel is available to create the stoma without tension and by preparing a large enough opening in the abdominal wall, this difficulty can be avoided.

If the bowel looks ischemic, it probably is ischemic. The optimal time to redo the stoma is at the time of the laparotomy. The treatment of stomal problems is addressed in Chapter 31.

### Intestinal Obstruction

Small bowel obstruction is not uncommon following abdominoperineal resection. Some element of ileus is normally present for a few days following surgery, but if flatus fails to pass by the sixth or seventh postoperative day, entertain the possibility that obstruction is present. The incidence of obstruction is approximately 3% in patients having this operation.

Obstruction is most commonly caused by adhesions between loops of bowel, a complication that can occur after laparotomy for any purpose, but two specific situations are directly related to abdominoperineal resection: (a) herniation below the pelvic floor and (b) herniation through the lateral colostomy space. The former usually occurs when the suture breaks or pulls out of the peritoneum, leaving a hole through which a loop of small intestine descends and becomes entrapped. Repair requires liberation of the bowel and closure of the defect. Rarely, the loop of bowel descends to the perineal skin or actually through the wound. Gangrene can also occur, but this is also unusual.

Herniation of the small bowel through the defect in the lateral gutter can produce a small bowel obstruction. Although some recommend a purse-string, interrupted, or continuous suture to close the space, and others prefer an extraperitoneal approach, I like to leave the defect widely patent on the theory that entrapment is less likely to take place if the opening is sufficiently large.

If surgery is required, the bowel is reduced and the opening enlarged. If the gutter had been left open and herniation with obstruction did occur, it is probably wise to attempt closure of the defect.

### Urinary Retention and Infection or Bladder Dysfunction

Urinary tract infection and urinary retention are the most common complications following abdominoperineal or low anterior resection, with an incidence of 20% to 40%. Wide iliopelvic lymphadenectomy increases the risk of voiding difficulties. Urinary retention can be caused by injury to the sympathetic or parasympathetic nerves to the bladder, the result of postoperative distention, local trauma, prostatic hypertrophy, or prolapse of the bladder into the pelvis.

The most important preventive maneuver is that of retaining a Foley catheter in place for 5 to 7 days. The catheter is removed at 6:00 a.m. and the voiding pattern carefully observed. If the patient is unable to void or urinates frequently in small amounts, a residual urine determination should be made. If it is more than 300 mL, the catheter should be reinserted and left for an additional 2 or 3 days. During this interval, it is reasonable to place the patient on bethanechol chloride (Urecholine; 25 to 50 mg), four times daily. This is suggested in an effort to improve detrusor tone. Urodynamic studies are advised if the patient is unable to void after the catheter has been removed.

A cystometrogram usually will demonstrate a flaccid type of bladder, but the urethral pressure profile will probably be normal. It is important to determine the external sphincter electromyogram (EMG). Often, after an abdominoperineal resection, the internal pudendal nerve is compromised, and the patient loses the innervation of the external sphincter. Continence, therefore, is maintained by the internal sphincter or bladder neck mechanism only. The cystometrogram, urethral pressure profile, and external sphincter EMG should be correlated with the anatomic findings of cystourethroscopy. If the patient has an obstructed prostate and a normal sphincter EMG, then it is reasonable to carry out a transurethral resection. It is safer, however, to defer prostatectomy for 6 weeks in a patient who has recently had abdominoperineal resection, to minimize the risk of a urinary–perineal fistula. If the external sphincter EMG shows a flaccid external sphincter, it would be unwise to carry out a transurethral resection of the prostate or any form of prostatectomy for fear of making the patient incontinent. Under these circumstances, it is advisable to leave the catheter in place for 6 weeks to 2 months, or to instruct the patient in the use of intermittent catheterization. It is hoped that this respite will allow the bladder residual urine to be of small enough volume to avoid overdistension of the bladder and decompensation of the detrusor musculature. Intermittent catheterization is preferable to patient incontinence.

Current urologic practice discourages clamping and unclamping the catheter in an attempt to restore detrusor tone. If the goal of keeping the bladder empty is achieved, the detrusor tone will ultimately return.

In women, the procedure is essentially the same as that described above. If the woman has difficulty voiding after an additional period of catheter drainage and treatment with bethanechol, she should be taught the technique of intermittent self-catheterization until the bladder tone returns and normal voiding occurs. Self-catheterization is an option in men also.

## Perineal Wound Sepsis

Perineal sepsis is not uncommon following abdominoperineal resection. It can be caused by contamination at the time of proctectomy from injury to the rectal wall, fecal spillage, the presence of a perforated carcinoma, an infected hematoma, or the presence of perineal disease (e.g., fistula or abscess). A prolonged operative time can also predispose to the subsequent development of sepsis.

Characteristically, the patient develops a low-grade fever on the third or fourth postoperative day, which progresses to a higher spiking fever elevation. In the absence of another obvious source for pyrexia, the perineal wound should be carefully explored with a gloved finger. Loculations should be broken and, if necessary, the wound reopened. Irrigating with one-half strength Dakin's solution (using a rubber catheter) is important to remove clot and debris.

## Abdominal Wound Infection and Intraabdominal Sepsis

Although wound infection alone is rarely fatal, it adds considerably to morbidity and prolongs the patient's hospital stay. The incidence of wound infection following abdominoperineal resection is the same as that for any colon resection (<5%).

The necessary ingredients of wound infection are contamination with pathogenic organisms and a susceptible host. Because of the nature of colonic and rectal surgery, some contamination is present in all patients, but a number of factors

**TABLE 23.1.** *Predisposing factors for the development of wound infections after colonic surgery*

| Factor | Infections (%) | Statistical significance |
|---|---|---|
| Preoperative irradiation | 22.2 | $p < 0.04$ |
| Serum albumin <2.9 g/dL | 20.1 | $p < 0.02$ |
| Preoperative stoma | 19.1 | $p < 0.001$ |
| Blood loss >2 U | 17.4 | $p < 0.03$ |
| Crohn's disease | 14.3 | $p < 0.002$ |
| Bowel preparation | | |
|   Other than mechanical preparation and nonabsorbable antibiotic | 14.1 | $p < 0.001$ |
|   Antibiotic other than erythromycin base and neomycin | 7.7 | $p < 0.001$ |
| Operative time >2 h | 11.7 | $p < 0.06$ |

From DeGennaro V, Corman ML, Coller JA, et al. Wound infections after colectomy. *Dis Colon Rectum* 1978;21:567, with permission.

are known to predispose to this complication (Table 23.1). Splenic trauma and the requirement for splenectomy concomitant with any colon operation increases the risk of infection in the early postoperative period. Combined spleen–colon trauma should be an indication rather than a contraindication for splenic salvage.

## Peripheral Neuropathy

The perineolithotomy position has been associated with a number of intraoperative and postoperative complications, especially as related to the compartment syndrome. As mentioned, it is for this reason that special care needs to be taken in positioning the patient to minimize the risk of vascular injury. Another complication that has been noted has been related to the self-retaining retractor, that of femoral neuropathy. This complication has been reported to be a consequence of a number of operations, most commonly inguinal hernia repair. In rare instances, this complication has been associated with the use of the self-retaining Bookwalter retractor. In a slender patient, the same phenomenon can occur if the Balfour retractor is used or if the O'Connor–O'Sullivan instrument is employed. With careful attention to the location of the retractor blades, this complication should be preventable.

## Impotence, Infertility, and Dyspareunia

Impotence following proctectomy for carcinoma of the rectum is the rule rather than the exception, especially in the older age group, and particularly when a wide iliopelvic lymphadenectomy is applied. The resection requires extensive pelvic dissection, which can result in injury to the parasympathetic nerves (nervi erigentes). Additionally, the patient's preoperative sexual function may have been less than adequate, and even minimal trauma may be sufficient to precipitate impotence. Preoperative libido may be the critical issue with respect to postoperative sexual function.

Women seem less likely to experience problems with orgasms, although most reports include a high number of widowed, elderly women who have no sexual partners. Retained menstrual blood, colpitis, chronic discharge from the vagina, and dyspareunia are not uncommon symptoms after proctectomy. In men, infertility can result even if tumescence is not impaired, because of injury to the sympathetic nerves and the consequence of retrograde ejaculation. Injury to the vas or seminal vesicles has also been reported and may be associated with infertility.

Preoperative discussion is probably wise, especially in a relatively young man having abdominoperineal resection. Such an individual may choose to "bank" his sperm before having this operation, or he may elect alternative therapy (e.g., local excision or electrocoagulation).

### Unhealed Perineal Wound and Persistent Perineal Sinus

The problem of delayed healing following proctectomy for cancer is unusual. This is in contradistinction to the frequency of the complication in individuals who have proctectomy for inflammatory bowel disease (see Chapter 29). However, with the increased use of preoperative and postoperative radiation therapy, more individuals are experiencing delay in perineal wound healing. This is a particular concern if the radiation dose approaches 6,000 cGy. A number of techniques have been used to ameliorate the condition and to effect healing, including reoperation and curettage, excision and grafting, muscle transposition, and the use of fibrin adhesive (fibrinogen concentrate and thrombin).

### Perineal Hernia

Symptomatic perineal hernia is a rare, late complication of abdominoperineal resection, with an incidence of less than 1%. The condition is much more common in women. Symptoms can include perineal pressure, fullness, pain, or feeling as if sitting on a lump. The hernia can cause skin breakdown or be associated with an evisceration.

Treatment should be directed to an abdominal or a combined abdominal and perineal approach. Attempting repair from the perineum alone is unlikely to be successful. In principle, the bowel must be delivered out of the pelvis and the pelvic floor reconstituted, usually with mesh such as Marlex. The pelvis should be drained and, if necessary, the redundant skin excised.

### Phantom Sensations

Phantom sensations are common after amputation of extremities, so it is not surprising that patients can experience feelings of an urge to defecate or to pass flatus after rectal excision. These symptoms can occur in up to two thirds of patients. Theoretically, such feelings are a normal response to removal of the rectum, because innervation is still represented at the level of the cerebral cortex. Reassurance and the passage of time usually alleviate patient anxiety.

### Perineal Pain

Intractable pain in the perineum in an individual who has had proctectomy for carcinoma of the rectum is caused by recurrent tumor until proved otherwise. However, patients occasionally complain bitterly of severe, deep-seated pain that is truly analogous to that of levator spasm (proctalgia fugax; see Chapter 16). This is a most difficult problem to treat. Inevitably, sitz baths and analgesic medications are used, with indifferent success. Perineal strengthening exercises and the use of muscle relaxants are more likely to be ameliorative. In a woman, a vaginal stimulating attachment of the electrogalvanic stimulator can be used. Injection with steroids is uniformly unsuccessful. Likewise, the injection of sclerosing agents is fraught with hazard. Despite every available study being negative, persistent pain, unresponsive to any of the above measures, will ultimately prove to be recurrent carcinoma in the vast majority of instances.

### Entrapped Ovary Syndrome

Patients with entrapped ovary syndrome can present with abdominal pain, a mass, or distension. If the ovary is to be preserved, excision of the cyst and oophoropexy is advised. Care should be taken at the time of the initial operation to be certain that the ovary remains as an intraperitoneal structure when the pelvic floor is closed, but because oophorectomy is recommended in all postmenopausal women, this should be a rare complication.

### Stomal Problems

Colostomy retraction, stenosis, prolapse, and hernia, as well as peristomal dermatitis and appliance management problems are discussed in Chapters 31 and 32.

## Results

### *Morbidity and Operative Mortality*

The operative mortality rate following abdominoperineal resection has essentially remained unchanged for more than 40 years, and ranges from 1% to 6.5%. Most institutions report a high complication rate of around 60% following this operation (Fig. 23.20).

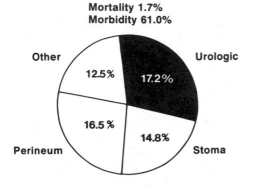

**FIG. 23.20.** Morbidity and mortality following abdominoperineal resection in 230 patients. (From Rosen L, Veidenheimer MC, Coller JA, Corman ML. Mortality, morbidity, and patterns of recurrence after abdominoperineal resection for cancer of the rectum. *Dis Colon Rectum* 1982;25: 202, with permission.)

## Long-Term Results

The 5-year survival in several large experiences is shown in Table 23.2 according to Dukes' classification. In my experience, the uncorrected 5-year survival rate approaches 90% for patients with Dukes' A lesions. This falls to 65% for Dukes' B and 23% for Dukes' C tumors. This is essentially the same as the uncorrected survival rate for colon resections during the same period. The uncorrected survival rate for all patients who had abdominoperineal resection was 54%. The 10-year survival rate is illustrated in Fig. 23.21. It can be appreciated that no significant falloff in survival occurs after 5 years. This implies that it is a rare patient indeed who dies of recurrent cancer of the rectum following this length of time.

Of patients, 40% to 45% develop recurrent cancer. In 25%, the first recurrence is local, whereas in 75%, the initial manifestation of the recurrence is in a distant location.

Patients with a Dukes' A lesion rarely develop a local recurrence. Local recurrence appears much earlier in patients with Dukes' C lesions than in those who initially harbor a Dukes' B tumor. However, once recurrence develops no statistically significant difference is seen in median survival time between the two groups of individuals. Furthermore, no statistically significant difference in survival time is seen, irrespective of whether the initial recurrence was local or distant.

**TABLE 23.2.** *Abdominoperineal resection: 5-yr survival rate*

| Author/Year | Dukes' lesion | A | B | C |
|---|---|---|---|---|
| Dukes/1940 | 93 | 65 | 23 | — |
| Gilbertsen/1960 | 80 | 50 | 23 | |
| Slanetz et al./1972 | 81 | 52 | 33 | |
| MacLennan et al./1976 | 91 | 59 | 25 | |
| Strauss et al./1978 | 82 | 40 | 15 | |
| Walz et al./1977 | 78 | 45 | 22 | |

From Rosen L, Veidenheimer MC, Coller JA, et al. Mortality, morbidity, and patterns of recurrence after abdominoperineal resection for cancer of the rectum. *Dis Colon Rectum* 1982;25: 202, with permission.

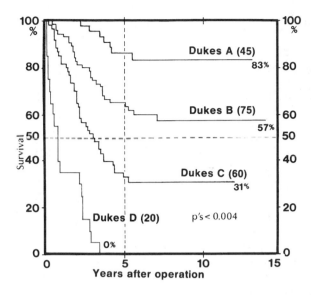

FIG. 23.21. Survival after abdominoperineal resection. (From Rosen L, Veidenheimer MC, Coller JA, Corman ML. Mortality, morbidity, and patterns of recurrence after abdominoperineal resection for cancer of the rectum. *Dis Colon Rectum* 1982;25:202, with permission.)

The incidence of recurrence increases with the length of the follow-up period. Completeness, longer follow-up, and an intensive search for recurrence, including a high autopsy rate, are some of the factors that inevitably yield higher recurrence rates.

### Follow-up Regimen

The appropriateness and timing of the follow-up regimen after resection for rectal cancer have been discussed in Chapter 22. As stated, the potential benefit for individuals from such evaluations following curative surgery has not been proved. Individuals subjected to intense follow-up have recurrence diagnosed earlier and have more operations for recurrence, but survival rates are not significantly improved. However, others have opined that a follow-up program based on carcinoembryonic antigen (CEA) tissue plasminogen activator and CA 19-9 assays is associated with an earlier diagnosis, with a good resectability rate for both metastatic disease and local recurrence.

### Palliative Abdominoperineal Resection

Palliative abdominoperineal resection has been advocated by a number of authors. Individuals who have extensive liver metastases, lung metastases, or disseminated disease (e.g., bone, brain) are poor candidates for this type of resection. Those with ascites or multiple peritoneal implants are also extremely high operative risks. Because of the mean survival time in patients with Dukes' D lesions approximates 1 year, some should be considered for a palliative resection; these include patients with perineal pain, tenesmus, or hemorrhage. If the tumor can be extirpated, a better quality of life may be anticipated.

The fact that there are long-term survivors when so-called "palliative" procedures are performed, implies that some individuals may still be well managed surgically, even though they have locally advanced disease. Extended resection in these patients, if feasible, has the potential of providing excellent palliation and even, occasionally, a cure.

## HARTMANN RESECTION

Occasionally, a patient with metastatic disease can be adequately treated by the so-called "Hartmann resection." The procedure certainly has the potential advantage of removing the symptomatic tumor mass, an important objective in a palliative resection. Unfortunately, when the operation is undertaken in an attempt to cure the patient, the colostomy is often permanent. Despite newer techniques devised to reestablish intestinal continuity, a major procedure is still required. It is for this reason that I do not recommend the Hartmann resection for patients whose disease is potentially curable.

## TREATMENT OF LOCAL RECURRENCE

The treatment of metastatic disease following resection of colorectal carcinoma is presented in Chapter 22. The discussion that follows is limited to the specific problem of recurrence following abdominoperineal resection.

### Symptoms and Diagnosis

One of the concerns expressed with laparoscopic-assisted colon resection for cancer is the apparent increased incidence of trocar site recurrence (see Chapter 27). However, remember that wound recurrence *does* develop following conventional surgical treatment of colorectal cancer, albeit rarely. As with perineal recurrence in general, its presence usually implies more extensive disease.

With perineal recurrence, patients complain of a painful mass. This can be the result of implantation in the skin, but more commonly is a consequence of downward extension of pelvic tumor. Biopsy usually confirms the diagnosis. With pelvic recurrence, the patient may be asymptomatic, but usually will report perineal, pelvic, or low abdominal pain, and the feeling as if sitting on a lump. The pain may radiate to the back, to the buttock, or have a sciatic distribution. If the tumor involves the bladder, prostate, or urethra, urinary symptoms (including hematuria) may develop.

The diagnosis can be made without special studies and without positive biopsy evidence of recurrence, so characteristic is the syndrome. Knowledge of a previously "unfavorable" pathology report is helpful. A mass may be felt in the perineum or in the vagina. CT has been used successfully to delineate both the presence of a tumor mass and the extent of pelvic spread, as well as evidence of ureteral obstruction. It has also been suggested as a potentially valuable study for follow-up evaluation to anticipate recurrence before symptoms appear. CT-guided percutaneous biopsy has been demonstrated to be a particularly useful tool for establishing the histologic diagnosis of recurrent carcinoma in the pelvis. But, as implied, histologic confirmation should not be needed to implement therapy. Elevation of the CEA level is certainly suggestive of recurrent disease, but all too often this laboratory study is within the normal range if the recurrence is confined to the pelvis. This is in contradistinction to those patients who have involvement of the liver or another organ (see Chapter 22). An intravenous pyelogram can be performed, especially if concern exists for impingement on the ureters on the basis of the CT study.

## Surgical

Extensive preoperative investigation is mandatory—including CT. $T_1$- and $T_2$-weighted imaging is important to exclude bony erosion or pelvic side wall involvement. Presence of such tumor extension implies nonresectability and contraindication to exploratory surgery. A list of recommendations follows:

Conduct colon study for local and remote metastases.
Provide ureteral stents.
Schedule case early in the day.
Anticipate need for other specialists.
Ensure availability of experienced assistance.
Plan incision carefully.
Allow for steep Trendelenburg position.
Position patient's arms at the sides.
Use lighted instruments, head lights, or both.
Anticipate excessive blood loss.

This list is only a means for preoperatively reminding the surgeon of the magnitude of reoperative cancer surgery. It is by no means exhaustive.

## Results

Unfortunately, no truly satisfactory treatment is available for perineal or pelvic recurrence. There is, however, the rare instance when perineal (the equivalent of suture line) recurrence develops secondary to implantation or to an inadequate skin excision. It still may be possible to cure the patient by reexcising the perineal wound. However, with recurrent pelvic malignancy, rarely can resection be successfully effected. The only patients likely to have a survival benefit from reoperative pelvic surgery for rectal cancer are those whose disease can be completely resected (an uncommon situation). In a review of more than 200 patients from the Mayo Clinic, 3-year, 5-year, and median survival rates were approximately 57, 34, and 45 months, respectively. Cumulative probability of local failure was 24%, 41%, and 47% at 1, 3, and 5 years, respectively. Others have observed that pelvic recurrence can be safely resected with expectation of long-term survival in approximately one third of cases. Selective application of the approach is strongly recommended to identify those individuals based on known risk factors.

## Radiotherapy

Surgical extirpation for pelvic recurrence has been used for palliation. But radiation therapy has been and continues to be the most effective treatment for palliating symptoms of locally recurrent disease, with palliative benefit lasting from several months up to 10 years. Although most studies demonstrate no significant difference in length of survival, little controversy exists concerning improvement of symptoms. Radiation therapy is effective in the treatment of pain for approximately three fourths of patients. It can also decrease the size of a mass, and for an ulcerating lesion, the amount of perineal or vaginal drainage.

Radiotherapy can be administered to a total of 60 Gy (depending on whether the patient received preoperative treatment; see later). Although some groups recommend short treatments of 20 Gy when symptoms develop rather than a large-dose course, others note no significant difference in response to the three dose levels—40, 50, and 60 Gy. Patients who are severely debilitated can be treated by so-called "hypofractionation"—the delivery of a single large dose (10 Gy) once a month for 3 months.

One of the burdens which the patient and the surgeon may be forced to deal with is the radionecrosis that develops after high-dose radiation therapy for extensive primary or recurrent rectal cancer. Associated complications, such as enterocutaneous fistula, urinary fistula, pelvic abscess, osteomyelitis, and persistent sinuses, further complicate the picture. Treating the foul-smelling discharge, alleviating the pain, and addressing the need for frequent dressing changes are of paramount concern.

### *Intraoperative Radiotherapy*

Intraoperative radiotherapy is discussed later in this chapter as applied to resection of a lesion with sterilization of any residual cells. The procedure is also of value in those individuals who have fixed, unresectable rectal or rectosigmoid lesions. A third application is that of combined management of recurrent cancer.

## Chemotherapy

Other treatment modalities include radium implantation and chemotherapy. Systemic chemotherapy as conventionally administered has not proved beneficial. However, some palliation has been achieved by pelvic intraarterial perfusion of 5-FU. In one study, the percutaneous placement of catheters in the internal iliac arteries, administration of 5-FU and mitomycin-C, and the application of whole-body hyperthermia have been reported to offer better pain relief than that of perfusion chemotherapy alone. Radiosensitizers (5-FU and mitomycin-C) also have been suggested to improve the response to radiotherapy (see later).

## Pain Management

For pain that cannot be effectively treated by radiotherapy and which is no longer responsive to narcotic analgesics, neurosurgical consultation is advised. Placement of epidural, intrathecal, and intraventricular catheters for narcotic drug delivery as well as the use of intrathecal alcohol or chordotomy may be appropriate alternatives in an intractable situation.

## COLOSTOMY OR ILEOSTOMY

A diversionary procedure without resection for cancer of the rectum is applied most frequently when the patient presents with obstruction or an impending obstruction. But the difficult question is whether to perform a rectal excision at that time. The answer depends on a number of factors: (a) the degree of bowel dilatation; (b) whether opportunities exist to "prepare" the colon or to effect an anastomosis; (c) whether the tumor is resectable and supplementary radiotherapy is contemplated; and, of course, (d) the condition of the patient. In general, when the surgeon is confronted with an obstruction, it is probably wiser to perform a colostomy and to return another day. An alternative approach is to consider the methods of antegrade irrigation discussed in Chapter 22, and to resect (with or without an anastomosis). Further options are the use of a Wallstent, other prostheses, and endoscopic, palliative approaches (see later). The techniques of stomal construction are discussed in Chapter 31.

If the patient's primary complaint is bleeding, colostomy is notoriously ineffective. Despite diversion, the bleeding often persists. Palliative abdominoperineal resection is one option and electrocoagulation and laser photocoagulation therapy others (see later). Radiotherapy has not proved to be of benefit in this situation. Another possibility for establishment of hemostasis is the application of gauze soaked in a 1% solution of alum (aluminum ammonium sulfate/aluminum potassium sulfate) as a styptic agent.

## LOW ANTERIOR RESECTION

The first resection of the sigmoid colon was performed in 1833 by Reybard of Lyons, but for the next 100 years practically all operative approaches to the treatment of carcinoma either involved extirpation of the rectum or another sphincter-saving procedure, such as the various modifications of the pull-through operation. It was not until the 1940s, that conventional anastomotic techniques were felt safe enough to be used for most cases of carcinoma of the rectum when intestinal continuity might be reestablished.

### Indications

The most important factor that determines the likelihood of performing an anastomosis is the level of the lesion. Although favorable factors (e.g., good differentiation, diploid histogram, limited bowel wall penetration with endorectal ultrasound, small size, and polypoid configuration) can safely reduce the distal margin of resection to 1 or 2 cm, it is the rare patient who should be considered for a low anterior resection when the tumor is less than 7 cm from the anal verge. When compared with other resective sphincter-saving operations, the low anterior resection is the one that is preferred.

## Technique

The patient can be positioned in the perineolithotomy (Lloyd-Davies) position or supine on the operating table when the surgeon feels confident that an anterior abdominal approach will permit anastomosis by a conventional suture method. An exploratory laparotomy is performed and a determination made of the possibility and advisability of resection.

The initial steps of the procedure are identical to those described for abdominoperineal resection; the splenic flexure is not routinely mobilized. I also do not believe in the so-called "high tie" of the inferior mesenteric artery. Having been satisfied that an anastomosis can be performed, the surgeon's next task is to divide the mesorectum. Right-angle clamps are placed posteriorly and the mesentery divided above the clamps. Tension on the proximal bowel permits separation of the mesentery from the posterior rectal wall. With a very low anastomosis, there is usually little or no mesentery to divide.

### *Total Mesorectal Excision*

Although tumor at the margin of resection and a second primary lesion are potential sources of recurrent disease, in all probability, these are uncommon causes of recurrence. It is generally believed that most suture-line recurrences are caused by residual tumor left in the pelvis (the so-called tangential or lateral margin) that subsequently grows into the lumen through the anastomosis.

A number of reports have emphasized the importance of mesorectal spread of the tumor in determining the risk of recurrence and survival. Emphasis has been placed on removing the *tongue* of mesorectum, with total mesorectal excision, to reduce the incidence of recurrence. In theory, failure to excise the mesorectum completely has the potential to leave gross or microscopic residual disease, which can predispose to local failure.

One of the concerns that has been expressed is the increased morbidity associated with removing the mesentery to the rectum distal to the anastomosis. Devascularization can be a consequence, with an increased incidence of anastomotic leak. Others express enthusiasm for the technique, commenting also that the procedure is compatible with autonomic nerve preservation as well as sphincter preservation.

The problem remains: When an abdominoperineal resection is performed (removing all of the mesorectum), the risk of recurrence in the pelvis is significantly greater than that reported by investigators who advise total mesorectal excision. For me, this is a conundrum that defies explanation. The fact is, local recurrence has been demonstrated to be closely related to tumor at the lateral rectal margins. As with abdominoperineal resection, total mesorectal excision adds nothing to the conventional operation when a surgeon is faced with lateral tumor spread.

### *Lymphadenectomy*

A number of surgeons continue to recommend systemic lymphadenectomy with lateral node dissection to minimize the likelihood of recurrence. With respect to inguinal node metastases from rectal adenocarcinoma, an unusual manifestation indeed, 5-year survivors are rare, irrespective of the method of management.

### *Conventional Suturing*

A crushing clamp is applied, usually 5 cm below the distal margin of the tumor; an angled or curved clamp placed in the anteroposterior plane is preferred. Only one is used.

Anchoring sutures are placed, and the bowel is divided distal to the clamp. Long Allis clamps can be used to identify the cut edge of the rectum (Fig. 23.22). With the proximal bowel divided and the specimen removed, an open end-to-end anastomosis is performed. Interrupted no. 3-0 or no. 4-0 long-term absorbable sutures are recommended, but the type of suture material is of less importance

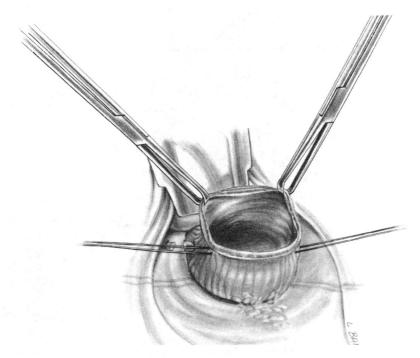

**FIG. 23.22.** Anterior resection. The open distal rectum is prepared for anastomosis. Allis clamps and guide sutures are helpful.

than is the meticulous approach to the technique used. Simple, interrupted sutures are placed as a single layer, taking deeper bites in the muscularis and minimal mucosa (the rectum has no serosa at this level). With a low anastomosis, it is easier to place all of the sutures into the posterior row initially, before tying (Fig. 23.23). The knots are then secured and the anterior row completed. The last suture is usually a horizontal mattress suture in order to invert the mucosa. A single layer is considered adequate, although the surgeon may prefer to pull the anterior peritoneum over the anastomosis with Lembert sutures. A continuous suture technique is also perfectly satisfactory. The floor of the pelvis is not reconstituted but is vigorously irrigated.

A useful step in the procedure is to place or secure omentum around the anastomosis. This can be done by freeing it from the transverse colon with care to avoid injury to the blood supply (Fig. 23.24). The appropriately tailored omen-

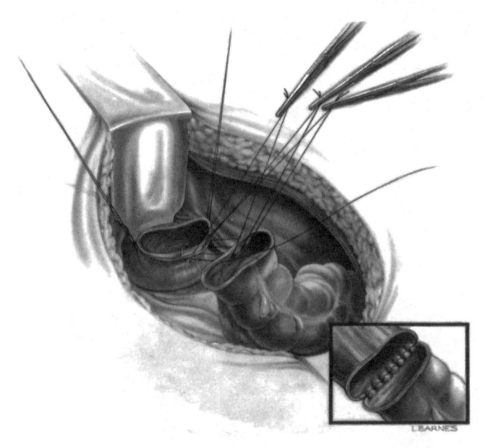

**FIG. 23.23.** Anterior resection. Sutures are initially placed in the posterior row but not secured. *Inset* demonstrates the posterior row completed.

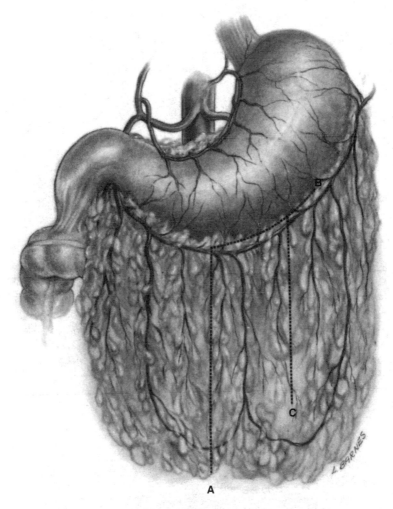

**FIG. 23.24.** Tailoring of the omentum. Adequate length can usually be achieved if the apron is divided along lines (**A** and **B**). If still more length is required, another incision (**C**) usually suffices.

tum is then brought down the lateral gutter into the pelvis, and an anchoring suture is placed below and posterior to the anastomosis to secure it.

### Use of Drains

The routine use of drains for pelvic anastomoses is not advised. The presence of a drain does not influence the postoperative morbidity or mortality. Furthermore, if the anastomosis leaks, the presence of a drain does not prevent the need for reoperation nor does pus or feces emerge from the drain in those individuals in whom a leak occurs.

### Stapled Anastomosis

The application of stapling instruments to effect colonic anastomoses is discussed in Chapter 22, but the creation of a low rectal anastomosis is usually not possible with the conventional instruments and maneuvers described in that chapter.

In 1978, the United States Surgical Corporation introduced a circular stapling device (similar to the Russian stapler, PKS) that is uniquely advantageous for effecting low colorectal anastomoses. The staplers create an inverted, circular anastomosis with two staggered rows of staples (Fig. 23.25), and remove tissue "doughnuts" (rings) of bowel from each end to create an adequate lumen. Cartridges are available in several diameters.

### Technique

A variety of stapling techniques have been suggested for performing an anastomosis in the rectum. The most commonly used is the end-to-end anastomosis using the circular stapling instrument passed transanally. The patient is placed in the perineolithotomy position to facilitate access to the anus and to the abdomen. After the bowel has been mobilized above and below the tumor and the blood supply has been divided, the proximal site for the anastomosis is prepared. In contrast to conventional suturing technique, the bowel must be meticulously debrided of all fat for 1.5 cm to 2 cm. A crushing clamp is placed distally, and a purse-string monofilament suture is placed proximally. The bowel is then divided between the clamps.

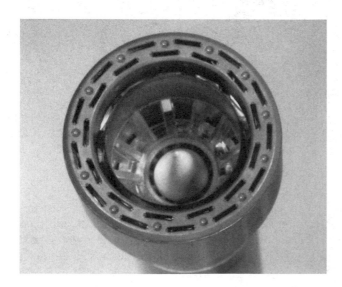

**FIG. 23.25.** Cartridge containing two staggered rows of staples. (Courtesy of United States Surgical Corporation.)

In like manner, the distal bowel below the tumor is freed and the mesentery debrided. A purse-string is placed an adequate distance below the tumor or, alternatively, a double-stapling technique can be used.

A crushing clamp is placed on the bowel distal to the tumor. It is helpful to apply a noncrushing intestinal clamp or vascular clamp on the distal rectal stump to use as a handle, or to place several guide sutures to elevate the rectum. The bowel is then divided, and the specimen is removed. Pressure on the perineum with the fist will often elevate the rectal remnant sufficiently to permit placement of the purse string.

An alternative technique involves inverting the rectal stump with the aid of guide sutures and passing the stump to the perineal operator. If the rectum is of sufficient length, it is sometimes possible to apply the purse-string device outside the anal verge. Realistically, although sufficient rectum remaining to permit this maneuver, it should be possible to apply the instrument through the abdomen. Occasionally, the situation occurs in which this can be a useful technique. After the suture has been placed, the rectum is returned to the pelvis.

Attention is then turned to the cartridge, the largest should be used whenever possible. The sigmoid colon usually has the smaller lumen, but with the aid of a sizer, the luminal discrepancy may be somewhat obviated.

The perineal surgeon gently dilates the anus, and the well-lubricated instrument is inserted into the rectum. The abdominal surgeon should guide the device anteriorly, because of a tendency for the perineal operator to direct the instrument into the sacrum. The anvil is advanced from the cartridge into the pelvis. The distal purse-string suture is then tied over the shaft (Fig. 23.26). Then, by using Allis or Babcock forceps, the proximal bowel is eased over the anvil and the proximal purse-string suture secured (Fig. 23.27). Both sutures are then cut.

The perineal surgeon then tightens the adjusting knob, and the bowel ends are approximated. The abdominal surgeon makes certain that no tissue comes between the anvil and the cartridge. The safety catch is released, and the handle grip is tightened to fire the staples and to cut the redundant bowel (Fig. 23.28). The anvil is advanced and, with a gentle rotational movement, the instrument is withdrawn with careful guidance by the abdominal operator.

Finally, the excised tissue "doughnuts," which are the cut edges of both ends of the anastomosis (with the purse-string sutures), are examined for the presence of intact rings. If the rings are not intact, the anastomosis will have to be redone or reinforced with sutures.

One of the concerns frequently expressed is the difficulty of passing the instrument through the anal canal without trauma. A number of suggestions have been made, including incorporating the anvil within a Penrose drain to permit smooth passage. Additionally, various anal retractors have been developed that allow passage of the instrument through them and into the pelvis.

The anastomosis can be inspected by placing saline solution in the pelvis and looking for bubbles when air is insufflated into the rectum and with the proximal bowel occluded with fingers or a noncrushing clamp (Fig. 23.29)

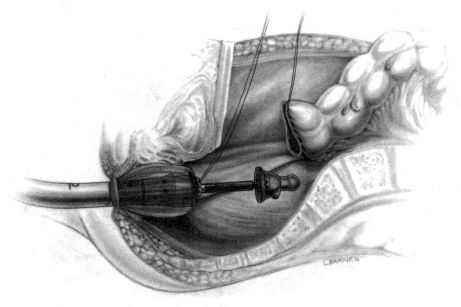

**FIG. 23.26.** Circular stapled anastomosis instrument is inserted through the anus, and the distal purse string is secured.

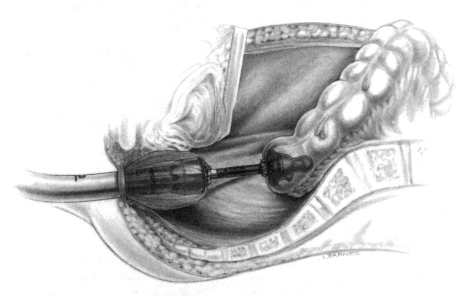

**FIG. 23.27.** Circular stapled anastomosis. Proximal and distal purse-string sutures are secured.

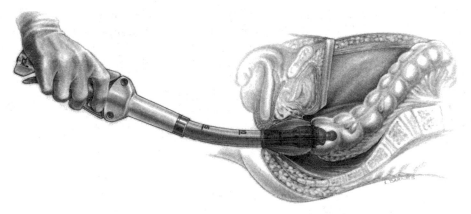

**FIG. 23.28.** Circular stapled anastomosis. The instrument is fired after the ends of the bowel have been approximated.

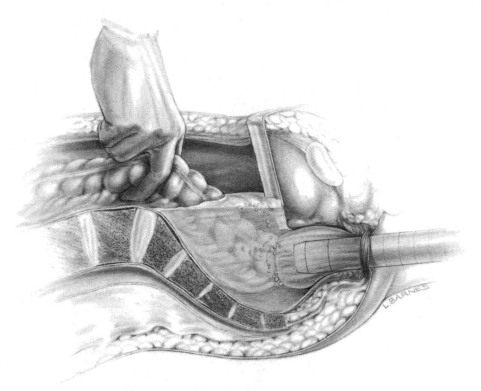

**FIG. 23.29.** Method of testing for integrity of low rectal anastomosis. Inspection can be achieved by means of the rigid sigmoidoscope. By compression of the proximal bowel with the fingers or a noncrushing clamp, and by the insufflation of air with saline in the pelvis, bubbles can be seen to escape from a leak. The site can then be identified and possibly repaired.

Proctosigmoidoscopic visualization of the adequacy of the lumen can also be helpful. If the technique has been properly performed and no evidence is seen of leak, no reinforcing sutures are necessary.

The method for performing the anastomosis with the detachable anvil is illustrated in conjunction with the double-stapling technique, but it is of equal applicability to the end-to-end standard approach just described.

### Double-Stapling Technique

An alternative to the placement of the distal purse string is to close the rectal stump by means of a linear stapler and to perform an end-to-end anastomosis using the so-called "double-stapling technique." It offers a relatively safe method of performing a low colorectal anastomosis, which might not otherwise be technically possible.

In this approach, the distal rectum is closed with a linear stapling instrument (Figs. 23.30 and 23.31). I prefer to use the 30-mm instrument for low-rectal double-stapled anastomoses. At this level, the rectal diameter is usually relatively

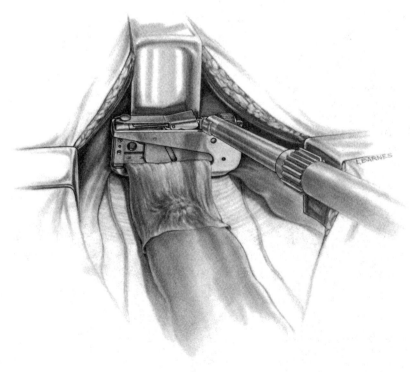

**FIG. 23.30.** Double-stapling anastomosis. Closure of the distal rectum with linear stapler (Roticulator). This instrument can be rotated in all three planes to permit accessibility to the low pelvis.

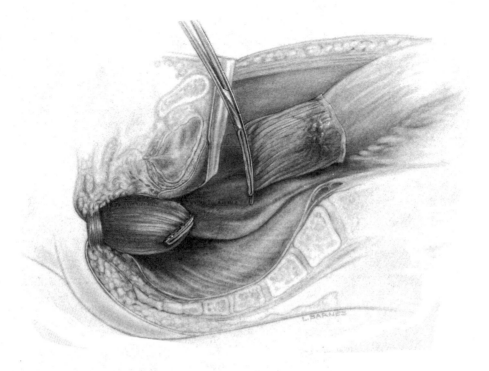

**FIG. 23.31.** Double-stapling anastomosis. Rectal stump is closed.

narrow, and minimal or no mesorectum needs to be dealt with. This permits the lowest application that I can achieve with the stapling device.

One final option is to apply the 30-mm stapler twice. This is especially useful when unable to incorporate the entire distal rectum with one application. Simply pass the pin through the rectum before firing the stapler and then reapply taking care to ascertain that the staple lines overlap (Fig. 23.32). Others have recommended an eversion technique (Fig. 23.33A). Incorporating a drain in the staple line facilitates pulling the bowel through (Fig. 23.33B, C).

After the anus has been dilated, the well-lubricated circular stapling device is inserted into the rectum with the trocar tip (Fig. 23.34). Alternatively, the center rod can be advanced with the EEA or ILS instrument and an incision made directly over the rod. The use of operating proctoscopes to facilitate insertion of the blunt-ended instrument helps prevent the stapler's sharp shoulders from impinging on the anal sphincter.

The center rod is passed through the closed rectum adjacent to or through the staple line, so that when the anastomosis is complete the linear row of staples will be partially excised (Fig. 23.35). Theoretically, if bowel wall between the circular and linear rows of staples is intact, the tissue might become ischemic and necrosis could result. A singular advantage of the detachable anvil and shaft

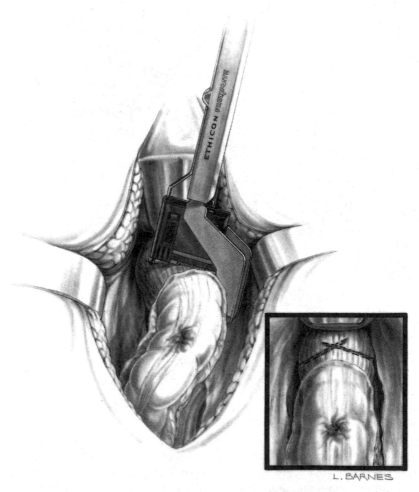

L. BARNES

**FIG. 23.32.** Application of 30-mm linear stapler to the distal rectum in preparation for a double-stapled anastomosis. The staple lines are overlapped. This can be accomplished by application from either side (*inset*), or the bowel can be divided part way before the second application.

is the ability of the surgeon to facilitate securing of the proximal purse string. A simple alternative for placing this purse string is to ligate the bowel around the center rod. Debridement of the mesentery can then be done expeditiously (Fig. 23.36). The extension is then reattached to the instrument shaft (Fig. 23.37), and the knob is turned in a clockwise fashion until the marking site appears on the handle, indicating adequate approximation of the two ends closed (Fig. 23.38). The stapler is closed and fired. The roentgenographic appearance of the staple

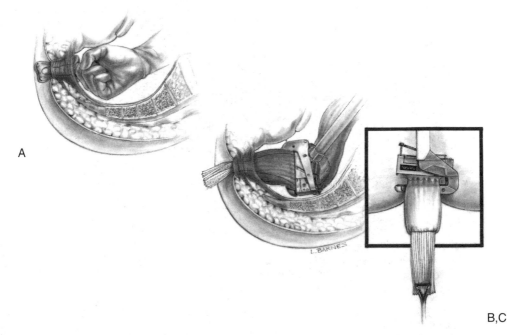

**FIG. 23.33.** Eversion technique to facilitate anastomosis using the double-stapling approach **A.** Manual eversion. **B.** Eversion after insertion of a corrugated rubber drain. **C.** Application of a linear stapler distal to the initial stapling to permit resection and low anastomosis. (From Scotté M, Téniére P, Planet M, et al. Eversion of the rectum: a simplified technical approach to ileoanal anastomosis. *Dis Colon Rectum* 1995;38:96, with permission.)

lines can be appreciated in Figure 23.39 as well as the findings on CT scan (Fig. 23.40).

The anastomosis is secure because of the fact that tissue and staple lines are held firmly in place before the staple-cutting stage. The intersecting staple is usually transferred to the removed doughnut; the knife will bend the intersecting staple rather than cut it.

### *Side-to-End and Side-to-Side Anastomoses*

A side-to-end anastomosis of the colon to the rectum has been advocated to deal with the disparity between the two lumens. Alternatively, a Cheatle cut can be added to deal with the luminal discrepancies or the circular stapling device can be employed.

One modification, however, is worth describing—restoring intestinal continuity by a double-stapling technique to create a side-to-end anastomosis (Fig. 23.41). The detachable anvil is inserted in the open proximal bowel, and the end is closed. Anastomosis is effected in the manner just described. Another method

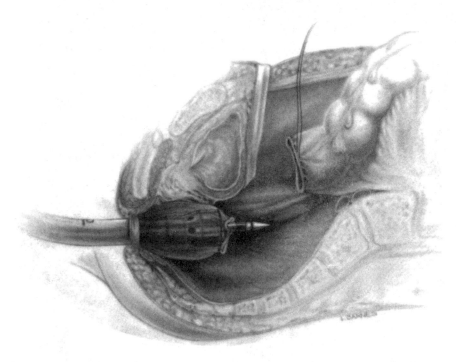

**FIG. 23.34.** Double-stapling anastomosis. CEEA with trocar tip penetrates the closed rectum at or adjacent to the linear staple line.

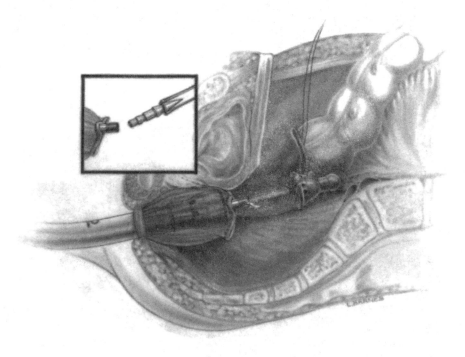

**FIG. 23.35.** Double-stapling anastomosis. The trocar tip is removed (*inset*), and the anvil with shaft is reattached. The anastomosis can then proceed in the standard manner.

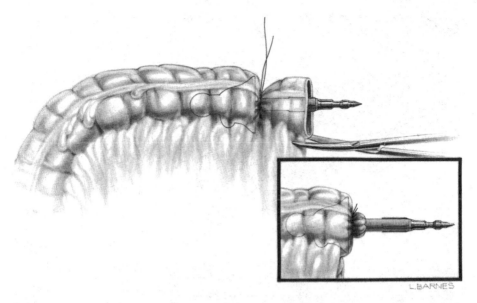

**FIG. 23.36.** Expeditious method for securing the proximal anvil with ligation of the bowel around the anvil, followed by debridement of the excess mesentery.

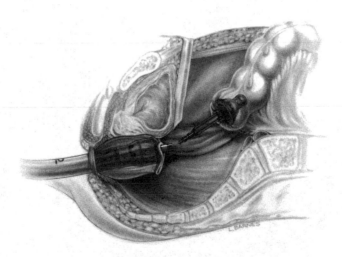

**FIG. 23.37.** Double-stapling anastomosis. Detachable shaft and anvil secured into proximal colon.

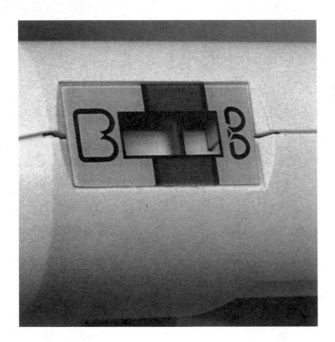

**FIG. 23.38.** Close-up view of gap-setting scale, which indicates the proper position of the ends of the bowel before firing the instrument. (Courtesy of Ethicon, Inc.)

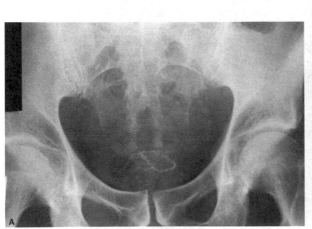
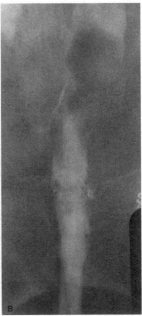

**FIG. 23.39.** Double-stapling technique. **A.** Intersecting staple lines can be seen on plain abdominal film. **B.** Barium enema study of another patient with anastomosis by this technique reveals neither narrowing nor extravasation.

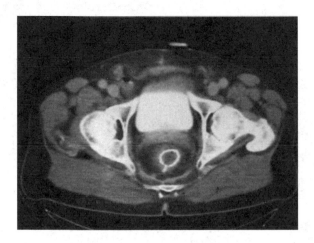

FIG. 23.40. Computed tomography of pelvis reveals linear and circular staples.

of accomplishing an anastomosis is to close the rectal stump and to perform what is essentially a low side-to-side anastomosis with the GIA or PLC instrument (Fig. 23.42).

*Comment*: Little doubt exists that the various stapling techniques can permit a secure anastomosis. The savings in time, albeit minimal, as well as the reduced risk of injury from needles in this acquired immunodeficiency syndrome (AIDS)-conscious environment will inevitably lead to almost complete replacement of conventional suturing for most surgeons. Fazio has outlined what are the important principles for minimizing complications related to the use of staplers. It is worth restating them here:

Use the largest caliber instrument that the anastomosis will accommodate.
Place the purse strings so that excessive bulk of tissue does not appear around the shaft.

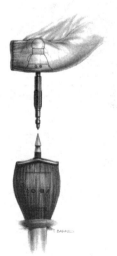

FIG. 23.41. Side-to-end ileorectal anastomosis by double-stapling method. Proximal anvil is inserted in open ileum and passed through the antimesenteric wall. The distal ileum is closed, and the stapling completed in the usual manner. The same principle can be applied to the colon, but this is rarely necessary.

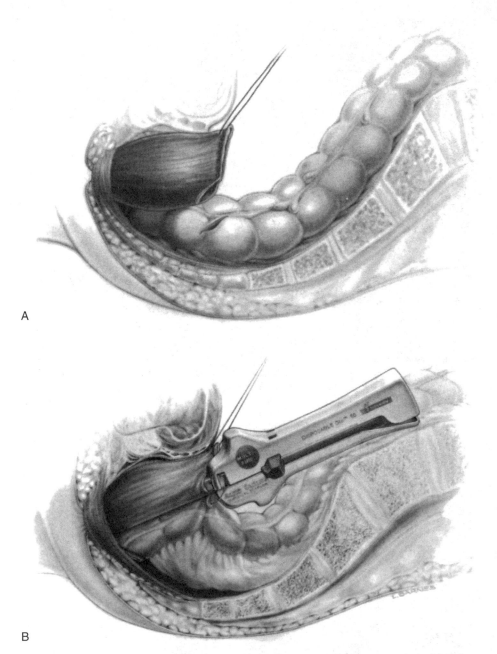

A

B

**FIG. 23.42.** "Bayonet" anastomosis. **A.** The proximal bowel is delivered low in the pelvis follow-ing closure of the rectal stump. Two small enterotomies are created. **B.** Each limb of the GIA instrument is inserted, and the instrument is fired.

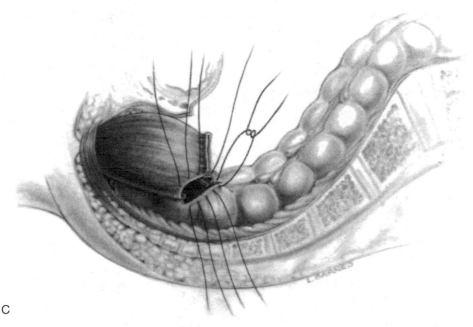

C

**FIG. 23.42.** (*continued*) **C.** The defect is closed by hand-sewing. (Adapted from Ravitch MM, Steichen FM. Staples and staplers. *Adv Surg* 1983;17:241.)

Ensure that the purse string can be snugged up close to the shaft.

Reinforce the purse string if concerned about the possibility of a gap.

Use the detachable anvil-shaft, especially if faced with a "formidable" pelvis.

Repair any identified defect.

Failure to effect a satisfactory repair mandates a diverting colostomy.

## Concomitant Colostomy

Probably the most common reason for subsequent anastomotic complications is tension on the suture line. This can compromise healing, not only because of distraction of the anastomosis itself, but because of vascular insufficiency. Although mobilizing the splenic flexure is rarely necessary in the performance of a low anterior resection, every effort must be made to free the proximal bowel so that no tension exists. Placing the omentum around the anastomosis also helps to minimize the risk of leak.

If the aforementioned precautions are taken, a transverse colostomy is usually unnecessary. Pelvic sepsis, blood loss, other systemic disease, and poor nutritional status, however, are relative indications for protecting the anastomosis. But if the patient is felt to have a limited survival, an abdominoperineal resection or a Hartmann resection is preferred. By creating a sigmoid colostomy rather than the more difficult to manage transverse colostomy, better palliation can be achieved in this situation.

**TABLE 23.3.** *Significance of related factors in anastomotic complications (i.e., obstruction, sepsis, and fistula) in 152 patients*

| Factor[a] | Significance |
|---|---|
| Atherosclerotic disease | $p < 0.001$ |
| Anemia | $p < 0.001$ |
| Anastomosis below the peritoneal reflection | $p < 0.001$ |
| Obstruction and perforation | $p < 0.001$ |
| Anastomosis below the closed peritoneum | $p < 0.005$ |
| Use of drains, anastomosis below the peritoneal reflection | $p < 0.01$ |
| Diabetes | $p < 0.019$ |
| Increased age | $p < 0.02$ |
| Use of drains, entire series | $p < 0.05$ |

[a]The following factors were not significant for anastomotic complications: operative transfusions, $p < 0.1$; abnormal serum albumin levels, $p < 0.2$; cancer in the margin of resection, $p < 0.3$; other organ involvement, $p < 0.3$; all other abnormal liver function tests, $p < 0.5$; other colonic disease (diverticulitis, diverticulosis) in specimen, $p < 0.5$; extent of disease (Dukes'), $p < 0.5$; operative blood loss, $p < 0.5$; anesthesia time, $p < 0.5$; gender, $p < 0.5$; abnormal prothrombin time, $p < 0.6$. Sample size for history of previous radiation therapy, for use of steroids, and for other debilitating diseases was too small for accurate calculations.
From Manson PN, Corman ML, Coller JA, et al. Anterior resection for adenocarcinoma: Lahey Clinic experience from 1963 through 1969. *Am J Surg* 1976;131:434, with permission.

It is generally believed that a temporary, diverting colostomy is avoided more often if a stapled anastomosis is created than if a hand-sewn technique is used. This may reflect a greater confidence in the uniform technique offered by a mechanical device as compared with the variability associated with the manual placement of each suture

Although the morbidity of colostomy closure is decreasing, it is still an important concern (see Chapter 31). Closure of the colostomy without resection produces the lowest incidence of complications when compared with other types of closure. If a colostomy is created, the interval between creation and closure should be at least 6 weeks. The longer the subsequent closure is deferred, the safer the procedure will be.

Obstructed or perforated tumors are associated with a high incidence of anastomotic breakdown. Therefore, the advisability of performing a proximal colostomy or delaying the anastomosis to a later time should be considered. Preoperatively, determining the factors that contribute to the subsequent development of anastomotic leakage will facilitate the intraoperative decision (Table 23.3). The techniques for creating and closing a transverse colostomy are discussed in Chapter 31.

## Postoperative Care

Postoperative care following low anterior resection is essentially the same as that for any operation on the colon. Prophylactic use of a nasogastric tube is not advised. An indwelling urinary catheter, however, is suggested for approximately 6 or 7 days. The amount of manipulation necessary to excise the rectum and effect a low anastomosis is equivalent to that required for an abdominoperineal resection. A progressive diet is instituted after the patient has passed flatus, or sooner, at the surgeon's personal preference. Discharge follows toleration of the diet, and after bowel and bladder functions are relatively normal. This usually requires about 7 days.

## Complications

### *Intraoperative Complications*

With the exception of the problems resulting from the creation of a stoma and with respect to the perineal wound, the intraoperative complications encountered with a low anterior resection by conventional suture technique are identical to those of abdominoperineal resection. Specific intraoperative difficulties related to the use of the stapler include serosal tears, incomplete "doughnuts," instrument failure, and difficulty extracting.

### *Postoperative Complications*

#### *Anastomotic Bleeding*

Hemorrhage from the anastomosis, seen in about 1% of patients, can be caused by inadequate hemostasis at the suture line, itself, or by rupture of a hematoma in the pelvis through the posterior wall of the anastomosis. The former situation usually presents within the first 48 hours, whereas the latter may not become apparent for 7 days or more. The problem can be managed expectantly, although exercise concern about an anastomotic dehiscence. Endoscopic electrocoagulation can be used effectively in the early postoperative period to control anastomotic bleeding. The frequency of this complication is probably more common than is evident from the literature, but the fact that most spontaneously cease and do not go on to anastomotic leak implies that this is a relatively minor concern.

#### *Obstruction at the Anastomosis*

Obstruction at the anastomosis without evidence of sepsis is not commonly seen, but when colonic ileus is associated with an "intact" ileocecal valve, perforation can result. Usually conservative treatment (nasogastric tube) will suffice; rarely, is it necessary to perform a laparotomy. Digital rectal examination may be helpful, but the use of a rectal tube is relatively contraindicated because of the danger of perforating the anastomosis. If unrelieved, this can be one of the few indications for cecostomy.

#### *Sepsis and Anastomotic Leak*

Anastomotic sepsis and fecal fistula, among the more serious concerns in the postoperative period, are the primary causes of operative mortality. A number of factors have been associated with these complications, including disease of the bowel itself (inflammation), inadequate blood supply, tension on the suture line, inaccurate suture placement, trauma, and failure to obtain a watertight seal. Diseases that affect local blood flow and response to infection (anemia, atherosclerotic disease, and diabetes) are important risk factors (see Table 23.3). Others have demonstrated that factors predictive of anastomotic leaks include chronic obstructive pulmonary disease, peritonitis, bowel obstruction, malnutrition, use of corticosteroids, and perioperative blood transfusion. When a leak occurs, it is usually located on the posterior aspect of the anastomosis.

The complication rate of anastomotic leak following anterior resection has been variously reported to be from 15% to 77%. More recently, however, studies seem to indicate a trend to lower rates (<10%), which may be caused by the more frequent use of the transanal circular stapling device, in addition to the implementation of intraoperative air testing and direct visualization by means of the sigmoidoscope.

*Management of the Anastomotic Leak.* The presence of fever, leukocytosis, and peritoneal signs should cause the surgeon to consider performing abdominal drainage and proximal diversion. A contrast study with Gastrografin (the use of barium is contraindicated) may demonstrate a leak into the abdomen or into the presacral (retrorectal) space. At the time of reoperation, care should be taken to ascertain that drainage of the affected area is adequate, but the anastomosis, itself, should be left alone. Unless it is completely or almost completely disrupted, it is assumed that eventual healing will take place. Attempt at suture repair is usually an exercise in futility, but even if "successful," a proximal colostomy or ileostomy should always be performed.

Occasionally, a patient will have an anastomotic leak but fail to develop abdominal signs and symptoms suggestive of this complication. It is usually evident, however, that an uneventful postoperative course is not the case. Fever and leukocytosis should certainly arouse suspicion. Diarrhea, rectal pain, tenesmus, low back pain, and sciatic symptoms can result from an abscess in the presacral space, a consequence of an anastomotic leak. Rectal examination may demonstrate a mass, and cautious proctoscopy may confirm the breakdown or the presence of purulent material. CT usually will demonstrate the abscess; the procedure can also be used to guide the placement of a transgluteal or transabdominal catheter in the hope that laparotomy and colostomy can be avoided.

*Colostomy Closure.* The question of when to close the colostomy often arises, especially if evidence of a small leak remains. I close the colostomy if the tract, as demonstrated on the water-soluble enema, is relatively short, and at least 2 months have elapsed since the original procedure. No argument is seen with the concept of delaying closure for another 4 to 6 weeks and repeating the study. But it is inappropriate to compel the patient to tolerate a difficult stoma for a longer time; the leak may never completely heal and, therefore, the colostomy should be removed. If the tract is long or if it communicates with the abdomen, and if such a radiologic appearance fails to improve, reresection is advised. The technical details of closing the colostomy are discussed in Chapter 31.

### Pelvic Abscess

In the absence of an anastomotic leak and if the pelvic floor has not been reconstituted, a pelvic abscess should be a rare complication. Additional treatment may be unnecessary if the abscess spontaneously drains through the anastomosis or through the vagina. If surgical drainage is required, it is usually done from below. CT-guided drainage is another possible option. If signs of peritonitis are present, laparotomy is required for drainage, and a concomitant colostomy should be performed.

### Fecal Fistula

Fecal fistula can develop early in the postoperative period as a consequence of an anastomotic leak (see earlier discussion). Usually, this complication requires abdominal drainage and a diversionary procedure. However, if the fistula arises at a later time, perhaps following drainage of an abdominal abscess, and connects with the abdominal wall, it can usually be treated expectantly in the absence of sepsis and the patient continues to have bowel movements. Without distal obstruction or persistent tumor, the fistula will usually close within a matter of a few weeks. If drainage is considerable, a colostomy appliance may be used.

### Late Complications

*Stricture.* Benign stricture following anterior resection is usually a consequence of an anastomotic breakdown with subsequent fibrosis (Fig. 23.43). With dehiscence of 50% or more of the circumference, healing will usually result in stricture formation. Stricture has been shown to develop more frequently following a diversionary colostomy, even in the absence of a leak, if a stapled anastomosis has been performed. Apparently, a stapled anastomosis may "need" the effect of dilatation by the passage of stool; the conventional suture technique appears to be associated with stenosis less commonly if a diversionary operation is done. Preoperative risk factors for development of this complication are obesity and abscess. Anastomotic leak, incomplete tissue "doughnut," postoperative radiation, and pelvic infection are also felt to be contributing factors.

*Management.* Nonsurgical treatment of an anastomotic stricture consists of the use of stool softeners, enemas, or suppositories. Dilatation can be performed manually if it is within reach of the finger. For higher strictures (viz., at a level of 8 to 12 cm) a double-ended Hegar's dilator (17 to 18 mm) or a flexible bougie can be used. Another alternative is to pass a narrow (1.1 cm) sigmoidoscope with

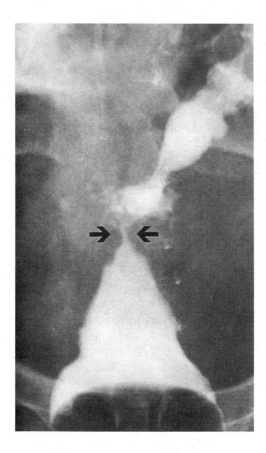

FIG. 23.43. Barium enema reveals rectal stricture (*arrows*) following anastomotic leak. This proved to be benign.

its obturator through the stricture, gradually dilating the opening with serial passage of instruments of increasing diameter. For higher level strictures, a curved metal dilator has been recommended, modeled after the Lister urethral dilator, because the curvature of the sacrum and the angulation of the bowel may make passage impossible. The application of the technique of endoscopic balloon dilatation, with or without the use of a guidewire has also been reported. Most patients require two to four dilatations, repeated at 3-month intervals. A risk exists of perforating the bowel, a particular concern if the stricture is above the level of the peritoneal reflection.

If a symptomatic stricture persists, transanal lysis with sharp knife or electrocautery in the posterior midline may ameliorate the condition (Fig. 23.44A). The use of the optical urethrotome knife has also been described, as well as a device called a "staple cutter" (a variation of a bone cutter). Following the procedure, frequent office visits with dilatation, as necessary, is recommended for a number of weeks. Alternatively, if possible, a proctoplasty is preferred, closing the proctotomy in a transverse fashion (Fig. 44B). Analogous to the Heinecke–

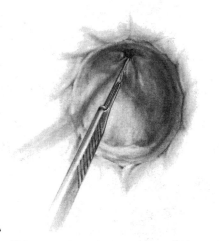
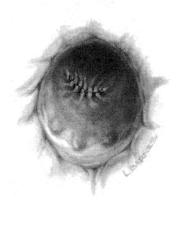

A

B

**FIG. 23.44.** Rectal stricture at site of low colorectal anastomosis. **A.** Lysis is performed posteriorly. **B.** Ideally, a proctoplasty is accomplished by means of transverse closure of the longitudinal proctotomy.

Mikulicz pyloroplasty as applied to the rectum, it is hoped that the diameter can be maintained without recurrent stenosis. The technique used for endoscopic papillotomy has also been suggested for the treatment of stricture, as has Eder Puestow dilatation over a guidewire, the technique used for the management of esophageal strictures. Another option is the use of an endo-stapler (Fig. 23.45). The Wallstent prosthesis has also been advocated for relieving obstruction, not only for malignant tumors, but also for benign stricture.

If all such treatments are of no avail, reresection may be indicated. An alternative to a standard resection is to pass the circular stapling instrument transanally without the anvil, with the center rod traversing the stricture. An enterotomy is created proximal to the strictured anastomosis, and the rod is visualized (Fig. 23.46). The anvil is replaced and the instrument closed and fired (Fig. 23.46, inset). A single tissue "doughnut" is created, which is the actual stricture. The enterotomy is then closed.

Always keep in mind that the cause of the stricture may be recurrent tumor. Evaluation by means of CT scan may be helpful, but biopsy or cytologic study is mandatory for establishing the diagnosis. Obviously, the use of dilatation as a palliative tool has some merit, but most successful reports employ cutting and ablating tools (e.g., the laser and electrocoagulator) for malignant disease (see later).

Virtually all of the reports concerning the management of rectal strictures are essentially individual case studies. The long-term effectiveness of the various modalities has not been subjected to critical analysis.

*Incontinence and Irregular Bowel Function.* Low anterior resection, irrespective of anastomotic technique, can be associated with control problems and other bowel management difficulties. One concern about the stapling technique is the

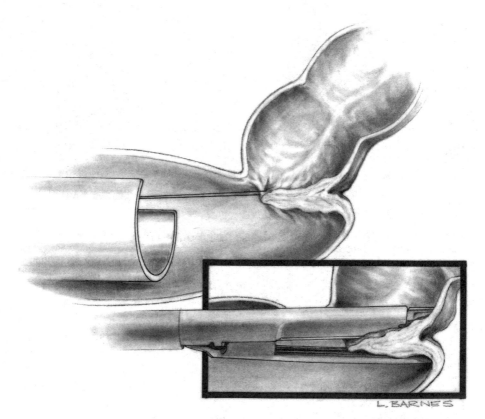

**FIG. 23.45.** Technique of division of anastomotic stricture as performed through a Faensler rectoscope using an endoGIA stapler. (From Pagni S, McLaughlin CM. Simple technique for the treatment of strictured colorectal anastomosis. *Dis Colon Rectum* 1995;38:433, with permission.)

fact that sphincter disruption can occur from dilatation associated with the passage of the instrument. The issue of stretching the internal and external sphincters has been addressed in the section on anal fissure in Chapter 3. Long-term functional outcome can also be impaired as a consequence of anastomotic leakage.

Most patients who have low anterior resection with anastomosis by the circular stapling device have had frequent bowel actions and soiling. These symptoms improve to a virtually normal state by 6 months, as do rectal sensation and reservoir capacity in most patients. However, abnormal rectoanal inhibitory reflex, anal canal resting pressure, and maximal squeeze pressure can persist.

Inflammatory reaction, narrowing at the anastomosis, sensory impairment, and bowel denervation all can contribute to impairment of control and irregular bowel habits. However, as long as the anal canal and sphincter muscles have been preserved and no anatomic abnormality is present, the symptoms usually resolve in a matter of a few months. "Slowing" medications should rarely be used because

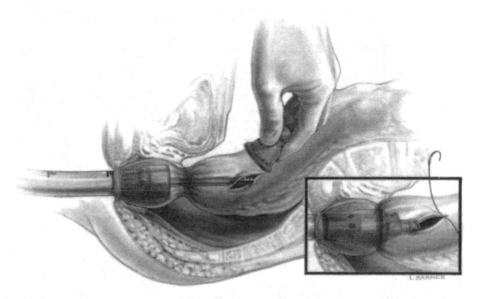

**FIG. 23.46.** Excision of strictured anastomosis with CEEA. Enterotomy in proximal bowel permits replacement of anvil. The enterotomy is then closed (*inset*).

of the risk of precipitating a fecal impaction. Most patients can regulate themselves by paying slightly more attention to their diet than had been their custom. Eventually, in most instances, all such restrictions become unnecessary.

### Recurrence and Survival Results Following Anterior Resection

In our experience with anterior resection in 152 patients, two in-hospital deaths occurred, a mortality rate of 1.3%. Survival data according to Dukes' classification is shown in Table 23.4. No statistically significant difference was seen in survival rates between abdominoperineal resection and anterior resection

**TABLE 23.4.** *Rates of 5-year survival for anterior resection according to Dukes' classification*

| Dukes' stage | Patients (n) | Series (%) | Survivors (n) uncorrected | 5-year survival (%) | Actuarially corrected 5-year survival (%) |
|---|---|---|---|---|---|
| A | 49 | 32.2 | 37 | 75.5 | 86.1 |
| B | 45 | 29.6 | 31 | 68.8 | 78.8 |
| C | 39 | 25.7 | 20 | 51.3 | 57.0 |
| D | 19 | 12.5 | 0 | 0.0 | 0.0 |
| A, B, C | 133 | 87.5 | 88 | 66.2 | 71.7 |
| All stages | 152 | 100.0 | 88 | 57.9 | 72.8 |

From Manson PN, Corman ML, Coller JA, et al. Anterior resection for adenocarcinoma: Lahey Clinic experience from 1963 through 1969. *Am J Surg* 1976;131:434, with permission.

**TABLE 23.5.** *Anastomotic recurrence after anterior resection: related factors*

| Factor[a] | Significance |
|---|---|
| Penetration of coats of bowel by cancer | $p < 0.003$ |
| Increased dedifferentiation | $p < 0.005$ |
| Ulcerating cancer | $p < 0.005$ |
| Tumor below peritoneal reflection | $p < 0.01$ |
| Distal margin of resection | $p < 0.01$ |
| Distal margin of resection of <6 cm | $p < 0.05$ |

[a]The following factors were not significant for anastomotic recurrence: lymph node involvement, $p < 0.07$; size of lesion, $p < 0.3$; proximal margin of resection, $p < 0.3$; previous colonic cancer, $p < 0.5$; polyps in specimen, $p < 0.5$; extent of disease (Dukes'), $p < 0.5$; other organ involvement, $p < 0.5$; blood vessel invasion, $p < 0.5$; age, $p < 0.5$; gender, $p < 0.6$.

From Manson PN, Corman ML, Coller JA, et al. Anterior resection for adenocarcinoma: Lahey Clinic experience from 1963 through 1969. *Am J Surg* 1976;131:434, with permission.

in those with Dukes' A and Dukes' B lesions. However, patients with Dukes' C tumors who had abdominoperineal resection had a significantly poorer survival rate than those who had a lesion sufficiently proximal to permit an anterior resection.

The most difficult problem following anterior resection is the management of locally recurrent disease. A dramatic decrease in the frequency of recurrence is seen when the lesion is more than 13 cm from the anal verge. Furthermore, it has been shown that most recurrences involve tumors that initially penetrated the rectal wall and extended into the surrounding tissue.

To minimize the risk of recurrence and the necessity of performing additional surgery, it may be possible to identify preoperatively the individual at a high risk. Table 23.5 lists those variables that are statistically significant in their association with increased risk of anastomotic recurrence. Table 23.6 shows the incidence of recurrence versus the histology. Table 23.7 compares the recurrence rate with Dukes' classification, and Table 23.8, the recurrence rate versus the distal margin of resection.

The incidence of anastomotic recurrence in our experience is summarized as follows:

- Increases with more distal lesions
- Increases with resection margins of less than 6 cm

**TABLE 23.6.** *Anterior resection for carcinoma: anastomotic recurrence versus histology*

| Type | Patients (n) | Recurrence (n)/(%) |
|---|---|---|
| Well differentiated | 107 | 5/4.7 |
| Moderately differentiated | 33 | 6/18.2 |
| Poorly differentiated | 5 | 4/80.0 |
| Villous | 7 | 3 (2 benign)/42.9 |
| Total | 152 | 18/11.8 |

From Manson PN, Corman ML, Coller JA, et al. Anastomotic recurrence after anterior resection for carcinoma: Lahey Clinic experience. *Dis Colon Rectum* 1976;19:219, with permission.

**TABLE 23.7.** *Anterior resection for carcinoma 5-yr survival (uncorrected)*

| Dukes' stage | Patients (n) | Survivors (n)/(%) |
|---|---|---|
| A | 49 | 38/77.6 |
| B | 45 | 30/66.6 |
| C | 39 | 19/48.7 |
| D | 19 | 1/5.3 |
| All stages | 152 | 88/57.9 |

From Manson PN, Corman ML, Coller JA, et al. Anastomotic recurrence after anterior resection for carcinoma: Lahey Clinic experience. *Dis Colon Rectum* 1976;19:219, with permission.

- Is higher with ulcerating tumors
- Is low with exophytic lesions
- Is prohibitively high with poorly differentiated growths
- Is low with well-differentiated tumors
- Is low when the tumor does not penetrate the bowel
- Is high with Dukes' B and C lesions
- Is high in the presence of metastatic disease

Therefore, in selecting patients for sphincter-saving procedures, the preoperative assessment is most important. If the tumor is low-lying (<8 cm from the anal verge), but especially if it is poorly differentiated, fixed, infiltrative or ulcerating, then a sphincter-saving operation is relatively contraindicated. Still, controversy concerning the ideal distal margin for anterior resection is unresolved.

Recurrence has been attributed to (a) unresected tumor (in the pelvis or the bowel wall itself); (b) a zone of potentially malignant mucosa; (c) a new primary tumor; (d) spillage of viable malignant cells; and (e) implantation by suture material. It has been also demonstrated that recurrence rates are higher for the same stage of lesion in men when compared with women. This is presumably because the pelvic anatomy is such that the operation can be performed with a greater distal and lateral margin in women than can be accomplished in most men.

**TABLE 23.8.** *Anterior resection for carcinoma: anastomotic recurrence versus distal margin of resection*

| Distal margin (cm) | Patients (n) | Recurrences (n)/(%) |
|---|---|---|
| 0 | 2 | 0/0 |
| 1 | 10 | 1/10.0 |
| 2 | 17 | 3/17.6 |
| 3 | 23 | 2/8.7 |
| 4 | 24 | 3/12.5 |
| 5 | 31 | 6/19.4 |
| 6 | 16 | 2/12.5 |
| 7 | 14 | 1/7.1 |
| >7 | 15 | 0/0 |

From Manson PN, Corman ML, Coller JA, et al. Anastomotic recurrence after anterior resection for carcinoma: Lahey Clinic experience. *Dis Colon Rectum* 1976;19:219, with permission.

### Results with Stapled Anastomoses

Because it is possible for surgeons to effect reestablishment of intestinal continuity for relatively low-lying lesions, concern has been expressed about the risk of tumor recurrence following stapled anastomosis. A case has been reported of tumor implantation in the anal canal, possibly as a consequence of trauma from the insertion of the circular stapler. Malignant cells have also been demonstrated in up to 90% of tissue doughnuts. But the real question is whether surgeons are compromising on the adequacy of the distal margin, and the corollary question, is it truly important. Most reports reveal no increase in local recurrence when the stapler is used, and some believe the incidence is actually reduced. A number of studies have demonstrated no statistically significant correlation between the incidence of recurrence and the length of distal margin when controlling for the other variables, unless the margin is minimal (<2 cm). In general, local recurrence rates following low anterior resection are essentially the same as the rates for abdominoperineal resection when comparing the same degree of differentiation and stage of tumor.

### Significance of Mucus Production

A differential pattern of mucus production in patients who develop recurrence exists, compared with those who remained tumor free. Mucus from tumors and the adjacent area is composed mainly of sialomucins, whereas normal mucus is composed predominantly of sulfated mucins. Several authors have observed that the presence of sialomucin is the optimal prognostic variable for anticipating local recurrence, but is not as accurate in its predictive ability for subsequent death or other recurrences; Dukes' classification was better for those patients. As of this writing, the only proved, effective method to limit the likelihood of local recurrence is to select those patients who are at an increased risk and either to perform an abdominoperineal resection or to consider the possibility of adjuvant radiotherapy (see later).

### Management of Recurrence Following Anterior Resection

When anastomotic recurrence develops, it usually presents within 2 years following resection. The patient may be without symptoms, but a suspicious area is identified, either by palpation (digital examination) or by proctosigmoidoscopy as part of the cancer follow-up. Many patients who present with recurrent cancer in the pelvis do not have disseminated disease, and under these circumstances the CEA is often not elevated. When symptoms develop, they can include bleeding, change in the caliber of the stool, and pelvic, abdominal, or sacral pain. Biopsy or scrapings for cytologic examination usually will confirm the diagnosis, but barium enema examination and CT scan also may be helpful (Fig. 23.47). Positron emission tomography (PET) has been used to follow up individuals with colorectal malignancy to differentiate between recurrent tumor and scar. The method uses the injection of fluorine-18-labeled deoxyglucose

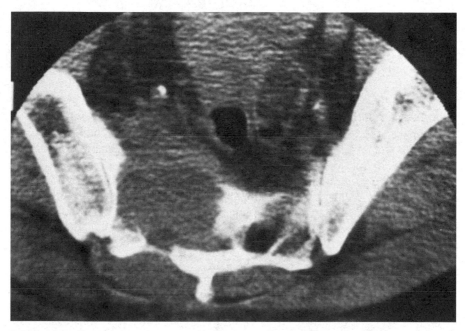

**FIG. 23.47.** Recurrent rectal cancer. Computed tomography scan shows marked bony erosion.

(FDG) to assess tumor metabolism. The application of monoclonal antibody scanning is discussed in Chapter 22.

The only hope for cure is reresection; this usually involves an abdominoperineal resection. Before undertaking reoperation, however, it is imperative to determine whether the patient has evidence of disseminated disease. Because of the possibility of retroperitoneal extension of the tumor and the likelihood of urinary tract involvement, a CT scan or intravenous pyelogram is mandatory.

### Surgical Principles

See earlier discussion, *Treatment of Recurrence.*

### Results of Reoperation

Studies of abdominoperineal resection following anastomotic recurrence have limited numbers of patients and are difficult to interpret. Overall cure rates are certainly less than 25% in those considered resectable for cure.

*Comment:* I feel that cure is rarely achieved except in those situations where a second primary lesion is found rather than recurrent disease, or when the pathologist reports that the recurrence is confined to, but does not breach the bowel wall. This may be the rare circumstance when mucosal seeding produces the recurrence rather than inward growth of residual pelvic disease.

## OTHER ANASTOMOTIC TECHNIQUES

### Transanal or Coloanal Anastomosis

An alternative technique for reestablishing intestinal continuity is the transanal or coloanal anastomosis. A hand-sewn technique is usually employed, using a round-bodied modification of a Turner-Warwick urethroplasty needle, or a long-term absorbable suture on a ⅝ circle needle. Using a Parks self-retaining, three-bladed anal retractor, paired Gelpi retractors placed at right angles to each other, a Lone Star Retractor, or a Bookwalter rectal kit (Codman, Randolph, MA, USA), a transanal anastomosis can be effected (Fig. 23.48). This is the technique used to reestablish continuity after colectomy, proctectomy, and ileal pouch for inflammatory bowel disease (see Chapter 29). The sutures incorporate the full thickness of the colon with the anal canal and the underlying internal sphincter. An alternative approach is to use a double-stapling technique.

### *Results*

It is recommended that every patient have a temporary diverting colostomy and that the left colon be completely mobilized to avoid tension on the anas-

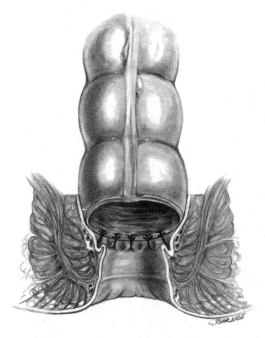
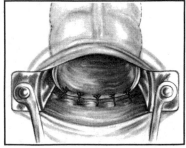

**FIG. 23.48.** A Parks retractor facilitates the insertion of sutures (*inset*) coloanal anastomosis.

tomosis. A more recent report from the same institution (Memorial Sloan-Kettering Cancer Center) involved 134 patients. Actuarially corrected 5-year survival for all patients was 73%. Mesenteric implants, positive microscopic resection margin, T3 tumor, perineural invasion (PNI), blood vessel invasion, and high tumor grade were associated with increased risk for pelvic recurrence. They and others report at least a satisfactory experience both in terms of bowel function and of recurrent disease, with a median stool frequency of two per day, with 22% of patients reporting four or more stools in 24 hours. Stool frequency tends to decrease with time, with the use of postoperative adjuvant radiotherapy influencing the frequency and difficulty with evacuation. All authors agree that the surgical morbidity is significantly higher than that of low anterior resection.

### Transanal or Coloanal Anastomosis with Colonic Reservoir

A J-shaped colonic reservoir has been used to supplement the coloanal anastomotic option described above in an effort to improve bowel function. The technique is essentially the same as that for a J-shaped ileal reservoir (see Chapter 29), except that the colon is used. Ideal pouch dimensions are 6 to 7 cm of undistended bowel circumference, with limb lengths of 8 to 10 cm. All investigators emphasize the importance of mobilizing the splenic flexure and preserving the first branch of the inferior mesenteric artery.

### *Results*

In the experience from both Mayo and Cleveland Clinics, involving 117 patients most of whom had a straight coloanal anastomosis, satisfactory fecal continence was achieved in 78%. No patient with a J-pouch had frequent incontinence. Five-year survival was 69%, but 62% had complications (anastomotic leak, 18%). Stool frequencies are fewer with this method, especially during the first year, than with patients having reconstruction without a reservoir, but others note that approximately 25% of individuals must evacuate with a small enema. Others have demonstrated that at 1 year, the patients with pouch had significantly fewer bowel movements in 24 hours and less nocturnal evacuations, urgency, and incontinence. Those familiar with the technique report no increase in morbidity or mortality attributable to the reservoir itself.

### Intraluminal Bypass

The indications and method for performing the so-called "intraluminal bypass" for effecting a colorectal anastomosis are discussed in Chapter 15.

## Abdominoanal Pull-through Procedures

An alternative method for reestablishing intestinal continuity following rectal resection is the pull-through procedure. The operation was initially described by Maunsell in 1892 and supported by Weir in 1901. It was developed primarily as an alternative to the transsacral excision of Kraske (see *Transsacral Resection*) and the Murphy anastomotic button (see Chapter 22). Pull-through procedures, in general, are applied for anastomoses below 7 cm, but are relatively infrequently used today because of the preference for other techniques (*viz.*, circular stapling, coloanal, and abdominosacral anastomoses) and other treatment modalities (e.g., local excision and electrocoagulation). As with other esoteric sphincter-saving alternatives, the surgeon should be wary of using the pull-through procedure for malignant disease. Several methods are used for accomplishing anal anastomosis by the pull-through approach.

### *Eversion Techniques*

The patient is placed in the perineolithotomy position if consideration is to be given to performing a pull-through procedure. The operation proceeds as if for a low anterior resection. However, when a pull-through operation is undertaken, greater length of proximal colon needs to be liberated. In virtually every instance, the splenic flexure requires mobilization. The bowel is divided as low as is possible and the specimen resected.

The safest anastomosis and the one that offers the best functional result is accomplished with the Weir procedure; the rectal stump is everted, the proximal bowel "pulled-through," and the anastomosis performed by the perineal operator with interrupted no. 3-0 long-term absorbable sutures (Fig. 23.49). The anastomotic area returns to the pelvis spontaneously. The pelvic peritoneal floor is left open; no drains are usually used, but a proximal colostomy is advised.

A modification of the Weir technique has been described by Turnbull and Cuthbertson and by Cutait and Figliolini. The rectal stump is everted, but the bowel is pulled through and left to project on the perineum for 7 or 8 cm. The cut edge of the rectum is sutured to the seromuscular surface of the intussuscepting colon, but not penetrating the lumen (Fig. 23.50). A catheter is secured into the protruding bowel. After 10 days to 2 weeks, the redundant colon is amputated and the anastomosis resutured; the rectum retracts into the pelvis.

### *Delayed Union–Amputation Techniques*

A more distal pull-through anastomosis can be effected using the Babcock, Bacon, or Black techniques. Babcock described his method of one-stage

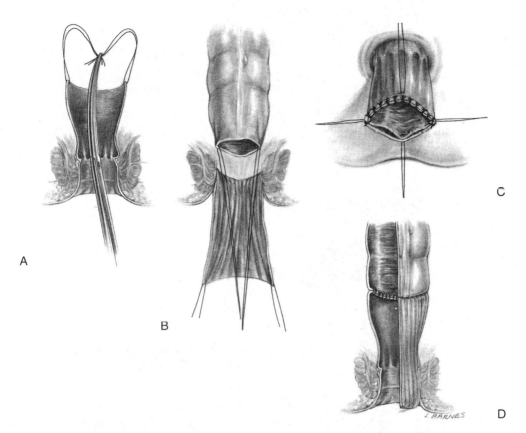

**FIG. 23.49.** Weir pull-through technique. **A.** Guide sutures evert the rectal stump. **B.** The proximal bowel is delivered through the everted rectal stump with guide sutures. **C.** The anastomosis is performed in one layer by the perineal surgeon. **D.** The bowel returns to the pelvis.

abdominoperineal proctosigmoidectomy with perineal anus in 1939. After a generous posterior sphincterotomy has been performed, the bowel is amputated at the top of the anal canal and pulled through. This allegedly reduces the risk of necrosis of the exteriorized colon. Healing takes place between the cut edge of the anorectum and the serosa of the colon. The stump is amputated performed 2 weeks later. In the Black modification, no sphincterotomy is undertaken.

Bacon first described his alternative in 1945. He removed the anal canal by way of the perineal route, dividing the bowel at or above the levatores. This permits a wider surface area to come in contact with the pulled-through bowel, a theoretic advantage in that healing may be more effective. As with the other procedures, the redundant bowel is amputated approximately 2 weeks later.

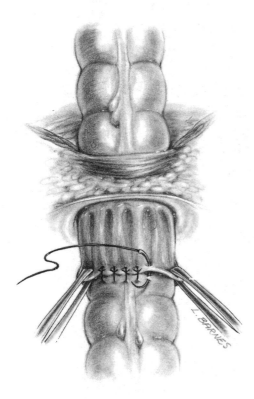

**FIG. 23.50.** Pull-through by eversion and seromuscular suture (first stage).

*Comment*: The delayed union–amputative techniques permit a lower anastomosis than can be achieved through eversion. Hence, an anastomosis can be effected in situations when an anterior abdominal approach with any suture technique is impossible. However, the anastomosis may be less secure, and subsequent continence may not be as satisfactory as with the former methods. With the temporary, perineal "colostomy," a proximal diversion, however, should be unnecessary.

One problem in my experience has been that of the wet anus. The mucosal ectropion associated with nonanastomotic pull-through procedures can be a source of considerable discharge and discomfort.

The advantage of the Weir (Maunsell) procedure is that it is tidier, because an anastomosis is performed per primam. The staging method, however, creates an uncomfortable, often frightening, foul-smelling, necrotic, perineal protrusion, but it can accomplish an anastomosis safely, without the need for a diversionary procedure; hence, it has this advantage. The fact of the matter is that both procedures are rarely useful alternatives to low anterior resection with or without the stapling instrument. To create an eversion of sufficient length to deliver the rectum to the perineum, a minimum of 6 cm of residual rectum is required. With less rectum available, eversion is virtually impossible; the tethering of the levatores tends to draw the bowel back into the pelvis. Most patients are able to have continuity reestablished by more conventional means (if reestablishment is considered advisable).

These operations should be performed rarely for any indication. Essentially, it should be relegated to the realm of historical curiosity, resurrected only when a surgeon wishes to apply it as an alternative to one of the esoteric sphincter-saving procedures, and when no other resective or local operation is appropriate, an extraordinarily unusual situation indeed.

## Transsacral or Transcoccygeal Resection

Sacral excision had been performed by Kocher in 1875. However, it has been associated with the name of Kraske ever since he described the technique in detail to the Fourteenth Congress of the German Association of Surgeons in 1884. Interestingly, in the classic description of the procedure, the bowel was brought out by establishing a sacral anus at the posterior end of the wound, and amputating the entire distal rectum. This, in essence, was a sacral colostomy. Others, such as Turner, modified the operation by performing an end-to-end anastomosis to the residual anorectum.

### *Technique*

Routine bowel preparation is carried out as if for an anterior resection. The operation is performed with the patient in the prone position and with the buttocks taped. An incision is made in the midline from just above the anal verge to the lower sacrum and carried through the subcutaneous tissue to expose the levator ani muscle and coccyx. The levator ani muscle is then divided, exposing the posterior wall of the rectum. The coccyx is then freed from its muscular attachments, disarticulated, and removed. If further exposure is necessary, the lower portion (two sacral segments) is excised using a Gigli saw. It is imperative when dividing the sacrum that the third sacral nerve on one side be preserved to avoid problems with incontinence.

The rectum is then completely mobilized. Care must be taken to avoid injuring the anterior rectum where it is adherent to the vagina or to the prostate. A Penrose drain is placed around the rectum for traction and the dissection is completed. The peritoneum can be opened on the anterior rectal surface. The bowel is then drawn downward as far as is possible and the superior hemorrhoidal vessels divided. The bowel is divided at the desired level and an anastomosis is effected with interrupted no. 3-0 long-term absorbable sutures as a single layer. The circular stapling technique has also been recommended (Fig. 23.51). A silastic drain is placed through a stab wound of the buttock into the presacral space and connected to suction. It is usually left in place for 48 to 72 hours or until drainage ceases.

Postoperatively, the treatment is essentially the same as that for a low anterior resection. When flatus is passed, a progressive diet is instituted. During the time of convalescence the patient is instructed on perineal strengthening exercises (see Chapter 13). A degree of incontinence occurs for several days to a few weeks; in all cases, however, virtually normal control will be restored eventually, assuming that the nerve supply has been preserved. Results of this operation in contemporary writings are essentially anecdotal.

*Comment:* Sacral excision rapidly had become the most popular modality of treatment for carcinoma of the rectum by the end of the 19th century, but the problems of anastomotic breakdown, fecal fistula, wound sepsis, and tumor recurrence have since caused the procedure to fall into disrepute. The Kraske operation usually permits resection of 8 to 10 cm of rectum

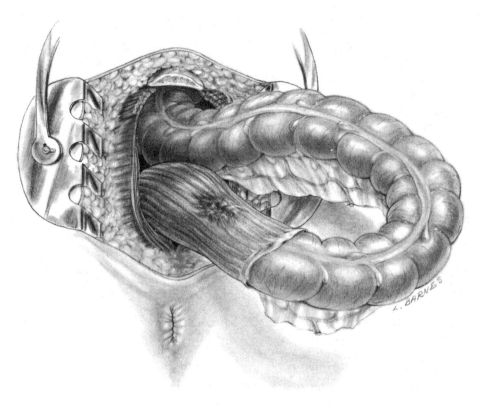

**FIG. 23.51.** Circular-stapled anastomosis by transcoccygeal approach. Note coccyx has been removed.

without difficulty. However, by contemporary standards, the operation must be regarded as inadequate for the management of rectal cancer because it fails to remove the "zone of upward spread."

Some surgeons, however, still recommend this alternative for small malignant tumors, but I believe that better local procedures are available for most such conditions (see later). The operation does, however, have application in carefully selected patients with benign disease: villous adenoma, benign rectal stricture, rectovaginal fistula, and rectoprostatic fistula.

## Abdominosacral Resection

Kraske was the first to suggest a combined abdominosacral resection to overcome the disadvantage of failure to remove the lymphatics of the rectum and rectosigmoid.

### *Technique*

In the modification described by Localio and Stahl, access to the abdomen and the sacrum is achieved simultaneously by placing the patient in the right lateral position. Two teams can then operate independently on the abdomen and over the sacrum. I have found this approach cumbersome, however, and much prefer the patient to be placed in the perineolithotomy position and the abdominal phase completed as if for a low anterior resection. The lateral stalks are divided, and the surgeon then decides on the advisability of reestablishing continuity and the choice of operation to accomplish this. If the sacral approach is elected, the abdomen is closed. It is important to fully mobilize the entire left colon and splenic flexure so that the bowel can be easily delivered and so that no tension is found on the subsequent anastomosis. The bowel is not divided during the abdominal phase of the procedure. A transverse loop colostomy or ileostomy is routinely performed.

The patient is then placed in the prone jackknife position, and the Kraske approach is used (see Figs. 21.13 through 21.15). With the rectum already fully mobilized, the bowel containing the tumor can be delivered through the incision and resected (Fig. 23.52). Anastomosis is accomplished with an interrupted sin-

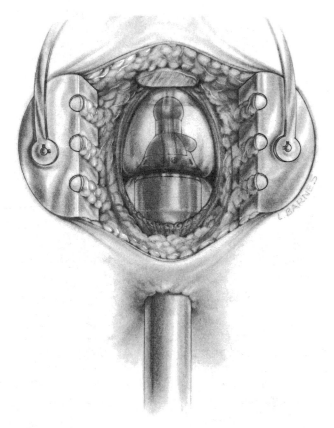

**FIG. 23.52.** Abdominosacral resection. The colon is delivered through the sacral defect and resected. Anastomosis is readily performed through the sacral wound.

gle-layer technique or, alternatively, by the circular stapling instrument (see Fig. 23.51). The muscles are repaired with heavy, long-term absorbable sutures, and a silastic drain is placed into the hollow of the sacrum and brought out through a stab wound in the buttock.

## Results

Localio et al. have probably had the most experience with this operation, reporting the results of 427 patients with carcinoma of the rectum. Preoperative assessment was made to determine the type of operation that the patient would require: abdominoperineal resection, anterior resection, or abdominosacral resection. A total of 100 abdominosacral resections were performed. Although recurrence rates and mortality rates were comparable for the three procedures, the morbidity of abdominosacral resection was much higher. Of the patients, 12% developed either a fecal fistula or peritonitis. Because of these complications, the authors advise that a colostomy should always be performed.

*Comment*: Although I have had only a limited experience with this operation, primarily for benign conditions, I am not enthusiastic about its value in the treatment of rectal cancer. It is true that the procedure effectively removes the cancer-bearing segment and lymphatics and that a low anastomosis can satisfactorily be achieved, but a candidate for its application is infrequent indeed. The fact that the patient must contend with a sacral wound as well as an abdominal incision causes me to look for an alternative operation for preserving the anal sphincter when such an approach is desirable.

## TRANSSPHINCTERIC EXCISION

Transsphincteric excision was resurrected about a quarter of a century ago by Mason as a way to remove selected low-lying cancers of the rectum. The procedure, however, is not new, having been advocated by Bevan in 1917 for "small carcinomas of the rectum without any radical involvement." Interestingly, however, the author did not seem to repair the sphincter, simply stating, "I do not hope to attain anything like complete continence," nor did he comment about the risk of the development of a fistula.

### Technique

With the patient in the prone jackknife position, the levator ani and external sphincter muscles are completely divided in the posterior midline. The bowel is opened, offering excellent exposure of the low and mid rectum (Fig. 23.53). Although tumors on the anterior wall are the easiest to demonstrate, those on the posterior or lateral walls can be brought into view by fully mobilizing the rectum.

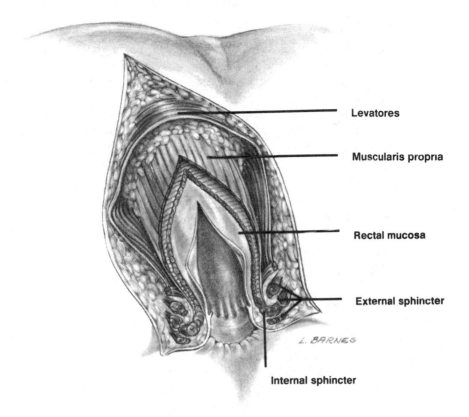

Levatores

Muscularis propria

Rectal mucosa

External sphincter

*L. BARNES*

**Internal sphincter**

**FIG. 23.53.** Transsphincteric excision. The rectum is opened like a book, posteriorly.

*Comment*: Although I have had no experience with this technique, the obvious criticism of failure to remove the associated lymphatics would relegate this procedure to one of palliation in the patient at poor risk. However, one could certainly consider this option as an alternative to local incision or transanal excision (see later). Yet, I cannot see why one would have to divide the sphincter muscles to accomplish this. I have no reservations, however, about dividing the sphincter muscles, because good functional results can be expected with direct repair. It may be useful to include the procedure in one's "repertoire of operations on the rectum," but it is doubtful that the treatment of cancer should be one of the indications.

## ABDOMINOTRANSSPHINCTERIC RESECTION

Mason reported an alternative means of effecting an anastomosis following an abdominoanal pull-through. By dividing the sphincter muscles as described in the preceding section, an anastomosis can be performed readily at the anal verge. As with other esoteric sphincter-saving approaches, it is not difficult for me to control my enthusiasm.

## LOCAL PROCEDURES

A number of local procedures can be used both for palliation and as curative approaches for the management of carcinoma of the rectum. With respect to cure, extensive preoperative evaluation should be obtained to be certain that a curative approach can be reasonably achieved through some form of local treatment. Individuals who are poor candidates for curative attempt at local incision include those with transmural involvement, poorly differentiated tumors, evident lymph node metastases, and those in whom a sphincter-saving operation can be carried out by conventional means and those who can tolerate a major operation. Five histopathologic characteristics have been identified as risk factors for lymph node metastases:

1. Small clusters of undifferentiated cancer cells ahead of the invasive front of the lesion ("tumor budding")
2. Poorly demarcated invasive front
3. Moderately or poorly differentiated cancer cells in the invasive front
4. Extension of the tumor to the middle or deep submucosal layer
5. Cancer cells in lymphatics

Investigators have concluded that those individuals with three or fewer risk factors had no nodal spread, whereas the rate of lymph node involvement with four or more risk factors was 33% and 67%, respectively. Such a classification may be useful in determining those individuals who might be preferred candidates for local excision. Others suggest that the incidence of lymph node metastases is higher for lesions more than 1 cm in diameter, for those showing massive submucosal invasion, and for moderately differentiated adenocarcinomas.

Despite all efforts for preoperative evaluation of lymph node metastases from rectal carcinomas, lymph node-clearing techniques may demonstrate tumor in lymph nodes as small as 1 mm, suggesting that even the best methods for preoperative assessment may miss tumors that are theoretically beyond surgical curability by simply local excision. The implication of this observation is that one should consider supplementary radiotherapy, either preoperatively or postoperatively, whenever a local procedure is recommended or performed.

### Electrocoagulation

Destruction of tumors by electric current has been reported virtually since electricity was harnessed. In 1913, Strauss advocated electrocoagulation for palliation in patients at poor risk with carcinoma of the rectum and in those individuals with extensive lesions. His indications were gradually broadened to include almost all stages of carcinoma of the rectum. Subsequent reports advocating electrosurgical destruction have dotted the literature, but their authors emphasized that the primary value of the procedure was in those patients who had incurable carcinoma or in those who refused colostomy. Despite Strauss' results, which were reported to be at least as satisfactory as those for surgically resected carcinomas, the value of this technique failed to have any significant impact on surgical thinking until Madden and Kandalaft reported their series in 1967. Subsequently, they updated their study in 1971, and Crile and Turnbull reported a series with favorable results in 1972. As a consequence, others have been encouraged to selectively apply this technique. Because of these reports, many surgeons have begun to use this treatment not only for palliation, but also for the potentially curable lesion.

### Indications

Electrocoagulation can be considered when (a) the tumor encompasses less than 50% of the bowel wall circumference; (b) the lesion is exophytic and well differentiated (or of a low-grade malignancy); (c) a patient with known metastases can have symptoms effectively palliated by this means; (d) debilitating disease is present; or (e) the patient refuses or cannot manage a colostomy. Relative contraindications to the procedure include a circumferential lesion, a poorly differentiated or highly anaplastic tumor, a deeply ulcerating growth, an anterior lesion in a woman, or a tumor that extends above the peritoneal reflection. Certainly, if the growth is high enough to be removed by anterior resection, this is the treatment of choice.

If electrocoagulation is contemplated, the importance of close follow-up examination and the possibility of readmission to the hospital must be stressed. It is much easier for a surgeon to perform an abdominoperineal excision knowing that little more can be offered the patient from the surgical point of view if the tumor recurs. However, if tumor recurs following electrocoagulation, it is extremely difficult to judge when this approach should be abandoned and when abdominoperineal excision should be done. Even after unsuccessful electrocoagulation, the patient may be cured by radical surgery many months after the initial therapy.

### Technique

All patients are treated in the hospital unless dealing with a very small lesion. Regional or general anesthesia is required. The patient is placed in the prone position if the tumor is primarily anterior, and in the lithotomy position if the tumor is essentially posterior. Following sphincter stretch, a plastic operating anal retractor of appropriate diameter and length is inserted. Local infiltration with bupivacaine and epinephrine can improve anal relaxation and limit the depth of anesthesia required.

The goal of electrocoagulation is to destroy by coagulating current the entire tumor and a margin of normal tissue, both deep to and around it. A standard electrocautery unit is used with the needle tip adapter, and only coagulating current is employed. The area for electrocoagulation is outlined by means of the needle

(Fig. 23.54A). The tip is then plunged into the tumor while the current is applied, and the process is repeated until the entire area has been treated (Fig. 23.54B). Necrotic tissue is removed by scraping, with the aid of an electrified wire loop or endometrial curette (Fig. 23.54C). When normal tissue is encountered (muscular wall or perirectal adipose tissue) the procedure is terminated. The operative time varies according to the size of the lesion and the degree of penetration; it can be as long as 2 hours. By no means should it be considered a minor undertaking. For larger tumors, more than one session may be required, each necessitating hospitalization and an anesthetic.

After a large tumor has been ablated, the patient, ideally, is confined in the hospital for several days, at which time further biopsies are taken, and a repeat coagulation is performed if necessary. The patient is seen at monthly intervals for the first 6 months and readmitted to the hospital (if possible) for biopsy and

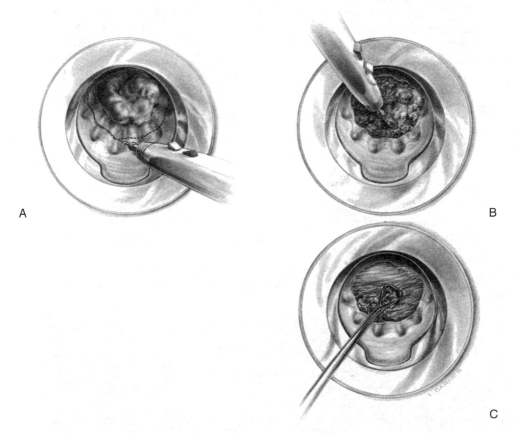

A

B

C

**FIG. 23.54.** Electrocoagulation of rectal cancer. **A.** The area of excision or electrocoagulation is outlined with the needle-tip electrode. **B.** Using the needle, the entire tumor mass is electrocoagulated. **C.** With an endometrial curette, the coagulum is scraped off and the process repeated. When only normal tissue remains, the operation is complete.

electrocoagulation if a recurrent tumor is suspected. After 6 months without evidence of tumor, the intervals between office visits are gradually lengthened to approximately four times a year.

## Complications

The most common postoperative complication is pyrexia. An oral temperature of 103°F (39.4°C) on the evening after surgery is not uncommon. It is because of this problem that broad-spectrum antibiotic treatment is recommended preoperatively and postoperatively for 24 hours. Pelvic peritonitis can occur without rectal perforation, but abdominal exploration, drainage, or colostomy is rarely indicated.

Hemorrhage at the time of surgery may necessitate multiple blood transfusions. All patients should have blood available when electrocoagulation is performed for large lesions. This can be a time-consuming operation, a procedure during which blood loss may seem minimal, but is indeed persistent. Late hemorrhage can occur up to several weeks after the procedure, probably secondary to sloughing of the eschar. This often requires readmission to the hospital and transfusion, and has been reported to occur in as many as 22% of patients who have electrocoagulation.

Rectal stricture can result from electrocoagulation if more than 50% of the bowel wall is involved by tumor. Repeated procedures increase the risk of this complication and impede the ability of the surgeon to visualize the area for possible recurrence. Benign stricture can be treated by lysis and the frequent insertion of a Hegar's dilator by the patient.

In women, rectovaginal fistula can result from vigorous burning of an anterior lesion. Electrocoagulation, therefore, should be performed only for small, exophytic lesions when they occur in this location.

## Results

Madden and Kandalaft updated their experience in 1983 to include a total of 204 patients treated by electrocoagulation. Their 5-year survival rates, even with ulcerating tumors, were impressive (57% with lesions of >3 cm and 63% if <3 cm). Patients with polypoid tumors had a 70% 5-year survival rate for the smaller tumors and a 64% rate for the larger ones.

Salvati et al. reported 81 patients who had electrocoagulation for cure and in whom at least a 5-year follow-up was available. The criteria for selection were essentially the same as those previously discussed. The overall 5-year survival rate was 47%, but 38% required conversion to an abdominoperineal resection. This last group had a 29% 5-year survival. The morbidity rate for electrocoagulation was 21%. Others have also become advocates of the judicious application of this technique. The subsequent colostomy rate, however, has been reported to be as high as 25%.

## Sequential Treatment

Eisenberg combined electrocoagulation with subsequent resection in the treatment of 250 patients, preferring to do low anterior resection, which calls into question the issue of performing this sphincter-saving alternative in the first instance. The survival results were exceptionally good: 85% following low anterior resection and 61% after abdominoperineal resection. Despite these favorable results, no one has been able to emulate the experience.

*Comment*: For electrocoagulation to be successfully employed, careful preoperative assessment must be made, including, ideally, transrectal ultrasound. Tumors should be mobile, exophytic, and well differentiated or moderately well differentiated. Flow cytometric evaluation may be helpful. The chance of lymph node metastases is considerably reduced if this protocol is followed.

Probably the most important criticism of this method is the failure to obtain a total pathologic specimen. Only biopsy can be depended on to determine histologic grade, and evidence obviously may be incomplete.

An additional concern is what to do if the tumor recurs. When should this treatment modality be abandoned? The answer, in my experience, lies in the quality of the doctor–patient relationship. The patient who accepts electrocoagulation in the first instance will often help to guide the surgeon in making future operative decisions. Finally, it is important to recognize that 5-year survival figures of 50%, 60%, 70%, or even 80% may not be laudatory, especially if the patients who were being selected for this treatment harbored the most favorable tumors (i.e., Dukes' A lesions).

## Transanal Excision

Transanal excision has been advocated by a number of surgeons for the definitive treatment of small (<3 cm), exophytic, movable, well-differentiated lesions. As with electrocoagulation, the preoperative evaluation should include histopathologic confirmation, especially the degree of differentiation, as well as endorectal ultrasound. The policy of less than resection is based on the knowledge that only a 10% risk of synchronous metastasis to regional lymph nodes exists when the cancer is confined to the rectal wall. The singular advantage of this technique over that of electrocoagulation is that it offers the opportunity for histologically evaluating a "total biopsy." Theoretically, if local excision is judged by the pathologist to be "complete," and the tumor is well or moderately well differentiated, reasonable recommendation is that no additional surgical treatment is required. The essential variable, therefore, is the capability and the interest of the pathologist. It is also extremely important to accurately orient the specimen for histologic examination. The following criteria have been suggested to help identify which neoplasms are theoretically suitable for transanal excision:

- <4 cm
- Confined to less than one quadrant

- <9 cm from anal verge
- Mobile
- Well-differentiated
- Absence of lymphovascular invasion
- Absence of PNI
- Ultrasonographic $T_1$, $T_2$, $N_0$ lesion
- On CT scan, no metastases

Unfortunately, no statistically meaningful studies are available concerning the risk of harboring additional tumor, and no prospective randomized clinical trials have been done.

## Technique

Transanal excision can be done through an operating proctoscope, but, more commonly, it is accomplished by dilating the anus and inserting retractors. As with electrocoagulation, proper positioning is crucial. Anterior lesions are best managed with the patient in the prone jackknife position, and posterior lesions are best treated with the patient in the lithotomy position. Ideally, an attempt should be made to achieve a 1-cm margin, but smaller margins may be as satisfactory. The tumor is outlined with this adequate margin by means of the needle tip electrocautery. Some individuals prefer injection of saline with or without epinephrine to facilitate hemostasis and to aid in the dissection. Generally, it is easier to begin the dissection from below the tumor using a clamp to hold the specimen as the dissection proceeds cephalad. Full-thickness rectal wall excision is performed; no attempt should be made to preserve part of the bowel wall.

## Results

The 5-year survival rate for tumors confined to the mucosa and submucosa is approximately 90%, and 75% when the cancer invades the muscularis propria. Three pathologic features have been identified that correlate with a high risk of recurrence and a poor outcome: positive surgical margins; poorly differentiated histology; and increasing depth of bowel wall invasion. Local control can be improved if postoperative radiotherapy is given for more invasive tumors and for those more than 3 cm in diameter. Others report a reasonably satisfactory experience in a highly selected group of patients.

*Comment*: The advantage of having a pathologic specimen to evaluate has caused me to utilize excision as the primary technique for those patients who are to have a local procedure. In essence, I use electrocoagulation primarily for palliation in those individuals who have larger lesions and who are not candidates for or refuse to have abdominoperineal resection. As discussed in the section on electrocoagulation, the major problem is what to do with an unfavorable pathology report and with subsequent recurrence.

At present, I recommend chemoradiation therapy for lesions that are subsequently found to be transmural or in cases of lymphatic or vascular invasion. Following completion of the treatment, the patient is reevaluated and a decision made whether a radical operation is appropriate. However, no meaningful statistics exist to determine whether additional surgery is necessary. But, certainly, ample evidence suggests that chemoradiation therapy can control local disease and downstage tumors (see later). If a resection is recommended, it should be performed not sooner than 3 weeks following completion of the chemoradiation therapy. I do not recommend proceeding immediately to resection with an unfavorable pathology report before adjuvant therapy has been tried. It is technically impossible to remove the rectum without entering a contaminated field, thereby increasing the risk of infection, and perhaps even jeopardizing the potential for cure through implantation of malignant cells.

### Transanal Endoscopic Microsurgery

Because of the technical problems associated with attempts at local excision of lesions at higher distances from the anal verge, Buess et al. developed a minimally invasive technique by means of a resectoscope. The procedure permits a stereoscopic, magnified view of a gas-dilated rectum, a feature that allows precise surgery to be performed in a difficult-to-reach area. The rectoscope has a diameter of 40 mm, with lengths available in either 12 or 20 cm (Fig. 23.55). All

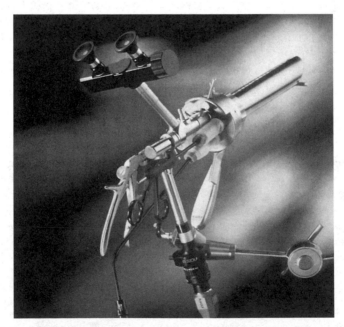

**FIG. 23.55.** Transanal endoscopic microsurgery system. The stereoscopic system permits excellent visualization. Up to four surgical instruments can be inserted at the same time. The assistant can follow the procedure through the use of a fiberoptic channel or through a video monitor. (Courtesy of Richard Wolf Medical Instruments, Inc. Vernon Hills, IL, USA.)

instruments are designed for endoscopic work, and include scissors, angled forceps, needle holder, suction device, and clip applicator.

## Results

The results are comparable to that of other local procedures that have been discussed. Remember, however, that the technique is often used for higher level lesions than could be attempted by conventional transanal excision or electrocoagulation. Others strongly advocate this procedure because of the excellent visualization obtained with this instrument. Winde et al. reported a 5-year survival rate of 96% in their 50 patients. Only 4.2% experienced a local recurrence. Others report comparable success with this technique. All conclude that the results are superior to alternative local approaches in the mid and upper rectum. One particular concern that has been expressed is the adverse effect of prolonged anal dilatation with the 4-cm diameter instrument.

*Comment:* Transanal endoscopic microsurgery is an exciting modality for satisfactorily performing local excision. However, two major disadvantages or concerns exist: First, the cost is considerable. Because of the limited applicability of this technique, it is doubtful whether many surgeons or institutions can justify the expense associated with this particular investment. Certainly, for distal rectal lesions, no significant advantage is seen to the technology when the option is available of merely using anorectal retractors. The other issue is the questionable application of this method for higher lesions, because these can often be resected by conventional means, with reestablishment of intestinal continuity. Therefore, although the instrument is indeed impressive and offers beautiful visualization, I do not see it entering the mainstream for most specialty surgeons in the management of carcinoma of the rectum.

## Laser Photocoagulation

Essentially, three methods are used for palliative endoscopic treatment of malignant strictures of the rectum–laser therapy, and its use in combination with either implantation of plastic prostheses or self-expanding metal stents. These have been discussed previously in this chapter and in Chapter 22. The advantage of stent placement is to maintain luminal patency to prevent the need for repetitive laser treatments. Many groups have used the Nd-YAG laser (see Chapter 1) for the palliative treatment of rectal cancer. As of this writing, however, no one is advocating this approach for the management of curable cancers of the rectum. For the unresectable tumor or when bleeding is a problem, the laser can restore luminal patency and achieve at least temporary hemostasis. When compared with other local procedures, laser therapy is unique in that it is of equal applicability to tumors above the peritoneal reflection as it is to those below. The Nd-YAG laser can also be used as a preresectional treatment for obstructing rectal carcinoma. Recanalization by this method permits primary resection and anastomosis to be accomplished.

Laser photocoagulation can be performed selectively on an outpatient basis, but it usually requires hospitalization. Standard bowel preparation is done; sedation alone may be adequate. Concern has been expressed that the energy delivered by the laser can be misleading. The actual tissue effect is as much related to the technique of application as it is to the laser power settings. Although laser endoscopy permits change of these settings to enhance a hemostatic or vaporizing effect, this must be recognized to avoid excessive cavitation.

Initial relief of symptoms has been reported to be approximately 90% in several published series; after a few months, however, individuals may require an additional treatment. The primary aim is to avoid a colostomy, and this is usually successful because patients are not expected to survive for very long. Perirectal abscess and bowel perforation, reportedly, are infrequent complications.

Self-expanding metal stents have been successfully used in combination with palliative laser therapy. Some authors have reported serious complications or signs of re-obstruction to be uncommon before the patient's death, with survival time up to 25 months. Others report a less favorable experience with this approach, with two thirds of those with large tumors requiring an alternative surgical approach.

*Comment*: The application of the laser in the treatment of benign and malignant neoplasms of the colon and rectum is a relatively recent phenomenon. However, with the increased use of endorectal ultrasound and other staging techniques, it is not unreasonable to expect that, at some point, patients with potentially curable cancers will be offered this alternative. This option, however, does require special expertise, and the equipment is expensive. Whether one is justified in becoming proficient with this technique at this time, is a matter of conjecture. Regardless, it is doubtful that laser photocoagulation will prove to be more advantageous than the other methods available for nonresectional treatment.

## Cryosurgery

Fritsch treated 219 patients with cryosurgery, but only for palliation. At 6 months to 7 years following treatment, local tumor was eradicated in 30% and reduced in size sufficiently to relieve symptoms in 24%. Fourteen percent experienced hemorrhage, and 26% developed stenoses; other major complications (e.g., peritonitis) were seen in 8%. Disadvantages included frequent discharge of necrotic tissue and malodorous secretions, as well as costly equipment. In other large series, colostomy was avoided in 80% (mean observation time, 2.3 years). The experience of others suggests that the cryosurgical technique provides therapeutic benefits for selected patients with advanced rectal cancer and for those who cannot tolerate a major operation.

## Endocavitary Irradiation

Radium needles and radiation therapy has been used in the palliative treatment of incurable or recurrent rectal cancer for almost 50 years. In fact, Sir Charles Gordon-Watson presented a paper on the use of radium in the treatment of rectal cancer as early as 1927. However, it was not until Papillon reported his experience in 1973 that radiation was applied as an alternative to surgery for a potentially curable lesion.

## Technique

The procedure requires a special device that can be inserted through a large-diameter proctoscope. The contact unit develops a high-radiation output (10 to 20 Gy/min) with low-voltage (50 kV) x-rays. The effective area is about 3 cm in diameter, with absorption of the x-rays essentially limited to a depth of 2 cm. Papillon recommends 25 to 40 Gy at each treatment, administered within 3 minutes. Treatments are repeated from 1 to 3 weeks later, for a total dose of between 80 and 150 Gy over a period of 4 to 10 weeks. Most patients can be managed outside a hospital setting, and no anesthesia is usually required.

In a later publication, Papillon suggests that, for patients younger than 60 years of age, a perirectal lymphadenectomy be considered. He has also added a combination of external beam radiation (30 Gy in 12 days), followed by iridium-192 implant 2 months later, to extend the field of radiation in the patient at poor risk in whom one wishes to use a "conservative treatment."

## Patient Selection

A number of criteria must be met if a patient is to be considered for this treatment:

- Accessibility of the entire lesion
- Small size (<4.5 cm)
- Noninfiltrating
- Histologically well-differentiated
- Palpable
- Movable
- Absence of palpable mesorectal nodes

## Results

Papillon initially reported on 106 patients, 70% of whom were alive and free of disease after 5 years. Local recurrence developed in 14 individuals (13%). Sixteen patients (15%) died of malignant disease. A more recent report from his center included 245 patients followed for more than 5 years. A local failure rate of 5.3% was noted. The death rate from cancer was 8.9%, and the 5-year survival rate, 76%.

From the Cleveland Clinic comes a report of 199 patients treated by endocavitary radiation, 126 of whom were managed with curative intent. Of these, 29% had a recurrence. With additional treatment, 11% were rendered free of disease. With more than 5 years of follow-up, 91% had no evidence of disease with additional treatment, but only 68% were cured on the basis of endocavitary irradiation alone.

## Complications

Very few complications were attributable to treatment with endocavitary irradiation. Jelden reported mild proctitis of short duration and occasional bleeding. Rectovaginal fistula has also been seen. Deaths directly related to the therapy have not been reported.

*Comment*: As with electrocoagulation, it is difficult to assess the results of endocavitary radiation by comparison with standard resective treatment. Only those who have the most favorable prognoses are selected. A patient who has abdominoperineal resection for a Dukes' A lesion has a chance of cure that approaches 90%. As with electrocoagulation, are some patients being deprived of the only possibility for cure if they harbor lymph node metastases? Even with careful patient selection, the decision to use any of the local treatments or procedures requires considerable preoperative counseling and close follow-up care.

## RADIOTHERAPY

The use of external beam radiotherapy in the management of rectal cancer as an adjunctive treatment to surgery, either preoperatively or postoperatively, has received considerable attention in recent years. In theory, preoperative treatment should decrease the size and the extent of tumor invasion and permit complete removal as well as minimize the risk of local recurrence. Preoperative treatment can also limit the likelihood of dissemination of viable tumor cells during surgical manipulation.

Postoperative therapy offers the distinct advantage of having a pathology report in hand; thus, the known extent of disease determines the field of treatment. In the postoperative patient who is known to have a less favorable lesion (Dukes' B or C), radiotherapy might reduce the risk of pelvic recurrence.

### Preoperative Radiotherapy

The rationale of the preoperative radiotherapy approach to the adjunctive management of rectal cancer is to alter the viability of cancer cells so that they are no longer capable of local implantation. Although the initial studies indicated improved survival, prospective evaluation has demonstrated that the overall survival rate is not better, but that the incidence of failure from local recurrence is reduced.

Numerous papers have attested to the success of the treatment either in reducing the size of the tumor or in decreasing the risk of local recurrence. Some have stated that survival rates are better. However, considerable disagreement remains to whether preoperative radiation therapy has any affect on survival. But few question that the technique is of demonstrable benefit in the management of "unresectable" tumors.

Considerable controversy remains to what the optimal dose for preoperative radiation treatment should be. Some have recommended a short course of high-dose therapy, whereas most centers in the United States suggest 40 to 45 Gy, delivered in 4 to 6 weeks. Surgery is recommended approximately 4 to 6 weeks after the completion of the treatment, because tumoricidal benefits can continue for some time. Data show no increased morbidity or mortality associated with supplementary treatment.

The largest prospective, randomized trials come from Sweden (the Stockholm Rectal Cancer Study Group and the Swedish Rectal Cancer Trial). In the Stockholm trial, the most recent publication analyzed postoperative morbidity, mortality, local recurrence, and death from rectal cancer in 1,399 patients who were prospectively randomized to preoperative radiotherapy or no radiotherapy. Those allocated to preoperative radiotherapy received a total dose of 35 Gy in five fractions over 1 week, with surgery performed within 1 week thereafter. Interestingly, patients operated on by surgeons who were certified specialists for at least 10 years had a lower risk of local recurrence and death from rectal cancer. A significantly reduced risk of local recurrence was observed, but no clear improvement in survival. However, the investigators also found that the postoperative mortality rate may be increased in the radiotherapy group.

In the Swedish Rectal Cancer Trial involving 1,168 patients (as of the most recent date), preoperative radiation was accomplished through 25 Gy and five fractions in 1 week, also followed by operation within 1 week. In this randomized, prospective study, the local recurrence rate during a period of 2 years was reduced by about 65%. Furthermore, this short-term regimen of high-dose preoperative radiotherapy was found to improve survival. The overall 5-year survival rate was 58% in the radiotherapy plus surgery group and 48% in the surgery-alone group ($p = 0.004$). This truly appears to be the first clear demonstration of improved survival by means of preoperative radiotherapy. Another prospective, randomized trial, by the Medical Research Council Rectal Cancer Working Party from Birmingham, England, used 40 Gy given in 20 fractions of 2 Gy over 4 weeks in those individuals randomized to preoperative radiotherapy. At 5-year follow-up, those who were randomized to radiation therapy had a statistically significantly lower incidence of local recurrence as well as fewer distant metastases, but survival results were equivocal. However, the numerous prospective, randomized trials that have been undertaken thus far suffer from several shortcomings. None uses standard dosages of radiation therapy. Second, the interval between the completion of radiation and surgery is generally considered to be inadequate. Most recommend 4 to 6 weeks following completion of the treatment to achieve maximal downstaging and tissue recovery. Finally, using anterior-posterior or posterior-anterior portals, rather than multiple-field techniques, predisposes to increased morbidity associated with the radiation.

Most experienced surgeons are well aware of the problem of delayed healing of the perineal wound when preoperative radiation is performed. Furthermore, an inherent problem concerns the well-controlled, randomized trial with this group of patients. Stratification by the usual criterion, namely depth of invasion (e.g., Dukes' classification) cannot be applied; other, less well-defined criteria, such as clinical judgment, must be used. Endorectal ultrasound is of help for staging the depth of penetration, and DNA ploidy seems to be an independent factor for predicting response to radiotherapy, but currently we must await the results of the studies currently in progress.

The safety of performing anastomosis in the rectum following radiation therapy has been a matter of some conjecture. A number of studies, however, have demonstrated that colorectal anastomoses can be performed without concern for an increased risk of complications if the radiation dose does not exceed 45 Gy.

Preoperative radiation therapy has minimal immediate effect on the anal sphincter and is not a major contributing factor to postoperative incontinence after sphincter-saving operations for rectal cancer. However, preoperative radiotherapy alters endosonographic staging and interferes with the endosonographic interpretation of the anastomotic area.

## Postoperative Radiotherapy

As stated, the primary advantage of postoperative radiotherapy is that selected patients can be offered this additional treatment based on their "unfavorable" pathology reports. For example, those individuals with Dukes' B and C tumors have a high incidence of local recurrence following resection. Conversely, disadvantages of this alternative include the risk that cells may be seeded outside the treatment area, wound healing can be delayed, and the physiology of residual tumor can be altered by the reduction in the vascular supply.

In patients with Dukes' B and C lesions, the local recurrence rate appears to be 8% to 10%. Generally, the perception is that postoperative radiotherapy is not as well tolerated as preoperative treatment. Anastomotic strictures have been reported to occur as a consequence of this regimen. Also the concern is seen for delay in commencement of the therapy because of problems with wound healing and other factors.

*Comment*: Until the results of controlled studies are available, my attitude is to advise supplementary radiotherapy for patients who are at a high risk of recurrence: those with poorly differentiated tumors and those with Dukes' B or C lesions. The treatment should begin not sooner than 1 month following the operation (to avoid problems with wound healing) or later than 2 months (to limit the likelihood of spread). The dosage to the tumor bed should be approximately 60 Gy. Radiotherapy is not without significant complications: urinary tract infection, diarrhea, small bowel injury, and skin and wound breakdown. Therefore, before embarking on such treatment consider other factors, such as the age of the patient and the quality of life anticipated.

## Palliative Radiotherapy

Radiotherapy can be uniquely beneficial in the treatment of patients with recurrent disease who have pelvic pain. This has been discussed earlier in this chapter. It has also been suggested for use in those patients with locally advanced lesions, in combination with chemotherapy, surgery, or both. Kodner et al. definitively treated by means of external radiation 84 patients with invasive rectal carcinoma. The use of external radiation before endocavitary radiation achieved local control in 93% of patients with favorable lesions. However, the investigators found little place for nonresective management of aggressive rectal cancers, even for palliation, unless an individual's life expectancy was less than 6 months.

## Hyperthermochemoradiotherapy

Mori et al. reported the application of a multimodality approach in the management of patients with rectal cancer—hyperthermochemoradiotherapy (HCR). This approach consists of a preoperative combination of hyperthermia at 42°C to 45°C for 40 minutes (two times per week for 2 weeks), intravenous 5-FU, and a total of 30 Gy irradiation. Reduction in tumor size was evident in their 11 patients with either no or only a few viable cancer cells present in the resected specimen. A later report from the same institution involving 36 patients revealed that 5-year survival rates were 91% compared with historical controls of 74% in those not receiving HCR. Whether this approach will prove to have merit in the management of patients with rectal cancer remains to be determined.

## Intraoperative Radiotherapy

Intraoperative radiotherapy (IORT) is a technique by which a resectable lesion is removed and the remaining cancer cells sterilized at the time of the operation, with the patient's abdomen open. The procedure has been reported to be of particular value for those who are found to have fixed, unresectable rectal or rectosigmoid lesions. The following criteria have been suggested to identify patients who may be suitable for IORT:

Tumor must be localized.
Tumor must be accessible to treatment applicator and in an area from which normal tissue can be displaced.
The patient's condition must be potentially curable, yet the tumor cannot be controlled by surgery alone.

Usually, the patient receives external beam radiation of 45 to 50 Gy. Four to 6 weeks following completion of the therapy, and after CT evaluation is performed to ascertain that no evidence of disseminated disease exists, the patient has reexploration and resection. If microscopic residual tumor is found, as determined by frozen-section examination, or if it is felt that cure is unlikely, an appropriate-sized Lucite "radiation applicator" is selected. Few institutions have dedicated IORT operating suites, so it may be necessary to transport the patient to the radiation therapy unit for "booster therapy." A dose of 15 to 20 Gy is then delivered as a single treatment.

As of this writing it is difficult to offer firm conclusions about the relative merits of this approach. Three to 5-year results from a number of centers for marginally resectable disease are approximately 50% and, for recurrent disease, about 40%. An overall 5-year survival of approximately 40% is reported, even in those with locally unresectable primary rectal cancer.

## CHEMOTHERAPY

The role of chemotherapy in colorectal cancer is discussed in Chapter 22.

## COMBINED CHEMOTHERAPY AND RADIOTHERAPY

### Preoperative

A number of published reports have been encouraging regarding the use of a modality combining chemotherapy and radiotherapy (see earlier and Chapter 22). The technique of using chemosensitized irradiation has succeeded in down-staging tumors (with respect to Dukes' classification) and in reducing tumor size. Unfortunately, until recently no data had appeared which indicated an increased cure rate.

### Postoperative

In 1991, Krook et al. demonstrated encouraging results with postoperative chemoradiation therapy. A total of 204 patients with rectal carcinoma that was either deeply invasive or metastatic to lymph nodes were randomly assigned to postoperative radiation alone (45 to 50 Gy) or to radiation plus fluorouracil. This treatment was both preceded and followed by a cycle of systemic therapy with fluorouracil plus semustine (methyl-CCNU). After a median follow-up of more than 7 years, the combined regimen reduced the recurrence rate by 34%. Initial local recurrence was reduced by 46% and distant metastasis by 37%. Additionally, the combined treatment reduced the rate of cancer-related deaths by 36% and the overall death rate by 29%.

O'Connell et al., reporting from the Mayo Clinic, administered 5-FU by protracted infusion throughout the duration of radiation therapy in 660 patients with Dukes' B and C tumors. With a median follow-up of 46 months among surviving patients, those who received the infusion had a significantly increased time before relapse as well as an improved survival. Others confirm that 5-FU combined with irradiation appears to maximize control of both local and distant metastatic disease. A 1-month protocol reported on behalf of the Norwegian Adjuvant Rectal Cancer Project Group, the use of 5-FU reduced local recurrence rate, increased recurrence-free survival and overall survival, without serious side effects when compared with those who did not have such treatment.

*Comment*: The implications of these studies are such that any individual with pathologic confirmation of a Dukes' B or C lesion should be considered for a postoperative protocol.

# 24

# Malignant Tumors
# of the Anal Canal

Carcinomas of the anal canal and perianal skin are uncommon clinical entities, accounting for 2% to 4% of all colorectal carcinomas. Anal canal cancer is almost three times more common than carcinoma of the anal margin. If the dentate line is taken as the distal limit of the anal canal, nearly 70% of all anal tumors will occur in the anal canal. However, if the anal canal is assumed to extend from the anorectal ring to the anal verge (the junction of modified squamous epithelium with the hair-bearing, keratinized perianal skin), 85% of anal tumors will arise in the anal canal. Anal canal tumors are more frequently seen in women (3:2), whereas carcinoma of the anal margin is more common in men (4:1), although the median age for both genders at presentation is the same (57 years).

## ANATOMY AND HISTOLOGY

Some controversy exists about the anatomic limits of the anal canal, although it is generally agreed that the proximal extent corresponds to the anorectal ring. The distal end has been variously proposed to be the dentate line, Hilton's line, and the anal verge. I believe it is that portion of the intestinal tract that lies between the termination of the rectal mucosa above and the beginning of the perianal skin below (Fig. 24.1). It is divided into a proximal transitional zone encompassing the columns and sinuses of Morgagni and a distal zone lined by squamous epithelium. The transitional zone is derived from the embryonic cloaca and separates the rectal mucosa from the squamous epithelium of the distal anal canal. The anal glands and ducts arise from this area and are lined by stratified columnar epithelium. The median number of anal glands is six, with 80% extending to the submucosa, 8% to the circular internal sphincter, 8% to the longitudinal internal sphincter, 2% to the intersphincteric space, and only 1% penetrating the external anal sphincter. The anal glands have definite secretory activity and are presumed to be responsible for lubricating the anal canal.

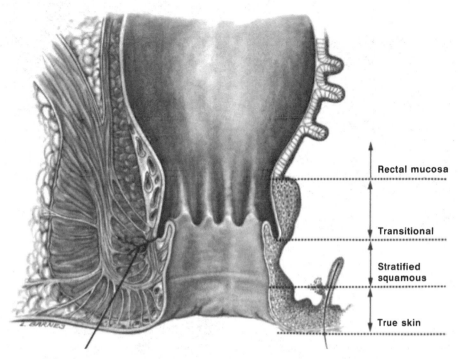

**FIG. 24.1.** Anatomy of the anus with histologic pattern schematically illustrated.

The transitional zone contains epithelium resembling that found in the urethra, but much variability exists in the region; patches of squamous epithelium are frequently present, especially over the crests of the columns of Morgagni. The junction between the transitional zone and squamous mucosa, which lies at the inferior limit of the columns of Morgagni, has been referred to as the "dentate" or "pectinate" line. However, some authors place the dentate line at the proximal limit of the anal canal, at the junction between the rectal mucosa and transitional zone. The more distal zone of the anal canal is lined by stratified squamous epithelium and can be differentiated histologically from perianal skin by the absence of the epidermal appendages found in the skin. Separating tumors that arise in the anal canal from those of the perianal skin is important because their biologic behavior and, consequently, treatment is distinctly different.

## CARCINOMA OF THE PERIANAL SKIN AND ANAL MARGIN

Neoplasms of the anal margin and perianal skin include squamous cell carcinoma, Bowen's disease, Paget's disease, and basal cell carcinoma. It is generally accepted that wide surgical excision is adequate treatment for lesions of the perianal skin (Fig. 24.2). Carcinomas of the anal margin have a better prognosis than

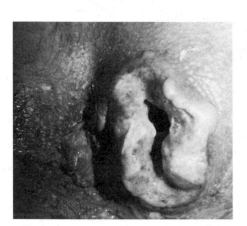 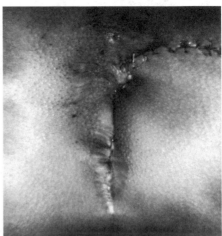

**FIG. 24.2.** Ulcerating squamous cell carcinoma of the buttock.

that of tumors of the anal canal. Superficial, well-to moderately differentiated T1 cancers of the anal margin can be successfully treated with radiotherapy alone or by local excision. However, because stage T2 lesions have an increased risk for lymph node metastases to the groin, radiotherapy to the primary tumor in conjunction with elective inguinal lymph node radiation is recommended. Furthermore, abdominoperineal resection is reserved for those who have complications secondary to the radiation therapy or locally recurrent disease. Local excision is associated with a corrected 5-year survival rate of 88%.

## Recommendation

It is self-evident that any suspicious lesion around the anus should be biopsied. If it is confirmed to be a malignant neoplasm, the usual treatment is to perform wide local excision, because these lesions tend not to metastasize. The defect created by excision can be left to granulate, covered by a split-thickness skin graft or closed by rotating a flap of adjacent skin.

## CLASSIFICATION OF ANAL CANAL TUMORS

Three histologic types of tumors are identified in the anal canal: (a) epidermoid (squamous cell) and mucoepidermoid carcinoma; (b) transitional–cloacogenic carcinoma; and (c) malignant melanoma. Some physicians regard transitional–cloacogenic carcinoma as a manifestation of epidermoid carcinoma because of some overlap with standard epidermoid carcinomas, whereas others believe it is a distinctly separate entity that arises from the transitional zone of the anal canal with different morphologic and clinical features. With the exception of melanoma, the clinical behavior of carcinoma of the anal canal appears to be relatively independent of the morphologic subtype when compared stage for stage and grade for grade.

Epidermoid (squamous cell) carcinoma account for two thirds of the tumors of the anal canal, transitional–cloacogenic carcinomas comprise approximately one fourth, and melanomas make up the remainder (15%).

## EPIDERMOID OR SQUAMOUS CELL CARCINOMA OF THE ANUS

### Incidence

Epidermoid carcinoma of the anus can be multifocal in the anal canal as well as in the perianal skin, perineum, and vulvar areas. They account for 1.5 to 4% of all carcinomas of the colon, rectum, and anus.

### Age and Gender

Epidermoid carcinoma can occur at almost any age but is usually found in the sixth and seventh decades. Most studies have shown a preponderance of carcinoma of the anal canal in women. The mean age of patients is 59 years. In Sweden, the annual age-adjusted incidence per 100,000 population for squamous cell carcinoma is 1.4 for women and 0.68 for men. However, in centers with a large patient population of men at high risk, the female:male ratio may approach unity.

### Predisposing Conditions

An increased incidence of anal cancer is seen with a number of anorectal inflammatory conditions (e.g., chronic anal fistula and anal condylomata). A possible relationship with human papillomavirus (HPV) types that are known to be associated with cervical and other genital cancers has been suggested. HPV-16 and -18 are involved in the development of anal and genital squamous cell carcinoma. Associations between positive herpes simplex virus 2 titer, cigarette smoking, a prior positive or questionable cervical Papanicolaou smear, and an increasing number of sexual partners have also been made with the development of anal cancer. An increased incidence of cancers in the anogenital region has also been observed in patients who have undergone renal transplant, presumably as a consequence of immunosuppression, and anal cancers have also occurred following radiation therapy for pruritus.

Several reports have suggested a significantly higher incidence in patients with Crohn's disease. Although it is unlikely that a patient with an anal fistula or condylomata would be treated with expectant observation, individuals with Crohn's disease are often managed in this way. Therefore, it is important to perform a biopsy of any unusual lesion; it may even be good counsel to suggest random anal biopsies at intervals for patients with this condition.

A relationship appears to exist between the human immunodeficiency virus (HIV) and squamous cell carcinoma. Because of the increased incidence of venereal disease in the homosexual population, increasing evidence suggests that gay men are at a particular risk for the development of anal cancer. Even in the absence of the acquired immunodeficiency syndrome (AIDS), anal canal carcinoma, Kaposi's sarcoma, and anorectal lymphoma are seen in younger patients and much more frequently than would be expected.

It can be appreciated, therefore, that a number of predisposing conditions are associated with the development of malignant anal canal tumors. This implies that the etiology probably represents an interaction between genetic as well as environmental factors. The genetic aspect may be related to changes in chromosome 11 (11q22) or the short arm of chromosome 3 (3p22).

In summary, therefore, the following variables are related to the development of anogenital carcinoma:

- Prior radiotherapy
- Chronic anal fistula
- Crohn's disease
- Smoking
- Positive Papanicolaou smear
- Cervical carcinoma
- HPV
- Hodgkin's disease
- Renal transplantation
- Promiscuity
- Positive herpes simplex virus II titer
- HIV
- Male homosexuality
- Anoreceptive intercourse
- Immunosuppression
- Positive serologic test for syphilis
- Anal condylomata

Current evidence suggests that the etiology of anal cancer is a multifactorial interaction among environmental factors, HPV infection, immune status, and suppressor genes.

## Signs and Symptoms

Symptoms of anal canal carcinoma include rectal bleeding, anal pain, pruritus, mucous discharge, tenesmus, the sensation of a lump in the anus, and a change in bowel habits. Rectal bleeding occurs in more than one half of individuals. The duration of symptoms is of little prognostic significance. Complaints such as discharge, incontinence, change in bowel habits, pelvic pain, or the passage of stool or gas through the vagina, suggest an advanced lesion. Tenesmus, the painful urgency to defecate, suggests invasion of the sphincter mechanism. Presentation is often late, with the mean size of tumor at diagnosis between 3 and 4 cm. Occasionally, a patient presents with a mass in the groin, a manifestation of a metastasis before the primary tumor causes significant symptoms. The condition can also be identified incidentally on review of the histology of a hemorrhoidectomy specimen.

## Examination and Biopsy

Rectal examination may reveal an ulcerating, hard, tender, bleeding mass in the anal canal or lower rectum. An advanced lesion may be excruciatingly tender at examination and require evaluation under an anesthetic. The lesion may fungate through the anal canal and appear on the perianal skin or present through a chronic draining anal fistula. Proctosigmoidoscopic examination usually shows that the tumor is confined to the anal canal. However, in far advanced cases, the lesion can extend upward to involve the rectum. Conversely, a carcinoma that seems to arise within the anal canal occasionally is a rectal cancer that has spread downward. Another possibility is implantation from a colon tumor, a particular concern if hemorrhoidectomy is performed at the time of a colectomy for cancer.

## Pathology

### *Epidermoid Carcinoma*

Epidermoid carcinoma originates from the stratified squamous epithelium of the distal anal mucosa and, therefore, morphologically resembles carcinoma arising from the buccal mucosa, esophagus, cervix uteri, and so forth. The tumor is composed of squamous epithelial cells that resemble normal anal mucosa to a varying extent, depending on the degree of differentiation (Fig. 24.3). The more differentiated tumors have readily apparent keratin formation, either as pearls or as individual cell keratinization. The lesions can be graded on the basis of the degree of keratinization and the nuclear morphology. This grade correlates with the behavior of the tumor: well-differentiated tumors tend to be less deeply invasive and are less likely to metastasize. More than 50% of anal canal tumors are nonkeratinizing, whereas 80% are poorly differentiated. This is in contrast to anal margin tumors, with 80% demonstrating keratinization and 85% being well differentiated.

A careful search using mucin stains may disclose a focus of mucin-producing cells in as many as 10% to 15% of patients. Such tumors have been classified separately as mucoepidermoid carcinomas, but little evidence exists that differences in the behavior of this subgroup warrant its separation. A spindle cell carcinoma (pseudosarcoma) has been reported to be another variant.

Squamous cell carcinoma antigen (SCC) has been shown to be a tumor marker that seems to be related to the histologic characteristics of differentiated epider-

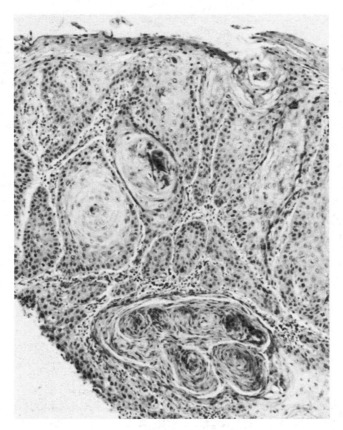

**FIG. 24.3.** This well-differentiated squamous cell carcinoma resembling normal squamous epithelium is producing keratin pearls (*bottom*). Less well-differentiated lesions lose their resemblance to squamous epithelium, lack keratin pearls, and behave more aggressively. (Original magnification ×100.)

moid tumors rather than to tumor site. No apparent prognostic value is seen for this study at the time of diagnosis, but the level of SCC may correlate well with the development of recurrence.

### Transitional–Cloacogenic Carcinoma

Transitional–cloacogenic carcinomas can resemble carcinomas of urothelium to a certain extent, or they can have patterns similar to those of basal cell carcinoma of skin—hence the term, *basaloid*, because the cells at the periphery are arranged in an orderly, palisaded fashion (Fig. 24.4). However, this variation in cell pattern must not be confused with basal cell carcinoma; the former is a malignant tumor that frequently metastasizes, whereas the latter is relatively benign.

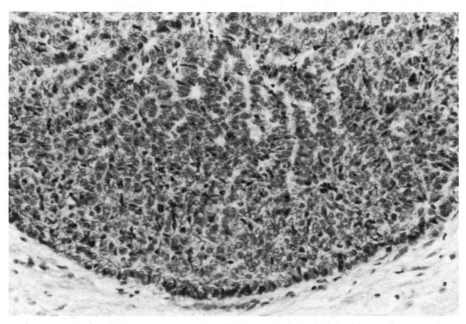

**FIG. 24.4.** Transitional–cloacogenic carcinoma. In this tumor, the cells at the periphery tend to arrange themselves in a palisade, thus resembling basal cell carcinoma of the skin. This variant of transitional–cloacogenic carcinoma is sometimes called "basaloid carcinoma." (Original magnification ×80.)

Those tumors resembling urothelial carcinomas are composed of islands or nests of cells that have indistinct borders and oval nuclei (Fig. 24.5). A focus of keratinization is often present. As stated, varying amounts of squamous elements produce a spectrum of lesions ranging from purely transitional through mixed varieties to purely squamous tumors. Some examples of transitional–cloacogenic carcinoma appear to arise in the lower part of the rectum above the transitional zone; others may not even involve the mucosa. The probable explanation for these phenomena is that such tumors can originate from the transitional epithelium that lines the anal ducts deep to the mucosa or in proximal ramifications of the ducts beneath rectal mucosa.

Transitional–cloacogenic tumors form a histologically recognizable subgroup of anal canal carcinomas, but on the basis of grade and stage of the lesions their behavior appears to be comparable to that of epidermoid carcinomas of similar grade and stage. Fewer studies of transitional–cloacogenic tumors have been published than for epidermoid carcinoma. Evidence, however, suggests sufficient overlap in the epidemiology (e.g., an increased incidence in anal-receptive homosexual men), the clinical presentation, and the results of classic treatment; thus, for the purposes of management, the two entities can be considered identical.

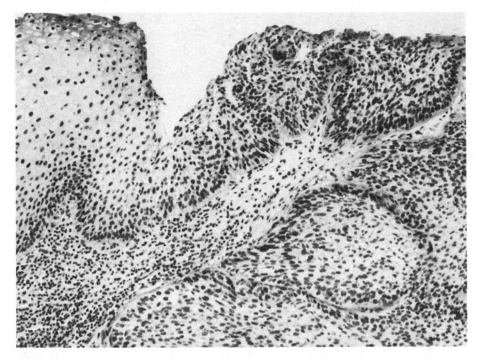

**FIG. 24.5.** Transitional–cloacogenic carcinoma. The tumor has an *in situ* component (*upper right*) resembling a transitional cell carcinoma of the urinary bladder, hence its name. (Original magnification ×125.)

### Melanoma

The histopathology of malignant melanoma is discussed later in this chapter.

### Adenocarcinoma

Adenocarcinoma of the anus is usually seen as a downward extension of a primary rectal tumor. However, glandular epithelium may be found on biopsy from ectopic glands of the anal wall, sebaceous glands of the perineum, tumors arising in anal glands or ducts, or from anal fistulas. As discussed in Chapter 19, the association with an underlying mucinous adenocarcinoma and Paget's disease has been well documented.

### Staging

No satisfactory method for staging anal canal tumors has been developed. Dukes' classification is not applicable, because invasion to groin nodes can occur when lymph node involvement is not evident in the resected specimen. The tumor, node, and metastasis (TNM) system has been criticized because it is difficult to distinguish tumor invasion limited to the internal sphincter from that involving the external sphincter, and because extension into the rectum or perianal skin does not necessarily imply a poorer prognosis. Histologic grade and clinical stage seem to be the best predictors of patient outcome.

## Treatment

Until the mid to late 1970s, abdominoperineal resection was felt to be the only curative approach to the management of anal canal carcinoma. However, even before the advent of multimodality therapy, basically two surgical approaches were used to the management of carcinoma of the anal canal: local excision and abdominoperineal resection. The choice of therapy depends on the stage of the tumor as determined by depth of invasion.

## Local Excision

For carcinoma confined to the mucosa (carcinoma *in situ*; see Fig. 24.5) and submucosa, wide local excision with or without anoplasty will usually be curative. For tumors invading the muscularis propria (the internal sphincter), local excision, including the internal sphincter, usually achieves cure. However, for tumors that invade more deeply than the internal sphincter, abdominoperineal resection has, historically, been the initial treatment of choice. These differences in therapy based on the stage of the tumor require precise preoperative evaluation, including careful digital examination to assess the depth of invasion, and also perhaps by endoanal ultrasound.

Other options in the management of small, superficial or minimally invasive anal canal cancers include cryosurgery, laser vaporization, and possibly the use of chemical or immunoablational topical agents (for intraepithelial neoplasia).

*Abdominoperineal Resection.* The technique of abdominoperineal resection is described in Chapter 23. An important principle to remember is that when the anal margin is involved by tumor, a wider excision of perianal skin is required than is customary for adenocarcinoma of the rectum.

## Results of Conventional Abdominoperineal Resection and Local Excision ("Historical" Data)

Five-year survival after abdominoperineal resection, reported to be between 20% and 70%, depends on tumor size, histologic grading, and depth of invasion. Pelvic or perineal recurrence accounts for 50% to 70% of failures, with only 10% of patients dying from disseminated disease. Of all surgical approaches, abdominoperineal resection with posterior exenteration had the lowest recurrence rate.

The Sloan-Kettering group observed that few patients with epidermoid cancer of the anal canal have been treated by local excision, and interpretation of the results can be somewhat confusing because these individuals may be combined with those who had tumors of the anal margin. At Memorial Sloan-Kettering Hospital, less than 10% of tumors were suitable for local excision; more than 60% of the patients so treated developed recurrence.

With lymph node involvement or invasion into the perirectal or perianal fat, the prognosis is much less optimistic. With lymph node involvement, a 29% 5-year survival rate is seen. It is generally agreed that the depth of invasion and the presence or absence of lymph node involvement are the major criteria for determining length of survival. The prognosis after resection for transitional–cloacogenic carcinoma is essentially the same as that for epidermoid carcinoma for the same depth of invasion. In analyzing survival with respect to cell differentiation, no relationship is apparent except that the more poorly differentiated lesions tend to present at a more advanced stage.

To all intents and purposes the above results are of historical interest, only. Today, it is not within the standard of care to go directly to abdominoperineal resection for carcinoma of the anal canal. This is because of the advances made with the use of combined therapy.

### Groin Dissection

Radical groin dissection had been advocated as a valuable adjunctive procedure in the primary treatment of carcinoma of the anal canal because of its possible spread to inguinal nodes. More recent reports are highly critical of this approach, however. Because of its high morbidity and because it is an unnecessary operation in the most patients, radical groin dissection as a therapeutic modality should be used only when adenopathy is subsequently discovered. For diagnostic and staging purposes, it seems reasonable to excise a large inguinal mass. Even though the cure rate is still low, some authors feel that this procedure reduces the risk of groin complications from tumor growth. However, these patients should probably be offered chemotherapy and radiotherapy in light of the responsiveness of this tumor to such an approach (see prior discussion).

### Pelvic Lymphadenectomy

Pelvic lymphadenectomy in conjunction with abdominoperineal resection can be performed relatively easily in some patients concomitant with abdominoperineal resection. The value of obtaining nodes to determine the prognosis and the advisability of adding other treatment may justify this approach, but it should not be performed if the dissection is difficult.

### Combined or Multimodality Therapy

In 1974, Nigro et al. reported dramatic results in the treatment of epidermoid carcinoma of the anus by means of preoperative radiation therapy and chemotherapy. Subsequent reports from Nigro's unit at Wayne State University School of Medicine revealed continued enthusiasm. The remarkable success of combined or multimodal therapy in the management of even locally extensive tumors or in individuals with regional node metastases has revolutionized the approach to the management of this condition.

The protocol initially consisted of preoperative radiation (a total of 30 Gy) to the tumor and to the pelvic and inguinal nodal areas in 15 treatments over a 3-week period (2 Gy/d, 5 days a week). The first day that radiotherapy is commenced, the patient is administered 5-fluorouracil in 5% glucose, 1,000 mg/m² per day, for 4 days as a continuous 24-hour infusion, and again from days 29 through 32. In addition, the patient is given mitomycin-C (15 mg/m²) as a single bolus on the first day. This protocol is usually associated with only a mild degree of thrombocytopenia and leukopenia. The most frequent side effects are low-grade stomatitis and moderate diarrhea. A number of variations of this radiation-chemotherapeutic scheme are currently available.

### Results

Analysis of the initial 45 patients treated under Dr. Nigro's protocol revealed that 38 of 45 patients (84%) were rendered free of cancer. Although the follow-up period of many patients was less than 5 years, 34 (89%) were alive and free of disease. All patients with residual tumor, even after abdominoperineal resection had been performed, died of disseminated disease.

Others have also reported favorable experience, even in patients with recurrent and locally advanced disease. Comparing the results of treatment by radical external beam radiation alone with the combined modality approach reveals an uncorrected 5-year survival rate for the two groups of approximately 70%. However, the primary tumor is better controlled with combination treatment (65% to 93%) than with radiation therapy alone (40% to 60%).

Most physicians today recommend that standard treatment should be a combined approach, and that surgery should be reserved for those who fail on this regimen. However, because of variable toxicity, it may be necessary to suspend or alter treatment for certain individuals.

### *Treatment and Results of Cloacogenic Carcinoma*

As with all invasive anal canal cancers, classic treatment has been abdominoperineal resection. Results following resection (without chemoradiation) have been essentially the same as that reported for epidermoid carcinoma, the 5-year survival rate being approximately 50%. However, the applicability of the combined modality approach, chemotherapy and radiation therapy, is as valid for this histologic type as it is for epidermoid carcinoma, and this should be the preferred approach. Statistics on survival rates should be the same as have been implied previously.

### Post-Therapy Evaluation and Treatment

The question of how to address the post-therapy evaluation is still a matter of some debate. Biopsy or local excision of the scar site can be performed 6 weeks after completion of the regimen. If no tumor is found, the patient is observed at intervals, perhaps every 2 to 3 months. Any suspicious area is subsequently biopsied. Some surgeons prefer observation without biopsy if no suspicious area is evident. Most clinicians believe that recurrent or persistent tumor following chemoradiation therapy mandates radical resection. An additional course of chemoradiation therapy is warranted in some cases, however.

Some authors have reported the application of SCC as a tumor marker for the follow-up of patients with carcinoma of the anal canal. The procedure was initially developed and used primarily for women with carcinoma of the uterus, but its applicability for epidermoid carcinoma of the anal canal has been proposed. The sensitivity of this antigen has been reported at 76%, specificity 86%, and positive predictive value at 62%. The implication of this is that with longer follow-up and greater accumulation of patients, SCC antigen may prove to be a valuable tumor marker in the long-term follow-up of individuals with squamous cell carcinoma of the anal canal.

More papers are now appearing with respect to the results of so-called "salvage" surgery following chemoradiation therapy—that is, abdominoperineal resection. The mortality rate at 3 years ranges from 50% to 70%.

### Radiation Therapy Alone

As stated, SCC is a radiosensitive tumor. The application of external beam radiation therapy as the sole method for the treatment of carcinoma of the anal canal, without chemotherapy, therefore, still has relevance. In patients treated with radiation therapy alone, with surgery reserved for those with residual carcinoma, survival rates of 50% to 60% have been noted. More than one half of the patients' tumors can be controlled by this approach. Three fourths of the long-term survivors may not require a colostomy. Five-year survival following this type of approach is 55% for squamous cancers and 60% for cloacogenic.

Some authors have advocated a treatment protocol that differentiates the approach according to tumor stage and tumor size. Radiation therapy alone is recommended for those individuals who harbor a tumor of 4 cm or less and chemoradiation therapy is limited to those with larger tumors or those that are fixed. One thing is clear; chemotherapy, when combined with radiation, reduces the amount of radiation required; hence, fewer late complications may be anticipated. As with chemoradiation therapy, the options following recurrence with radiation therapy alone are essentially the same—additional nonsurgical treatment, radical resection, and local excision.

## Interstitial Curie Therapy

In 1973, Papillon reported on epidermoid carcinomas treated by interstitial Curie therapy over a 20-year period. This was usually accomplished under general anesthesia, using radium needles inserted either through the skin or the anal mucosa. The dose was less than 40 Gy in 2 or 3 days. A second implant was usually performed for residual tumor 2 months after the first implant, and external irradiation might also have been given coincident with the implantation. The 5-year disease-free rate was 68%. Others have reported success rates ranging from 53% to 68%. The local control rate for patients with tumors smaller than 5 cm and with negative inguinal nodes was significantly better than that for patients with more advanced disease.

This treatment must be planned carefully to avoid radionecrosis. More recently, suggestion has been made for a split course of irradiation with cobalt 60 and iridium 192 with the addition of chemotherapy during the first few days. Results so far are encouraging and imply that this approach is worthy of further study.

## Carcinoma in a Hemorrhoidectomy Specimen

The problem of what to do when the pathologist reports a focus of carcinoma in a hemorrhoidectomy specimen is one of the quandaries that occasionally confronts the surgeon. However, the surgeon often wishes to not be aware of the focus of carcinoma, because it certainly imposes the burden of a difficult recommendation. However, if a pathology report is obtained that describes the presence of invasive carcinoma, the microscopic appearance should at least be confirmed and the depth of invasion ascertained. It is usually not helpful to examine the patient again until the wounds are healed. The following protocol is recommended:

Reexamine the patient under anesthesia in 4 to 6 weeks when the wounds are healed, and perform multiple biopsies, mapping the source in the anus from which the biopsies were taken. It is always impossible to know from which site the hemorrhoid tissue harboring the tumor was obtained.

If results of the biopsies are negative, follow the patient's status at 3-month intervals for 1 year and biopsy any suspicious areas.

If no recurrence develops by 1 year, the patient is considered cured. If a recurrence is identified, the patient can be considered for local excision or the standard chemoradiation therapy protocol for anal canal carcinoma.

*Comment*: The following protocol is recommended for management of carcinoma of the anal canal:

Local excision can be an adequate operation for patients with tumor invasion into the submucosa or the internal sphincter only. Endoanal ultrasound can be useful in staging the tumor.

Close follow-up evaluation should be pursued, and biopsies of suspicious areas should be done. Chemoradiation therapy should be considered for recurrent tumor, with abdominoperineal resection probably reserved for those who fail this therapy.

Those with suspected invasion into the muscle, or perirectal or perianal soft tissue should have preoperative chemoradiation therapy in accordance with the Nigro protocol.

Recurrent tumor following chemoradiation therapy can be selectively treated with additional chemoradiation therapy or by abdominoperineal resection.

If metastatic inguinal nodes persist or subsequently develop following chemoradiation therapy, interval radical groin dissection should be considered.

The Nigro protocol has clearly become the standard for the treatment of anal canal cancer against which all other options must be compared. However, the optimal dosage for radiation as well as the timing and choices of chemotherapeutic regimens are evolving. Despite this, results are so impressive that unless otherwise contraindicated, contemporary medical treatment mandates that this approach be used initially for all patients with invasive anal canal cancer.

## MALIGNANT MELANOMA

Although the anal canal represents the most common site for the development of malignant melanoma in the alimentary tract, it is an extremely rare condition, accounting for only 0.2% of all melanomas and 0.5% of tumors of the anorectum. The tumor is presumed to arise from melanocytes present in the squamous mucosa of the lower anal canal.

### Symptoms

Rectal bleeding is the most common complaint, occurring in one half of patients. Anorectal pain and change in bowel habits are also frequently reported. Many patients note a feeling of a lump or a "hemorrhoid," with the attendant discomfort. A mass in the groin may also be an initiating complaint. Approximately 1 in 10 will have the melanoma discovered on pathologic review of hemorrhoidectomy specimens.

### Physical Findings

Findings on physical examination vary from a small hemorrhoidlike, pigmented lesion to a deeply ulcerating or polypoid mass at or near the anorectal junction. Pigment may be readily apparent, but 29% are histologically amelanotic. In the Sloan-Kettering experience, an indication of the advanced stage of the disease and, therefore, the poor prognosis, was reflected by the fact that 75% of individuals harbored tumors more than 1 cm in diameter (average, 4 cm).

## Histology

The cells comprising the lesion usually assume either a polygonal or a spindle shape (Figs. 24.6 and 24.7) and are often arranged in nests to produce an alveolar pattern. If the mucosa overlying the lesion is not ulcerated, evidence of a junctional component (e.g., nests of melanoma cells within the squamous epithelium) may be found. This finding confirms the squamous mucosa of the anal canal as the primary site of origin. Melanin identified within the tumor cells permits diagnosis of the lesion as a melanoma rather than as a poorly differentiated carcinoma. Electron microscopy can be of value in identifying apparently amelanotic melanomas by demonstrating melanosomes within the tumor cells.

## Treatment and Results

Because anorectal melanoma is more likely to metastasize to mesenteric lymph nodes than squamous cell carcinoma of the anus, abdominoperineal resection has been the standard of treatment. This, and radical groin lymph node

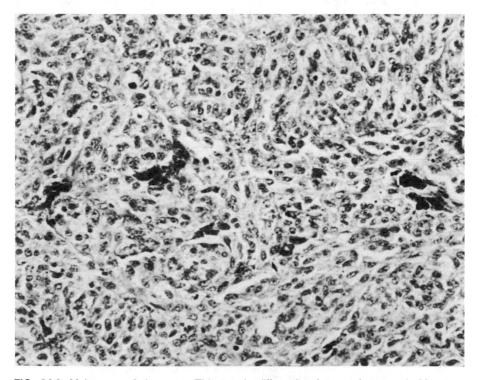

**FIG. 24.6.** Melanoma of the anus. This poorly differentiated tumor is recognizable as a melanoma only because of the black pigment being produced. (Original magnification ×250.)

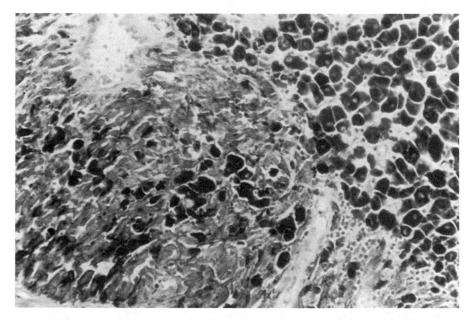

**FIG. 24.7.** Melanoma of the anal canal. Another variant displaying epithelioid pattern with extensive melanin pigment present. (Original magnification ×360.)

dissection, have been the mainstays of surgical therapies for this condition. However, because the prognosis has been so grim, a case has been made for either no treatment at all or for simply local excision. Several reports have noted no statistically significant difference in survival rate of patients treated for cure by local excision versus abdominoperineal resection. The major benefit of radical resection may be for controlling local and regional disease. Most series report either none or only the rare cure. Based on the Memorial Sloan-Kettering experience two conclusions are set forth:

1. Most patients with anorectal melanoma will die of their disease, regardless of therapy.
2. Surgical cure can be achieved in a small subset of patients with localized, relatively early disease or favorable tumor biology.

The Sloan-Kettering group, therefore, believe that abdominoperineal resection with pelvic lymphadenectomy is a reasonable alternative for those individuals without locally advanced tumors or evidence of regional lymph node involvement. In this group of patients, they emphasize the importance of pelvic lymphadenectomy. One pertinent observation is that all of the long-term survivors were women. It appears that female sex is a favorable prognostic factor in individuals with cutaneous melanoma as well. Women with operable melanoma of the anus according to the criteria set forth by the Memorial Sloan-Kettering group have a 29% survival following abdominoperineal resection.

Supplementary treatment with radiotherapy has been of no consistent benefit, nor have the various chemotherapeutic agents uniformly helped. Immunotherapy, usually with BCG vaccine, has been used for malignant melanoma in other sites, but recommendations concerning its value with malignant melanoma of the anal canal have been anecdotal and discouraging. Most investigators, however, recommend an aggressive multimodality approach, but no consistency was seen in patient selection, pathologic extent, or treatment employed with the few long-term survivors that have been reported.

## MISCELLANEOUS ANAL CONDITIONS

### Verrucous Squamous Carcinoma

A very rare tumor, verrucous squamous carcinoma, has come to be known as the tumor of Buschke and Löwenstein because of their description of it in 1925. The lesion is frequently confused with benign anal conditions, especially condyloma. It may appear as a pale, pink, cauliflowerlike mass on the perianal skin or in the anal canal.

Histologically, the tumor is so well differentiated that it closely resembles benign, proliferative lesions of squamous epithelium, and it may not be recognizable as a carcinoma until invasion of underlying structures can be identified. For this reason, superficial biopsies of verrucous squamous cell carcinomas are frequently not diagnosed as carcinoma; biopsies should be taken from the base of the lesion to demonstrate invasion.

Classic treatment consists of wide local excision or abdominoperineal resection for invasive tumors. However, the value of combined modality therapy needs to be explored (for additional discussion, see Chapter 19).

### Keratoacanthoma

Keratoacanthoma is an exophytic, benign skin tumor, usually with a central crater, 0.5 to 2.0 cm in diameter, that is most often associated with exposure to the sun. Only three cases involving the perianal skin and one in the anal canal have been reported. Local excision or electrocoagulation should be curative, although the histologic appearance can mimic that of squamous cell carcinoma.

### Pseudosarcomatous Carcinoma

Pseudosarcoma has been described in the esophagus, larynx, oral cavity, and other areas, but only one reported case of such a tumor in the anal canal. The patient presented with a pedunculated 4-cm mass. Microscopic examination of the locally excised specimen revealed epithelial elements in sarcomalike areas. No recurrence was noted after a 25-month follow-up.

### Carcinoma of the Anal Glands and Ducts

Colloid or mucinous adenocarcinoma of anal glandular or ductal origin is a rare entity, but may not be as infrequent as the literature suggests. This can be explained by the fact that the site of origin is destroyed early by the malignant growth. The most common symptoms are anal pain (58%) and rectal bleeding in 40%; 37% perceive a mass, whereas more than 50% present with a fistula.

Because this is a highly malignant variant, abdominoperineal resection is usually recommended. Local excision, however, can be considered for early lesions, but radical resection is generally required to control disease. The place of chemoradiation therapy is probably similar to that of conventional adenocarcinoma of the rectum, but this has not been clearly defined.

### *Results*

Median survival is 29 months, and three quarters develop recurrence, despite an aggressive surgical approach. It is evident that anal adenocarcinoma is associated with a poor prognosis despite radical surgery.

### Malignant Fibrous Histiocytoma

Malignant fibrous histiocytoma is a pleiomorphic sarcoma that classically arises in the extremities and metastasizes to the lungs and regional lymph nodes, but which also can occur rarely in the gastrointestinal tract. Only one case involving the anal canal has been identified. This was managed by abdominoperineal resection and radiotherapy.

### Inflammatory Cloacogenic Polyp

Inflammatory cloacogenic polyp is a nonneoplastic anal tumor that can be analogous to a prolapse in the area of the transitional zone. The primary complaint is usually that of rectal bleeding. The polyp is found primarily on the anterior wall of the anal canal, not unlike the distribution seen in solitary rectal ulcer (see Chapter 17). The cause of the condition is uncertain, but theories include ischemia, trauma (manual, stercoral), congenital, and early prolapse. Histologically, the lesion is characterized by a tubulovillous pattern of growth, superficial ulceration, displaced crypts, and extension of chronically inflamed fibromuscular stroma into the lamina propria (Fig. 24.8).

Treatment consists simply of local excision.

### Basal Cell Carcinoma, Bowen's Disease, and Paget's Disease

See Chapter 19.

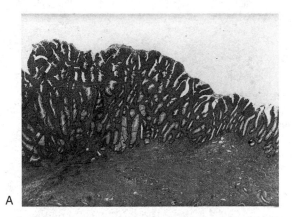

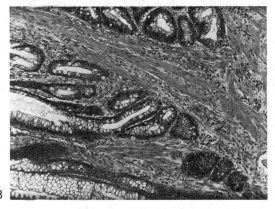

**FIG. 24.8.** Inflammatory cloacogenic polyp. **A.** Nonulcerated surface showing glandular hyperplasia with a thickened submucosa. (Original magnification ×20.) **B.** Higher power demonstrates colonic glands and inflammatory cells with muscle bundles extending between the glands into the submucosa. (Original magnification ×100.)

# 25

## Less Common Tumors and Tumorlike Lesions of the Colon, Rectum, and Anus

Although adenoma and adenocarcinoma constitute the most commonly seen neoplasms of the colon, rectum, and anus, many other tumors and tumorlike conditions in this anatomic region have been described. Of these, some represent extraordinarily rare lesions and may, thus, be the source of difficult decisions in the therapeutic approach to the patient. Others are important because they represent benign conditions that can be mistaken for malignant processes. Many lesions present a similar clinical picture, despite their diverse pathologic natures.

### CLASSIFICATION OF UNUSUAL TUMORS AND TUMORLIKE CONDITIONS

#### Tumors of Epithelial Origin

Carcinoid tumor
Neuroendocrine (NE) carcinoma
Bowen's disease
Perianal Paget's disease
Basal cell carcinoma
Cloacogenic carcinoma
Malignant melanoma
Squamous cell carcinoma
Adenosquamous carcinoma (adenoacanthoma)
Stem cell carcinoma

#### Tumors of Lymphoid Origin

Lymphoid hyperplasia (benign lymphoma, lymphoid polyp)
Malignant lymphoma
Extramedullary plasmacytoma

## Mesenchymal Tumors

Fibrous tissue origin
  Fibroma
  Inflammatory fibroid polyp (eosinophilic granuloma)
  Fibrosarcoma
  Malignant fibrous histiocytoma
Smooth muscle origin
  Leiomyoma
  Leiomyosarcoma
  Rhabdomyosarcoma
Adipose tissue origin
  Lipoma
  Liposarcoma

## Tumors of Neural Origin

Neurofibroma
Neurilemmoma (schwannoma)
Ganglioneuroma
Granular cell tumor

## Vascular Lesions

Hemangioma
Lymphangioma
Hemangiopericytoma
Malignant vascular tumors (angiosarcoma, Kaposi's sarcoma)

## Heterotopias and Hamartomas

Endometriosis
Hamartoma
Dermoid cyst and teratoma
Colitis cystica profunda (enterogenous cysts)
Ectopic tissue

## Exogenous, Extrinsic, and Miscellaneous Conditions

Metastatic tumor
Barium granuloma
Oleoma
Sarcoidosis
Wegener's granulomatosis

Amyloidosis
Malacoplakia
Sacrococcygeal chordoma
Ependymoma
Extramedullary (extraadrenal) myelolipoma
Pneumatosis cystoides intestinalis (*Pneumatosis coli*)
Duplication

## TUMORS OF EPITHELIAL ORIGIN

### Carcinoid Tumor

Carcinoids are slow-growing tumors of neuroectodermal origin that belong to the Amine Precursor Uptake and Decarboxylation (APUD) system. They are the most common NE neoplasms of the gastrointestinal tract. Although carcinoids occur most commonly as primary tumors of the gastrointestinal tract, they can also be found in such diverse locations as the bronchus, ovary, and kidney. Carcinoids arise from the Kulchitsky or basogranular enterochromaffin cells located in the crypts of Lieberkühn.

### *Classification and Diagnosis*

Current classification relates both to the anatomic site of the tumor and to the reactivity to silver incorporation by cytoplasmic granules. A positive argentaffin reaction (argentaffinity) involves the reduction of silver salts to metallic silver by strong endogenous-reducing substances. Argentaffinity usually implies that the argyrophil reaction will be positive, but the mechanism for the latter reaction is unknown. A positive argyrophil reaction occurs when metallic silver added in solution is precipitated on the cytoplasmic granules of the carcinoid cells. Two distinctive types of neurosecretory granules have been observed by electron microscopy: A relatively small granule appears to be associated with argyrophil carcinoids and a larger one with argentaffin.

Midgut carcinoids (mid duodenum to mid transverse colon) are usually both argyrophil and argentaffin positive; frequently, they are multicentric in origin and often associated with the carcinoid syndrome. The syndrome is characterized by a complex of symptoms thought to be related to overproduction of serotonin (5-hydroxytryptamine [5-HT]); however, less than 10% of all patients with carcinoid tumors exhibit this manifestation. Hindgut carcinoids have been reported to be rarely argyrophil or argentaffin positive; they are usually unicentric, and are not associated with the carcinoid syndrome.

Determination of urine 5-hydroxyindoleacetic acid (5-HIAA) excretion is not helpful in defining metastatic disease in rectal tumors, because hindgut lesions are generally argentaffin negative and do not produce a detectable increase in tryptophan metabolites. Table 25.1 summarizes the classic differences between carcinoids based on gut location.

**TABLE 25.1.** *Classic differences among foregut, midgut, and hindgut carcinoids*

Location
  Lungs, stomach, first part of duodenum
  Duodenum through right colon, appendix
  Transverse or left colon, rectum
Staining
  Nonargentaffin but argyrophilic
  Argentaffin + argyrophilic
  Nonargentaffin but argyrophilic
Bioactivity
  5-HT, ACTH, tachykinins, neurotensin, HCG; gastron; low 5-HT content; high MAO activity
    without DAO activity
  5-HT, tachykinins, rarely ACTH or 5-hydroxy-tryptophan; lower MAO activity than foregut
    carcinoids but higher DAO activity
  Low 5-HT or ACTH content; may secrete somatostatin, tachykinins, glicentin, PYY, 5-HT,
    neurotensin, pancreatic polypeptide, dopamine
Metastasis
  25%, particularly to bone; metastases not required for systemic symptoms
  60% to 80% (proportional to tumor size) to liver; rarely to bone
  5% to 40% to bone
Presentation
  Pulmonary obstruction, atypical neurohumoral symptoms
  Bowel obstruction, classic carcinoid syndrome (diarrhea and flushing) if metastatic
  Usually discovered by chance; rarely cause humoral symptoms

5-HT, serotonin; ACTH, adrenocorticotropic hormone; DAO, diamine oxidase; HCG, human chorionic gonadotropin; MAO, monoamine oxidase; PYY, peptide YY.
From Basson MD, Ahlman H, Wangberg B, et al. Biology and management of the midgut carcinoid. *Am J Surg* 1993;165:288, with permission.

## *Incidence, Distribution and Associated Conditions*

The incidence of gastrointestinal carcinoid tumors increases from duodenum to ileum, with more than 80% located in the distal small bowel. They arise most commonly in the appendix and are found in 0.26% of appendectomy specimens. The next most common location is the small intestine, followed by the rectum and stomach. Colonic involvement is infrequent, comprising 2.5% of gastrointestinal carcinoids. An incidence of 0.7 per 100,000 population is expected.

Carcinoid tumors, irrespective of their site of origin, are associated with an increased incidence of other malignant tumors, especially those of the gastrointestinal tract. In addition, an increased incidence of breast and uterine malignancies, as well as cancer of the hematopoietic system, have been described. Because of the possible association with myelofibrosis, evaluation of the bowel in an individual with hematologic disease can be useful. An association between ulcerative colitis and rectal carcinoid tumors has also been postulated.

## *Age and Gender*

The condition occurs most commonly in individuals in their sixth and seventh decades; the mean age is 55 years. The tumors are seen most frequently in women, at a 2:1 ratio.

### Signs, Symptoms and Diagnosis

#### Appendix

The presentation is usually that of an individual with right lower quadrant abdominal pain and signs and symptoms of appendicitis. The identification of the tumor, itself, usually awaits pathologic confirmation. This often is a fortuitous finding that presents somewhat of a controversy in subsequent management (see later). The prevalence of carcinoids has been estimated to be 0.26% to 0.32%. Most are present at the tip (67%), with the body comprising 21%, and only 7% seen at the base.

#### Small Bowel

Carcinoid tumors are frequently asymptomatic. The frequency of metastases at diagnosis depends on the clinical presentation. This ranges from approximately 33% to 64%; in asymptomatic individuals, 93% who are diagnosed with small bowel carcinoids harbor metastases.

Quantification of 5-HT and its metabolites, especially 24-hour urinary 5-HIAA has been found to detect up to 84% of carcinoid tumors. Unfortunately, small bowel carcinoids commonly present late because of the nonspecific signs and symptoms that occur. This leads to failure to pursue investigative studies that might identify the lesion at an earlier stage. The single most common presenting complaint is that of small bowel obstruction, but most have nonspecific gastrointestinal symptoms.

The most rewarding diagnostic study for the evaluation of a suspected small bowel carcinoid is enteroclysis. However, a routine small bowel series is usually sufficient. It is important to remember that small carcinoids are frequently multiple. Recommendation is for the use of computed tomography (CT) scan to evaluate the small bowel.

#### Colon

Colonic carcinoids usually grow to a large size before they become symptomatic. Even then, they are less likely to cause obstruction or rectal bleeding than adenocarcinoma of the colon; 33% are asymptomatic. When the lesion does produce symptoms, they are indistinguishable from those caused by adenocarcinoma (e.g., bleeding, change in bowel habits, abdominal pain). Colonic carcinoids have a similar 5-year survival to that of adenocarcinoma.

Radiologic evaluation of colonic carcinoids reflects the appearance of the clinically seen lesion. For larger tumors, it is virtually impossible to distinguish the pathology from that of an adenocarcinoma. This is true even on colonoscopy or direct visualization. Of colon carcinoids, 48% are located in the cecum, 16% in the ascending colon, 6% in the transverse colon, 11% in the descending colon, and 13% in the sigmoid. As mentioned, patients with carcinoid tumors have an increased incidence of gastrointestinal adenocarcinoma. Thorough evaluation of the gastrointestinal tract is, therefore, advised.

### Rectum

In the rectum, a carcinoid tumor usually is observed as a small, circumscribed, yellowish, submucosal nodule, 1 cm or less in diameter. It is often found incidentally, either at the time of pathologic examination of an excised rectum for another condition, or in the course of clinical examination for other complaints. One half of rectal carcinoids are discovered at the time of anorectal examination of asymptomatic individuals. The single most common complaint is that of anorectal discomfort, with rectal bleeding being the most second common. Other complaints include constipation, weight loss, change in bowel habits, rectal obstruction, "hemorrhoids," diarrhea, and the presence of an abdominal mass.

### Histopathology and DNA Ploidy

Microscopically, it is difficult to differentiate between benign and malignant carcinoid. The usual criterion of malignancy (e.g., mitotic activity or pyknotic nuclei) is often lacking. The incidence of malignancy varies from 8% to 40%, with the evidence based on the presence of local extension or metastasis. The tumor is composed of uniform, small, round, or polygonal cells with prominent, round nuclei and eosinophilic cytoplasmic granules (Fig. 25.1). Five carcinoid

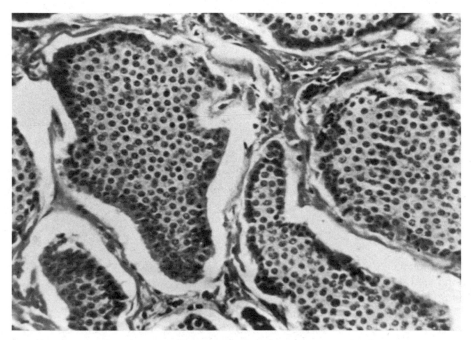

**FIG. 25.1.** Carcinoid. Uniform cells with minimal variation of cell nuclei in clusters within the lymphatic spaces. (Original magnification ×280; from Corman ML, Veidenheimer MC, Swinton NW. *Diseases of the anus, rectum and colon.* Part I: neoplasms. New York: Medcom, 1972.)

histologic growth patterns are generally accepted: insular, trabecular, glandular, undifferentiated, and mixed.

Aneuploidy appears to be associated with stage, size, and invasion by tumor. The data from one study, however, suggested that a near-hypertriploid pattern was the most precise and reliable parameter for predicting the prognosis of colorectal carcinoid tumors.

### Management

#### Appendix

Appendectomy, alone, is adequate treatment for appendiceal carcinoids less than 2 cm in diameter, even if lymphatic invasion is noted on subsequent histologic examination. A right colectomy is suggested for larger lesions in young patients, and for those tumors identified to have vascular involvement or to have invasion of the mesoappendix.

#### Small Bowel

As suggested, the major difficulty in managing patients with small bowel carcinoid is the fact that these individuals present late in the course of the disease. It is extremely important to examine the entire small bowel, looking for the presence of synchronous lesions. If at all possible, resection of obvious nodal involvement is encouraged, including removal of superficial hepatic metastases as well as performing a cholecystectomy. Performance of the last procedure is advised if prolonged somatostatin analogue therapy is anticipated.

#### Colon

Treatment for colonic carcinoid is resection. Because these tumors grow relatively slowly, metastatic disease is not a contraindication to resection of the primary lesion. Metastases occur more frequently with carcinoids of the large bowel than with carcinoids of the small intestine. Perhaps this can be explained by the fact that carcinoid tumors can attain a considerable size in the colon before they become symptomatic.

#### Rectum

In the rectum, the size of the carcinoid is the distinguishing feature that determines treatment. Most tumors less than 2 cm in diameter require only local, transanal excision. However, those that are demonstrably invasive or are 2 cm or larger in diameter should probably be treated by a cancer type of resection. Laparoscopic excision of a proximal rectal carcinoid has also been described. It is important to remember that 30% of patients present with synchronous or metachronous carcinomas, usually colorectal.

## Results

### Appendix

Less than 2.5% of patients will develop evidence of recurrent disease, and less than 1% will succumb to metastatic disease if the aforementioned guidelines are followed.

### Small Bowel

Cure following resection of carcinoid of the small bowel is unusual because of the frequent late stage at presentation. In the unusual circumstance of disease confined to the bowel itself, without lymph node involvement or metastatic disease, the likelihood of cure is excellent. For tumors 1 to 2 cm in diameter, 18% to 44% have been found to be metastatic to the liver, with spread to the lymph nodes in up to 85% of cases. Size appears to be the variable that correlates most closely with survival.

### Colon

The average length of survival after resection of colonic carcinoids is 26 months. When a distinction is made between cecal and other colonic sites, the former is found to be associated with a 71% incidence of metastasis, whereas the latter has a 33% incidence. Five-year survival rates of 37% have been described. Tumors larger than 2 cm metastasize in approximately 75% of patients, whereas only one of six less than 2 cm metastasize. Survival for carcinoids of the colon is significantly lower when compared with carcinoids of the rectum or appendix or with colonic adenocarcinomas. Tumor stage, histologic pattern, tumor differentiation, nuclear grade, and mitotic rate are found to significantly influence the survival rate.

### Rectum

All patients with lesions less than 2 cm can be expected to survive 5 years. The survival rate for patients with lesions measuring 2 cm or more in diameter is 40%. Rectal carcinoid tumors are probably cured only when they are discovered before the T3 stage, are less than 2 cm in diameter, and when lymph nodes are not involved.

### Adjuvant Therapy

Radiotherapy and chemotherapy have not proved to be effective in the treatment of carcinoid of the colon and rectum. Adequate surgical excision remains the treatment of choice. With respect to metastatic disease to the liver, drug combinations of 5-fluorouracil and streptozotocin have achieved high, albeit brief, response rates, whereas hepatic dearterialization and embolization are also useful palliative approaches.

The most efficacious program for the treatment of the carcinoid syndrome is to surgically remove (debulk) as much of the primary and secondary tumors as is possible to limit production of the polypeptides. In addition to chemotherapy, somatostatin (Sandostatin) use is advised, because it inhibits the severe diarrhea and flushing episodes associated with the disease. The suggested daily program during the first 2 weeks of therapy ranges from 100 to 600 µg/day, in two to four divided, subcutaneously injected doses. Somatostatin analogues (e.g., octreotide, and somatuline) have shown variable inhibition of tumor growth and therapeutic tolerance. Alpha-interferon has also been successfully used to control symptoms.

### Neuroendocrine Carcinoma

A type of neuroendocrine malignancy usually found in the lung (oat cell carcinoma, small cell carcinoma), on occasion, has been reported in extrapulmonary sites, including the colon and rectum. The so-called NE system includes endocrine cells distributed throughout the gastrointestinal tract, pancreas, lung, thyroid, adrenal gland, skin, and elsewhere, with intestinal NE cells being the largest component. Neoplastic proliferation of NE cells occurs primarily in the appendix, ileum, and rectum.

These tumors can be identified by immunohistochemical stains with application of a limited battery of available antibodies. Many of the so-called "poorly differentiated" gastrointestinal malignancies are probably NE tumors; however, by applying appropriate markers, the true incidence and distribution may become apparent, probably occurring in at least 4% of colon and rectal cancers. These cancers must be differentiated from other small cell cancers, such as lymphoma.

Generally, the tumors are extremely aggressive and associated with a poor prognosis. Extensive preoperative workup is suggested, because of the high rate of concomitant metastases, with the bone marrow frequently involved. Despite the aggressive clinical behavior that is characteristic of the tumor in the lung, one half of patients survive 5 years. Chemotherapy is often the same as that used for oat cell carcinoma of the lung.

### Bowen's Disease, Perianal Paget's Disease, and Basal Cell Carcinoma

See Chapter 19.

### Cloacogenic Carcinoma and Malignant Melanoma

See Chapter 24.

## Squamous Cell Carcinoma

Primary squamous cell carcinoma of the colon and rectum is an extremely rare tumor; approximately 70 cases have been reported. The incidence of this tumor is believed to be 1 per 3,000 malignant tumors of the bowel. These lesions tend to be distributed uniformly throughout the colon.

A number of theories have been postulated about the etiology and pathogenicity. These include metaplasia of glandular epithelium, embryonal rests, squamous metaplasia of existing adenoma or adenocarcinoma, damaged epithelium from toxic substances, and basal cell anaplasia. Specific predisposing factors that have been associated are ulcerative colitis, radiotherapy, colonic duplication, and schistosomiasis.

Symptoms are the same as those for adenocarcinoma, especially bleeding and change in bowel habits. Evaluation of the patient should proceed in the manner outlined in the chapters on cancer of the colon (Chapter 22) and rectum (Chapter 23). Total colonoscopy is suggested because of the not uncommon association of synchronous benign and malignant tumors.

Histologic examination may demonstrate squamous metaplasia of the colonic mucosa as well as the carcinoma.

In the absence of metastases, the lesion should be treated in the same manner as that for adenocarcinoma.

## Adenosquamous Carcinoma or Adenoacanthoma

Adenosquamous carcinoma of the colon is an extremely rare tumor. A number of authors believe that if careful review of the histologic pattern of tumors thought to be squamous carcinomas were undertaken, some of the lesions would prove to be adenosquamous cancers (adenoacanthomas), a mixture of both glandular and squamous features. These tumors appear to account for approximately 0.18% of adenocarcinomas.

Theoretic causes of this histologic manifestation include embryonal rests, indeterminate basal cells, squamous metaplasia, and a germ or pluripotential stem cell. An increased association with ulcerative colitis has been suggested.

Adenosquamous cancers, in general, are aggressive tumors and are associated with a less favorable prognosis than is adenocarcinoma. Most patients are stage III or IV on presentation. Median survival is only 23 months.

## Stem Cell Carcinoma

Another highly aggressive tumor of the colon and rectum may be a variant of adenoacanthoma, the so-called "stem cell" carcinoma. In theory, a pluripotential stem cell in the mucosa of the gastrointestinal tract may be capable of differentiation in several directions. Only a few cases have been reported.

## TUMORS OF LYMPHOID ORIGIN

### Lymphoid Hyperplasia; Benign Lymphoma; Lymphoid Polyp

Lymphoid hyperplasia is a benign, focal, or diffuse condition that typically occurs where clusters of lymphoid follicles are present (terminal ileum, rectum). Although the cause is unknown, the possibility of an inflammatory reaction as well as a hereditary predisposition has been suggested. In children, an infectious process is thought to precipitate the acute form of the disease.

The tumors are usually single and most frequently found in the lower one third of the rectum. They are seen in an individual at any age, but in adults are most commonly noted during the third and fourth decades. In children, the peak incidence is between 1 and 3 years; they are twice as common in boys as in girls.

It has been suggested that the lesions are congenital malformations or hamartomas, a hypothesis that is supported by their occasional familial occurrence. Others have observed an association with familial polyposis.

Lymphoid hyperplasia is characterized radiographically by small, uniform, localized, or generalized polypoid lesions. A fleck of barium can be seen in the center of the polyp on contrast study, representing umbilication at the apex of the lymphoid nodule. A central dimple in the nodule is considered good evidence for making the diagnosis. Endoscopic examination with biopsy confirms the nature of the lesion. The nodules are usually small, firm, and sessile but occasionally are large and can become pedunculated. When removed and sectioned, the tumors are found to be composed of well-differentiated lymphoid tissue with follicles separated by white fibrous bands and covered by a rather thin mucous membrane. The macroscopic and microscopic appearance can resemble malignant lymphoma or Hodgkin's disease. In fact, the condition has been regarded by some as a form of malignant lymphoma and has even been designated as pseudolymphoma. However, the lesion lacks the infiltrating and destructive characteristics of malignant lymphoma and does not become disseminated. The condition also can resemble leukemic infiltration of the bowel, but in leukemia the lesion tends to have a segmental distribution.

### Symptoms

Although no symptoms may occur if located in the rectum, a lymphoid polyp can cause considerable pain when it occurs in the anal canal. Colonic lesions can cause bleeding, abdominal pain, change in bowel habits, and symptoms related to intussusception, the last especially in children. Anemia and weight loss can be seen in the chronic form.

### Treatment

Local excision is indicated and adequate for isolated or scattered lesions. Removal is important to differentiate the condition from other neoplasms.

Recurrences are rare, occurring in approximately 5% even though a number of polyps may have been incompletely removed.

When the condition mimics acute appendicitis—a common presentation in children—appendectomy is performed. With chronic symptoms and extensive involvement of the terminal ileum, an ileocecal resection may be advisable. Adults with lymphoid polyposis have been treated by colectomy with and without ileorectal anastomosis. In other instances, less extensive bowel resections have been done in those with lymphoid hyperplasia who were misdiagnosed preoperatively.

Because radiotherapy and cytotoxic agents are often beneficial in the treatment of malignant lymphomas of the gastrointestinal tract, similar treatment has been proposed for benign lymphoid polyposis. In the absence of symptoms, management should be expectant; spontaneous regression can occur without treatment.

## Malignant Lymphoma

Malignant lymphoma, as a primary lesion or as part of a generalized malignant process, can involve the gastrointestinal tract. As a primary tumor, lymphoma comprises between 1% and 4% of all gastrointestinal malignancies but only 0.5% of colonic and 0.1% of rectal cancers. Gastric involvement is more common than that of small or large intestinal lymphoma and carries a better prognosis. Colonic lymphoma preferentially involves the cecum and the rectum; however, concurrent tumors elsewhere in the large bowel, the small bowel, and the stomach have been reported.

Malignant lymphoma of the colon has been reported in association with a variety of other entities, especially those of altered immune status (e.g., acquired immune deficiency syndrome [AIDS]). A high-grade B-cell lymphoma in an individual infected with the human immunodeficiency virus (HIV) is considered an AIDS-defining condition. Most intestinal lymphomas in the AIDS population are of the non-Hodgkin's type (NHL). Gastrointestinal NHL represents 17% of those with extranodal involvement.

Associations with macroglobulinemia, chronic ulcerative colitis, Crohn's disease, and celiac disease have been observed. With the concern for possible concomitant leukemia, total and differential white blood cell counts are mandated as part of an evaluation.

In most series, the incidence is greater in men than in women by a ratio of 2:1.282. Most patients are above 50 years of age at diagnosis, but the condition can occur at any age.

### Signs and Symptoms

Many individuals complain of "crampy," abdominal pain localized to the area of the tumor. Other prominent symptoms include weight loss, change in bowel habits, diarrhea, weakness, nausea, vomiting, anorexia, bleeding, and fever. Discrete intraabdominal masses are generally not appreciated until late in the course of the disease.

Symptoms produced by rectal involvement are variable and largely depend on whether the growth has become ulcerated. In early stages, with an intact mucosa, symptoms consist of a bearing-down sensation or a feeling of fullness in the rectum, with some rectal irritability and low backache. When ulceration of the overlying mucosa has developed, bleeding and mucous discharge may be noticed; later, pain and soreness are described if the growth begins to encroach on the anal canal. A high index of suspicion must be maintained in homosexual patients and, obviously, if AIDS is known or suspected. Obstructive symptoms are unlikely to occur because the primary growth often remains fairly localized to one quadrant and does not usually extend in an annular fashion, as is seen with carcinoma.

### Pathogenesis

It is thought that malignant lymphoma starts in the submucosal lymphoid tissue, which in places extends into the mucosa. It is not known whether it begins multicentrically or arises from a single area and later spreads by direct extension or through lymphatic channels. At presentation, a large segment of colon may be involved in a uniform and continuous fashion. Submucosal infiltration often extends beyond the area of obvious involvement, and additional lesions may be found apart from that region. Marked involvement is most common in the ileocecal or the rectosigmoid area, where tumors sometimes become confluent and form a large conglomerate mass. This can cause intussusception and intestinal obstruction. In the ileocecal region, the process usually extends into the appendix and into the ileum for a variable distance. When the rectum is the site of the tumor, inguinal nodes can be enlarged and palpable. Extensive serosal or retroperitoneal involvement is not characteristic of diffuse lymphoma.

### Endoscopy and Radiology

Clinical and radiographic diagnosis of colonic and rectal lymphoma can be obscured by the variety of appearances it can assume. The endoscopic appearance can resemble that of Crohn's disease, such as has been described for the extremely rarely reported cases of granulocytic sarcoma and malignant histiocytosis.

From the radiologic point of view, diffuse lymphoma of the colon must be differentiated from familial polyposis, ulcerative colitis with pseudopolyposis, granulomatous colitis, nodular lymphoid hyperplasia, and schistosomiasis. Although radiologic differentiation from carcinoma may be impossible, certain presentations strongly suggest lymphoma: presence of a bulky extracolonic component, concentric dilatation of the lumen, and a polypoid filling defect of the terminal ileum and ileocecal valve.

### *Histopathology*

Macroscopic examination of the tumor reveals a polypoid or ulcerated mass resembling carcinoma or a diffuse process extending over a large segment of colon, sometimes with numerous polypoid intraluminal excrescences. The bowel wall is thickened and rubbery in consistency, and its cut surface demonstrates a greatly thickened mucosa, often with prominent convoluted folds resembling the surface of brain and reaching a thickness of 1 or 2 cm. The submucosa is markedly thickened as a result of infiltration by closely packed tumor cells. In contrast to disease in the small bowel, deep ulceration and perforation are uncommon. However, superficial ulceration and necrosis may be seen.

A nonulcerated, submucous tumor in the rectal wall requires differentiation from benign lesions, such as lipoma, myoma, and nodular lymphoid hyperplasia, and also from an inflammatory condition, such as an intramuscular abscess. Thus, biopsy and histologic examination are crucial to the evaluation of such lesions (Fig. 25.2). Microscopic examination usually readily distinguishes lymphoma from other malignancies. However, a nonspecific lymphoid infiltrate in the mucosa and submucosa can present a problem with differential diagnosis. Under these circumstances, some have recommended immunocytochemical studies as well as gene rearrangement analysis with DNA probes to elucidate the precise nature of the process.

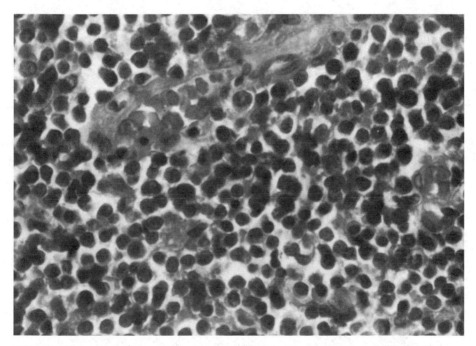

**FIG. 25.2.** Lymphoma of the cecum. Note the lymphoblasts in the wall of the bowel. (Original magnification ×600; courtesy of Rudolf Garret, M.D.)

Regional lymph nodes are involved in approximately one half of the patients at the time of laparotomy. Enlarged node presence may, however, represent reactive lymphoid hyperplasia and must be carefully examined histologically to document the presence of tumor. Because involvement beyond a single segment of bowel and its regional nodes excludes the diagnosis of primary lymphoma, a careful search for additional diseased nodes is necessary.

### Classification

Malignant lymphoma is classified on the basis of its cellular morphology and immunologic surface markers. Included are the following histologic types: lymphocytic lymphoma, lymphosarcoma, reticulum cell sarcoma, giant follicular lymphoma, and Hodgkin's disease—the rarest disease of the colon or rectum.

Tumors are also classified on the basis of extent of involvement:

Class I: confined to bowel wall
Class II: regional node involvement within drainage area of bowel primary
Class III: paraaortic node involvement; direct extension to adjacent viscera

The prognosis for primary extranodal lymphoma in the colon or rectum is not clearly related to cell type but is affected by stage.

### Treatment

If the lymphoma is confined to the rectum and the tumor is resectable, surgical excision should be followed by radiation therapy. In those tumors considered unresectable, radiation therapy is of definite benefit. A combined program with chemotherapy is recommended for systemic disease.

### Results

A 50% 5-year survival in those patients operated on for cure can be expected. When the tumor is confined to the bowel or involves only local nodes, the survival rate in both situations is also 50%. When regional nodes are involved, the 5-year survival rate falls to 12%.

The treatment of NHL in the setting of HIV infection has been much less effective than in individuals without immunodeficiency (see Chapter 20). The use of cytotoxic agents exacerbates the already existing immune impairment and leaves the person with prolonged neutropenia and at further risk for opportunistic infection. Survival time is generally less than 1 year.

### Extramedullary Plasmacytoma

Primary plasmacytoma is a localized plasma cell tumor that is most commonly found in the nasopharynx, although it has been reported in many other parts of the body. Plasma cell neoplasms are classified in five categories: multiple myeloma, solitary myeloma, extramedullary plasmacytoma (with multiple myeloma), plasma cell leukemia, and primary plasmacytoma.

The condition involves the colon extremely rarely, fewer than 10 cases having been reported as a primary disease; a number have involved the bowel secondarily. Primary tumors elsewhere in the gastrointestinal tract have also been noted. Disseminated multiple myeloma is often diagnosed in patients who have a localized plasmacytoma if these patients are followed for a long enough period. Therefore, a bone marrow examination should be performed at some point after an extramedullary plasmacytoma has been diagnosed. Primary and secondary colorectal plasmacytoma is more common in men than in women by a ratio of 3:2.

Presenting symptoms include abdominal pain, bleeding, anorexia, nausea, vomiting, and weight loss. The tumor can be single or multiple and consist of diffuse cellular infiltrates or of polypoid or nodular protrusions. Microscopic examination demonstrates the characteristic population of plasma cells; identification by means of immunoperoxidase stains has also been advised.

Treatment ideally consists of total excision, when possible. Metastasis to any organ other than lymph nodes is rare. Plasmacytomas that are not readily resectable might be responsive to radiotherapy. The use of chemotherapy is restricted to disseminated disease.

## MESENCHYMAL TUMORS

### Fibrous Tissue Origin

#### *Fibroma*

Fibroma of the colon is a very rare tumor belonging to the uncommon spindle cell group of benign tumors that also includes leiomyomas. Its incidence is only one tenth that of leiomyoma, however.

The tumor can originate in any layer of the bowel wall but arises most frequently in the submucosa. Fibromas have been reported in the appendicular stump and near the mesentery. Reports of fibroma of the colon are few. Abdominal pain and distension may be noted, and resection is the treatment of choice.

Fibroma of the anorectal region is very rare. It can arise from a hypertrophied papilla or by fibrous infiltration of a large prolapsing internal hemorrhoid, generally as a result of repeated attacks of thrombosis and strangulation without sloughing. It is encapsulated, firm, slightly movable, ovoid, of small to moderate size, and has little tendency to ulcerate. It is usually situated in the wall. In time, the covering of columnar epithelium becomes converted into squamous epithelium. A smooth, pale fibrous polyp results. The tumor can remain in the wall of the rectum or become polypoid and extend into the lumen. In general, it is single and of grows slowly. However, fibrous polyps can be multiple, so a careful proctoscopy is essential.

Symptoms include tenesmus and a sense of heaviness in the rectum. If ulceration has occurred (an exception), bleeding may be noted. The diagnosis is seldom made without microscopic examination. Transanal excision is the appropriate treatment.

### Inflammatory Fibroid Polyp or Eosinophilic Granuloma

Inflammatory fibroid polyp is a rare, focal lesion occurring in the submucosa of the gastrointestinal tract, least commonly in the colon. Only a few cases have been reported. Another term for the condition is "eosinophilic granuloma." Although the cause is uncertain, proliferation of submucosal mesenchymal fibrous tissue and variable eosinophilic infiltration suggests the effect of an inflammatory stimulus.

Rectal bleeding, tenesmus, change in bowel habits, and diarrhea are the most common symptoms. Obstruction caused by intussusception has also been reported. Radiographically, the impression may be that of a carcinoma. Because malignant degeneration has not been noted, however, endoscopic removal is suggested. A concern is that lesions may be sessile and submucosal, and have a tendency to bleed readily. If colonoscopic resection is unsuccessful or inadvisable, colectomy or colotomy and polypectomy should be performed.

### Fibrosarcoma

Of the sarcomas involving the gastrointestinal tract, fibrosarcoma is one of the rarest. Most tumors are situated in the rectum, within 10 cm of the pectinate line. Only two cases of fibrosarcoma of the colon have been reported. A single case of anal fibrosarcoma has been described.

The most common presenting symptom of fibrosarcoma of the rectum is difficulty with defecation. Pain is the second most common symptom, and bleeding, third. Proctosigmoidoscopic examination may reveal the tumor to be consistent with an adenocarcinoma, and only histologic determination can establish the definitive diagnosis.

Microscopically, the tumor is characterized by strands of fibrous tissue that infiltrate the adjacent structures of the bowel wall, but tend to spare the mucosa until late in the disease. The presence of mitoses is helpful in confirming the malignant nature of the lesion.

Treatment is essentially the same as that for adenocarcinoma: radical resection of the involved bowel with or without a sphincter-saving approach. Neither radiotherapy nor chemotherapy has been helpful in the management of this rare condition.

### Malignant Fibrous Histiocytoma

Malignant fibrous histiocytoma is an extremely rare fibrosarcoma variant in which histiocytelike cells are present. The lesion is usually found in the lower extremity.

Tumors tend to be large; they present with obstructive symptoms, and are thought clinically to be adenocarcinomas. Treatment is radical resection; prognosis is presumably poor. A partial response has been reported with chemotherapy.

### Smooth Muscle Origin

*Leiomyoma.* Smooth muscle tumors of the alimentary tract are rare, and benign smooth muscle tumors of the colon are exceedingly uncommon.

Smooth muscle tumors are found in patients of all ages with a gradual increase in frequency and malignant degeneration up to the sixth decade. The tumor is classified according to its appearance and direction of growth. The intracolonic type can be pedunculated or sessile. The extracolonic type grows away from the lumen of the bowel and lies in the abdominal cavity attached to the wall. The dumbbell type grows into the lumen and into the abdominal cavity simultaneously. This type of tumor accounts for 4% of all smooth muscle tumors of the gastrointestinal tract. These usually reach a much larger size than those with unilateral spread. The constrictive type encircles a variable length of bowel. The sigmoid and transverse colon seem to be the most common sites, with very few leiomyomas found in the cecum.

The tumor can be an incidental finding in an asymptomatic individual, or the patient may present with pain or a lump. Perforation, intestinal obstruction (secondary to the tumor itself or to intussusception), and hemorrhage have been reported.

Macroscopically, the tumor appears well encapsulated. On cross-section, leiomyomas have a fleshy appearance; because the tumor is under pressure, it tends to protrude. Histologically, a typical spindle cell neoplasm can be observed. Most investigators believe that the mitotic rate is the single most important criterion for diagnosis of malignancy. Other indicators are a variation in nuclear size and shape, hyperchromasia, frequent bizarre cells, and difficulty in identifying longitudinal myofibrils. Suspect malignant degeneration if the mitotic rate is high, growth is rapid, ulcer is present, or the lesion is more than 2.5 cm in diameter. Smooth muscle tumors are usually locally invasive, but metastasis from a primary tumor in the gastrointestinal tract has been described.

*Treatment.* Surgical excision results in cure unless the tumor is extraperitoneal or rectal. Complete removal should be attempted, regardless of the radiologic appearance or of probable inoperability. Because it is generally not possible to distinguish benign from malignant lesions preoperatively, a standard cancer operation should be performed under such circumstances.

*Rectal Leiomyoma.* Only a few cases of rectal leiomyomas have been reported. Approximately one third are found in men. The tumors often tend to arise from the internal anal sphincter. Smaller myomas, which usually cause no symptoms and can be found on routine rectal examination, are usually removed with a diathermy snare or by transanal excision. Large lesions can interfere with defecation, and cause a sense of fullness in the rectum and a frequent desire to defecate. Because of these distressing symptoms and the possibility of obstruction and malignant degeneration, removal of the growth is indicated. When the tumor is essentially extrarectal, it is best to excise it by an extrarectal approach rather than transanally.

Even large tumors can be treated by local excision, but if clinical suspicion of malignancy exists (e.g., ulceration, hemorrhage, or extrarectal fixation), radical surgical treatment by excision of the rectum is indicated. Biopsies can be difficult to interpret in such cases. Recurrence is common, occurring in slightly less than 50%.

*Leiomyosarcoma.*

*Colon.* Leiomyosarcoma of the large bowel is a very rare lesion; the total number of published cases is probably fewer than 100. No age predilection for this disease is apparent. It affects the genders equally and is more than twice as common in the rectum as it is in the rest of the colon.

Leiomyosarcoma arises from the smooth muscle of the bowel wall. An insidious disease, it can remain asymptomatic for a long period. Weight loss is almost never recorded, but pain is a common symptom. Tarry stools and the sequelae of anemia are the most frequent presentations. A palpable tumor is almost always present when the lesion occurs in the rectum, and in some instances, obstruction is also seen.

Diagnosis of this lesion preoperatively is extremely difficult because it resembles carcinoma of the colon in its radiographic appearance. The tumor can project into the lumen of the bowel, grow outward, or present as a dumbbell-type tumor. An interesting radiologic finding can be demonstrated when tracks of barium extend into a subserosal tumor. Sonographic features can include a thick echogenic rim with central cavitation. Colonoscopy and biopsy are useful in confirming the diagnosis.

Leiomyosarcoma is usually a tumor of low-grade malignancy. Patients who have been treated by resection have lived many years, despite residual tumor or metastases. The lungs and regional lymph nodes are rarely involved, but the tumor does have a tendency to metastasize to the liver.

*Rectum.* More than 100 cases of rectal leiomyosarcoma have been recorded in the literature. The tumor arises in the smooth muscle of the rectal wall. Most are seen in the lower one third of the rectum and are more commonly found in men than in women. The tumor can present as a nodular or protuberant swelling with some central ulceration that appears to arise in the deeper layers of the bowel wall. Most are large and consist microscopically of interlacing bands of well-differentiated, smooth muscle fibers and histologically of a low-grade malignancy. Extensive direct spread into the perirectal tissue is a characteristic feature. This can make surgical removal so difficult that local recurrence even after excision of the rectum is not uncommon.

Smooth muscle sarcomas of the rectum do not usually metastasize to regional lymph nodes unless they are poorly differentiated.

*Results.* Although most leiomyosarcomas are of a low-grade malignancy, the ultimate prognosis is very poor. This is essentially because of late diagnosis and extensive local spread by the time of surgery. Rectal disease has been shown to have an overall survival rate of 20%. Apart from local recurrence, metastasis to the liver and lungs is the most common cause of death. Local excision is liable to be followed by recurrence, although it can be delayed for some years. A standard cancer resection is the recommended treatment for all operable lesions. Although the tumor is not radiosensitive, chemotherapy with vincristine, cyclophosphamide, actinomycin D, and doxorubicin has been advocated because of the poor prognosis.

*Rhabdomyosarcoma.* Rhabdomyosarcoma is the most common soft-tissue sarcoma in children; it occurs most frequently in the head and neck, genitourinary tract, extremity, and trunk. A few cases have been reported in the perirectal area. Rhabdomyosarcoma has been classified into four types: pleomorphic, alveolar, embryonal, and botryoid. However, the histologic diagnosis can be confused with other mesenchymal lesions.

The patient usually presents with a mass in the perianal area. Current therapy should include adequate local excision, or resection followed by chemotherapy (vincristine, actinomycin D, and cyclophosphamide). Prognosis is generally poor.

## Adipose Tissue Origin

### *Lipoma*

Excluding hyperplastic polyps, lipoma is the second most common benign tumor of the colon (after adenomatous polyp) and the most common intramural tumor; however, it is still a relatively rare entity, with an incidence of 0.2% to 0.3%.

Colonic lipomas are well differentiated, benign, fatty tumors arising from deposits of adipose connective tissue in the bowel wall. Malignant change has not been reported. Approximately 90% are submucosal and 10% subserosal. The submucosal lipoma is covered by mucosa and, occasionally, by muscularis mucosae; it grows toward the intestinal lumen. The mucosa covering the tumor can become atrophic, congested, ulcerated, or even necrotic, or it can retain its normal yellowish appearance. The subserosal type usually originates from the appendices epiploicae and grows toward the peritoneal cavity.

Colonic lipomas usually occur in patients between the ages of 50 and 70 years with about an equal gender distribution. The average age is similar to that of individuals with colonic carcinoma. However, patients with colonic lipoma do not appear ill nor do they experience anorexia, weight loss, or anemia. Most colonic lipomas are asymptomatic and are found at autopsy or incidentally during an operation for some other problem. However, with size in excess of 2 cm, approximately one third will give rise to some symptom, which can include constipation, diarrhea, abdominal pain, and rectal bleeding. The presence of a palpable mass may be the lipoma, itself, impaction of fecal material, or intussuscepted bowel.

The most common sites for lipoma are the cecum, ascending colon, and sigmoid colon. Lipoma or lipomatosis of the ileocecal valve is characterized by diffuse submucosal adipose infiltration of the valve; most occur in the right colon. Multiple lipomas can be found in more than one quarter of patients who have intestinal lipomas.

Barium enema examination can usually distinguish a lipoma from that of another type of tumor. A water enema with low kilovoltage technique takes advantage of the different absorption coefficients of fat and water: fat-containing lesions will appear relatively radiolucent. The shape of the mass may be observed to change during fluoroscopic examination as a consequence of peristalsis or of manual pressure, the so-called "squeeze sign."

Mucosal lipomas can also be diagnosed with the colonoscope. A number of endoscopic features suggesting lipoma have been described, including the "cushion sign" (identification of the lipoma with pressure from a biopsy forceps), the "tenting sign" (elevation of the overlying mucosa with the biopsy forceps), and the "naked fat sign" (extrusion of fat following biopsy). Not uncommonly, they can be removed by means of this instrument. However, this approach is usually limited to symptomatic patients and those in whom the lesion is somewhat pedunculated. The microscopic appearance is that of mature adipose tissue surrounded by a fibrous capsule.

Colonic lipomas do not require treatment except when they ulcerate. Once the diagnosis has been established and carcinoma has been ruled out, the patient need only be reassured. However, in the symptomatic patient, a limited resection or colotomy and lipomectomy is usually advised.

Lipoma of the rectum is extremely rare. When it can be reached with the finger, it usually is felt as a soft, smooth, lobulated mass. Pedunculated lesions can prolapse and present a slight problem of differential diagnosis, especially if hemorrhagic or necrotic. If it is seen with the aid of a proctoscope, the yellow color of the fat of which it is composed is usually apparent through the mucosa. The most frequent site in the rectal area is the perianal region, in which case the tumor develops from the subcutaneous tissue.

A lipoma in the perianal region or buttock usually causes no symptoms, unless it becomes large and the overlying skin becomes irritated. When situated in the rectum or the sigmoid or when traumatized, it can produce symptoms because of its size. Tenesmus can result when the growth is in the lower rectum and involves the internal sphincter.

Ligation of the base and removal can be done when the tumor is pedunculated. Incision and enucleation can be done if the lipoma is confined to the rectal wall.

## Lipomatosis

Several cases have been reported of lipomas throughout the colon, numbering in excess of 100 lesions. Radiographically, colonic lipomatosis must be differentiated from numerous benign and malignant conditions. "Pseudolipomatosis," which has also been described, is felt to be caused by entrapment of gas in the lamina propria.

## TUMORS OF NEURAL ORIGIN

### Neurofibroma, Neurilemmoma or Schwannoma, and Ganglioneuromatosis

Von Recklinghausen first described multiple subcutaneous neurofibromas (neurofibromatosis) in 1882. The condition has since been known as "von Recklinghausen's disease." Visceral involvement in disseminated neurofibromatosis is considered rare. The possibility of this disease should be considered if gastrointestinal bleeding or intestinal obstruction occurs in a patient known to have generalized neurofibromatosis. It can be seen, however, in the alimentary tract and nowhere else.

The lesions in the intestinal tract arise in the submucosa or muscularis. As the tumor enlarges, the overlying mucosa becomes ulcerated and bleeds. Intussusception can produce intestinal obstruction. Sarcomatous degeneration is a recognized complication.

Local excision is preferred unless a large cluster is noted in one segment; under these circumstances, resection may be advisable.

Ganglioneuromas are neuroectodermal tumors that are rarely found in the colon. They are composed of nerve fibers, Schwann sheath elements, and ganglion cells. When solitary, they can resemble a carcinoma radiologically. Treatment is local excision or resection. Anorectal neurilemmoma, reported uncommonly, also should be adequately treated by excisional biopsy.

Neurogenic tumors have been reported to be the cause of masses in the presacral space. They can be identified by palpation on rectal examination and confirmed by CT. Treatment is local excision or resection, usually by a transcoccygeal approach.

### Granular Cell Tumor

Granular cell tumor is an uncommon tumor of uncertain histogenesis, although electron microscopy and histochemical studies suggest a definite neural pattern most closely resembling a damaged Schwann cell.

Usually the tumor involves the tongue (33%), skin and subcutaneous soft tissues (10%), and skeletal muscle (5%). About 50% of the tumors occur in the oral cavity and nasopharynx. However, it has also been reported found in most other organ systems. Involvement of the gastrointestinal tract is rare. In a review of the literature, less than 20 cases involving the large intestine were identified, mainly in the proximal portion of the colon, and only two tumors were identified in the rectum. Anal and perianal lesions have also been reported.

In the colon, granular cell tumors appear as yellowish white submucosal nodules, usually less than 2 cm in diameter. Most are found incidentally, but abdominal pain and bleeding can occur. Malignant degeneration can result, but this is unusual, and the possibility of such an association is still controversial.

Treatment has been local excision, if it is possible, or resection. Success with colonoscopic removal may prove to be the optimal therapy for most lesions.

## VASCULAR LESIONS

### Hemangioma

Hemangioma, although found in virtually every organ of the body, is one of the rarer tumors found in the colon. The pathogenesis of these tumors is not well defined. However, they are generally agreed to be congenital, with their origin in embryonic sequestrations of mesodermal tissue. Enlargement occurs by projection of budding endothelial cells. Whether these growths are neoplastic or congenital is a matter of some controversy.

The capillary hemangioma consists of small, thin-walled, closely packed vessels with a well-differentiated, hyperplastic endothelial lining. These tumors are distributed equally throughout the gastrointestinal tract. They represent 6% of benign vascular tumors, arise from the submucosal vascular plexus, and are often encapsulated. Mucosal ulceration occurs in one half of these lesions.

The cavernous hemangioma is composed of large, thin-walled vessels that are much larger than those of the capillary hemangioma. The supporting stroma contains scant connective tissue and, possibly, smooth muscle fibers. These lesions can be of the "multiple phlebectasia" type, characterized by a multitude of discrete tumors of less than 1 cm in diameter. Although they represent one third of all the benign vascular tumors of the gastrointestinal tract, they are frequently overlooked. The simple polypoid type of cavernous hemangioma constitutes 10% of benign vascular intestinal malformations and is usually of sufficient size to produce such symptoms as obstruction and hemorrhage. The diffuse, expansive type varies widely in shape and size, and often involves 20 to 30 cm of intestine, occasionally in multiple locations. Diffuse cavernous hemangiomas, which produce severe symptoms at a relatively early age, account for 20% of intestinal angiomas.

Venous angiomas are often confused with cavernous hemangiomas. Both are composed of large, thin-walled vessels with large lumens. However, the walls of venous angiomas contain varying amounts of smooth muscle and usually resemble veins. Many of these tumors are extensive, especially those found in the extremities. Thrombosis is common in venous as well as in cavernous hemangiomas; calcification frequently occurs in these thrombi and in the surrounding interstitial tissue.

Enlarged hemangiomas can produce symptoms of obstruction or hemorrhage. The obstructive symptoms can be caused either by the tumor, volvulus, or intussusception. The most common complication of hemangioma of the colon is bleeding; the incidence in colorectal hemangioma is 60% to 90%. Early onset and frequency of hemorrhage often lead to a diagnosis in adolescence or early adulthood. Characteristically, colonic hemangiomas bleed episodically, slowly, and persistently. The symptoms are melena and the results of anemia: fatigue and weakness. Cavernous hemangiomas tend to bleed massively much more frequently than capillary hemangiomas. Melena begins in childhood, is recurrent throughout adolescence, and results in intermittent symptomatic anemia. Bleeding tends to become more severe with each recurrent episode. Although early onset of bleeding with recurrence usually leads to a definitive diagnosis and treatment during adolescence, hemangiomas of the colon can be difficult to confirm before laparotomy. A positive family history may be helpful.

Physical examination is often unremarkable, but the presence of hemangiomas of the skin or mucous membrane should raise a suspicion that a similar lesion might be present in the colon.

Barium enema may reveal a filling defect, and phleboliths may be noted within the filling defect. The occurrence of multiple, calcific, well-circumscribed densities, probably related to thrombosis within the tumor, is seen particularly with cavernous hemangioma of the colon. CT has been shown to demonstrate characteristic findings—a thickened mesentery containing large vacuoles, and transmural thickening of the involved segment. Selective angiography may also reveal a vascular malformation, particularly in the late vascular phase, although the differential diagnosis between angioma and arteriovenous malformation (AVM) is often confusing. Injection of the resected specimen with contrast material may be useful for assuring adequacy of the margins.

Endoscopic diagnosis usually is not difficult; the tumor will appear deep red or purple. If colonoscopic resection is considered, be wary of the possibility of inducing uncontrolled hemorrhage.

Resection of a bleeding colonic hemangioma is the optimal treatment. If the benign nature of the tumor can be determined at laparotomy and confirmed by adequate frozen section examination, local excision of the hemangioma is sufficient. If malignancy cannot be excluded, the involved segment should be resected.

Only 75 cases of hemangioma of the rectum had been reported in the world literature before 1978. It seems reasonable to attempt a sphincter-saving operation, if hemorrhage can be controlled and no evidence of malignant change is seen.

### Lymphangioma

Lymphangioma of the gastrointestinal tract is a very rare lesion, and the colon is the least frequent site involved. The lesion originates in the lymphatic plexus within the submucosa into which the lacteals of the villi empty.

Lymphangiomas of the colon can be submucosal or pedunculated. The small number of documented submucosal lymphangiomas of the gastrointestinal tract does not permit satisfactory analysis of the radiologic characteristics.

The presence of blood vessels within many lesions designated as lymphangiomas is well recognized and has been taken as evidence that these lesions actually represent vascular malformations or hamartomas rather than true neoplasms. Differentiation from hemangioma may be impossible in lesions that lack abundant intraluminal and interstitial lymphocytes as evidence of their lymphatic origin.

Apart from lymphangioma, the histologic differential diagnosis includes lesions that may produce cystic spaces in the submucosal region of the bowel. The epithelial lining of colitis cystica profunda usually permits its easy recognition. However, the giant-cell lining that remains behind after dissolution of the oils in an oil granuloma (oleoma) may be more difficult to recognize. Gas cysts of recent origin may lack a lining. Whenever chronic, they are lined by giant cells similar to those of the oil granuloma.

None of the reported lymphangiomas of the colon and rectum has infiltrated the muscularis propria. However, such infiltration has occurred in lymphangioma of the small bowel.

Excisional biopsy with careful visualization under suitable anesthesia is the recommended procedure for rectal lesions. Colonoscopy is a valuable adjunct in the diagnosis of more proximal lesions. Colonoscopic polypectomy for pedunculated lymphangiomas appears to be a satisfactory treatment, but a limited resection should be considered for all sessile or infiltrative tumors.

### Hemangiopericytoma

Hemangiopericytoma, an extremely rare tumor that arises from pericytes, is usually found in the soft tissue of the trunk and extremities. Review of English-language publications revealed only two cases involving the colon, the small intestine being the most common gastrointestinal site. Abdominal pain, intestinal obstruction, intussusception, and rectal bleeding are associated with intestinal tumors. Malignant degeneration is usually based on the clinical course (recurrence or metastases) rather than the histologic picture. Microscopically, the tumor appears as multiple endothelial-lined capillaries or capillary buds. Resection is the treatment of choice.

### Malignant Vascular Tumors

Malignant vascular tumors include hemangioendothelioma, angiosarcoma, Kaposi's sarcoma, and benign metastasizing hemangioma. They represent approximately 13% of all vascular lesions of the colon and rectum, but with AIDS becoming epidemic, and the association of this condition with Kaposi's sarcoma, many more cases can be anticipated.

#### *Angiosarcoma*

Angiosarcoma is a malignant tumor of the vascular endothelium that is thought to arise from a hemangioma. The histology is characterized by varying degrees of endothelial proliferation and the formation of anastomosing vascular channels. Only three cases have been described involving the colon. Treatment is resection.

### *Kaposi's Sarcoma*

See Chapter 20.

## HETEROTOPIAS AND HAMARTOMAS

### Endometriosis

Endometriosis is a disorder resulting from the presence of actively growing and functioning endometrial tissue, both glandular and stromal, in sites outside the uterus.

### *Pathogenesis*

The pathogenesis of this common disorder is not clearly understood. Many theories have been proposed to explain the disease. One theory suggests fragments of endometrium are regurgitated with the menstrual blood through the oviducts in a retrograde fashion and implanted onto peritoneal surfaces and pelvic and abdominal structures. These would then erode into the subserosal tissues with viable cells growing and functioning, and ultimately lead to further implantation.

Another proposal is that of coelomic epithelial metaplasia. This assumes that dormant, immature cellular elements of Müllerian origin are known to persist into adult life, particularly throughout the central region of the pelvis. After menarche, repeated cyclic ovarian stimulation of these elements, with their totipotential capacities for differentiation, could result in the metaplastic formation of functioning endometrial tissue in ectopic sites.

Other theories have been suggested, including lymphatic dissemination of endometrial cells and deportation of normal endometrium by way of venous channels. These do not seem to offer a satisfactory explanation for the pathology.

### *Incidence*

Endometriosis occurs almost exclusively in women; in 75%, the condition develops between the ages of 20 and 40 years, and in 25%, up to the age of menopause. Isolated case reports have also appeared of endometriosis in men with prostatic cancer who are receiving estrogen therapy. The incidence of intestinal endometriosis among patients known to have endometriosis has been reported to be 5.4%.

### Symptoms and Signs

The classic history is one of acquired or secondary dysmenorrhea. The pain is related to, but does not necessarily occur simultaneously with each menstrual period. Pelvic discomfort associated with endometriosis is more likely to begin a day or two before the onset of menstrual flow, although its intensity can increase during the early days of menstruation. It tends to be a deep-seated ache or bearing-down pain in the lower part of the abdomen, posterior pelvis, vagina, or back, and often radiates into the rectal and perineal areas with tenesmus and symptoms suggestive of an irritable bowel. When, as is often the case, an endometrioma of one or both ovaries is present, dull, unilateral or bilateral lower abdominal pain, often with radiation to the thighs, may be noted.

The discomfort tends to abate after 2 or 3 days, subsiding completely toward the end of or just after the menstrual period. The patient will then be comfortable once more until a day or two before the onset of the next menstrual flow. However, as the disease progresses, pain tends to become more severe and can last most of each cycle.

Not all patients with endometriosis have pain, however. Despite extensive disease that may be palpable on pelvic examination or found at laparotomy, 15% to 20% of patients report no discomfort whatsoever. They can harbor other manifestations of the pathologic process, notably infertility or the presence of a mass. Other symptoms include dyspareunia, cyclic bowel disturbances with painful defecation, rectal bleeding, and intestinal obstruction. Although rectal bleeding is an uncommon presenting symptom of endometriosis, colon endometriosis should be considered when bleeding is associated with the menses. Leakage or rupture of an enlarging ovarian endometrioma can produce generalized peritonitis and an acute abdominal problem. Spillage of the contents of a "chocolate" endometrial cyst produces an intense local irritation and inflammatory response that results in chemical peritonitis.

A characteristic, almost diagnostic, physical finding is the hard, fixed, fibrotic nodule in the uterosacral ligaments, cul-de-sac, or posterior surface of the lower uterine wall and cervix. This nodularity is almost universally present in patients with endometriosis and is pathognomonic for the disease. In endometriosis of the rectovaginal septum, bidigital rectovaginal examination helps to define the pathologic condition.

### Diagnostic Studies

If the history is characteristic but the physical findings minimal or equivocal, laparoscopy or culdoscopy can prove valuable in establishing a definitive diagnosis. Other diagnostic tests include barium enema, intravenous pyelography to determine location and degree of obstruction (if involvement of the ureters or periureteral tissue is suspected), and cystoscopy (during the menstrual period) to reveal the characteristic bluish black, submucosal, cystic lesions if endometriosis of the bladder is suspected. Ileal endometriosis, especially, can present some confusion in differential diagnosis with Crohn's disease. Both conditions produce local inflammation and stricture. Preoperative endorectal ultrasound is also reliable for assessing rectal wall involvement.

### *Histopathology*

The three diagnostic histologic features of endometriosis are endometrial glands, endometrial stroma, and evidence of fresh hemorrhage (red cells and hemosiderin pigment) or old hemorrhage (hemosiderin-laden macrophages).

Because of its microscopic resemblance to normal endometrium and its known response to ovarian hormonal stimulation, the functioning epithelium of an endometrioma sometimes closely duplicates phases of the normal intrauterine endometrium, showing proliferative changes in the preovulatory or progestational phase. However, more often, the ectopic endometrial tissues are out of phase with the normal endometrium and are found in the proliferative stage, even during the secretory phase of the normal menstrual cycle. This may be caused by the difference in blood supply and the effects of increasing tissue fibrosis surrounding the endometriosis.

In the ovary, the process is almost always bilateral. The tendency is for the formation of cystic structures, varying from tiny bluish or dark brown blisters to large "chocolate" cysts. Usually present are considerable fibrosis and puckering of the ovarian surface in the region of the cyst, and adherence to neighboring structures.

### *Treatment*

Treatment of endometriosis is often based on the patient's age, severity of symptoms, hormonal status, and desire for childbearing.

### *Medical*

Endometrial implants disappear after administration of large doses of progestins and estrogen, but recurrence is seen in some instances. The action of these therapies has not been completely elucidated. The use of progestin alone or in combination with estrogen has become the standard method of hormonal treatment of endometriosis.

A more recent addition to the medical management of endometriosis has been danazol (Danocrine). Its efficacy is based on the fact that it creates a hypoestrogenic–hyperandrogenic state, which is detrimental to the growth and function of endometrial tissue. In doses of 200 to 800 mg/d, the pituitary inhibiting action results in suppression of ovulation, abolition of the mid-cycle increase of luteinizing hormone, and amenorrhea. The recommended dosage schedule for danazol in the treatment of endometriosis is 200 mg four times a day for at least

6 months. A maintenance dose of 200 to 400 mg daily may control pain after the initial treatment. Menstruation ceases with the commencement of therapy and returns promptly after the treatment has been discontinued. The pain of endometriosis is usually relieved in at least 80% of patients. Unfortunately, danazol has major side effects in nearly 85% of women treated with the drug, including weight gain, edema, acne, hirsutism, oily skin, deepening of the voice, clitoromegaly, and menometrorrhagia.

Most recently, the use of gonadotropin-releasing hormone (GRH) agonists has proved to be beneficial for the treatment of endometriosis. GRH is a hypothalamic decapeptide that controls pituitary secretion of luteinizing hormone and follicle-stimulating hormone. When administered by nasal spray (400 to 800 µg/d) and compared with danazol, the drug is as effective and has fewer side effects other than hypoestrogenism.

## Surgical

Endometriosis involving the small or large bowel can be preferentially excised. However, caution is suggested against extensive dissection beneath the peritoneal reflection, in the posterior cul-de-sac, or in the rectovaginal septum. Fistula complicating low anterior resection for endometriosis is not an uncommon occurrence. With respect to fertility, of those who tried to become pregnant following resection, almost 50% have gone on to successful delivery. After a mean follow-up of 60 months, 100% note relief with respect to cyclic bleeding, and 91% are free of rectal pain.

If pelvic endometriosis is so extensive that complete resection or fulguration is impossible or inadvisable and if childbearing has been completed, bilateral oophorectomy is curative, because recurrence or progression depends on cyclic ovarian hormone production. Natural menopause, if imminent, can also be relied on to cure the process.

After surgical castration for relief of endometriosis, estrogen replacement therapy should be instituted to prevent menopausal symptoms. Medroxyprogesterone acetate used for the first 6 to 9 months after operation alleviates menopausal symptoms and promotes further necrobiosis of any residual endometriosis.

## Management to Maintain Reproductive Capacity

The most difficult therapeutic decisions arise when young women with extensive disease would like to retain reproductive capability. Reasonable efforts should be made to eradicate the disease surgically in these individuals. Postoperatively, patients should be advised to commence childbearing as soon as possible. Because pregnancy eliminates menstruation for a period of 9 months, some therapeutic benefit can be expected. When childbearing is completed, definitive surgical therapy is less traumatic.

If childbearing is not a practical alternative, the patient should be given hormone therapy designed to prevent menstruation. Oral contraceptive pills given in a cyclic manner to allow intermittent withdrawal bleeding are not beneficial therapeutically. Birth control pills given daily and in sufficient potency to prevent breakthrough bleeding will result in softening, resorption, and necrobiosis of the endometrial glands. Medroxyprogesterone acetate (100 to 150 mg), given by intramuscular injection every 2 to 3 months, will suppress menstruation. Its main disadvantages are occasional troublesome breakthrough bleeding requiring the addition of estrogen for control, and in a small percentage of women, permanent anovulation and resultant sterility. Medroxyprogesterone acetate is not generally recommended for patients who are interested in further childbearing; danazol is the treatment of choice.

In the experience of most physicians, hormone therapy does not always cure the process, but it gives the patient time to consider alternatives and to complete childbearing before progression of the disease or before increased symptoms and complications require the absolutely successful therapy: bilateral oophorectomy with hysterectomy.

### Perineal Endometrioma

Perineal endometrioma is a special situation in which implantation of viable endometrial cells occurs in episiotomy incisions. A tender nodule producing cyclic symptoms at the site of an episiotomy is highly suggestive of the diagnosis. Local excision is the treatment of choice, although suppressive therapy may be employed.

### Hamartoma

Hamartomas are tumorlike malformations that result from inborn errors of tissue development; they are characterized by abnormal mixtures of mature tissue indigenous to that area. Hamartomas can be derived from any of the germinal layers, and any type of tissue can predominate. The nomenclature depends on the tissue type that predominates: with vascular predominance, it is angiomatous; with fatty tissue, it is lipomatous; and with lymphoid tissue, it is lymphomatous.

Hamartomas should be differentiated from teratomas and dermoids. The term "teratoma" describes a spontaneous, autonomous new growth derived from pluripotential tissues. It is foreign to the region in which it occurs and is composed of elements of all three germinal layers. A dermoid tumor has the same histogenesis but differs in that it is usually cystic. Unlike a teratoma, it originates from only two germinal layers: the ectoderm and the mesoderm. Clinically, it is difficult to differentiate between teratomas, dermoids (especially when small), and hamartomas.

Suspicion of hamartoma can arise by a small but definite funnel-shaped dimple in the posterior midline at the anal margin or the mid-anal level. This anal dimple associated with a higher lesion has been reported only once, although it must have been encountered many times.

Complete surgical removal is the only effective treatment for retrorectal cystic hamartoma. The surgical approach can be either through the anal canal or posteriorly, transcoccygeally. However, in those instances in which a large cyst lies at a very high level, an abdominal approach is indicated.

## Dermoid Cyst and Teratoma

Dermoid cysts are tumors of epithelial origin believed caused by faulty inclusion of ectoderm when the embryo coalesces. They generally do not appear until adult life and are more common in women than in men.

Patients can be asymptomatic but are usually found to have an extrarectal mass as an incidental finding on rectal examination. Endoscopic examination is usually unrewarding. As mentioned, a cyst can become infected and mimic an anorectal abscess or fistula. A plain abdominal radiograph may be helpful, but a CT scan should be done with any question of malignancy (e.g., chordoma). Preoperative biopsy is unnecessary and should not be performed.

The mass can frequently be resected by a posterior approach, with or without removal of the coccyx. An abdominal or abdominosacral operation may be required for a more extensive or more proximal lesion. Prognosis is excellent; recurrence after surgery, however, is possible if the lesion is incompletely removed.

Dermoid cysts can also occur within the rectum, but this is even more unusual than the postanal or presacral locations. In this situation, intraluminal cysts can produce varied rectal symptoms, including hair protruding from the anus, rectal bleeding, or prolapse of the mass. With this type of presentation, transanal excision is the recommended approach. Endoscopic resection has also been described.

## Colitis Cystica Profunda or Enterogenous Cysts

Colitis cystica profunda is a rare, nonneoplastic condition characterized by the presence of mucous cysts deep to the muscularis mucosa and usually confined to the sigmoid colon and rectum. The most common symptoms are rectal bleeding, passage of mucus, diarrhea, and rectal pain. The primary diagnosis from which it must be differentiated is mucus-producing adenocarcinoma.

Colitis cystica profunda can be categorized into two groups: localized, in which the cysts are confined to a distinct area of the rectum; and diffuse, in which the cysts are located in extensive areas. The histogenesis of this benign condition remains in dispute.

Colitis cystica profunda of the localized type can protrude slightly into the lumen of the bowel as a polypoid mass and, thus, mimic carcinoma of the rectum. Because it is usually located on the anterior rectal wall—the most common site for solitary ulcer—considerable confusion can exist.

The cause of the condition is unknown. However, a number of patients give a history of prior rectal trauma, especially the removal of a large polyp. Correlation between anorectal dysfunction and this disease has been described. Others have theorized that, most probably, the primary factor is a weakness or defect in the muscularis mucosa resulting in mucosal herniation. Certainly, the fact that resolution has followed the successful management of internal procidentia and rectal prolapse implies a causative or an associative role with these conditions.

Differentiation by biopsy can be difficult. To establish the diagnosis with certainty, an adequate tissue biopsy must be obtained that reveals submucosal cyst formation. Lesions can have histologic appearances suggestive of both solitary ulcer and colitis profunda.

Although successful medical management by the use of steroid enemas has been reported, transanal excision of the lesion is the optimal therapy, if it can be performed. A transcoccygeal approach is another alternative. Not uncommonly, the lesion is unresectable, except by radical abdominoperineal resection. Such treatment is contraindicated, however, for this benign condition. Another option is mucosal sleeve excision with coloanal pull-through. Reassurance and periodic proctosigmoidoscopy are suggested for those not amenable to complete removal.

## Ectopic Tissue

Besides ectopic gastric or pancreatic mucosa in a Meckel's diverticulum, ectopic tissue in the intestine or colon is unusual. Two types have been reported: gastric mucosal replacement of the rectal mucosa and salivary gland tissue in the submucosa. It has been suggested that the cells lining the primitive gut have the capacity to differentiate into any epithelial type that would normally be present at another level. This would not, however, explain the presence of salivary gland tissue; perhaps the presence of stem cells lining the cloacal zone may account for this rare observation.

Review of the literature on heterotopic gastric mucosa producing rectal "peptic" ulceration found fewer than 30 reported cases. Analysis reveals the main features to be as follows:

All but one were diagnosed in infants or in adults younger than 26 years of age.
Rectal peptic ulceration was identified in only one half of cases, but almost all exhibited rectal bleeding.
Rectal duplication was present in 21%.
Limited excision is generally successful.

Protrusion of tissue can occur in a child, raising the suspicion for the presence of a juvenile polyp. Patients may be asymptomatic or complain of mucous discharge, change in bowel habits, or rectal bleeding.

The true pathologic nature of the lesion is usually not suspected at the time of removal but is confirmed by histologic examination. Transanal local excision is the appropriate treatment.

Six documented cases of heterotopic gastric mucosa have occurred in the large bowel, proximal to the rectum. Most have been managed by resection, because bleeding identified by means of angiography or radioisotope scan leads to surgery. It is only when the lesion has been submitted to histologic evaluation that the actual cause is confirmed. Reports now exist of successful management by a H2 antagonist.

## EXOGENOUS, EXTRINSIC, AND MISCELLANEOUS TUMORS

### Metastatic Tumor

Metastatic tumor to the colon and rectum can cause symptoms of abdominal pain, bleeding, and change in bowel habits. Life-threatening emergencies, in the form of massive gastrointestinal hemorrhage, obstruction, and perforation have been reported. Although usually producing extrinsic compression of the bowel on barium enema examination, ulceration can mimic primary carcinoma of the colon. Tumors of adjacent organs that can invade the colon and rectum include prostate, uterus, ovary, kidney, stomach, duodenum, and pancreas. Metastatic disease can occur from breast, malignant melanoma, hypernephroma, and pulmonary origins. Palliative resection or bypass is usually advised for symptomatic tumors. Certainly, the possibility for cure exists if the site involved represents a solitary lesion.

### Barium Granuloma

A submucosal rectal nodule that can be confused with a neoplastic condition, especially a carcinoid, may be caused by a barium granuloma. Such lesions appear in the lower rectum, usually as submucosal white or yellowish plaques, and they are frequently asymptomatic. A break in the continuity of the rectal mucosa is the probable initiating factor. Transanal excision is mandatory for diagnosis.

Histologically, the presence of barium produces a typical foreign body granulomatous reaction. The barium crystals lie in a pool in the submucosa in early lesions, but macrophages rapidly accumulate and phagocytose the crystalline barium sulfate.

Care in the introduction of the enema catheter and caution with use of the balloon tip are clearly indicated to prevent barium granuloma. A number of cases of rupture of the bowel with barium peritonitis have been reported when barium enema examination has followed rectal biopsy. Optimally, if a polyp excision or electrocoagulation is contemplated on an individual who is to have barium enema examination, the patient should complete the contrast study and then return for the other procedure. Barium granuloma of the more proximal colon is usually related to inflammatory bowel disease.

### Oleoma, Eleoma, Oil Granuloma, and Paraffinoma

Oleoma, also known as oleogranuloma or paraffinoma, is a rare entity that occurs in the gastrointestinal tract or skin as a result of an injection of mineral oil (paraffin) for the treatment of hemorrhoids, or enema or vegetable oil in the management of constipation. The lesion can be defined as an intramural pseudo-tumor that develops as a foreign body reaction. The "tumor" is occasionally cystic and can be termed an "oleocyst." The differential diagnosis must be confirmed by biopsy to rule out other neoplastic and inflammation conditions.

The clinical manifestations can develop rapidly or may not present for many years after oil enters the tissue. The injection site usually appears as one or more irregular, firm nodules. In the gastrointestinal tract, oleomas are usually found proximal to the dentate line in the lower portion of the rectum.

An oleoma is usually localized to the submucosa. However, considerable inflammation of the mucosa and even the perianal skin may be present. The appearance of the lesion depends on the oil present: vegetable oils produce the least reaction, animal oils a greater one, and mineral oils the most severe changes.

Histologically, oleomas appear as large, mononuclear phagocytes; epithelioid cells; eosinophilic leukocytes; and multinucleated giant cells of the foreign body type, surrounding large, clear spaces that give the tissue a Swiss cheese or spongiform appearance under low-power amplification. Histologic staining with oil red 0 verifies the presence of the lipid. The reaction usually remains localized to the submucosa, but not infrequently involves the lamina propria of the mucosa and may extend into the perirectal fat.

### Sarcoidosis

Sarcoidosis is a generalized, granulomatous disease with protean manifestations. The condition usually creates restrictive lung disease but can occasionally involve the gastrointestinal tract. In the limited number of cases reported, patients usually do not have symptoms referable to the bowel. When symptoms are present, they can include anorexia, nausea, vomiting, abdominal pain, and gastrointestinal bleeding. Proctosigmoidoscopic examination may reveal mild inflammatory changes or a submucosal rectal nodule.

The characteristic noncaseating granuloma of sarcoidosis may be seen on biopsy or excision of a lesion. Histologic examination may confirm a granuloma composed primarily of histiocytes; no evidence is found of caseous necrosis.

Differential diagnosis must include Crohn's disease, but the presence of a lesion in the lung usually clarifies any possible confusion.

## Wegener's Granulomatosis

Wegener's granulomatosis, a necrotizing vasculitis associated with granulomatous lesions of the upper and lower respiratory tract and the kidney, has been reported in one instance to present as a perianal ulcer. Treatment was by immunosuppressive therapy.

## Amyloidosis

Amyloidosis is a pathologic condition caused by the deposition within tissues of a fibrillar protein known as amyloid. The Third International Symposium on Amyloidosis recommended the following classification:

Primary amyloidosis: no evidence of preceding or coexisting disease, except multiple myeloma
Secondary amyloidosis: coexistence of other conditions
Localized amyloid: single organ rather than generalized involvement
Familial
Senile amyloid

Involvement of the gastrointestinal tract is reported in 70% of patients with primary amyloidosis and 55% of those with the secondary form. Amyloidosis not uncommonly affects the colon in association with a number of systemic diseases, particularly pulmonary, renal, hematologic, and arthritic. Symptoms include malabsorption, diarrhea, bleeding, vomiting, abdominal pain, and, rarely, signs of peritonitis.

### Rectal Biopsy

The value of rectal biopsy for establishing the diagnosis of systemic amyloid has been a matter of controversy. In patients with known amyloidosis, a positive result from a rectal biopsy is found in 33% to 90%. It is imperative that adequate submucosal tissue be obtained to confirm the diagnosis. Although some authors have advocated a suction biopsy forceps, I prefer to use the ordinary rectal biopsy instrument. Because no sample of tissue is being taken from an exophytic lesion, the biopsy should be obtained from a valve of Houston or from the posterior rectal wall. If bleeding is encountered, slight pressure with an epinephrine-soaked cotton swab is advised. Electrocoagulation should be avoided because of the risk of perforating the bowel.

An interesting diagnostic observation is the "postproctoscopic periorbital purpura." The hydrostatic forces imposed on the delicate periorbital vasculature when the patient is placed in the prone, jackknife position for biopsy can precipitate rupture of the vessels whose walls are compromised by amyloid deposition.

Special stains are important for the identification of amyloid. A homogeneous eosinophilic substance can be seen by means of Congo red stain; this material can be overlooked if the standard hematoxylin and eosin technique is used.

### Response to Treatment

Another purpose of rectal biopsy is to evaluate the success of different modalities of treatment. Penicillamine therapy results in improvement that can be observed by serial histologic examination. Melphalan and prednisone have been used with limited benefit to possibly decrease immunoglobulin production and prevent progressive amyloid deposition. Colchicine has also been reported to have some therapeutic value.

### Amyloid Tumor

Localized amyloid tumors of the gastrointestinal tract are extremely unusual. All reported cases involving the large bowel presented with lower gastrointestinal bleeding. A colonic perforation has also been observed. Rarely, amyloidosis of the colon produces a mass lesion or obstructive symptoms. Resection should be considered for a symptomatic, well-defined tumor.

### Malacoplakia

Malacoplakia is a rare, chronic inflammatory disorder most commonly affecting the urinary bladder and other portions of the genitourinary tract. Clinical presentation is varied, but rectal bleeding, diarrhea, and obstructive symptoms are most commonly described. The lesion may be observed as an incidental finding. A preponderance of women is seen among patients with the genitourinary lesion, but this is not the case with those who have colonic involvement.

No characteristic radiologic changes of malacoplakia are seen. The barium enema may be indistinguishable from carcinoma or from granulomatous colitis.

The macroscopic lesion appears as a mucosal thickening or plaque and can assume a polypoid configuration. Histologically it is seen as a proliferation of eosinophilic, coarsely granular histiocytes often containing laminated calcific concretions—the so-called "Michaelis-Gutmann bodies" that are virtually pathognomonic of this entity. The histiocytic proliferation is accompanied by a chronic inflammatory infiltrate and sometimes by fibrosis.

Although the pathogenesis is not fully understood, ultrastructural evidence suggests that altered heat response to certain species of gram-negative bacteria may be involved. Sound ultrastructural evidence implies that the Michaelis-Gutmann body is a morphologic byproduct of impaired lysosomal function. An immunologic association may exist as well, because the condition has been identified in a patient with hypogammaglobulinemia, and a genetic predisposition has also been observed.

Although, for the most part, the lesions are self-limited or responsive to antibiotic therapy, occasionally resection is necessary because of bleeding, the development of nonhealing fistulas, or localized anatomic complications. Biopsy and histologic examination are necessary to differentiate this lesion from carcinoma, which it can resemble clinically. It is of interest that malacoplakia has been associated as an incidental finding with colonic carcinoma.

## Sacrococcygeal Chordoma

Sacrococcygeal chordoma, a rare tumor of the fetal notochord, is characterized by a slow but inexorably progressive growth that usually spans a period of years. It invades by direct extension. Irrespective of the method of treatment chosen, the prognosis is poor. This tumor has been reported to demonstrate distant metastases in more than 40% of patients. The usual sites of distribution of chordoma are sacrococcygeal, 50%; sphenoccipital, 35%; and vertebral, 15%. Rare examples are of extranotochordal origin.

### *Signs, Symptoms, and Findings*

Symptoms are produced as the tumor proliferates, often reaching considerable size before the diagnosis is made. Surrounding soft tissue and viscera are at first simply displaced, but eventually adjacent bone is gradually eroded. The most common initial symptom is pain; it is so gradual in onset and of such indefinite character that patients with this complaint often experience a delay in diagnosis of months to years. Constipation is the second most common presenting complaint.

The most significant physical finding is a firm, smooth, presacral mass, with overlying intact rectal mucosa. The history may contain prior treatment for a neurologic, orthopedic, or urologic disorder.

### *Studies*

Bone destruction, a soft-tissue mass, and anterior rectum displacement are the characteristic radiographic signs. These tumors often involve far more soft tissue than the osseous deformity would imply and at operation, bone destruction is likely to be more extensive than had been evident from the radiographic studies.

Radiographic examination, including CT scan and magnetic resonance imaging, is the only investigative procedure necessary for making the diagnosis of chordoma. Needle biopsy is to be condemned because of the likelihood of implanting viable tumor cells.

### *Treatment*

Cure of sacrococcygeal chordoma depends on complete extirpation of the tumor, ideally by *en bloc* removal of the coccyx and the lower sacral segments with the lesion. The limiting factor of the extent of resection performed is the need to preserve the $S_2$ nerve roots, because their removal will lead to permanent neurologic damage and fecal and urinary incontinence. In addition to neurologic impairment, resections beyond the lower three sacral segments can result in instability and collapse of the pelvis and descent of the lumbar spine.

Some surgeons favor a radical approach, including abdominosacral resection or even posterior exenteration and sacrectomy. Exposure of the sciatic and pudendal nerves is required if a large growth that extends into the buttocks must be extirpated. High sacral resections can be done by dividing the fused sacral laminae with fine rongeurs, opening the sacral canal, exposing the dural sac and sacral roots, and dividing the sacral bodies with an osteotome.

Radiation therapy is controversial, because the tumor has not been proved to be radiosensitive. It is often used, however, when surgical excision is impossible. No chemotherapeutic regimen, thus far, has proved beneficial. If recurrence develops following resection, debulking may palliate pain symptoms. If radiotherapy has been used, subsequent healing can be considerably delayed or the wound may not heal at all.

For unremitting pain, uncontrolled by medication, chordotomy may be necessary.

## Results

Results of surgical treatment for chordoma are difficult to interpret, because patients often live a long time, even with persistent localized or disseminated disease. Furthermore, many publications are based on only one or two cases, with only a few months of follow-up. The overall 5-year survival appears to be around 75%. However, only 30% will be considered cured. The average disease-free survival was 63 months.

## Ependymoma

Ependymomas are the most common tumors of glial origin in the spinal cord, especially in the region of the cauda equina. Clinically, a mass, which is thought to be a pilonidal cyst or sinus, is a common presenting feature. Ependymomas occur mainly in patients during the third decade of life and present either in the soft tissue posterior to the rectum or in the pelvis. Patients whose tumors are located in the pelvic region present with sphincter dysfunction attributable to sacral nerve involvement.

Histologic examination reveals a papillary neoplasm, with cells containing relatively regular nuclei without significant mitotic activity. Conventional and CT studies may reveal erosion of the sacrum, and myelography will demonstrate an extradural mass indenting the fecal sac from below.

Wide excision is the preferred treatment, but as with chordoma, recurrence is common. A combined posterior and anterior approach with the goal of complete tumor removal is ideal, when possible. If this is not feasible, radiation therapy should be considered as palliative treatment. Because of the increased incidence of systemic metastases, the average postoperative survival is about 10 years.

### Extramedullary (Extra-Adrenal Myelolipoma)

Myelolipomas are usually found in the adrenal glands, but rarely can be seen in other sites. These include intrathoracic, paravertebral, retroperitoneal, intracranial, and presacral locations as well as the liver, stomach, and iliac fossa. The most frequent extraadrenal site is the presacral area.

Symptoms include low back pain, rectal fullness, pain on sitting, and urinary symptoms. Rectal examination may reveal an anterior sacral mass. Because of the benign nature of the disease, radiologic studies do not demonstrate bony invasion.

Myelolipoma is characterized histologically by the presence of active hematopoietic elements intermixed with fat.

Treatment consists of a standard transcoccygeal approach. Anticipate a complete cure for this benign process.

### Anterior Sacral Meningocele

Anterior sacral meningocele is a congenital cystic structure that can appear as a presacral mass. Located in the presacral space, it communicates with the dural sac through a narrow neck that passes through a much larger, smooth, sacral bony defect. Radiography of the pelvis may demonstrate the characteristic "scimitar sign."

The treatment approach is via a posterior sacral laminectomy.

### Pneumatosis Cystoides Intestinalis or *Pneumatosis coli*

Pneumatosis cystoides intestinalis (*Pneumatosis coli,* when the condition is confined to the colon), is a relatively uncommon disease of unknown cause. It is characterized by the presence of gas-filled cysts within the wall of portions of the gastrointestinal tract. It most commonly occurs in the jejunum and ileum, with only 6% of cases being seen in the colon. The disease is noted usually in the older population, but it can occur at any age. Its relationship with other conditions has been well documented, most frequently, pulmonary disease is associated (e.g., chronic obstructive lung disease). It can also be seen with peptic ulcer, pyloric stenosis, collagen disease, acute gastroenteritis, nontropical sprue, intestinal obstruction, mesenteric occlusion, ischemic colitis, inflammatory bowel disease, and carcinoma of the colon; following abdominal trauma, as a result of endoscopic maneuvers (especially colonoscopy); with steroid therapy and exposure to organic solvents (e.g., trichloroethylene); following organ transplantation; and after surgical procedures on the bowel.

The reasons for the occurrence in association with such diverse entities are unclear. One possibility is that increased intraluminal pressure may force the gas into the wall of the bowel. This may account for its association with certain primary diseases of the gastrointestinal tract. However, on close inspection of the bowel in such patients, it does not appear that the integrity of the mucosa is breached.

The theory for the condition occurring in association with chronic obstructive pulmonary disease is that a pulmonary bleb ruptures and dissects retroperitoneally along the vessels, reaching the bowel wall. In support of this postulate is the fact that segmental distribution of the blebs usually is observed. A third theory, which may be more relevant in infants with severe gastroenteritis, speculates that gas-forming bacteria account for the formation of the cysts. Another possible implicating factor is the suggestion that the condition may be caused by an abnormal H2 metabolism.

Many patients who harbor this condition do so without symptoms. The lesions may be noted on radiographic examination or at the time of endoscopy. When symptoms are present, they can be vague, or they can include abdominal pain, diarrhea, and the passage of mucus and blood in the stool.

Physical examination is usually not revealing. Rarely, is abdominal tenderness or distension present. Digital examination of the rectum may reveal an extramucosal mass, if the cysts indeed extend into that area.

Barium enema examination usually reveals well-demarcated, lucent wall defects of varying size, usually grouped in clusters with an intact overlying mucosa (Fig. 25.3). The condition can be confused with inflammatory bowel dis-

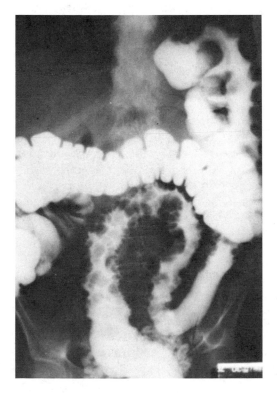

**FIG. 25.3.** *Pneumatosis coli.* Multiple lucent cystlike defects throughout the left colon.

ease, multiple polyposis, or carcinoma. Definitive diagnosis can be established by means of colonoscopy; some have advocated this technique for confirming the presence of the benign cysts.

Histologic examination of the biopsy specimen reveals normal mucosa beneath which are seen cystic spaces lined by endothelium. A mild inflammatory infiltrate may be present; multinucleated giant cells are noticed frequently.

### *Treatment*

By administering oxygen at relatively high concentration, resorption of the gas in the cysts (which are mostly nitrogen) should occur. Although no consistent recommendation can be made about its administration, most authors believe that it is necessary to reach an arterial $Po_2$ in excess of 300 mmHg to achieve the desired results. A concentration of oxygen between 55% and 75% is generally used in the inhaled gas. A minimum of 48 hours of therapy is recommended for up to 5 days. Exercise concern, however, about the possibility of oxygen toxicity. In fact, I treat only those patients who have symptoms. In these individuals, the ameliorative effect of oxygen therapy usually is apparent within 1 or 2 days. A report of successful treatment with metronidazole lends credence to the theory that anaerobic bacteria, in some manner, are responsible.

Surgery is usually reserved for those with localized disease and when hemorrhage, obstruction, or perforation supervenes. Treatment of obstruction by means of endoscopic puncture and sclerotherapy of the cyst walls has been described.

### *Pneumoperitoneum*

Pneumoperitoneum can supervene in a patient with pneumatosis. Abdominal signs and symptoms are usually absent. If the patient has been known to harbor cysts, a trial of conservative therapy is advocated. Usually, no communication with the gastrointestinal tract exists; therefore, do not treat the radiographic finding. Expectant management will usually be followed by gradual disappearance of the free gas. In the rare situation in which the disease continues to cause symptoms and the cysts are localized to a limited segment of the bowel, consider resection.

### **Duplication**

### *Colonic*

Colonic duplication is an uncommon congenital anomaly that usually occurs during infancy or early childhood. However, occasional cases can present in the older age groups. Obstruction and the presence of an abdominal mass are usually the signs and symptoms apparent in infancy. Progressive abdominal pain, bleeding, an abdominal mass, and rarely perforation are characteristic of child-hood or adult onset. Diarrhea, constipation, distension, and obstruction are additional symptoms, and an intussusception is sometimes observed.

True intestinal duplications must be distinguished from enteric cysts. Characteristics of this anomaly include intimate attachment to some part of the alimentary tract, a smooth muscle coat, and a mucosal lining similar to that of the stomach, small bowel, or colon. Four subtypes have been described:

1. A tubular duplication branching into the mesenteric leaves
2. A double-barreled, communicating structure (Fig. 25.4)
3. A free-lying, cystic duplication connected to the alimentary tract by a thin mesenteric stalk
4. A cystic duplication attached to the bowel by a common wall

Plain abdominal x-ray films may demonstrate a soft-tissue mass, evidence of small or large bowel obstruction, and the presence of a gas-filled structure with an air–fluid level on the erect film. Barium enema examination may demonstrate displacement of the bowel, compression by the mass, or, in the case of a communicating lesion, an irregular double lumen. The condition is not uncommonly associated with other congenital anomalies, such as malrotation, Meckel's diverticulum, lumbosacral spine deformities (e.g., double vertebrae), and genitourinary abnormalities (double uterus, double vagina, double bladder, and double

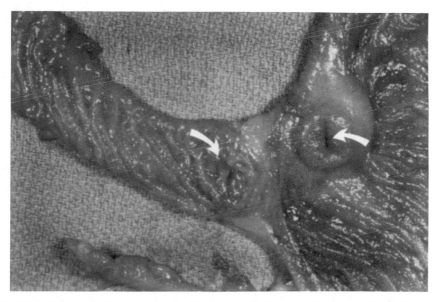

**FIG. 25.4.** Colonic duplication. Note two distinct lumina (*arrows*). (Courtesy of Rudolf Garret, M.D.)

urethra). CT and an intravenous pyelogram should be part of the evaluation of any individual found to harbor a colon or rectal duplication.

Treatment can involve excision of the mass, with preservation of the normal colon (a communication is usually not demonstrable), although ischemia of the bowel wall and perforation are potential hazards if this approach is used. Alternatively, an *en bloc* resection with anastomosis may be required when in cases of a double-barreled, communicating lesion.

## Rectum

As suggested, all regions of the gut can be associated with a duplication, but the rectum is the least common location. It is likely that many remain asymptomatic, unless complicated by infection, bleeding, or malignant degeneration. A number of reports of carcinoma arising in a rectal duplication suggest that all should be treated by surgical excision, even if they appear benign. Care must be taken to remove the cyst and still preserve integrity of the rectum, but the possibility of recurrence from multiple satellites in the wall of the duplication should be recognized.

# 26

# Diverticular Disease

Diverticular disease (diverticulitis and diverticulosis) was rare before the end of the 19th century. However, the disease has become progressively more pervasive in the 20th century and virtually epidemic in Western countries. Today, a person's risk for the development of diverticular disease by age 60 in the United States approximates 50%. However, probably not more than 10% of persons with colonic diverticula have symptoms, and only a small proportion of these ever require surgery.

## PATHOGENESIS

Diverticula occur most commonly on the antimesenteric surface of the bowel, usually in the sigmoid colon, between the taeniae at the points where the blood vessels penetrate the wall. The tunnels formed by the blood vessels weaken the muscle, and presumably the diverticula become manifest as a result of high intra-colonic pressure impacting on these areas. This is an important anatomic fact that can also be relevant to the complication of hemorrhage from diverticula (see Chapter 28).

### Physiology

Normal colonic motility is discussed in Chapters 2 and 6. Motor studies in patients with diverticular disease reveal an exaggerated response to pharmaco-logic stimuli, increased intraluminal pressures, and faster frequency waves and rapid contractions (more than five per minute).

Increased pressure is brought about through progressive colonic narrowing and segmentation. When contraction occurs in a segment that is relatively nar-rowed, considerable intraluminal pressure develops, causing the colon to hyper-trophy. The pressure is greater when the lumen is narrowed, which explains the increased likelihood that diverticula will develop in the sigmoid colon, the nar-rowest segment. The thickened colonic muscle becomes uneven, with resultant herniation through the weakened parts of its wall. The problem is exacerbated by the fact that the tensile strength and elasticity of the colon decline with age; this is most marked on the left side. Additionally, the sigmoid must propel the most formed fecal material, which contributes further to the problem in this area.

## Histology

Microscopically, the diverticula are of the pulsion type, consisting only of mucous membrane and peritoneum. In the absence of complications, particularly inflammation, the lining is entirely normal except for an increase in the size and number of lymphoid follicles. The muscle shows thickening but no evidence of cellular hypertrophy or hyperplasia. Antimesenteric diverticula have only a thin layer of investing longitudinal muscle, mucous membrane, and muscularis mucosae separating the fecal contents of the bowel from the peritoneal cavity.

## ETIOLOGY, EPIDEMIOLOGY, AND DIET

The increasing incidence of diverticular disease over the past 100 years has coincided with a reduction in the amount of cereal fiber consumption to as little as one tenth of that previously eaten. Because of this sudden change, diverticular disease has become epidemic in Western countries within approximately 40 years. In fact, with economic development, affluence, and westernization of diet, an increased incidence of diverticular disease has been noted among native Africans.

A high-fiber diet produces a large, bulky stool that requires less "effort" by the bowel to propel the contents. Fiber increases stool weight, decreases whole-gut transit time, and lowers colonic intraluminal pressure. Muscular hypertrophy does not occur, and segmentation is much less likely to develop.

The addition of fiber has been shown to be effective in the treatment of many symptomatic patients with uncomplicated diverticular disease. Fiber can be obtained by eating certain vegetables and fruits that are high in fiber, or alternatively, by using one of a number of proprietary preparations, the so-called "bulk laxatives," made from the outer covering of the psyllium grain or from sterculia- and ispaghula-derived hydrophilic colloids. Preparations include Konsyl, Citrucel, FiberCon, Metamucil, among others.

## Age, Sex, and Heredity

Most studies report that diverticular disease is more common in women; the incidence increases with advancing age. However, the correlation between the incidence of the condition and the presence or duration of symptoms is less clear. For example, young men are more likely to require surgical intervention for complications than are elderly patients, some even during the initial attack.

## Relationship to Nonsteroidal Antiinflammatory Drugs

A number of studies have suggested an association between nonsteroidal anti-inflammatory drugs (NSAIDs) and the development of complications of diverticular disease. Possible explanations include a direct effect on the bowel wall through inhibition of prostaglandin synthesis itself, or the inhibitory effect of leukocyte function with failure of the immune system to localize the process. Case-control studies have consistently found that more individuals with complicated diverticulitis were taking NSAIDs than were randomly selected other groups.

## Other Relationships

Alcoholism is a risk factor for the development of diverticulitis. Those who smoke are also at an increased risk for suffering a complication during an episode of acute diverticulitis.

## SYMPTOMS AND FINDINGS

### Irritable Bowel Syndrome

The irritable bowel syndrome is estimated to affect up to one quarter of the population of Western countries. Basically, the diagnosis of irritable bowel syndrome is a diagnosis of exclusion. Diagnostic criteria include the continuous or recurrent presence of the following symptoms for at least 3 months:

- Abdominal pain relieved by defecation or associated with a change in frequency or consistency of stool
- Disturbed defecation at least 25% of the time and three or more of the following:
  - Altered stool frequency
  - Altered stool form
  - Altered stool passage (straining, urgency, or tenesmus)
  - Passage of mucus
  - Abdominal distension

The term *irritable bowel syndrome* suggests that these patients have an abnormality in the intestine, but the symptoms can develop without any anatomic defect and certainly in the absence of diverticulosis. The regimen for therapy often includes dietary modification, antidiarrheal medication (if appropriate), anticholinergics, and possibly antianxiety compounds.

### Diverticulitis

#### Symptoms

Patients with diverticulitis complain primarily of abdominal pain. Pain is usually located in the left lower quadrant and tends to be constant rather than colicky in nature. The pain can radiate to the back, left flank, groin, and leg, although these observations can also be seen with an irritable bowel. The duration and severity of symptoms are variable, depending on whether the patient has a localized or diffuse process. Nausea and vomiting are uncommon complaints unless some element of intestinal obstruction is present. A change in bowel habits is frequently observed—an absence of bowel movements or diarrhea.

Patients with acute diverticular disease often mention urinary problems (dysuria, urgency, frequency, nocturia), which may be attributable to impingement of the inflammatory mass on the wall of the bladder. A urinary tract infection may imply communication with the bowel (see later). Passage of gas in the urine or through the vagina is diagnostic of a fistula (see later).

Fever is also commonly observed in patients with acute diverticulitis. It is usually low grade, but if peritonitis develops or if an abscess is present, the temperature can be considerably elevated.

Massive lower gastrointestinal bleeding is not felt to be a complication of diverticulitis. This problem is dealt with in Chapter 28.

### Physical Examination

Physical examination may reveal localized to generalized tenderness reflecting the severity of the process. Tenderness and a mass in the pelvis from a sigmoid phlegmon may be noted on rectal or vaginal examination. An abdominal mass can occasionally be felt. Extraperitoneal infection can present with back, buttock, and hip and leg pain; a positive psoas sign; perineal and scrotal pain and swelling; and subcutaneous, mediastinal, and cervical emphysema. Perforation below the peritoneal reflection can lead to a buttock abscess and a consequent anorectal fistula (see Chapters 10 and 11).

### Endoscopy

The surgeon must weigh the risks of the procedure against the potential benefit of the information gleaned. A theoretic risk exists of disturbing a walled-off perforation with the instrument itself, or more likely by the insufflation of air. Although rigid proctosigmoidoscopy can be carried out with minimal use of air, considerable caution should be exercised with air insufflation when the flexible instrument is used. Despite the risks, direct visualization can be helpful in distinguishing between diverticulitis and other pathologic conditions (e.g., ischemic colitis, carcinoma, inflammatory bowel disease; see later).

### Contrast Studies

The most valuable and most commonly employed study to evaluate patients with diverticular disease is the barium enema examination. However, this should not be performed in the acute situation, because barium peritonitis, an often fatal complication, may result. A gentle, water-soluble enema (e.g., Gastrografin) is a safer alternative.

### Computed Tomography

More recently, a number of articles have appeared suggesting that computed tomography (CT) should be the initial imaging technique, because of the superior definition of bowel wall thickness and the extent of extraluminal disease. Often, accurate diagnosis of fistulas can be made through the intimate association of the inflamed segment to other organs. This investigation is thought to be particularly valuable in the diagnosis of right-sided diverticulitis.

Computed tomography is also useful as a *therapeutic* modality, through the application of CT-guided drainage to avoid surgical intervention in the acute setting (see later).

### Ultrasonography

Ultrasonography in the diagnosis of acute and complicated colonic diverticulitis has been reported to be accurate in 88% to 98% of patients. Unfortunately, the examination in the acutely tender patient is extremely uncomfortable and may not be possible. This modality can be helpful when the clinical findings are equivocal.

## MEDICAL MANAGEMENT OF ACUTE DIVERTICULAR DISEASE

The American Society of Colon and Rectal Surgeons has established a Standards Task Force to identify guidelines in the management of a number of conditions. Such "parameters" have been produced for sigmoid diverticulitis.

Patients who present with tenderness and the suggestion of a sausagelike mass in the left lower quadrant, in the absence of systemic signs and symptoms, can be initially treated on an outpatient basis. A low-residue diet is suggested during the acute phase of the illness to allow relative bowel rest. A broad-spectrum antibiotic is advised; this should be continued for 10 days. If the symptoms continue to improve, elective evaluation is undertaken when the acute process has resolved. If the patient's symptoms fail to improve, inpatient therapy is recommended.

For a person who has more severe abdominal signs and symptoms, has pyrexia, is immunocompromised, or appears systemically ill, hospitalization is indicated. Medical management includes the usual supportive measures. No oral intake is advised unless the patient's symptoms fail to suggest the need for imminent operation; under such circumstances, clear liquids are permitted. It is usually unnecessary to use a nasogastric tube unless intestinal obstruction or vomiting is evident. In the inpatient setting, systemic antibiotics are warranted. These are given intravenously and should include an agent to which anaerobic organisms are sensitive. As the symptoms improve, a progressive diet is insti-tuted, supplemented by a stool softener. With aggressive medical management, the patient's symptoms should improve considerably within 24 to 48 hours. As long as consistent improvement is observed, investigation can be deferred until the acute process has been largely ameliorated. However, if the patient's symp-toms persist unchanged for a period of 2 days, radiologic investigation is neces-sary to try to confirm the diagnosis (see later).

### DIFFERENTIAL DIAGNOSIS

### Carcinoma

The most important differential diagnosis is the possible identification of a cancer as the cause of the patient's symptoms. If a carcinoma is present, surgical intervention will be required within a relatively short period of time, irrespective of the fact that the symptoms may not have completely resolved. Conversely, if satisfied that the patient's findings point to diverticulitis, surgery can be delayed as long as the clinical condition improves. Unfortunately, differentiation between sigmoid diverticulitis and carcinoma is not always readily established.

Investigations to help make the diagnosis are contrast enema, CT, and flexible sigmoidoscopy or colonoscopy. An intact colonic mucosa, the length of the nar-rowed segment (in carcinoma, the stricture is usually short, whereas with diver-ticulitis, the stricture usually tends to be longer), and a mass in the wall of the bowel with mucosa intact all are helpful in differentiating the two diagnoses.

An associated diverticula within or around the segment of narrowing has also been thought to be reasonable circumstantial evidence for the presence of benign disease. However, because carcinoma of the colon and diverticular disease are fre-quently seen concurrently, too much emphasis should not be placed on this finding.

Flexible sigmoidoscopy and colonoscopy are useful in differentiating between diverticulitis and carcinoma. The surgeon can feel assured only if the entire mucosa has been visualized and appears intact. Erythema and edema of the bowel wall may be seen, and, occasionally, pus may be observed to exude from one of the orifices. Real concerns in the acute setting are injury to the bowel from the instrument, or air pressure causing perforation through a thin-walled diverticulum or walled-off abscess. For these reasons, only the most courageous or foolhardy endoscopist would embark on this procedure in an acutely ill patient. Examination under such circumstances is probably contraindicated, but as the individual's symptoms improve, endoscopic evaluation should be consid-ered if the differential diagnosis is still in question.

Computed tomography can be helpful in making the diagnosis. Signs of local-ized wall thickening, increased soft-tissue density in the pericolic fat, and large soft-tissue masses related to the colon are helpful, as well as is the presence of divertic-ula. Perforated carcinoma, however, may exhibit the same changes on CT. If the inflamed segment is long (>10 cm), and no enlarged lymph nodes visualized, the CT scan is more likely to provide the correct diagnosis (i.e., diverticulitis).

## Polyps

Some concern has been expressed about the differential diagnosis between sigmoid diverticulosis and a concomitant polyp. It may be difficult to distinguish between the two with a contrast enema, but once the acute episode has resolved, an endoscopy is the preferred investigation to establish the diagnosis with certainty.

## Other Diseases

Other diseases can demonstrate signs, symptoms, and findings that mimic diverticulitis. These include Crohn's disease, ulcerative colitis, acute appendicitis, ischemic colitis, pelvic inflammatory disease, and conditions affecting the urinary tract (e.g., infection and nephrolithiasis).

## Crohn's Disease

It is sometimes difficult to differentiate Crohn's disease from diverticulitis. Several symptoms, however, can lead the surgeon to suspect the possibility of the former, especially if the patient complains of diarrhea and rectal bleeding. The presence of anal inflammation (e.g., fissure or fistula) is also suggestive of Crohn's disease (see Chapters 11 and 30). Sigmoidoscopic examination reveals a normal rectum in diverticulitis, whereas with Crohn's disease, the rectum may or may not be spared. Extracolonic manifestations (e.g., pyoderma, arthritis) should lead the surgeon to suspect Crohn's disease. At the time of laparotomy, it may still be impossible to distinguish between the two conditions. With diverticulitis, the mucosal surface, although edematous, is usually normal. Special technical difficulties in performing the resection, on opening the resected specimen and failure of decompression to result in resolution of the colonic inflammatory process, and evidence of granularity or ulceration are all indicative of inflammatory bowel disease.

## Ulcerative Colitis

The distinction between acute diverticulitis and a complication of ulcerative colitis should not be difficult. Proctosigmoidoscopic examination virtually always reveals disease in the rectum in patients with ulcerative colitis (see Chapter 29). The suggestion of inflammatory bowel disease would certainly dictate different medical management or an alternative operative approach.

## Ischemic Colitis

Ischemic colitis can pose a problem in differential diagnosis. However, patients who have disease limited to the sigmoid colon usually present with frequent bowel movements and rectal bleeding. Abdominal pain is often not helpful in distinguishing the two diagnoses (see Chapter 28).

# COMPLICATIONS

## Free Perforation

Free perforation with generalized peritonitis is an uncommon complication of diverticulitis. Patients are critically ill and demonstrate the usual signs and symptoms of septicemia. The history can be one of a rather sudden onset of abdominal pain, usually in the lower abdomen, progressing to generalized involvement. Marked abdominal distension may be noted. Abdominal rigidity is usually observed. An upright film of the abdomen or a lateral decubitus x-ray film will reveal the presence of free gas. The amount of gas present on the roentgenogram is thought to help differentiate a colonic from a gastroduodenal perforation: the more gas present, the greater the likelihood of a colonic perforation. CT may also demonstrate a perforation or free gas in the peritoneal cavity.

## Phlegmon or Abscess

The most common complication of sigmoid diverticulitis is a walled-off perforation or abscess; the acute inflammatory reaction usually involves the sigmoid colon and its mesentery. Signs and symptoms are most often confined to the left lower quadrant of the abdomen. Treatment is usually by the medical measures previously mentioned, but the presence of an abscess should be suggested for patients who continue to have pain, fever, white blood cell count elevation, or failure to tolerate oral alimentation.

## *Computed Tomography-Guided Percutaneous Drainage*

Patients who fail to respond despite vigorous medical management, and who are found to have a localized abscess, should be considered for CT-guided percutaneous drainage of the septic process. Success depends on the ability to find a safe, direct route to the abscess cavity. If initial percutaneous drainage cannot be performed successfully, pelvic or intraabdominal abscess usually requires a staged surgical procedure.

## Fistulas

The most common cause of internal fistulas is diverticulitis. Others include malignant tumors from several organs, nonspecific inflammatory bowel disease (in particular, Crohn's disease), and the sequelae of radiation therapy. Rarely, injury to the urinary tract or kidney, nephrolithiasis, chronic suppurative processes, tuberculosis, and tumors of the kidney can lead to an enteric communication.

Although a fistula is relatively infrequently seen, colovesical fistula is the most common internal fistula complicating diverticulitis. Others include colocutaneous, colovaginal, coloenteric, and other unusual manifestations (e.g., coloureteric, colouterine, and colosalpynx).

### Colovesical Fistula

Pneumaturia is the most frequent complaint, followed by urinary frequency, dysuria, fecaluria, and hematuria. Complaints unrelated to the urinary tract included lower abdominal pain and fever.

Studies used to evaluate patients suspected of having colovesical fistula include urinalysis, urine culture, barium enema, cystoscopy, cystography, intravenous pyelography, and endoscopy. The intravenous pyelogram is almost routinely performed as part of the diagnostic evaluation, but it will virtually never identify the presence of a fistula. The major benefit of the study is detection of ureteral involvement, particularly by extrinsic compression (see Chapter 23). Some feel that cystoscopy is most likely to identify the fistula, but this is usually inferred by the visualization of an inflammatory reaction in the bladder mucosa. The test that most frequently actually identifies the communication is the barium enema. No articles support flexible sigmoidoscopy or colonoscopy to help diagnose a fistula. CT is probably the most accurate diagnostic tool for confirming that a communication exists between the urinary and gastrointestinal tracts by revealing a close association between inflamed colon and bladder.

Despite intensive radiologic and endoscopic studies, it may not be possible to identify a fistula with certainty. An operation can still be recommended, although on the basis of clinical suspicion, without the requirement for such confirmation. Surgery can be performed almost as a one-stage resection of the inflamed segment. The bladder is not closed, but a Foley catheter is left in place for approximately 7 days.

### Colovaginal Fistula

Colovaginal fistula virtually never occurs in a woman who still has her uterus. Conversely, the most common cause of a high rectovaginal fistula is injury as a consequence of hysterectomy. Discharge of feces, blood, pus, mucus, or gas is the usual complaint. Barium enema may identify the communication by revealing a fistula or by demonstrating a loop of sigmoid colon in the pelvis. Another method is to place the patient in lithotomy position, and fill the vagina with water. A sigmoidoscope is placed into the rectum, and air is insufflated. Bubbles appearing in the vagina establish the presence of a colo-vaginal fistula. Management is the same as that for colovesical fistula.

### Ureterocolic Fistula

Ureterocolic fistula is extremely rare and is usually caused by urinary calculi. Symptoms include urinary tract infection, fecaluria, and abdominal or flank pain. Barium enema is the most reliable diagnostic rest for demonstrating the fistula.

## Thigh Abscess

Enteric infections, on rare occasions, can spread to the thigh. The most common routes by which the infection could develop in this area are as follows: (a) via the neurovascular bundles that penetrate the muscle and fascia of the abdominal wall; (b) through the inguinal rings; and (c) through the pelvic floor along the rectum.

## Hemorrhage

See Chapter 28.

## SURGICAL TREATMENT OF ACUTE DIVERTICULITIS

When patients fail to respond to medical measures or their condition is deteriorating, urgent surgical intervention is required. Obviously, in someone with generalized peritonitis and a pneumoperitoneum, emergency operation is indicated.

Essentially, seven operations are available for the treatment of sigmoid diverticulitis in the acute situation.

1. Transverse colostomy and drainage of the perforation
2. Exteriorization of the involved segment
3. Resection: sigmoid or descending colon colostomy and mucous fistula
4. Resection: end-colostomy and closure of rectal stump (Hartmann)
5. Resection: primary anastomosis and protecting transverse colostomy
6. Resection: primary anastomosis and intraluminal bypass (no colostomy)
7. Resection and primary anastomosis (no stoma)

### Transverse Colostomy and Drainage

A three-stage operation had been recommended for the treatment of acute diverticulitis for many years. However, it is a suboptimal alternative because it does not deal with the primary process, and the patient must suffer with an unsatisfactory stoma (a transverse colostomy). Consequently, other surgical options are preferred.

### Exteriorization and Resection with Colostomy and Mucous Fistula

Colonic exteriorization has been advocated for cancer since the end of the 19th century. Traditionally, resection was done subsequently and anastomosis was effected, often with some form of spur-crushing clamp. This operation succeeds in removing the nidus of sepsis from the peritoneal cavity, the single most important aim of surgery for complicated sigmoid diverticulitis. Today, however, it is considered neither appropriate nor necessary to delay resection until the peritoneal cavity has "sealed." The bowel is now removed at the time of stomal construction. Currently, other methods are used to treat acute sigmoid diverticulitis, which have a reduced morbidity and mortality, thus relegating this option to one of historical interest only.

### Resection with Sigmoid Colostomy and Closure of Rectal Stump; Hartmann Procedure

It is generally agreed that if the source of infection can be removed at the initial operation, the Hartmann procedure would be the most satisfactory operative approach.

The operation involves resection of the inflamed bowel, and an end-sigmoid colostomy with closure of the rectal stump. The procedure effectively removes the source of sepsis from the peritoneal cavity, creates a most satisfactory stoma, and obviates the risk of anastomosis under septic conditions. It does, however, have one major disadvantage: the second stage of the operation, performed 6 or more weeks later, requires a major abdominal procedure. At that time, the colostomy must be excised and the proximal bowel liberated. This often necessitates mobilizing the splenic flexure, a procedure that poses some risk for splenic injury. The so-called Hartmann pouch can be difficult to identify and may be considerably retracted. Because of the advent of the stapled anastomosis by circular stapler, however, it is no longer necessary to mobilize it to the extent that was previously required for conventional suture anastomosis. Because the operation is of some magnitude, many patients at high risk have been deprived of the opportunity of having intestinal continuity reestablished. Occasionally, therefore, the Hartmann operation results in a permanent stoma.

#### *Anastomosis Following the Hartmann Procedure*

The use of the circular stapling instrument is strongly advised because it permits a technically simple anastomosis. The instrument is introduced into the rectum to the apex of the rectal stump, at which the spike is extended through the wall. The proximal bowel segment is drawn over the anvil, and the previously applied proximal purse-string suture is tied. The parts of the instrument are then reconnected and the stapling gun is fired, creating an end-to-end anastomosis without rectal mobilization.

The laparoscopically assisted approach has been advocated for reestablishing intestinal continuity following the Hartmann procedure. This technique is discussed in Chapter 27. Basically, the results are comparable with those of the open procedure.

#### *Timing of Reversal of Colostomy*

The question of timing of the reanastomosis following Hartmann's resection is a matter of some controversy. The interval between the primary and secondary operation is the most important factor in predicting the safety of the second operation. Authors advise waiting from 15 weeks to 3 months before embarking on the reversal, but most surgeons are willing to accept the somewhat increased morbidity and intervene sooner.

### Results

In analyzing the results of the Hartmann resection for acute or perforated diverticular disease, it is inadequate to talk merely in terms of the first stage. In calculating the overall morbidity and mortality, consider the subsequent procedure or procedures. Unfortunately, much of the literature fails to deal with the entire spectrum of surgery required to effect complete resolution of the disease process, including reestablishment of intestinal continuity.

Some investigators compared their experience with the three-stage procedure and the Hartmann resection in patients with colon perforation secondary to diverticular disease. An overall morbidity of 71% was noted after the three-stage operation, and of 37% after the Hartmann procedure. Wound infection was the major morbidity. The operative mortality in the former was 5%, versus approximately 6% in the latter. Only 4 additional surgical procedures were required in the Hartmann group, whereas 34 additional operations were required in the three-stage group. Others also have reported favorable results with Hartmann's operation for perforated diverticulitis. No question remains that the Hartmann procedure is the preferred option if an anastomosis is deemed unsafe.

### Resection and Anastomosis with or without Transverse Colostomy

#### With Transverse Colostomy

The primary disadvantages of the Hartmann operation are the potential difficulty and risks involved in subsequently reestablishing intestinal continuity. An alternative approach is to effect an anastomosis at the initial operation and protect it with a transverse colostomy or ileostomy. The second-stage procedure therefore is simplified, although it too is not without morbidity. The resection and anastomosis can be performed in accordance with the principles outlined, with the recognition that virtually always a rim of relatively uninvolved rectum will permit a safe anastomosis.

A transverse colostomy should not be done whimsically; considerable morbidity is associated with its creation as well as its closure (see Chapters 23 and 31). Furthermore, it is not a stoma that is convenient to manage. A left transverse colostomy is performed as far to the left as is possible, so that the splenic flexure tethers the efferent limb to reduce the risk of prolapse. This form of stoma, however, does adequately divert the fecal stream if properly constructed. Alternatively, an ileostomy can be fashioned. This is a better stoma, but is further from the anastomosis, and the problem of stool between the ileostomy and the anastomosis is still present. However, once the surgeon has embarked on this approach, the colostomy should remain at least 6 weeks.

Before stoma closure, the anastomosis should be examined by means of the rigid proctosigmoidoscope, flexible instrument, or water-soluble contrast enema to ensure that the anastomosis is intact.

### *Primary Resection and Anastomosis without Colostomy*

The treatment of perforated diverticulitis of the sigmoid colon by primary resection and anastomosis but with no colostomy was advocated by Madden and Tan in 1961.

### *Results*

Evaluation of reported series is difficult. With generalized peritonitis or fecal contamination, a colostomy is mandatory. Others have advised that patients who are receiving steroids should have a protective colostomy created. The need remains for a large, prospective, randomized, controlled clinical trial to assess the place of the various options in the management of acute diverticulitis.

### Intracolonic Bypass

In 1984, Ger and Ravo presented an experimental technique whereby a safe colorectal anastomosis could be performed by implanting a latex (Silastic) sheeting within the lumen of the bowel, even in the presence of massive contamination. The principle of the so-called "intracolonic bypass" involves suturing a specially prepared soft tube within the lumen of the proximal bowel; it conducts the fecal flow into the distal bowel without fecal contact of the anastomotic site.

### *Results*

When used in a clinical setting in individuals who were not ill with complicated diverticulitis, no clinical leaks occurred and only one radiologic leak was seen in the bypass group, whereas five clinical leaks and eight radiologic leaks were seen in those given a conventional anastomosis. The difficulty remains, however, in honestly assessing the results, as it is not always clear whether patients truly qualify as candidates for urgent or emergency operation. The point is moot, however, because the device is no longer available for implantation.

*Comment*: I prefer to manage acute diverticular disease by removing the inflammation at the first operation. Ideally, an anastomosis should be effected at the initial procedure. The Hartmann resection is used if technical factors preclude satisfactory anastomosis or if the patient's condition is tenuous.

A protecting colostomy is usually not used if the bowel is relatively well prepared (a not uncommon situation when the patient has been hospitalized for a number of days before operation). Also, if the perforation is into the mesentery or if the abscess is relatively small and localized to the pelvis, a colostomy is not a requisite. However, with peritonitis, a poorly prepared bowel (fecal loading), obstruction, or fecal contamination, the Hartmann operation should be performed, or a loop, left transverse colostomy should be done concomitantly with resection and primary anastomosis.

Drainage is recommended if an abscess is present. Irrigation with large volumes of Ringer's lactate solution is advised for fecal peritonitis. Broad-spectrum, systemic antibiotic therapy that addresses anaerobes, as well as gram-negative, and gram-positive organisms is suggested.

## ELECTIVE RESECTION

### Natural History of Complicated Diverticular Disease

The decision when to intervene surgically in a patient with uncomplicated sigmoid diverticular disease is a matter of considerable controversy, and is always a cause of debate and conflict between internists and surgeons. The antecedent history of a complication of diverticulitis somewhat simplifies the operative recommendation, but many patients who might benefit from resection do not have such a history. Radiologic evaluation that reveals narrowing, deformity, or even partial obstruction may help decide in favor of a procedure, but one can never be certain that symptoms will resolve following resection unless acute disease is found at laparotomy. If colonoscopy reveals edema, stricture, or pus, resection at some point would seem indicated. Conversely, if colonoscopic evaluation is unremarkable, resection of the sigmoid colon is less likely to resolve the patient's complaints.

### Technique

The technical details of elective resection of diverticulitis are essentially the same as those of carcinoma of the sigmoid colon, with minor variations.

Resection should be performed with the anastomosis placed into the rectum. Attempt at removal of all diverticula is meddlesome and unnecessary. Splenic flexure mobilization may be required if all the inflamed colon is resected, especially in cases of hypertrophy of the muscular layers of the bowel. A review from the Mayo Clinic noted recurrent diverticulitis in 12.5% of the patients in whom the sigmoid colon had been used for the distal anastomosis, but in only 6.7% of those when the rectum had been used.

Elective resection for diverticular disease has been described by a laparoscopic approach. In the experience at the Lahey Clinic, elective laparoscopic resection was found to be as safe as the conventional, open operation and was associated with a shorter hospitalization with more rapid recovery. However, the authors caution that the higher cost of operating room time may make it difficult to justify the procedure economically. The laparoscopically assisted technique is discussed in Chapter 27.

### Recommendations for Elective Resection

Elective resection is advised for patients who have had one or more attacks of left lower quadrant pain associated with fever, leukocytosis, and radiologic evidence of diverticulitis, especially if any of the following apply:

- The patient is younger than 55 years of age (<40 years for men).
- Radiologic evidence of leak is seen.
- The patient has urinary tract symptoms (suggestive of impending fistula).
- Evidence of obstruction is found.

If radiologic and endoscopic changes that cannot exclude cancer are present, resection is mandated.

## MYOTOMY

Reilly recommended sigmoid myotomy in the treatment of long-standing, uncomplicated diverticular disease. The procedure involves division of the antimesenteric taenia and underlying circular muscle from the rectosigmoid junction for "whatever distance is necessary," sometimes as much as 60 cm.

*Comment*: It is difficult to interpret Reilly's experience. In the uncomplicated group, it would appear that the procedure, in actuality, was being performed for irritable bowel complaints. In fact, Reilly observed that the indications for application of the procedure seem to be diminishing.

The application of myotomy for an irritable bowel, the "prediverticular state," and for diverticulosis may prove useful and is worthy of further investigation. Physiologic evaluation (motility and pressure studies) may permit identification of patients who will benefit from this approach. Certainly, we feel this operation has little to offer in the treatment of diverticular disease.

## COLONIC COMPLICATIONS OF ORGAN TRANSPLANTATION AND RENAL FAILURE

Patients who have undergone transplantation are susceptible to the development of a variety of colonic complications, including prolonged ileus, colonic dilatation, intestinal obstruction, ischemic colitis, necrotizing enterocolitis, ulceration, hemorrhage, and perforated diverticulitis.

The percentage of free perforations is much higher in renal transplant patients, whereas mesenteric abscess or walled-off perforation is more common in individuals who have not had transplantation. The use of immunosuppressive agents and steroids is believed to be responsible. Even when a person does not manifest systemic signs and symptoms, surgical intervention should be done early and should always include a resection. Because of diminished host resistance, it is extremely unlikely that a demonstrable perforation or abscess will resolve with conservative therapy. Early intervention has been shown to improve survival.

## GIANT COLONIC DIVERTICULUM

Giant colonic diverticulum is a rare clinical entity. The disease most frequently involves the sigmoid colon, solitary giant diverticula have been found in other areas of the bowel. All described cases originate from the antimesenteric border of the colon, with the lesion usually representing a pseudodiverticulum, or less commonly, a true diverticulum.

Theories include distension of a diverticulum by gas-forming organisms after the neck has been occluded, and a ball-valve mechanism that causes trapping of gas in the abscess cavity when the intraluminal pressure of the bowel increases.

Patients may present with perforation, sepsis, intestinal obstruction (resulting from compression by the mass), and rectal bleeding. Most complain of abdominal pain or the presence of a lump. Differential diagnosis includes congenital duplication of the colon, colonic volvulus, emphysematous cholecystitis, infected pancreatic pseudocyst, pneumatosis cystoides intestinalis, giant duodenal diverticulum, intestinal obstruction, intraabdominal lipoma, and intraabdominal abscess. Treatment is removal of the diverticulum by resection of the sigmoid colon.

## DIVERTICULAR DISEASE OF THE RIGHT COLON

### Pathophysiology and Epidemiology

Diverticula that involve the right colon can be solitary or multiple. They should be distinguished from right-sided diverticula that exist concurrently with extensive diverticulosis throughout the colon. The former type of diverticulum traditionally has been thought to be congenital; most were believed to be true diverticula, although others suggest that the cause is the same as that of left-sided diverticular disease—abnormal thickening of the muscle in the wall of the colon.

Right-sided diverticular disease is more common in Asia than elsewhere. At least in this population, adoption of a Western diet may influence the prevalence of diverticular disease, but the site at which diverticula tend to occur is probably determined more by race or by genetic predisposition.

### Signs and Symptoms

The symptoms and signs of right-sided diverticulitis mimic those of appendicitis. Patients can complain of epigastric pain, nausea, and vomiting, with migration of the pain into the right iliac fossa. Depending on whether the process is localized or diffuse, low-grade fever, moderate tenderness, guarding, and rebound may be noted. The leukocyte count is usually elevated.

### Radiologic Studies

Radiologic findings consistent with right-sided diverticulitis include the presence of a paracolic mass, a calcified fecalith, and a distended loop of small bowel near the mass. However, these findings are also seen with acute appendicitis, so unless the patient has had the appendix removed, this triad of radiologic observations is not particularly helpful.

Computed tomography has been shown to be beneficial in diagnosing acute diverticulitis. Consequently, CT can be of value primarily for patients with atypical findings of acute appendicitis, especially in the older age group, and for those who have had appendectomy. The potential for CT-guided drainage further justifies selective application of this modality. However, the success of resection without concern for a temporary stoma makes CT a less attractive consideration.

## Treatment

Surgical treatment should include excision of the involved diverticulum and closure. However, because the inflammatory mass usually involves a large portion of the cecum or right colon, a resective procedure is usually required. Resection is probably advisable whenever an inflammatory mass is present, because of the difficulty in distinguishing the lesion from a perforating carcinoma.

## DIVERTICULAR DISEASE OF THE TRANSVERSE COLON

Reports of acute diverticulitis of the transverse colon are extremely rare. As with right colon diverticulitis, individuals tend to be younger and, most commonly, thought to have acute appendicitis or cholecystitis. Resection is the preferred treatment.

## SOLITARY CECAL ULCER

Solitary cecal ulcer is a condition of uncertain cause. A number of theories have been postulated to explain its occurrence, including drugs (especially corticosteroids), stasis with stercoral ulceration, diverticulitis, inflammatory bowel disease, foreign body, arteriovenous malformation, infection, ischemia, and a genetic predisposition. In the more recent literature, solitary cecal ulcer seems to be frequently associated with end-stage renal disease.

Patients may present with signs and symptoms suggestive of acute appendicitis. Massive hemorrhage is not an uncommon consequence.

The surgical treatment for perforation requires a resection of the involved segment, especially the diagnosis of malignancy cannot be excluded.

# 27

# Laparoscopic-Assisted Colon and Rectal Surgery

I have asked Dr. Jonathan M. Sackier, Professor of Surgery at The George Washington University School of Medicine and Health Sciences, and Director, Washington Institute of Surgical Endoscopy, to give his perspectives on this new technology. His opinions are especially valued because, at the time of this writing, he is one of the most experienced with laparoscopic bowel surgery. He has authored an important book on the subject of minimally invasive surgery.

The advent of videoendoscopy has facilitated the implementation of laparoscopy in the practice of the general surgeon and has stimulated an avalanche of technological advances to facilitate the undertaking of major operative procedures through minimal incisions. Published reports have included techniques for diagnostic laparoscopy, appendectomy, lysis of adhesions, colotomy and removal of a polyp and lipoma, rectal suspension, cecopexy, creation of a loop colostomy, cecostomy, resection for endometriosis, and colectomy for other benign conditions as well as for cancer. Because of the large numbers of colon operations that are performed in the United States, it seems natural that much of the recent laboratory and clinical efforts have been to develop the techniques for accomplishing bowel resection and even anastomosis, intracorporeally. Whether efforts to perform the procedures laparoscopically prove merely to be the situation of technology in advance of an application or truly represent a singular advance in the management of individuals with colorectal disease remains to be proved.

But a concern is the loss of one's tactile sense; exploration with the hand is not possible. It is probably a requisite that, with the availability of computed tomography and abdominal ultrasonography as well as transcolorectal endosonography (TES), complete preoperative assessment be undertaken before surgery for a malignant process.

At the 90th Annual Convention of the American Society of Colon and Rectal Surgeons (1991), a resolution was adopted by the Fellows of the Society. The following statement was the result of the consensus:

WHEREAS new technology is evolving to remove intra-abdominal organs with less invasive methods, and

WHEREAS the efficacy of this technology is unproven, and

WHEREAS the complications of the use of this technology, including morbidity, mortality, and inadequate treatment, are unknown and may exceed traditional therapies, and

WHEREAS it is important to encourage and foster the development of this technology, therefore be it

RESOLVED that the American Society of Colon and Rectal Surgeons regards laparoscopic colectomy as an unproven technology, and that it is only appropriate to perform laparoscopic intestinal resections in an environment designed to meaningfully evaluate patient safety and efficacy of this technique.

As a consequence of this action, the Society established a registry for laparoscopic colon operations, the appropriate forms for which are available from the Society's office (American Society of Colon and Rectal Surgeons, 800 E. Northwest Highway, Suite 1080, Palatine, IL 60067, USA).

## INTRODUCTION

Georg Kelling, a young German physician whose doctoral thesis was entitled *On Measuring Stomach Capacity,* was the originator of laparoscopy. What he succeeded in accomplishing was to apply the earlier work of Robert Simons of Bonn who, at the inspiration of Von Recklinghausen, had written a dissertation on the effects of pneumoperitoneum (1870). This phenomenon was originally called "abdominal emphysema" by Wegner, but curiously was not seen to cause inflammation. In 1882 von Mosetig-Moorhof instituted the concept of pneumoperitoneum for the treatment of tuberculosis with apparent cure. This work was confirmed by another German physician, Willem Nolen. In 1901, Kelling established that an intraabdominal pressure of approximately 50 mmHg could arrest intraabdominal hemorrhage. Over the ensuing years, he devoted himself to the development of equipment for this area of investigation. Although some of his experiments were successful, a number of the animals used for these procedures died, presumably as a result of the high pressures used.

On the basis of these experimental data, Kelling introduced a Nitze cystoscope to observe the effects that air tamponade produced on the abdominal viscera and presented his work to the 73rd Congress of German Natural Scientists and Physicians in Hamburg in 1902. That same year, Dimitri Ott, a German gynecologist, also succeeded in viewing the abdominal cavity, but he used an incision in the posterior fornix of the vagina. He also succeeded in bringing light into the abdomen through the use of head mirrors.

Credit for the first true human celioscopy is usually given to Jacobaeus (1912), who promoted the procedure for the treatment of ascites. The following year, Bernheim published his experience with *Organoscopy,* and Kelling reported his initial laparoscopic series in 1923. In 1929, another German physician, Heinz Kalk, published an article on the use of the laparothorascope with which he had performed 41 examinations of 36 patients. He credited Jacobaeus for being the major contributor to the development of laparoscopy and felt that the technique held its primary application for that of the evaluation of liver disease. An Irish immigrant to the United States, John Ruddock, was another proponent of peritoneoscopy. In 1934, he also commented on the value of performing laparoscopy in patients with ascites. Additionally, he introduced a number of instruments and developed the concept of retrieving biopsies under laparoscopic control.

Over the past several decades, important technological advances have been made in the management of colon and rectal diseases. In the late 1960s and early 1970s, the development of the flexible endoscope resulted in the ability to manage colonic neoplastic disease noninvasively. Later in the 1970s, the development of stapling devices radically altered the way surgeons reestablished intestinal continuity. And then, in the late 1980s and the beginning of this decade, we have witnessed the development of videoendoscopy, a consequence of which has been the promotion of laparoscopic surgery. Colonoscopy and stapling devices, without question, have reduced operative morbidity, mortality, and cost. This has been accomplished without sacrificing the long-term benefits of surgical treatment.

The first application of laparoscopy to general surgery was to that of appendectomy. This was initially performed by Semm in the early 1980s, although DeKok had performed a laparoscopically assisted procedure in 1977. But, it was the introduction of video-assisted endoscopy that permitted the surgeon to share the intraoperative view with assistants, as well as the development of improved hand instrumentation, which led to the explosion in laparoscopic technology in the late 1980s.

The introduction of laparoscopic cholecystectomy in Europe and in the United States led to numerous other investigators using the technique for virtually every operation. As of this writing, the laparoscope has been the eyes for some surgeons for essentially every known colorectal procedure.

## LAPAROSCOPIC TEAM

### Operating Room

The operating room needs to be large enough to accommodate all of the equipment necessary for performing complex procedures. Ideally, ceiling-suspended television mounts reduce the need for floor space to accommodate the monitors. Ordinary operating rooms have insufficient electrical outlets, so supplementary ones may need to be created. Furthermore, the use of a C-arm may be required, so consideration should be given to the space needed. Because the patient's abdomen is continually being perfused by cooling gases, special attention needs to be paid to keeping the room temperature at an appropriate level.

## Anesthesia

The anesthesiologist must understand potential complications of laparoscopy that are either unique to this procedure or are at an increased risk with this operation. These include gas embolism, cardiac dysrhythmia, carbon dioxide retention, and oxygen desaturation, as well as the potential for pneumothorax and pneumomediastinum. Another concern is the use of nitrous oxide, which can lead to intestinal distension. Additionally, the requirement for changing the patient's position can interfere with venous return and oxygenation, and possibly increase intracranial pressure.

At the completion of the operation, leakage of carbon dioxide into the preperitoneal or retroperitoneal spaces can result in profound subcutaneous emphysema. The decision must be made whether to keep the patient intubated to allow sufficient time for the carbon dioxide to be resorbed. Failure to do this can lead to carbon dioxide retention, which in the recently anesthetized patient can have dire consequences. Finally, care must be taken with patient positioning to avoid nerve compression injury. Special warming devices are usually required, especially if the procedure is anticipated to take a relatively long time. As mentioned, gas flow within the peritoneal cavity can lead to hypothermia, with profound pejorative effects on a patient's metabolic balance.

## Nursing

One nurse should be given the responsibility for all of the laparoscopic equipment. A checklist should be prepared before each operation. This includes such important issues as ensuring sufficient spare gas cylinders, bulbs for light sources, tape rolls for digital image capture units, and so on. Obviously, the nurse must ensure that all equipment is functioning properly. The nurse is also responsible for setting the room up with all the equipment in the appropriate position for each operation. Finally, it is mandatory to have the required equipment available for conversion to an open procedure should the need arise. Usually, this consists of having available a scalpel and laparotomy pads on the Mayo stand, as well as standard open surgical equipment in the room and available.

## TECHNIQUE—GENERAL PRINCIPLES

### Pneumoperitoneum

To obtain the space needed to perform surgery, gas must be introduced into the abdomen. This is usually accomplished by means of a Veress needle, which is introduced through a small puncture wound. The needle is available in either a reusable or disposable form. The Veress needle consists of a sharp outer trocar with a blunt, hollow, spring-loaded inner obturator. When inserting the needle, the obturator is pushed back into the trocar until the peritoneal cavity is entered. The obturator then springs back to prevent trauma to any underlying structures.

To avoid injury, the surgeon lifts up the abdominal wall and uses a second finger to prevent the inadvertent introduction of the needle too far and to avoid pointing the needle in the direction of a major vessel. Having entered the supposed peritoneal cavity, the needle should be aspirated with a syringe. If blood is obtained, the needle should be repositioned. If a gush of blood is found, the surgeon must consider that the aorta, vena cavae, or iliac vessel has been entered. There should be no hesitation in converting to an open laparotomy at this point.

If intestinal contents are noted in the syringe, the planned laparoscopic surgery can be continued, and subsequently the nature of the injury evaluated. This is most commonly a small hole in the bowel, which can be sutured. Having aspirated the needle, the surgeon should then inject saline and aspirate again. If in the peritoneal cavity, fluid cannot be retrieved. Conversely, if in the preperitoneal space, the saline will be aspirated. Under these circumstances, the needle needs to be repositioned. Another useful test is the hanging drop technique. A drop of saline is placed at the open end of the needle while lifting up the abdominal wall; if the peritoneal cavity has been entered the fluid will disappear.

An alternative to the Veress technique for entering the abdomen was described initially by Hasson in 1978. The abdominal cavity is entered through a small incision under direct visualization. This is most commonly done under the umbilicus through the raised up linea alba, entering the abdomen at the thinnest point of the anterior wall. The Hasson cannula has a blunt tip and wings, to which stay sutures may be attached. The Hasson technique should be used routinely if laparoscopic surgery is planned for the individual who has had prior abdominal surgery, who harbors an umbilical hernia, or if a Veress penetration has failed.

Having introduced either a needle or Hasson cannula, gas should then be pumped into the abdomen. A high-flow insufflator attached to a carbon dioxide cylinder is normally used. The use of other gases has been suggested, including nitrous oxide and helium, but carbon dioxide is familiar, inexpensive, and readily available; hence it is preferred.

The gas should be introduced no faster than 1.5 L/min to prevent the potentially fatal complications of diaphragmatic rupture and dysrhythmia. Additionally, the pressure should not exceed 15 mmHg to minimize the risk of impeding venous return, to avoid vagal stimulation by diaphragmatic stretching (leading to postoperative pain), and to limit the likelihood for pneumothorax and pneumomediastinum. Furthermore, be aware that pneumoperitoneum will cause acidosis from carbon dioxide absorption. Finally, the peritoneal surface may appear inflamed because of vascular dilation which, in patients at higher risk, might lead to vascular collapse. Finally, if the needle is inadvertently introduced into a vessel or a solid organ, the potential exists for producing a carbon dioxide gas embolism. This may be recognized by drastic alterations in the patient's hemodynamic state and the production of the characteristic mill wheel cardiac murmur.

Some have suggested that laparoscopic surgery can be performed without a pneumoperitoneum, by creating space through elevation of the abdominal wall. Such gasless laparoscopy has yet to achieve popularity or, indeed, prove to have any benefit when compared with conventional open operations.

## Operative Ports

In common parlance, the words "trocar" and "cannula" have become inter-changeable. The word "trocar" probably emanates from *trochartor trois-quarts*, a three-sided sharp perforator within a metal cannula. The original trocars for laparoscopy consisted of a hollow, three-sided, sharp blade with a metal sheath and a flap or button valve. If adequately maintained and frequently sharpened, they are still an effective means for performing laparoscopy. The best way to ensure that no harm is caused is to judiciously introduce subsequent trocars under direct visualization. If a larger port is required than had previously been created, a dilating obturator can be inserted. Trocar size is dictated by the instruments to be used. Currently, trocars are available in a range of sizes from 2.7 to 33 mm.

Because the pneumoperitoneum is usually created through the umbilicus, the first trocar is usually positioned at this site, and the camera introduced here. Subsequent ports should be placed in accordance with the following principles:

The instruments introduced through them must be able to reach the target organ.

The instrument tip should not point toward the camera because this impedes depth of field perception.

The tips of the instruments should not be working parallel with the line of sight, because this prevents visualization of the working mechanism.

The instruments should not be close together, because this leads to what has been termed "fencing."

The cannulae should not rest directly on the iliac crest or costal margin, because this leads to postoperative pain.

The cannulae should not be inserted directly through visible vessels in the abdominal wall or the known location of the epigastric vessels.

Ideally, instruments should be brought in to 60 to 120 degrees from the line of site (Fig. 27.1). An additional innovation has been proposed: the use of gas-impermeable envelopes to allow hand-assisted laparoscopy.

## Light Sources

Lighting of the abdomen is optimally achieved by means of a 300-watt Xenon cold light source. However, if only a diagnostic laparotomy is intended, a 150-watt halogen source may be sufficient. Furthermore, it may be necessary to have additional light sources available in the room should ancillary equipment be required (e.g., an illuminated ureteral stent). An additional light source may be

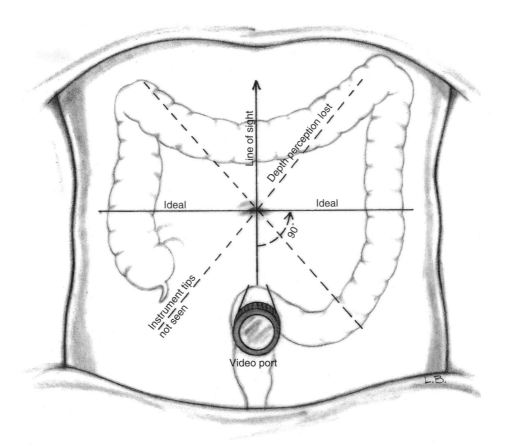

**FIG. 27.1.** Schematic port selection. The line of sight dictates what angles of introduction will best serve the surgeon. If too acute, the tips of the instruments will not be observed; too obtuse and depth of field perception will be impaired.

required if the surgeon intends to perform intraoperative colonoscopy to identify the location of a lesion or if a gastroscope is required to view the duodenum when performing a right colectomy.

### Visualization

A large range of laparoscopes is available, varying in size from 2.7 to 10 mm, in disposable or reusable forms, and with a variety of viewing lenses. A zero-degree optic provides a straight view and is easier to manipulate. However, angled telescopes with either a 30-degree or 45-degree optic have the advantage of permitting the surgeon to view a structure from several perspectives. Flexible tip laparoscopes are also available, but they have failed to gain popularity. A means of preventing fogging of the tip of the telescope is necessary.

The older laparoscopes follow the Palmar-Jacobs design, wherein the beam is split to provide an offset viewing channel and with a lumen for introducing instruments. Modern laparoscopes do not use this construction, and a television camera attaches directly to the eyepiece. The cameras are either one- or three-chip instruments. Although the latter provides better color definition, because conventional 420-line televisions are used, the advantage is lost. With the introduction of high-definition television, the addition of digital enhancement technology may increase the popularity of the three-chip cameras.

## Documentation

It is often useful to obtain a permanent record of the procedure to augment the patient's chart, to provide the surgeon with a mechanism for communicating operative findings to other physicians, and, regrettably, for medicolegal purposes. Capturing images on video is certainly feasible but has a number of practical drawbacks. First, the storage is costly. Second, is the question of who is the legal owner. Third, whom does it benefit: the patient, the surgeon, or the legal community? For teaching purposes, however, video images are ideal. Super VHS and three quarter inch format are excellent and ideal for later editing. Hard-image capture with either digital or analog technology provides high-quality pictures that are well suited to teaching or to publication. Some systems enable images to be incorporated into the operative report much as that which has been used by flexible endoscopists.

## Energy Sources

Most laparoscopic procedures can be safely performed by monopolar or bipolar electrosurgery, a modality with which most surgeons are familiar. The generators for electrocoagulation and cutting are readily available and extremely efficient. Furthermore, many hand instruments now incorporate electrosurgery, some providing additional suction and irrigation, which eliminate the number of instrument changes required. Bipolar electrosurgery has the theoretic advantage of limiting energy spread, but it is certainly slower and more cumbersome.

A newer alternative is the harmonic scalpel device, which limits heat spread and has the capability of coagulating relatively large blood vessels. It has been demonstrably effective for taking down the mesentery in laparoscopic colectomy. With respect to lasers, they are an expensive means to achieve the same end.

## Robotic Control

A major drawback to laparoscopic surgery is the requirement for someone to hold the camera. Most surgeons use another physician, nurse, technician, or medical student for this purpose. The slightest tremor, physiologic or even as a consequence of the magnification produced by working close to a structure, can cause intense nausea for the entire operating team. Furthermore, the inability to follow the movement of every instrument in and out of the abdomen can lead to iatrogenic injury.

The development of the automated endoscopic system for optimal positioning (AESOP) robot has solved much of the problem. The system, which provides effective and predictable camera control, has achieved widespread popularity. A number of interfaces for controlling this device are available, including foot and hand control. More recently, a voice-activation system has been instituted.

## Hand Instruments

Most laparoscopic instruments are clones of the standard open varieties and include most of the familiar patterns. Special purse-string devices have been developed specifically for laparoscopic surgery as well as deployable bowel clamps to obviate the need for using ports with every single instrument. Stapling devices are also available, analogous to the instruments for open surgery. The requirement for occluding vessels has led to the development of a wide range of clip appliers, pretied suture loops, and sewing machines. It is necessary, however, for the serious laparoscopic surgeon to develop the necessary skills to perform intracorporeal suturing and knotting. Specially designed needle holders and sutures are available for this purpose. Laparoscopic instruments, in fact, are being applied to open abdominal operations and to transanal surgery. The added length and excellent construction provide particular advantages in certain situations.

## Intraoperative Ultrasound

Ultrasound has become a familiar part of the practice of many colon and rectal surgeons through its transanal application for the evaluation of rectal cancer. With the development of laparoscopic probes, a whole host of indications have been proposed. It is of obvious importance to evaluate the liver in patients with malignancy, a task that is impossible in the absence of tactile sensation. Intraoperative ultrasound is an extremely important adjunct for assessing liver metastases in this situation. Furthermore, the use of Doppler signals assists in locating vessels within a fatty mesentery and can identify lymph nodes inside the peritoneal cavity.

## LAPAROSCOPIC-ASSISTED COLECTOMY

### Background

Laparoscopic surgery has not attained the level of popularity in the management of colorectal disease as it is has for hepatobiliary surgery. Reasons for this include (a) the need for frequent repositioning; (b) multiple large vessels requiring ligation, which can be time consuming and hazardous; (c) the retrieval of the specimen mandates laparotomy, essentially defeating the whole laparoscopic philosophy; (d) an anastomosis must be fashioned, which can be awkward to accomplish intracorporeally; and (e) the potential benefits of laparoscopic surgery—reduced pain, reduced length of hospitalization, earlier return to normal activity, and a better cosmetic result are insignificant if the primary concern is treating malignancy.

Despite these concerns, the popularity of laparoscopic cholecystectomy and the fanfare of media attention that accompanied its introduction, laparoscopic-assisted colectomy has numerous supporters within the medical profession and is being increasingly applied to a host of colorectal problems. Still, it has been virtually impossible to conduct a meaningful evaluation of the true benefit. A number of benefits have been suggested, including reduced pain, improved cosmetic result, earlier discharge, and earlier return to work in those individuals who have had a laparoscopic procedure. Immune function may be less compromised by laparoscopic surgery. One other possible benefit is the reduction of adhesion formation, an observation that has been described by gynecologists for a number of years. Theoretically, this would certainly limit readmissions for intestinal obstruction. However, data following laparoscopic-assisted colectomy concerning adhesion formation currently are absent.

The issue of cost with laparoscopy is extremely difficult to analyze. In the current healthcare environment within the United States, it is difficult to amortize cost across the broad spectrum of reimbursement plans—fee-for-service, contractual arrangements, and the indigent patient. What does seem likely, however, is that whatever savings are achieved through reduction in hospital stay will be more than eliminated by the increased operative time and the requirement for expensive equipment.

## Patient Preparation

Preparing a patient for laparoscopic colorectal procedures is essentially the same as that for conventional, open surgery. However, in certain areas potential differences occur.

In addressing the patient's history, knowledge of prior surgical procedures will help the surgeon evaluate the likelihood of finding intraabdominal adhesions, which might render a laparoscopic operation difficult or impossible to accomplish with safety. A special note should be made of a history of bleeding tendency or likelihood of liver disease; portal hypertension and varices can cause massive hemorrhage. Be aware of the possibility of respiratory problems, because the use of carbon dioxide pneumoperitoneum can lead to impaired gas exchange. Consider using either a gasless laparoscopic approach or falling back on an open procedure. Knowledge that the patient harbors a hiatal hernia can pose a problem in and of itself. A large hernia filled with carbon dioxide can impair respiration.

Physical examination should note any evidence of inguinal hernias. Some surgeons recommend placing a truss perioperatively to prevent massive distension of a hernia sac, a consequence of gas insufflation.

The usual preoperative studies are done, but the threshold for performing pulmonary function evaluation should be lower, especially in older patients undergoing laparoscopy. The use of ultrasound has been recommended to map intra-abdominal adhesions preoperatively, which helps to determine whether the abdomen is entered using a Veress needle or by the Hasson cannula (see earlier discussion). This use of ultrasound for this indication requires the radiologist to be familiar with the visceral slide technique.

## Consent

As with all operations, appropriate informed consent is considered mandatory. This communication should include a comprehensive discussion of the alternatives and the possibility of conversion to an open procedure. A discussion of the risks should include the possibility of needle or trocar injury, problems with insufflation, the possibility of postoperative subcutaneous emphysema, and the standard complications usually addressed when obtaining consent for the open procedure. Every consent form should carry the phrase "Laparoscopic . . . , possible open." I also believe that, when possible, this conversation should take place in the presence of the next of kin and that a detailed record be kept of this communication.

## Indications

The indications for laparoscopic colectomy are essentially the same as for conventional operations on the bowel. It should be clearly understood, however, that the application of this modality in no way changes traditional surgical judgment nor should it lead to a compromise in technique. This technology should be an alternative to traditional surgical techniques, but should not be viewed as an exclusive one. The patient must not be subjected to a procedure that compromises the effectiveness of what could have been accomplished by conventional means, nor should there be an increased risk. If, during the course of the operation, the surgeon believes that efficacy or safety is being compromised, then it is appropriate, or even requisite, to abandon laparoscopic surgery and return to one of the standard open methods. Conversion to an open procedure should never be viewed as a failure.

## DIAGNOSTIC LAPAROSCOPY

### Elective

#### Cancer

Some have recommended the performance of a diagnostic laparotomy to evaluate the liver and peritoneal surfaces before undertaking a resection for colorectal cancer. However, with the current controversy concerning cutaneous implantation (see later), one must question whether this is an appropriate indication. That aside, an excellent view can certainly be obtained. In fact, occasionally, the staging of the patient's disease may be altered through this investigation. No question, laparoscopic assessment is an extremely effective method for evaluating patients following resection and with CT, or monoclonal scan evidence suggestive of recurrent disease. Biopsies can be taken from areas of the liver that are inaccessible to the percutaneous approach as well as from the serosal surface of the bowel, omentum, and peritoneum. A second-look procedure has been used for many years by gynecologists for follow-up evaluation of individuals who were diagnosed with ovarian cancer.

### Pain

The use of laparoscopy for the evaluation of an individual with abdominal pain has been well documented in the literature, both gynecologic and general surgical. A thorough evaluation of the abdominal contents can be achieved by this method. Ultimately, however, a diagnostic laparoscopy for pain often leads to the performance of an appendectomy or to lysis of adhesions.

### Inflammatory Bowel Disease

In circumstances where the diagnosis is in question, or to evaluate another aspect of the condition (e.g., concomitant liver disease), a laparoscopic approach may be useful.

### Fever

Occasionally, patients will present with fever of unknown origin in whom all other tests fail to locate a source. Laparoscopic evaluation may identify tuberculosis, brucellosis, inflammatory bowel disease, lymphoma, or abscess.

## Emergency

### Pain

It is not uncommon for diagnostic confusion to arise in a patient with abdominal pain, especially in women of reproductive age. Whereas gynecologists have used laparoscopy for this indication for many years, general surgeons have begun to apply it with increased frequency for this indication. If the diagnosis of appendicitis is made, the surgeon can proceed with appendectomy. It should be noted, however, that laparoscopy is not a substitute for clinical examination and appropriate judgment. Other conditions (e.g., diverticulitis) can cause the surgeon either to continue the procedure with laparoscopic guidance or to convert to open surgery, depending on experience and the nature of the disease.

## Obstruction

Use of laparoscopic guidance in the patient with intestinal obstruction must be applied with particular caution for obvious reasons, which is why it has not been widely used to assess the source and location of intestinal obstruction. The distended bowel, as well as concern for creating additional trauma from trocar placement, has dissuaded many otherwise experienced laparoscopic surgeons from adopting this approach. However, it is possible that with judicious application of the technique, the cause of obstruction and the relief of the source may be undertaken laparoscopically.

## Ischemia

Patients with mesenteric ischemia are most often elderly and have concomitant, significant disease. Such individuals tolerate major surgical procedures poorly. A diagnostic laparoscopy, which can even be performed at the bedside in the intensive care unit or emergency room, can clarify any confusion about the diagnosis. If gangrene affecting a large segment of the bowel is identified, no surgical intervention can be considered. If the bowel is viable, the surgeon can elect to maximize oxygen delivery and improve hemodynamic status by means of a cannula left *in situ*. Following completion of an open procedure for ischemia, the surgeon might leave a cannula in place with a purse string tied around the fascia. The tip of the cannula can be buried in a pocket of peritoneum to enable bedside second-look laparoscopy.

## Diverticulitis

Whereas the primary means of staging for diverticulitis is computerized tomography, laparoscopy may permit assessment of the disease and, in certain circumstances, assist in the placement of a drain.

## Trauma

Laparoscopy has been effectively applied for triaging of patients with blunt abdominal trauma. The procedure can be carried out in the emergency room in a similar manner to that of diagnostic peritoneal lavage (DPL). The limitation of DPL is that false-positive determinations are not uncommon. The consequence of an incorrect evaluation is to perform an unnecessary laparotomy, an occurrence in up to 25% of patients. In the absence of multisystem injury, laparoscopy can be performed in the emergency room under local anesthesia. Under these circumstances, one simply attempts to grade the pathologic findings.

If intestinal contents are seen within the abdominal cavity, it is evident that major intestinal damage has occurred. A laparotomy, therefore, is mandatory. If blood is identified, consider the following categories:

Minor: A small amount of blood is seen, which can be irrigated away; it is not seen to recollect. No source is identified. Such patients can have their other injuries attended to and be reevaluated later.

Moderate: Blood is seen along the paracolic gutters or between loops of intestines. It is irrigated away, but reaccumulates. If a bleeding source is seen, the surgeon may decide whether it requires immediate attention or other injuries should be attended to first.

Major: On inserting the Veress needle, frank blood is obtained, or when inserting the laparoscope, the intestines are seen to float on a pool of blood. Such patients require immediate laparotomy.

Obviously, knowledge of the mechanism of injury is important. For example, deceleration accidents are much more likely to be associated with tears to the bowel or mesentery.

Penetrating trauma to the colon from knife wounds, not only to the abdomen but also to the perineum, can be evaluated by laparoscopy. The skin entrance wound should be closed before the laparoscope is inserted. If no breech of the peritoneum can be seen, then assume that no interperitoneal injury has occurred. Conversely, if the peritoneum has been lacerated, search for an injury and ascertain whether the patient requires open surgery or simply further observation. Also, consider the possibility of using laparoscopy to assess the occasional gunshot wound, especially when the bullet seems to take an oblique course or perhaps with smaller caliber weapons. Obviously, a bullet wound of the colon must be treated by open surgery.

## THERAPEUTIC LAPAROSCOPY

### Appendectomy

Laparoscopic appendectomy was first described by Semm, a gynecologist, in 1983. Many of the early reports of this operation involve primarily removing normal appendices in individuals with abdominal pain. Many now believe that laparoscopic appendectomy should be the standard of care for all patients presenting with appendicitis, be they women of reproductive age, children, or adult males.

### *Technique*

The surgeon stands on the patient's left, the television is placed by the patient's right foot, and the operation is performed with the table tilted right side up and head down to permit abdominal contents to fall away from the right iliac fossa. The laparoscope is introduced through a port at the umbilicus, and two additional ports are placed—one in the right upper quadrant and one in the left iliac fossa (Fig. 27.2). I prefer to use only large ports so that the telescope can be moved from position to position. The appendix is grasped, and if not clearly visible, the cecum is mobilized from its retroperitoneal attachments by the use of monopolar electrocautery. The blood supply should be divided by means of electrocautery (monopolar or bipolar), the harmonic scalpel, individual clips and scissors, or a stapling device. Ligatures can be used, but this tends to be rather time-consuming. The junction of the appendix with the cecum is then clearly identified. The appendix is then removed following division at the base after Roeder loops are applied, and individual staples or a linear stapler used. The appendix is then placed in a bag or withdrawn through a metal reducer tube.

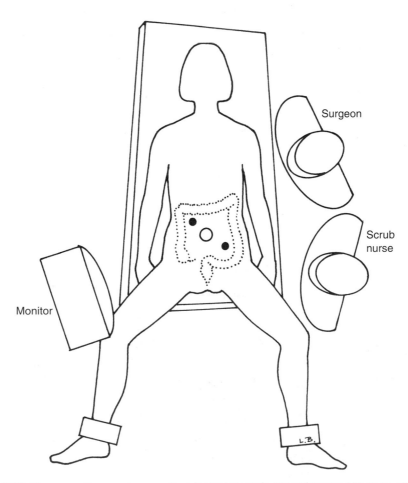

**FIG. 27.2.** Trocar positions and room set-up for laparoscopic appendectomy. Lithotomy stirrups allow access to the vagina for uterine manipulation.

## Colon Resection

### *Indications*

#### *Inflammatory Bowel Disease*

Because surgery for inflammatory bowel disease is often performed in young patients, the concern for a good cosmetic result has been suggested as an important reason for laparoscopically assisted colectomy. Furthermore, individuals with Crohn's disease must often have repeated operations because of complications and recurrence. These patients may benefit from a laparoscopic approach because a reduction in adhesions seems to be associated with this method. Whether tissue handling with laparoscopic instruments is associated with a higher recurrence rate in patients with Crohn's disease or a higher rate of complications has not been determined. However, laparoscopic surgery is an effective and reasonable alternative for such patients.

#### *Volvulus*

It has been mentioned that laparoscopy in the presence of an obstructed, distended colon is challenging and potentially hazardous. However, in a patient who has had successful reduction of a volvulus and who requires resection, use of a laparoscopic approach is reasonable. The resection can be performed close to the bowel wall, thereby minimizing the risk of ureteral injury. Furthermore, no need is seen to identify the major vessels to that segment of the colon, and often very little mobilization is required.

#### *Diverticular Disease*

With respect to elective resection for diverticular disease, the same principle holds as has been mentioned for volvulus. With a benign process, one may stay close to the bowel wall, thus limiting the risk of injury to retroperitoneal structures and major blood vessels. However, the role of laparoscopic surgery in the treatment of acute diverticulitis is less clear.

#### *Cancer*

The appropriateness of performing laparoscopic surgery for malignant disease of the colon is the single greatest question facing surgeons using this technique. Certainly, from the technical perspective, none doubt that laparoscopically guided colectomy is feasible for this indication. The real question is whether the theoretic reduction of days in the hospital, the apparent decreased pain, and the possibility of returning to work earlier are worthwhile objectives. The most important concern is the possibility of increased risk of recurrence.

The American Society of Colon and Rectal Surgeons has issued the following statement:

> The absence of 5-year survival data makes it premature to endorse laparoscopic colon resection for cancer. If laparoscopic colon resection is performed, it is important to follow traditional surgical principles and standards. It is appropriate to continue to perform all laparoscopic resections in an environment where the outcomes can be meaningfully evaluated. The American Society of Colon and Rectal Surgeons encourages the development of randomized, prospective studies to evaluate the safety, efficacy, and benefits of this alternative.

The American Society of Colon and Rectal Surgeons, the Society of American Gastrointestinal Endoscopic Surgeons, and the American College of Surgeons Commission on Cancer have jointly sponsored a registry to identify as early as possible the patterns of practice and acute complications of laparoscopic colectomy. No question, potentially curative oncologic resections can be performed. Early outcomes are comparable to conventional therapy: the ability to obtain appropriate resection margins, harvest large numbers of lymph nodes, and succeed in performing high ligation of blood vessels. Some studies show less consistency with a laparoscopic approach than would be preferred. For example, concern is expressed about the variability in the distal margin that can be obtained at laparoscopic resection. Also, the possibility exists that adequate removal of the mesorectum for low rectal resections may not be as thorough, an important consideration as expressed by some. Others believe that laparoscopic abdominoperineal resection can be performed according to oncologic principles with proximal vascular ligation of the inferior mesenteric artery, wide clearance of pelvic side walls, and complete removal of the mesorectum. Inadequate lateral or radial margins in individuals having laparoscopic abdominoperineal resection have also been reported. The issue of the lack of tactile sensation for exploring the abdomen is also an expressed concern. In fact, a dexterity arm has been developed that allows the surgeon to place his or her hand and arm into the insufflated peritoneum through an incision, securing the arm with a sealed sleeve with a Velcro strap. Although it is certainly true that one of the pitfalls of laparoscopic colectomy is missing significant intraabdominal pathology, the concept of creating a wound sufficiently large for a surgeon to pass an arm into the abdomen is certainly against the concept of minimally invasive surgery.

The concern about the number of reports of port site recurrence following laparoscopic-assisted colectomy has stimulated significant discussion. Some have opined that, except for controlled, clinical studies, laparoscopic colectomy for malignancy should be abandoned. Still, the incidence appears low. Furthermore, when compared with the incidence of wound seeding with the open procedure, the statistics are no more meaningful than with laparoscopic surgery. Only two published series have addressed wound seeding before the laparoscopic era, with an actual incidence of isolated wound recurrence of 0.4%. From the literature, it is certainly clear that, for tumors other than the colon, port site recurrence has been a concern. Laparoscopic cholecystectomy has been associated with port site recurrence when an unsuspected gallbladder cancer has been removed. Although wound recurrence may be excused in advanced cancers, a report of port site recurrence with a Dukes' A lesion is most disturbing. Clearly, the issue of port site recurrence needs to be resolved before surgeons begin performing laparoscopic colectomy for cancer in the absence of prospective clinical trials.

## Polypectomy

Some have proposed that a laparoscopic approach is appropriate for the removal of large polyps. Be concerned, however, that this might represent a compromise of adequate cancer surgery. Certainly, most benign polyps can be removed colonoscopically, and those that are too large merit formal resection. In other words, if an abdominal approach is indicated, the same principles discussed in Chapter 21 concerning resection must be applied.

Minimally invasive surgery has been applied to the repair of colonoscopic perforations of colon. The approach is recommended on two fronts. Rather than observe the patient to see whether he or she develops signs and symptoms of peritonitis, consider laparoscopic exploration to see whether a free perforation actually exists. Additionally, direct suture repair of colonic perforation can be accomplished. The technique permits early direct assessment of the extent of injury and, theoretically, prevents delay in the identification of the source.

## Pull-Through Procedures

Pull-through operations for Hirschsprung's disease have been described in the pediatric population. This approach appears to be gaining popularity among pediatric surgeons.

## Technique

### Stomal Construction

In the usual manner, the telescope is introduced through the umbilicus. A site that has been preselected for the stoma is used for a large trocar opening. A 12-mm opening is ideal for an ileostomy, whereas a 15-mm is recommended for a colostomy. The selected loop is held by graspers that have been introduced through an appropriately positioned trocar site, and a window is made in an avascular portion of the mesentery. A Penrose drain is introduced into the abdomen, passed through the window, and grasped with a secure instrument placed through the cannula at the proposed stoma site (Fig. 27.3). The pneumoperitoneum is released and the bowel brought up through the incision. If one wishes, slow introduction of a pneumoperitoneum will allow the surgeon to secure the mesentery to the peritoneal surface by sutures. The cannulae are then withdrawn and the stoma matured in the usual fashion.

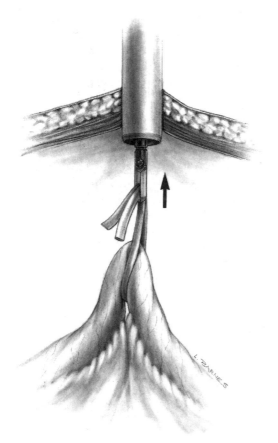

**FIG. 27.3.** The chosen loop of bowel is isolated, and a Penrose drain is placed through an avascular mesenteric window. The drain is grasped via a cannula passed into the abdomen at the selected stoma site.

### Closure Following Hartmann Operation

Reestablishment of intestinal continuity can be achieved following the Hartmann procedure by laparoscopic means. The technique involves mobilization of the stoma with placement of the anvil into the proximal bowel with a pursestring suture by the usual means. The abdomen is then insufflated following closure of the stomal wound. The rectal stump is identified and an intracorporeal anastomosis created. Successful laparoscopic reestablishment of intestinal continuity can be impeded, however, because of dense adhesions from the original inflammatory reaction.

### Rectopexy

Rectal prolapse is a condition that lends itself to a laparoscopic approach. Trocar sites are created at the umbilicus and in the left and right upper quadrants of the abdomen. If necessary, an additional trocar site can be placed in the substernal region if cephalad traction on the rectum is required. The patient is placed in a steep Trendelenburg position. An oblique-viewing laparoscope facilitates visualization for mobilizing the rectum. Then a standard suture rectopexy can be performed, or a mesh may be inserted. If the latter is used, a tacking technique is advised. This facilitates the problems associated with a laborious and time-consuming suture method. Obviously, a suture technique must be used to secure the mesh to the rectum, itself.

## Cecopexy

The application of cecopexy for the treatment of cecal volvulus by conventional, open technique is discussed in Chapter 28. The benefits of this approach are problematic. The fact that the operation can be performed laparoscopically does not increase the likelihood of success. As has been stated, a laparoscopic approach should not be applied to the treatment of the condition if it in any way compromises the likelihood of a successful result. But, if the indications are appropriate, two trocar sites are positioned in the midline, one above and one below the telescope insertion site. Additional traction can be supplied by a cannula positioned in the right upper quadrant. The patient is rolled with the right side up and head down to provide optimal access to the cecum. Sutures are then placed from the taenia of the right colon into the peritoneal surface.

## Laparoscopic Colectomy

Some surgeons prefer to place the patient in the supine position on the operating table for colectomy, but the perineolithotomy position is routinely suggested. This permits an assistant (or surgeon) to be placed between the patient's legs, if necessary, but more importantly, enables synchronous colonoscopy to be performed should it be necessary to corroborate the area of disease. Hemodynamic monitoring is a requisite for all laparoscopic procedures, but with the generally longer period of time required for laparoscopic colectomy, this is an especially important issue. The measurement of arterial blood gases is necessary to limit the likelihood of complications resulting from acidosis, a particular concern in individuals with a marginal cardiopulmonary status.

A number of operating room configurations are advised, but with experience, it is common for each surgeon to adopt an approach not only for the placement of the surgeon, assistant, camera operator, and nurse, but also for the locations of the various ports. Although many surgeons prefer to place the video camera in the umbilicus, others do not believe that this is always optimal, because it fails to permit identification of all areas of the colon (see earlier discussion). Requisite principles require flexibility, innovativeness, and a willingness to move the ports around or to create new ports as necessary.

Once the abdomen is entered and the abdominal cavity is visualized, additional ports can be placed. If a larger port is required than had previously been created, a dilating obturator can be inserted. At the site of the camera placement, 10- to 12-mm ports are used; however, regardless of the planned application of the port site, smaller sizes than these should rarely be considered. The upper portal permits visualization of the lower two thirds of the abdomen, but when it becomes necessary to visualize either the flexures or the transverse colon, the camera can be moved to one of the hypogastric ports. Generally, the operating surgeon uses the suprapubic port plus another port on the side of the abdomen opposite from which the bowel is being mobilized or resected. Conversely, the assistant employs the operative port on the same side that is being dissected, and an additional port is used if the assistant is capable of performing a two-handed technique. In contrast with laparoscopic cholecystectomy, the patient is placed in a steep Trendelenburg position and rotated away from the side of the colon being resected, to allow the small intestine to be moved out of the operative field. The importance of patient position, with lateral rotation to either side, cannot be overestimated, because these maneuvers are essential for providing the optimal possible exposure. The dissection can now be commenced.

### Right Hemicolectomy

Because the small bowel cannot be manually retracted with ease during colon mobilization, patients having right hemicolectomy are optimally positioned in the left lateral decubitus position. I prefer to use the port positions described for cecopexy (Fig. 27.4). Should conversion to open colectomy be necessary, either a midline incision joining the cannula insertion sites or a right transverse incision can be made. During the dissection of the ileocecal region, the patient is placed in the Trendelenburg position and in the reverse Trendelenburg position during the dissection of the hepatic flexure. The right colon is mobilized in the usual manner with the endoscopic electrocoagulation system. The right colic vessels are dissected and coagulated with electrocoagulation forceps, and ligated with an endoclip applicator. The technique for resection and anastomosis is discussed in the following section. Currently, no method is available for withdrawing the specimen without creating an incision. Therefore, it is appropriate to perform the mobilization intracorporeally with internal division of the vessels and then to exteriorize the specimen for resection and anastomosis.

### Left Hemicolectomy and Anterior Resection

Trocar positions are essentially the mirror image of those that were recommended for right hemicolectomy (Fig. 27.5). The patient is rolled with the left side up and the head down. The small bowel is then gently teased toward the right upper quadrant. The colon is mobilized in a similar manner described previously and the vessels divided. The surgeon can then effect an anastomosis by one of several means, but the major differences are with respect to the performance of either an extracorporeal or an intracorporeal anastomosis.

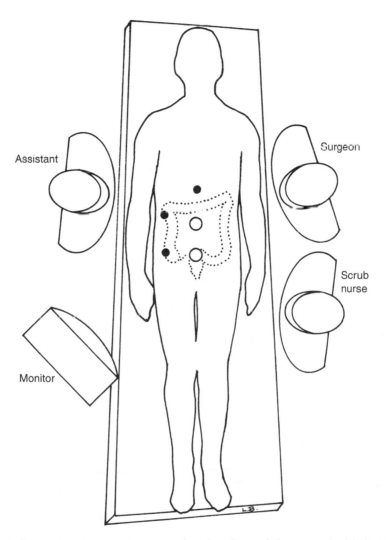

**FIG. 27.4.** The position for trocars, personnel, and equipment in laparoscopic right hemicolectomy.

### *Extracorporeal Anastomosis*

It is usually unnecessary to skeletonize the bowel wall when an extracorporeal anastomosis is contemplated. The bowel is exteriorized in continuity, resected, and anastomosed externally. A major advantage of performing an extracorporeal anastomosis is to ascertain that the diseased segment of bowel has been identified and eliminated. Conversely, if an intracorporeal anastomosis is contemplated, the option of intraoperative colonoscopy is available to make certain that the proper segment of bowel is being removed.

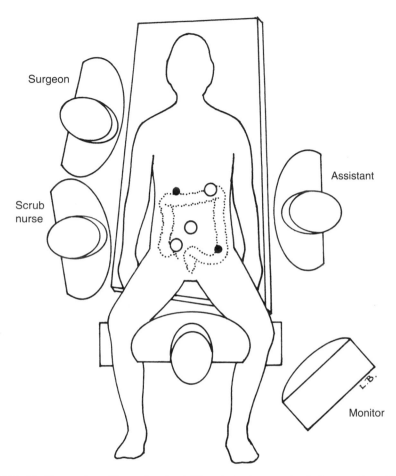

**FIG. 27.5.** Position preferred for performing left hemicolectomy and anterior resection of the rectum.

## Modified Extracorporeal Technique

Once the mobilization has been completed, the bowel is grasped through the nearest operative port. For right colon surgery, this usually means a port in the right lower quadrant. For sigmoid lesions, this can mean the midline suprapubic port, and for left colon operations, the left lower quadrant port. A small incision is made adjacent to the site, and the bowel is visualized. It is then grasped and drawn into the wound. A 5-cm incision is usually adequate to accomplish the task, unless a larger mass is present. A finger can be inserted through the incision and passed through the window in the mesentery. With appropriate traction, the mobilized bowel is drawn into the incision, and the mesentery is identified, clamped, and divided, as required. The anastomosis is completed once the pathology has been confirmed. The bowel is then replaced in the abdomen and the incision closed. A pneumoperitoneum is then reinstituted and the abdomen carefully inspected for hemostasis. The cavity is copiously irrigated, and any clots are removed. The ports are withdrawn under direct visualization and the sites closed.

This method effects a compromise between a total extracorporeal resection and anastomosis and that of a total intracorporeal resection and anastomosis. The bowel is divided internally using a linear stapler or cutter or by applying bowel clamps. The colon is divided and the proximal end brought out through a large trocar insertion site. Then, one can suture the anastomosis by using a biofragmental anastomosis ring, the anvil of the stapling gun, or by returning the proximal end to the abdominal cavity after the resection has been completed. However, this last approach is challenging and time-consuming.

### *Intracorporeal Anastomosis*

Although technically feasible, the completion of a total intracorporeal anastomosis is a highly advanced laparoscopic technical concept. It can be regarded as a less than satisfactory approach for reestablishing intestinal continuity for many patients and, indeed, for most surgeons familiar with laparoscopy. Still, its application is valid, and it is worth discussing the technical approaches to accomplish this. One obvious concern is the risk for fecal contamination when the bowel is divided.

The generally recommended technique is as follows: The proximal resection margin is identified and divided with a linear stapler. I prefer to leave the proximal bowel clamped but unstapled. The distal margin to be resected is then divided. A plastic bag is introduced through the rectum and the specimen retrieved and extracted transanally. Alternatively, the specimen can be removed through a small incision, which is then closed before effecting an anastomosis (Fig. 27.6). A sutured anastomosis can then be performed by whatever technique the surgeon selects, or a stapling technique used.

If a stapling option is elected, the following approach is used: The anvil of the circular stapling device is detached from the stapling gun, and a suture is tied to the prong on the anvil and wrapped around it. It is then reattached to the gun, introduced into the anal canal, and the anvil retrieved within the abdominal cavity. The anvil is then placed inside the proximal colon, and the needle with the suture is brought out through a tenia, close to the edge of the bowel. The proximal colon is then stapled closed, thereby entrapping the anvil inside. A small incision is made at the staple line on the proximal bowel. Traction on the suture allows the center rod to be brought through this opening. The rectum is then closed with a linear stapler. An end-to-end circular stapled anastomosis is then effected in the usual double-stapled fashion. Figure 27.7 illustrates the technique as described for performing a complete intracorporeal anastomosis.

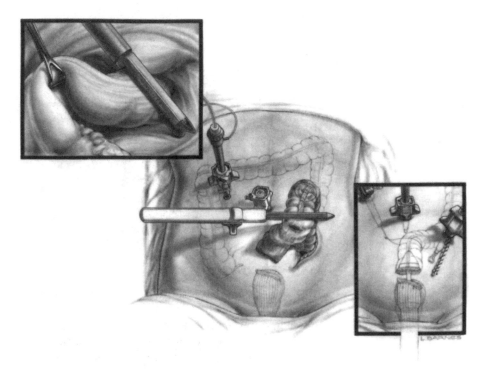

**FIG. 27.6.** Anastomosis is effected by means of a double-stapling technique. The proximal anvil had been placed extracorporeally (not shown).

## Total Colectomy

Laparoscopic total colectomy obviously implies not only the mobilization and resection of the right and left colons, but removal of the transverse colon. This is undoubtedly the most difficult part of the operation, because it involves either separation of the omental attachments or inclusion of the omentum in the resected specimen. This is a much more cumbersome undertaking in that it is necessary to move the television monitors, depending on the surgeon's position and the section of the colon being mobilized. As mentioned, when working on the patient's right, the surgeon stands on the left side, and the television is placed at the patient's right hip. The opposite is true if the left colon is being mobilized. If the ultimate goal is to perform an ileorectal anastomosis, such as in an operation for colonic inertia, the specimen can be extracted through the rectum and a sutured or stapled anastomosis done in accordance with the principles previously discussed. However, if the operation is being performed for inflammatory bowel disease and a reservoir-anal procedure is contemplated, an extracorporeal pouch construction is usually performed.

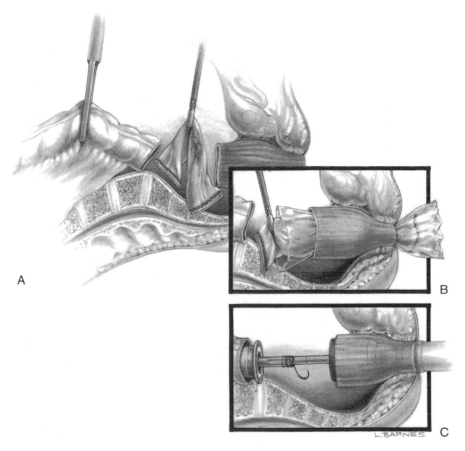

**FIG. 27.7.** Intracorporeal anastomotic technique. **A.** The proximal bowel is occluded, and the specimen stapled at both resection margins. **B.** A plastic bag is introduced through the rectum. It is then opened to receive the specimen, which is then withdrawn. **C.** The circular stapler is inserted into the rectum. A suture is secured to the anvil.

## Abdominoperineal Resection

Removing the specimen presents no problem because one merely needs to excise the rectum through the perineal incision. The laparoscopic approach is used to mobilize and divide the bowel as well as to create the colostomy.

The patient is placed in a steep Trendelenburg position, rotated to the right or left, depending on which side of the rectum is being dissected. Following complete mobilization, the perineal dissection is carried out as has been described in Chapter 23. The rectum is then delivered and the perineal wound closed, with drainage effected either through the perineum or through the abdomen.

*Comment*: The introduction of laparoscopic techniques has been a recent phenomenon. The explosion in the technology and equipment has been remarkable, with proliferation of training opportunities enabling many surgeons to embark on the various laparoscopic approaches to the treatment of colon and rectal disease. Inevitably, improvement in visualization and tissue manipulation will permit an increased number of procedures to be performed in this manner, but it is incumbent on all of us to approach this new technology in a way that does no harm to the patient. Although the issue of patient discomfort and perhaps earlier discharge are worthy objectives, it will only be through carefully controlled trials that the complications and results will enable us to make reasoned, appropriate decisions on behalf of our patients.

# 28

## Vascular Diseases

### Hemorrhage, Mesenteric Occlusive and Nonocclusive Disease, Ischemia, Radiation Enteritis, and Volvulus

#### HEMORRHAGE

Gastrointestinal (GI) bleeding can result from numerous causes. Conditions such as colorectal cancer, inflammatory bowel disease, hemorrhoids, infectious colitides, ischemia, radiation, Meckel's diverticulum, and virtually every disease that affects the mucosa of the intestinal tract can be associated, at some time, with bleeding. Other causes include immunosuppression, coagulopathy, Osler-Weber-Rendu telangiectasia, Dieulafoy's disease, blue rubber nevus syndrome, Behçet's disease, aortoduodenal fistula, rupture of a splenic artery aneurysm, rupture of a pancreatic pseudocyst into the colon, angiosarcoma, and variceal bleeding. Those with the acquired immunodeficiency syndrome (AIDS) can present with GI tract hemorrhage from a number of causes: colitis from cytomegalovirus, herpes simplex virus, or bacteria; lymphoma; idiopathic proctocolitis; and Kaposi's sarcoma. For our purposes, four specific conditions will be discussed in this section: diverticulosis, angiodysplasia, colorectal varices, and Meckel's diverticulum.

#### Diverticulosis

Massive lower GI bleeding has been generally attributed to diverticular disease, usually without evidence of diverticulitis.

The problem is that most lower GI hemorrhage comes from the right side of the colon, wherein are few or no diverticula. Recent evidence suggests that unexplained vigorous lower intestinal bleeding, even in the presence of known diverticulosis, is likely caused by an arteriovenous malformation (vascular ectasia, angiodysplasia). With the availability of angiography and scintigraphy, and the ability to identify preoperatively the site of bleeding, arteriovenous malformations have not uncommonly been observed in areas where diverticulosis is present.

### Angiodysplasia or Vascular Ectasia

The contemporary attitude is that most lower GI bleeding originates from a vascular malformation, which is most commonly seen in the right colon, although malformations can occur throughout the colon and rectum. This condition appears to be caused by degenerative lesions from an acquired and progressive dilatation of previously normal blood vessels. Muscular contraction or increased intraluminal pressure produces obstruction of the perforating veins. These submucosal structures then become dilated and tortuous, with an associated arteriovenous communication.

Pathologically, angiodysplastic lesions appear to be ectasias, or dilatations of vascular structures. They represent collections of thin-walled, dilated vessels (either capillaries or veins) usually lying in the submucosa. Rarely, the condition can be associated with vascular malformations elsewhere in the GI tract (e.g., Osler-Weber-Rendu disease).

### *Relationship to Calcific Aortic Stenosis*

A mechanism for the association and the ameliorative response to cardiac surgery is not clear. It may be a consumption phenomenon or a qualitative alteration of platelet function produced by the roughened stenotic valve in the area of greatest pressure and velocity of the bloodstream. This subtle coagulation defect, combined with a thin-walled vascular lesion, may tend to promote the hemorrhage. Another contributing factor may be the abnormal arterial inflow pulse wave. Be aware of this relationship so that an earlier diagnosis may spare these patients from multiple hospitalizations and transfusions. Certainly, correction of aortic stenosis, not only corrects the cardiac hemodynamic instability, but also stops the GI hemorrhage.

### Meckel's Diverticulum

Meckel's diverticulum is generally acknowledged to be the most prevalent congenital anomaly of the GI tract.

The rule of "2's": 2% of the population, about 2 inches long, and approximately 2 feet proximal to the ileocecal valve is a helpful reminder. The diverticulum contains all layers of the bowel wall but, in some cases, it can harbor heterotopic gastric, pancreatic, biliary, or even colonic tissues. The two most frequently observed complications are intestinal obstruction, caused by intussusception, and hemorrhage, usually because of peptic ulceration. Hemorrhage occurs most frequently in children between the ages of 10 and 15, but it is not unusual to observe this presentation in adults.

### Diagnostic Studies

The preferred test for evaluating bleeding when Meckel's diverticulum is suspected is 99m technetium $^{99m}$Tc-scintigraphy. This study has an accuracy rate of approximately 83%. Selective mesenteric angiography can also be helpful in making the correct diagnosis.

### Treatment

Treatment is by resection of the diverticulum, possibly with a portion of small bowel, especially if the base of the diverticulum is broad. Because of the risk of complications, when found incidentally, resection is not recommended.

## Colorectal Varices

Colorectal varices—a rare cause of lower intestinal hemorrhage—is almost always associated with cirrhosis with resultant portal hypertension, or as a consequence of portal venous obstruction. Even more rare are colonic varices of the so-called familial or idiopathic variety.

The condition can present at any age, including the first decade of life. To conclude that the problem truly represents idiopathic colonic varices, liver disease and portal venous obstruction must be excluded.

Generally, if the bleeding is in a patient whose colonic varices are secondary to liver disease, treatment parallels that of the management of bleeding esophageal varices from portal hypertension. Conversely, in those individuals whose colonic varices are attributed to a congenital cause, favorable prognosis has been associated with colonic resection.

## Symptoms of Hemorrhage

Patients usually present with no antecedent history, and they frequently have no abdominal pain. Blood from the rectum can be bright red or maroon and can contain clots. If the bleeding is severe enough, hypotension can ensue, with the requirement for resuscitative measures. Usually, however, the individual's condition is relatively stable, permitting time for evaluation.

## Evaluation of Hemorrhage

An organized approach to the evaluation of the patient with massive hemorrhage of presumed colonic origin is suggested. An algorithm is presented in Figure 28.1 that provides an overview for carrying out the proper sequence of investigations in the hemorrhaging patient.

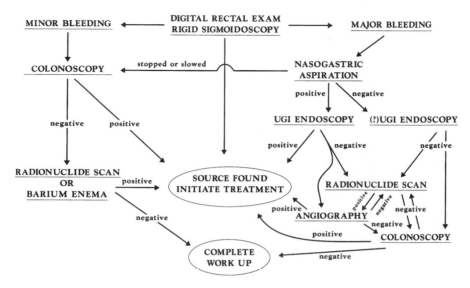

**FIG. 28.1.** Recommended algorithm for the management of gastrointestinal bleeding.

Physical examination of the massively bleeding patient is usually unrewarding. Perform a digital rectal examination and a limited rigid sigmoidoscopy initially. If the source is found, appropriate therapy can be implemented. To exclude an upper GI source, placement of a nasogastric tube is helpful.

### Colonoscopy

If the source is not identified by initial investigation, then proceed to more invasive procedures as will be discussed.

The American Society for Gastrointestinal Endoscopy published a series of statements discussing the use of endoscopy in clinical situations, using these guidelines to aid the physician in the appropriate use of this modality in various clinical situations.* It was concluded that emergency colonoscopy has the advantages of disclosing a bleeding lesion in 50% to 70% of patients examined and that definitive treatment of an identified lesion by snare cautery, fulguration, or laser photocoagulation may be possible. Furthermore, massively bleeding lesions that have stopped may be more readily identifiable by colonoscopy than by other means (e.g., angiography). Disadvantages of colonoscopy under these circumstances include the following:

The need for available and skilled endoscopists
An increased risk of perforation
Delay to adequately prepare the bowel (1 to 3 hours)

---

*American Society for Gastrointestinal Endoscopy, 13 Elm St., Manchester, MA 01944.

The possibility of unsuccessful diagnosis or treatment because of technical problems or massive bleeding

## Therapeutic Colonoscopy

For the treatment of angiodysplastic lesions, sclerotherapy, electrocoagulation, and, more recently, endoscopic GI laser therapy have been used successfully (see Chapter 4). The recommended technique is to treat the periphery initially and the center last, to reduce the vascular supply to the lesion and to diminish the potential for later bleeding.

## *Angiography*

If the source of bleeding has been identified by rectal examination, sigmoidoscopy, upper GI endoscopy, or colonoscopy (if attempted at all), therapy can be instituted. Unfortunately, in patients who bleed massively from the colon, these studies are usually not helpful except to eliminate another cause. The next investigative procedure that should be performed is either selective angiography or radionuclide scan. Unless angiography is not available at the hospital, the patient should not be taken to the operating room without this radiologic investigation. Direct selective catheterization of the mesenteric vessels, should be initiated with the superior mesenteric artery, because of the higher incidence of colonic bleeding from the right side. The standard sensitivity that most publications suggest identifying blood loss by means of angiography is 0.5 mL/min. However, bowel gas, the presence of fluid within the lumen, body habitus, and other variables can make it difficult to identify extravasation, unless the rate of bleeding is as much as 5 mL/min (300 mL/h).

Injection of the major blood vessel in the resected specimen with silicon rubber compound and clearing with methyl salicylate may reveal a vascular tuft or dilated blood vessels. The potential value of the technique is to permit the pathologist to identify the lesion macroscopically.

## Therapeutic Angiography

If the bleeding point is identified, it may be possible to control the hemorrhage by either an embolization technique or by the infusion of vasopressin (Pitressin). Vasopressin causes contraction of smooth muscle, especially the capillaries, small arterioles and venules, with less effect on the smooth musculature of the larger veins. Vasopressin use has several disadvantages. Side effects of the drug include decreased cardiac output, hypertension, and arrhythmias. Also concern is seen related to prolonged catheter use: embolism, hemorrhage around the puncture site, hematoma, and limitation of activity.

Diagnostic angiography can be followed by selective embolization with Gelfoam strips or by autologous clotted blood through the same catheter.

Embolization can also lead in some patients to postembolic colonic ischemia and, possibly, even to infarction. Not every patient is suitable nor is every lesion amenable to such therapy. However, for those deemed appropriate and who achieve a satisfactory response, operative intervention can be avoided or at least delayed so that it can be undertaken at an elective time.

### *Nuclear Medicine Techniques*

#### *Technetium Sulfur Colloid Scintigraphy*

Localizing the site of acute GI hemorrhage has been attempted using technetium ($^{99m}$Tc) sulfur colloid scintigraphy. The imaging agent used for conventional liver scans is injected into the venous circulation and, with the abdomen of the patient under the gamma camera, a radionuclide angiogram is obtained. The principle of the study is that the labeled colloid is rapidly cleared from the bloodstream by the reticuloendothelial system, but an active site of bleeding appears as a "hot spot," because the extravasated isotope is no longer recirculating and cannot be cleared by the system.

The problem is that the isotope is cleared so rapidly that bleeding must be very active at the time of the scan for results to be positive.

#### *Tagged Red Blood Cells*

Another alternative is the use of $^{99m}$Tc- tagged red blood cells. This technique permits identification of a bleeding point caused by hemorrhage of a lesser magnitude. In contrast to technetium sulfur colloid scintigraphy, the labeled red cells are not cleared rapidly and are available to produce a positive scan through repeated periods of imaging, even if the extravasation occurs over a number of days. This technique can be successful in detecting the presence of continuing hemorrhage with transfusion requirements as little as 500 mL within 24 hours. The scan is most accurate within the first 2 hours following administration.

### Estrogen-Progesterone Therapy

In recent years, a number of papers have appeared indicating that estrogen-progesterone therapy may be effective in controlling severe, recurrent bleeding from GI vascular malformations. The mechanism of action of hormonal therapy to control bleeding with this condition is not clearly understood. Theories include an effect on coagulation, induction of stasis in the mesenteric microcirculation, and improvement in the integrity of the vascular endothelial lining. Side effects include thromboembolic disease, an increased risk for the development of malignancies, nausea, vomiting, loss of libido, and gynecomastia. Still, hormonal therapy should be considered in situations when prolonged, obscure GI bleeding thought to be caused by angiodysplasia cannot adequately be managed by other means.

## Surgical Treatment

If the bleeding point is identified by angiography, endoscopy, or nuclear medicine techniques, appropriate therapy can be instituted: medical management or resection, depending on the nature of the lesion and the patient's clinical course. If, however, the patient continues to bleed, and the source has not been identified, most surgeons today believe that subtotal colectomy is the preferred procedure.

### *Operative Colonoscopy and Enteroscopy*

Another option for operatively identifying the source of bleeding involves a combination of laparotomy and colonoscopy, using a two-team approach. Intraoperative cleansing of the bowel can be effected through a small cecostomy. The abdominal surgeon can assist the colonoscopist in the passage of the instrument to make one final attempt to identify a discrete bleeding point. If one is seen, it can possibly be dealt with through the instrument, or it can be effectively treated by a less-than-total abdominal colectomy.

Intraoperative enteroscopy can be done with the colonoscope passed per orum, guiding the instrument through the duodenum and into the small bowel. Segmental visualization can be accomplished by occluding the bowel at intervals to avoid overdistension. In recent years, Sonde enteroscopes have been developed to assist in the performance of small bowel endoscopy. Although containing no therapeutic channel, this instrument can help identify obscure causes of bleeding.

### *Operative Arteriography*

Intraoperative localization of vascular ectasias can be accomplished by placing the bowel to be examined on a sterile cassette cover and injecting the segmental arterial branch with methylglucamine diatrizoate (Renografin 76), or by using highly selective angiographic catheter placement combined with intraoperative methylene blue dye injection. Ideally, the surgeon might be able to resect a limited amount of small intestine.

*Comment*: With the diagnostic studies available, the surgeon should rarely have to resort to blind resection. It is axiomatic that if a lesion is clearly demonstrated on angiography, a limited resection is appropriate. However, without complete certainty about the source of the bleeding, the few minutes necessary to remove the remainder of the bowel should add very little risk. Furthermore, in the absence of blood in the small bowel, the maneuvers associated with operative colonoscopy and operative angiography truly prolong the surgical time with its attendant risks, and have the potential hazards of contamination with the former technique and toxicity with the latter.

## MESENTERIC OCCLUSIVE AND NONOCCLUSIVE DISEASE

The gut receives 20% of resting and 35% of postprandial cardiac output, of which 70% supplies the mucosa. If the blood pressure falls below 70 mmHg, intestinal perfusion can be compromised. Below 40 mmHg, this mechanism fails and the bowel becomes progressively more ischemic, with anaerobic metabolism replacing aerobic. The nature and rapidity of the ischemic process are affected by the collateral circulation and by disorders of splanchnic autoregulation.

Major occlusive disease is usually caused by mesenteric vascular obstruction by atheroma, thrombus, or embolus. Other causes include dissecting aneurysm, arteritis, sepsis, intestinal obstruction, and trauma. Hypercoagulable conditions and the use of oral contraceptives can also precipitate intestinal vascular thromboses, often involving the venous circulation. Low flow states, including long-standing congestive heart failure, the prolonged use of diuretics, cardiac arrhythmias, recent myocardial infarction, hypovolemia, hypotension, burns, pancreatitis, and GI hemorrhage, also predispose to ischemia. These causes are found in most patients who develop ischemic changes of the small and large bowel, as a consequence of nonocclusive vascular disease.

### Signs and Symptoms

The most frequent symptoms of mesenteric occlusion are abdominal pain and rectal bleeding. Usually, a disparity is seen between the severity of the pain and the paucity of significant abdominal findings early in the disease course. However, with intestinal infarction, signs and symptoms of peritonitis rapidly ensue. Other complaints include back pain, nausea, vomiting, and diarrhea.

In patients with so-called "abdominal angina," abdominal pain is also evident, usually developing 15 to 20 minutes following the ingestion of food. Pain is characteristically epigastric or periumbilical; weight loss and malnutrition may ensue.

### Laboratory and Radiologic Studies

Laboratory investigations usually reveal an elevated white blood cell count, elevated hematocrit, and a metabolic acidosis. Determination of arterial blood gases confirms the base deficit and should serve to alert the physician to the severity of the illness.

Angiography and computed tomography (CT) are the preferred investigations to determine the presence of mesenteric ischemia. Plain films of the abdomen may demonstrate thickened bowel loops, a ground-glass appearance from ascites, the classic "thumb-printing," and gas in the bowel wall, portal vein, or peritoneal cavity. However, in one fourth of patients with mesenteric infarction a normal plain film of the abdomen is seen.

### Evaluation and Treatment Protocol

A comprehensive, algorithmic approach to the diagnosis and therapy of mesenteric occlusive and nonocclusive disease has been proposed. The protocol advocates initial treatment directed at correcting the predisposing or precipitating causes of the ischemia. Based on the angiographic findings and the presence or absence of peritoneal signs, the patient is then treated according to the protocol established (Fig. 28.2).

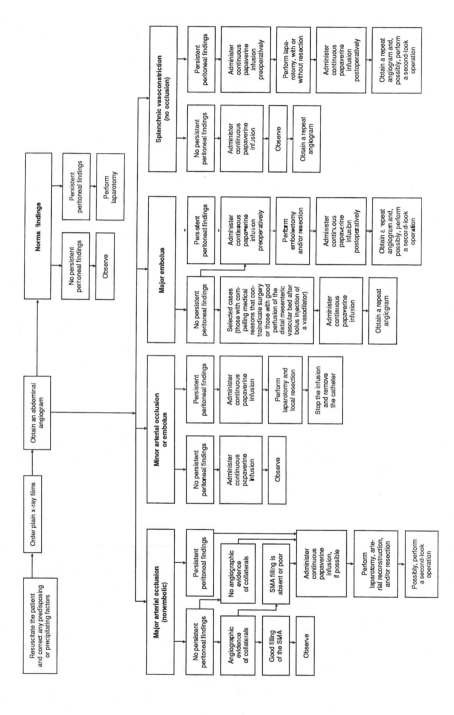

**FIG. 28.2.** Managing acute mesenteric ischemia based on the angiographic findings. (From Boley E, Boley SJ. Acute mesenteric ischemia: treat aggressively for best results. *Journal Critical Illness* 1986;1:54, with permission.)

How much intestine should be removed is always a source of concern. Visual appreciation of bowel damage based on capillary bleeding, color, and contractility is often misleading and commonly induces the surgeon to remove more bowel than is truly necessary. Doppler ultrasound has been compared with fluorescein in determining bowel viability in a prospective, controlled study of patients with intestinal ischemia. The fluorescein method has been shown to be superior.

### *Venous Mesenteric Ischemia*

Venous thrombosis is a rare cause of mesenteric infarction, but the diagnosis is notoriously difficult to make. Causes can be primary, such as those conditions that increase viscosity of the blood or its tendency to coagulate; or secondary, including portal hypertension, intraabdominal sepsis, pancreatitis, intraabdominal neoplasms, inflammatory bowel disease, abdominal trauma, and various types of gastroenterides. The condition is usually confined to a limited segment of the bowel, and, therefore, carries with it a better prognosis than that of arterial occlusive or nonocclusive disease. Contrast-enhanced CT may be helpful in making the diagnosis by revealing hypodensity in the trunk of the superior mesenteric vein, thickening of the intestinal wall and valvulae conniventes localized in a jejunoileal segment, as well as peritoneal fluid. Optimal treatment in those patients with reversible damage is anticoagulation. Intravenous heparin should be administered before the operation.

### Results

The best results are obtained in patients who are diagnosed within 24 hours of the onset of pain. If the patient undergoes laparotomy and resection, some investigators emphasize the importance of establishing double stomas whenever the viability of the remaining bowel is questionable. Despite aggressive surgical intervention, the mortality rate is high.

### ISCHEMIC COLITIS

Ischemic colitis is a term used to describe a syndrome caused by occlusive or nonocclusive vascular disease as it affects the large bowel. It is a condition that usually is found in the aging population, with an increased incidence in women, although the disease has been associated with hemorrhagic shock even in young patients. A number of conditions can produce ischemia. These include arteriosclerosis, emboli, myocardial infarction, vasculitis, colorectal neoplasms, portal hypertension, strangulated hernia, volvulus, periarteritis nodosa, systemic lupus erythematosus, rheumatoid arthritis, polycythemia vera, scleroderma, hemodialysis, anaphylactoid shock, and many others.

The blood supply comes mainly through the superior and inferior mesenteric arteries to the colon (see Chapter 1). The reduction of blood flow to the colon appears to have its clearest manifestation in two watershed areas: Sudeck's point and Griffiths' point (see Chapter 1). However, a number of factors, such as large and small vessel arterial disease, perfusion pressure, plasma viscosity, as well as the adequacy of collateral circulation, may combine to produce even total colonic ischemia.

### Classification, Symptoms, Findings, and Diagnosis

Ischemic colitis has been classified on the basis of its three general manifestations: gangrenous, strictured, and transient or reversible.

If gangrene of the colon develops, the patient may complain of severe abdominal pain, nausea, and vomiting. Bowel movements can be absent, or bloody diarrhea noted. Physical examination will reveal evidence of peritonitis if the bowel is involved by transmural disease, and certainly if a perforation has occurred. Plain abdominal x-ray study may demonstrate free gas under the diaphragm.

The development of an ischemic stricture probably is a consequence of an initial extensive inflammatory process, but not to the point of bowel perforation. Patients may have minimal symptoms, or nausea, vomiting, and abdominal distension may develop. Barium enema may reveal a lesion difficult to distinguish from carcinoma. If the patient has a symptomatic stricture and the diagnosis cannot be established with certainty, resection is indicated.

In patients who have reversible or transient ischemic disease, rectal bleeding may be the only complaint. Abdominal pain and tenderness on the left side are usually minimal or may not even be evident. With the exception of rectal sparing, it is essentially impossible to distinguish the changes observed on colonoscopy from that of nonspecific inflammatory bowel disease. However, endoscopic changes of pallor of the mucosa and hemorrhagic areas may help suggest the condition to be ischemic colitis.

A plain film of the abdomen may reveal characteristic "thumb-printing," usually in the region of the splenic flexure. In more advanced cases may be noted the presence of gas in the wall of the colon. Barium enema examination characteristically shows thumbprinting, edema of the bowel wall, and narrowing, primarily in the areas of the splenic flexure, the distal transverse colon, and the descending colon. However, in a patient who is suspected of having a bowel infarction, barium enema is contraindicated. An arteriogram can reveal helpful information even if only a flush study of the aorta is done. Occlusion of one of the major vessels or branches should lead the surgeon to suspect the cause of the patient's symptoms.

Pathologic changes of the colon can reveal disease limited to the mucosa and submucosa as the rich blood supply makes this area more sensitive to ischemic changes. The muscularis propria is relatively resistant to the effects of decreased perfusion, but transmural involvement can occur.

## Management and Results

Medical management includes intravenous fluid replacement, nasogastric suction, broad-spectrum antibiotic therapy, and the usual supportive measures. In most cases of colonic ischemia, signs and symptoms subside within a day or two, with resolution of the submucosal or intramural hemorrhage. Surgical intervention is indicated for signs and symptoms of peritonitis and for obstruction.

At operation, it is often difficult to determine the extent of colonic ischemia. Consequently, subtotal or total colectomy is the preferred approach if an anastomosis is contemplated, but resection with a diversionary stoma is probably safer.

Operative intervention required for ischemic colitis is associated with a very high mortality rate, probably because many of these patients are elderly and have multisystem diseases.

## Ischemic Colitis and Surgery of the Abdominal Aorta

Ischemic colitis can develop following resection of an abdominal aortic aneurysm. The incidence of this complication has been variously reported to be from less than 1% to more than 25%. The higher rates are usually associated with other factors (e.g., prolonged hypotension that often accompanies the management of ruptured aneurysm). The combination of intraabdominal sepsis with a prosthetic vascular graft is potentially catastrophic, with a mortality rate of up 75%.

### Diagnosis and Prevention

Recommendations for preventing ischemic colitis at the time of surgery have included reimplantation of the inferior mesenteric artery, if it is large, measurement of the stump pressure; Doppler ultrasound; indirect measurement of pH in the wall of the sigmoid colon; and preservation of the first branch of the vessel.

Rectal bleeding within the first 72 hours following aneurysmectomy is a characteristic symptom that mandates investigation. Colonoscopy is a particularly useful technique for establishing the diagnosis of ischemic colitis in the postoperative period.

### Treatment

When colonic ischemia occurs as a consequence of surgery on the abdominal aorta, a high index of suspicion is required, and treatment must be initiated promptly and aggressively. When the condition is recognized intraoperatively, the problem can be handled in one of two ways: One option is to remove the inferior mesenteric artery from its origin, along with a cuff of aorta, and to reimplant it into the aortic prosthesis. Also consider the possibility of vascular reconstruction by means of endarterectomy and angioplasty. The other obvious alternative is to resect the diseased segment of bowel when the lack of viability becomes apparent. Obviously, it is essential to ensure the colon is viable at the end of the operation.

### Ischemic Colitis: Collagen Vascular Diseases

The collagen vascular diseases represent a collection of conditions believed to be caused by pathologic alterations in the immune system. They can occur in any organ and may be associated with GI complaints. The conditions can affect the blood supply to the colon and produce ischemic changes, either isolated to this organ or as part of the systemic process: polyarteritis nodosa, cryoglobulinemia, Henoch-Schönlein purpura, Behçet's syndrome, systemic lupus erythematosus, polymyositis, and scleroderma. Colonic ischemia in the setting of collagen vascular diseases is usually caused by vasculitis or, less commonly, thrombosis. Deposition of immune complexes in blood vessel walls is the most widely accepted pathogenic mechanism. This can lead to hemorrhage, infarction with perforation, or problems with functional colonic disorders, such as inertia.

Medical management is usually the primary therapy; occasionally, however, a patient will require surgical intervention for hemorrhage, obstruction, necrosis, or perforation.

If surgery does become necessary for acute abdominal complications of polyarteritis nodosa, the prognosis is poor.

### Ischemic Proctitis

As discussed, generally the rectum is spared from ischemia because of the collateral blood supply. The implication of the manifestation in so distal a location is inadequate collateral circulation. Diagnosis is usually made by the characteristic appearance on proctosigmoidoscopy. When ischemia of the rectum occurs, the symptoms and pathologic changes are identical to that described for the colon.

## RADIATION ENTERITIS

Radiation injuries to the GI tract are among the most difficult management problems facing the surgeon. It is not uncommon for the patient to suffer the deleterious effects of ionizing radiation long after the primary disease process for which the radiation was used had been cured.

Radiation damage is cumulative and progressive. A finite amount of radiation is tolerable, beyond which additional radiotherapy at any time following the initial treatment can precipitate complications. Certain conditions (e.g., diabetes mellitus, hypertension, and previous abdominal surgery) are believed to predispose the bowel to radiation injury. Other factors that increase the risk include infection, poor design of radiation treatment approaches, inadequate vaginal packing during implants, the presence of intraabdominal adhesions (by fixing loops of bowel), concomitant chemotherapy, and overlooking signals of distress or masking them by overmedication.

Virtually all who have radiation to the abdomen will develop early symptoms of radiation injury to the bowel, and 5% to 20% will have long-term sequelae of radiation enteritis, particularly if receiving more than 50 Gy. Certain groups such as children, and people with light complexions are more sensitive to radiotherapy.

Although the small bowel is more sensitive to irradiation, the most common site of injury is the rectum, because of its fixity in the pelvis. Radiation injury may be a consequence of treatment for carcinoma of the endometrium, carcinoma of the bladder, carcinoma of the rectum or rectosigmoid, prostatic cancer, ovarian cancer, carcinoma of the anal canal, and carcinoma of the cervix.

The use of multidirectional, sharply collimated, high-energy photon and electron beams allows concentration of the radiation to the tumor rather than to normal structures. These advances, it is hoped, will reduce the incidence of radiotherapy enteritis in the future.

## Symptoms and Pathophysiology

The symptoms of radiation injury depend on whether dealing with the acute process, usually occurring during the course of the treatment, or with the result of therapy, weeks, months, or even years later. Three phases of radiation effects have been identified: (a) acute, primarily affecting the mucosa; (b) subacute, with predominant effects in the submucosa; and (c) chronic, generally affecting all layers of the bowel wall. Acute radiation enteritis is caused by destruction of the rapidly dividing cells at the base of the crypts of the GI mucosa. Destruction of cells that rapidly turn over and obliteration of blood vessels, combined with a fibroblastic response, are the events that produce the less acute and chronic manifestations. Progressive fibrosis and vascular lesions leading to ischemia, together with impaired regeneration of the irradiated mucosal epithelium, causes the pathology found.

Nausea, vomiting, diarrhea, and cramping abdominal pain are seen in 75% of patients who have radiotherapy. Radiation to the small intestine can result in malabsorption, partial intestinal obstruction, and severe diarrhea leading to malnutrition and fluid and electrolyte imbalance. Other complications include signs and symptoms of urinary fistula, vaginal fistula, and anorectal ulceration.

## Investigative Studies

For disease involving the rectum or rectosigmoid, proctoscopic examination may reveal loss of vessel pattern, edema, contact bleeding, telangiectasis, ulceration, and granularity. Later changes can include thickening of the rectal wall, stricture, or fistula into the vagina or into the bladder. Endoscopic evidence of injury includes pallor of the mucosa, prominent submucosal telangiectatic vessels, friability, erythema, and granularity.

Radiologic studies performed during the course of therapy are usually not helpful in identifying specific radiation changes. Months or years after the treatment, however, profound radiologic changes may be apparent on contrast study of the intestinal tract. Commonly involved areas include the sigmoid colon, rectum, and terminal ileum. Angiographic studies may reveal arterial and venous irregularity, beading and focal obstruction of the bowel wall vasculature, and crowding of vessels because of foreshortening of the intestine.

## Treatment

Before surgery, it is important to evaluate the entire intestinal tract for the presence of associated radiation-induced abnormalities and for the possibility of recurrent primary disease. The choice of procedure will depend on the level of the injury, the patient's prognosis, and the extent of radiation damage as determined at the time of exploration. Essentially five options are available for the surgical management of radiation enteritis: primary closure (of a fistula), resection, bypass, exclusion, and diversionary stoma (ileostomy or colostomy). It is generally agreed, however, that operations for radiation enteritis should be avoided, except when complications develop.

## Results

Characteristically, a tendency is to underestimate the amount of damage produced by the radiation when examining the serosal surface of the intestine. To anticipate a favorable result of the operation, all radiation-injured tissue must be adequately excised and an anastomosis effected in relatively normal bowel. A number of papers attest to the high morbidity associated with surgical intervention, with anastomotic leak rates of up to 65%, therefore, indicating the need for liberal implementation of a diversionary stoma. For those not considered candidates for surgical intervention because of extensive disease and poor nutritional state, home total parenteral nutrition (TPN) has been advocated by some, with mixed results.

## RADIATION PROCTITIS

As stated, because of its fixed position, the rectum is particularly vulnerable to the effects of radiation. Ulcerative proctitis secondary to radiation-induced injury can produce symptoms of rectal bleeding, abdominal pain, diarrhea, passage of mucus, rectal pain, incontinence, and tenesmus. Stricture, obstruction, and fistula formation into the bladder, urethra, or vagina are potential consequences of chronic radiation injury. It is an extremely troublesome condition to treat.

## Treatment

Management is usually directed to dietary measures, the addition of "slowing" medications for diarrhea, bulk agents, stool softeners, iron replacement (if anemia is a concern), and antispasmodics.

Topical approaches to the control of symptoms associated with radiation proctitis have been offered, including sulfasalazine, tranexamic acid, sucralfate enemas, and hydrocortisone enemas, but the efficacy of these approaches has not been well documented. Topical formalin has been used successfully for a number of years to control intractable hemorrhagic cystitis. In recent years, this agent has also been used to control rectal bleeding.

## Surgical Treatment

Those who fail to respond to noninvasive treatment can be offered the possibility of argon or Nd-YAG laser therapy to control symptoms of bleeding caused by radiation proctitis. This can be performed via the fiberoptic sigmoidoscope.

*Comment*: Intestinal complications of radiation therapy present difficult management problems. I attempt resection for patients who are symptomatic when the disease involves primarily the small intestine. Conversely, with rectal radiation injury, the functional outcome after resection may not warrant such aggressive intervention. Proximal diversion provides good palliation of symptoms without the risk associated with more radical surgery.

## VOLVULUS

### Sigmoid Volvulus

Sigmoid volvulus is a relatively rare condition that has been recognized since antiquity. Ballantyne stated that the authors of the Ebers papyrus from ancient Egypt wrote that either the volvulus spontaneously reduced or the sigmoid colon rotted. Detorsion was recognized even then as the requirement for ameliorating the condition. Whether this can be accomplished by medical or by surgical means has been the subject of a considerable body of literature. In the United States, sigmoid volvulus is an uncommon cause of intestinal obstruction, whereas in other areas of the world, such as Pakistan, Brazil, India, Poland, and Russia, it is the single most common cause.

### *Pathogenesis*

The pathogenesis of sigmoid volvulus is obscure. Most patients are elderly and have a high incidence of associated medical or psychiatric problems. In this group, chronic constipation is thought to be an important factor. However, the greater incidence of volvulus is found in eastern Europe, India, and Africa, which is thought to be related to a high-residue diet.

The anatomic conditions that predispose to sigmoid volvulus—a long, mobile sigmoid loop with close approximation of the afferent and efferent limbs, creating a short base of mesentery around which axis the volvulus occurs—is found in both Eastern and Western groups of patients. A genetic predisposition has been identified within families and within certain tribes.

### Signs and Symptoms

Patients with sigmoid volvulus usually present with the characteristic signs and symptoms of colonic obstruction. These include absence of bowel movements, failure to pass flatus, crampy abdominal pain, nausea, and vomiting.

Physical examination may reveal a distended abdomen; minimal to mild tenderness may be noted. Peritoneal irritation is usually absent, unless viability of the bowel is compromised. Rectal examination usually demonstrates an empty ampulla.

### Investigative Studies

The plain abdominal x-ray usually reveals a markedly dilated sigmoid colon and proximal bowel, with relatively minimal gas noted in the rectum.

Barium enema examination may demonstrate complete retrograde obstruction to the flow of barium at the level of the torsion or may reveal an area of narrowing with proximal dilatation, if the obstruction is incomplete or recently reduced.

### Treatment

#### Nonoperative

Initial management depends on whether the bowel is believed viable or nonviable. In the former circumstance, attempt at reduction should be made by means of proctosigmoidoscopy and insertion of a rectal tube. If the volvulus can be reduced, an explosive discharge of gas and feces will be immediately recognized. The rectal tube should be left in place for about 48 hours to avoid the possibility of immediate recurrence.

Colonoscopy has also been successfully used in the treatment of sigmoid volvulus. The technique has the advantage of permitting evaluation of the viability of a greater area of colonic mucosa, but the procedure must be performed with limited manipulation to minimize the risk of perforation of the distended and edematous bowel. An attempt at colonoscopic reduction should be considered if proctosigmoidoscopic manipulation has been unsuccessful.

Although nonsurgical reduction of the volvulus avoids an emergency operation, the recurrence rate is very high. Therefore, if the patient can possibly withstand an elective operation, optimally, it should be performed during the same hospitalization after the bowel has been adequately prepared. If the patient is not medically fit for surgery, then attempt colonoscopically to fix the colon to the anterior abdominal wall via several percutaneously placed tubes. This is akin to placing a percutaneous endoscopic gastrostomy in the stomach.

### Surgical Treatment

If the volvulus cannot be successfully reduced, laparotomy is indicated. The choice of procedure depends on whether the viability of the bowel is compromised. Possible surgical alternatives include resection and anastomosis (total or partial colectomy [with or without a proximal colostomy]), Hartmann resection, exteriorization resection, detorsion, and detorsion with colopexy.

Obviously, if the colon is demonstrated to be nonviable, a resection is indicated. This is done for the same reason and in the same manner that a resection would be done of a perforated colon for any other condition (diverticulitis, carcinoma). Whether to perform an anastomosis, a Hartmann procedure, or one of the other surgical options available is a judgment left to the surgeon. The pros and cons of the different operative approaches are discussed in Chapter 26.

### Results

Those with viable bowel have an overall operative mortality rate of approximately 12%, as compared with an operative mortality of up to 53% in those with nonviable bowel. Certainly, for those with viable bowel, the mortality rate is higher if resection is performed, but there is no recurrence. Detorsion alone, however, is associated with a significant recurrence risk.

*Comment*: I prefer to perform resection with or without a primary anastomosis, depending on the patient's condition and whether the operation is done on an elective or an emergency basis. Detorsion alone is not adequate long-term therapy.

### Sigmoid Volvulus in Children

Sigmoid volvulus has been infrequently reported in children. Volvulus in children is difficult to diagnose, the course tends to be rather fulminant, passage of a rectal tube or endoscope may be difficult or impossible, and early operative intervention is more often advised than in adults.

### Ileosigmoid Knotting

Ileosigmoid knotting is unusual in Western countries but is relatively common in Africa, Asia, and the Middle East. The condition is initiated by a loop of ileum wrapping around the base of a redundant sigmoid colon. The manifestation can be a variant of midgut volvulus. Approximately three fourths of the patients develop gangrene of the bowel requiring laparotomy and resection.

## Cecal Volvulus

Cecal volvulus is less common than volvulus of the sigmoid colon, representing approximately 25% to 30% of patients with this condition. Abnormal mobility of the cecum and ascending colon, which allows this condition to occur, has been estimated to occur in 10% to 20% of the population. The resultant vascular compromise leads to gangrene and to perforation.

Precipitating causes include distal obstruction, meteorism occurring from unpressurized air travel, pregnancy, prior abdominal operations (adhesions), congenital bands, violent coughing, intermittent positive-pressure breathing, mesenteric adenitis, prolonged constipation, a distal obstructing lesion, and colonic atony (adynamic ileus).

### Signs and Symptoms

Abdominal pain is usually the predominant complaint; it can be relatively low grade and colicky in nature. Frequently present is abdominal distension, which can be asymmetric, with a mass in the hypogastrium or on the right side. Bowel sounds are usually obstructive in nature. Some patients have more chronic manifestations, with intermittent, cramping abdominal pain and distension that usually resolves spontaneously.

### Radiologic Studies

Radiologic investigation usually reveals characteristic findings. The cecum and ascending colon can be found in any part of the abdomen, but the most common displacement is into the epigastrium and to the left upper quadrant. Classic x-ray findings include a "coffee-bean" shape and visible mucosal folds at the site of obstruction; usually, no gas can be seen distal to the point of obstruction. Barium enema may reveal the classic bird's beak deformity caused by obstruction in the region of the cecum.

### Treatment

Colonoscopy has been successfully employed to reduce volvulus of the cecum. Choices of surgical procedures for cecal volvulus without perforation or gangrene include detorsion (with or without appendectomy), cecopexy, cecostomy (or a combination of the two), and resection. Laparoscopic cecopexy by placement of anchoring sutures has also been reported. Obviously, if the viability of the bowel is compromised or if perforation is present, resection is required.

### *Results*

Detorsion alone or with appendectomy is generally felt to be associated with a high recurrence rate and is not advocated in any of the contemporary articles on the subject. Interpretation of the results of the other surgical alternatives is somewhat difficult, because most papers address mortality and recurrence, but not morbidity.

*Comment*: A safe and effective method for the management of the condition when the bowel is viable is cecostomy with cecopexy. However, resection of the right colon is a relatively safe procedure and the one I recommend. Laparoscopic cecopexy may be less invasive, but still suffers from its association with an increased risk of recurrence.

### Volvulus of the Transverse Colon

The transverse colon is the area of the colon in which volvulus least frequently occurs, representing less than 10% of all cases of volvulus. Usually, supporting tissues (e.g., gastrocolic omentum, lienocolic and phrenicocolic ligaments) are congenitally absent or may have been surgically removed. As with cecal volvulus, the condition can be associated with distal obstructing lesions, chronic constipation, prior abdominal surgery, or pregnancy. The condition is usually not diagnosed preoperatively. The radiologic findings are not truly characteristic, except for the demonstration of obvious colonic dilatation.

Simple colopexy is followed by a high incidence of recurrence. Therefore, the transverse colon should be resected by an extended right hemicolectomy or a partial left colectomy, depending on the presentation.

### Volvulus and Pregnancy

One of the predisposing factors for the development of volvuli of all types is pregnancy. Intestinal obstruction during pregnancy is extremely rare. However, in this group of patients, 25% of obstructions are caused by volvulus, almost the same incidence as that produced by adhesions. Because of the risk both to the mother and to the fetus, urgent surgical intervention is demanded.

# 29

## Ulcerative Colitis

The expression *nonspecific inflammatory bowel disease* (IBD) is used to describe two conditions of unknown cause: ulcerative colitis and Crohn's disease. The symptoms are frequently alike, radiologic investigation can pose confusion in differentiation, and even pathologic evaluation may reveal overlapping features, with an indeterminate colitis reported in 15% of patients. It has also been suggested that both conditions can coexist in the same individual. Because of the often diverse approaches to management and the fact that a vulnerable age group is often affected (young persons in their late teens and early twenties), these diseases are among the most challenging confronting the physician today.

### HISTORICAL PERSPECTIVE

Samuel Wilks is generally credited with coining the term *ulcerative colitis* in a letter to the editor of the *Medical Times and Gazette* published in 1859, in which he described the postmortem appearance of the intestine. Subsequently, the Surgeon General of the Union army after the Civil War referred to the disease "ulcerative colitis" and included photomicrographs of the condition. Other detailed descriptions followed, and by the early 20th century more than 300 case reports of ulcerative colitis had been collected for presentation to the Royal Society of Medicine.

### EPIDEMIOLOGY (INCIDENCE, PREVALENCE) AND ETIOLOGY

As suggested, the nonspecific IBD, especially Crohn's disease, have become pervasive worldwide. Unfortunately, our understanding of their pathogenesis still remains obscure.

Evaluation of the epidemiology of the two conditions is made difficult by the plethora of diarrheal states found throughout the world that may be infectious or parasitic in nature and that present with symptoms not unlike those of nonspecific IBD. Furthermore, because of international failure to classify the two diseases as distinct from the numerous specific inflammatory bowel problems, our ability to obtain meaningful data is compromised. Most of the information, therefore, has been accumulated from Western countries, where the diseases are relatively prevalent; in the United States, however, IBD is not even a reportable condition.

Available evidence suggests considerable variation in the incidence rates—common in developed countries and unusual in Asia, Africa, and South America. Because a true surveillance of prevalence requires an exhaustive clinical, endoscopic, and radiologic evaluation of all members of a sample population, the true prevalence is based on inference rather than analysis of well-established data. A seasonal variation even seems to appear, not only of onset, but also of relapse. A statistically significant increase has been observed in the months of August to January.

The incidence of ulcerative colitis and Crohn's disease in England, the United States, and Scandinavia is reported to be from 4 to 6 cases per 100,000 white adults per year, with prevalence rates of between 40 and 100 cases per 100,000. An increased incidence of Crohn's disease has been seen during the past 20 years. The condition is more common in whites, among Jewish people, and among those of Western origin (especially northern Europe and the northern part of eastern Europe). As with carcinoma of the colon, the prevalence of IBD in many industrialized countries, and the development of the conditions among those from low-risk populations who emigrate to higher-risk areas, suggest an environmental cause.

Investigative efforts to identify the causative agent responsible for the non-specific IBDs have thus far been unsuccessful. IBD that appears nonspecific in nature has been found in hamsters, horses, swine, and the canine population, but an experimental animal model for induction or transmission of the disease still eludes investigators. The two primary areas of investigation that continue to be pursued actively are immunology and infection.

## Genetics

A number of studies have shown the existence of family aggregations with the disease, implying that genetic factors also must play a role. There is a high degree of concordance in monozygotic twins. Although ulcerative colitis and Crohn's disease are not classic genetic disorders, a genetically mediated mechanism is suggested because of the following factors: (a) IBD in family members born in widely separated areas or living apart for long periods; (b) increased incidence among Jews; and (c) the tendency toward familial aggregation of cases with ankylosing spondylitis in Crohn's disease. Ashkenazi Jews with IBD, have a lifetime risk for the development of IBD in relatives to be 8.9% for offspring, 8.8% for siblings, and 3.5% for parents. Although the possibility of a common environment may contribute to the increased risk of IBD, the shared genetic pool is much more likely to be the primary factor. A familial occurrence has been noted in 17.5% of patients with IBD. The ethnic, familial, twin, disease association, and genetic marker studies of IBD are best explained by the concept that the conditions represent multifactorial diseases. Environmental and genetic factors probably contribute to disease susceptibility.

## Autoimmunity

The idea of circulating antiepithelial antibodies combining with antigens on the intestinal cell surface and damaging the cells seems a reasonable theory to explain the cause of IBD. However, despite the demonstration of anticolon antibodies in both blood and tissue of patients with IBD, current evidence seems to militate against the likelihood that these play a primary pathogenetic role in the two conditions.

Immune complex mediation of IBD has been felt by some to be a responsible factor, but studies have failed to corroborate a significantly increased frequency or concentration of these complexes, regardless of disease activity. Other immunologic mechanisms that have been investigated include abnormality and variability of circulating lymphocytes, lymphocyte cytotoxicity, defective cell-mediated immunity, immediate hypersensitivity, leukocyte chemotactic impairment, and immunoregulatory cellular imbalance. At the level of the immune response, a genetic influence is suggested by the association of ulcerative colitis with HLA-DR2 and by the occurrence of various autoantibodies in the unaffected relatives of patients with ulcerative colitis. Furthermore, studies of monozygotic twins have indicated that the altered mucosal production of IgG1 and IgG2 in ulcerative colitis can be genetically determined. A useful concept of the pathogenesis for IBD may involve an interaction between host responses, immunologic genetic influences, and external agents, but no definitive proof has yet been forthcoming.

## Infection

With respect to infectious agents, ulcerative colitis in particular has been attributed to bacterial causes for more than 60 years. Crohn's disease specifically was often confused with tuberculosis. This observation led Crohn and coworkers to suggest that a mycobacterial agent might cause the disease. Subsequent studies failed to demonstrate conclusively an association with an infective agent and, in fact, the incidence of IBD correlates inversely with that of the infectious dysenteries. However, the concept of a microbial infection as the offending agent has been resurrected with the recognition of new bacterial causes of enteritis and colitis (especially *Campylobacter jejuni* and *Clostridium difficile*). Other bacteriologic agents (*Shigella, Salmonella, Streptococcus faecalis, Pseudomonas* variant, *Chlamydia, Mycobacterium*, and many others) have been proposed, but their role has not been confirmed.

Considerable interest has been expressed in a possible viral cause of ulcerative colitis and Crohn's disease. Transmission of granulomatous lesions has been successfully carried out in experimental animals. Tissue culture and electron microscopic investigation have also suggested that a viral agent is present in tissue from patients with IBD. However, considerable controversy continues concerning the specificity of these findings.

## Diet

Dietary factors, especially cow's milk, have been implicated as possible causative agents for the development of IBD. Early studies seemed to demonstrate an elevated milk-protein antibody level in patients with ulcerative colitis in comparison with a control population. Subsequent studies in which milk was excluded from the diet failed to demonstrate an improvement in the clinical response, and later studies with milk and milk products failed to demonstrate any correlation. Other factors that have been under investigation include chemical food additives, mercury ingestion, inadequate fiber, excess intake of refined sugar, and even the increased consumption of corn flakes. No clear consensus suggests that dietary factors play a role in the cause of either ulcerative colitis or Crohn's disease.

## Oxidative Metabolism

Recent evidence suggests that abnormal oxidative metabolism may be of significance in the activity of IBD. Increased attention has been placed on the role of free radicals in both normal metabolism and defense against disease. A free radical is defined as any species capable of independent existence that contains one or more unpaired electrons. It appears that reactive oxygen metabolites are produced in excess in active IBD. The effects of specific antiinflammatory antioxidants (e.g., aminosalicylates) are compatible with the proposition that free radicals play a major role in the pathogenesis of IBD.

## Stool

Studies of the role of the fecal stream in causing an exacerbation of symptoms in Crohn's colitis have yielded confusing results. No definite conclusions can be made at this time regarding the role of the fecal stream in the development of these diseases, and controversy continues.

## Smoking

Two distinct patterns of cigarette smoking are seen in patients with IBD; those with ulcerative colitis are much less likely to smoke than those with Crohn's disease. Additionally, cigarette smoking has been found to have a negative correlation with ulcerative colitis. In some cases, complete remission of symptoms was obtained through the use of nicotine-laced chewing gum. In other cases, exacerbation of the disease was noted when patients ceased smoking. Conversely, Crohn's disease is more common in smokers than in those who have never smoked. The increased risk seems to be more apparent in women and may also be associated with a greater likelihood of recurrence.

## Oral Contraceptives

Both ulcerative colitis and Crohn's disease have been found to be more common among women using oral contraceptives than in those who do not. A possible vascular (ischemic) basis for this observation has been suggested. No information is currently available on the effect of stopping the contraceptive pill on the activity of IBD.

## Psychological Factors

The psychological aspects and the possible psychosomatic factors contributing to the onset and exacerbation of IBD, and of ulcerative colitis in particular, have been a subject of considerable debate since 1930. Although many articles have been published to support the description of the susceptible personality, opponents of the psychosomatic theory point out that the concept is based on either anecdotal or uncontrolled studies. A number of publications have compared patients with ulcerative colitis with normal subjects and those with other illnesses and have found no evidence of an increased frequency of psychiatric illness. Furthermore, those with ulcerative colitis who had a psychiatric illness did not appear to have more serious gastrointestinal involvement, nor did severity of the ulcerative colitis predict a more frequent or more severe psychiatric disorder. Furthermore, psychotherapy has not been effective in altering the disease course.

## Age, Sex, and Race

Ulcerative colitis and Crohn's disease occur at any age, but are most commonly seen in persons under 30 years of age. The incidence is highest among teenagers, but a small secondary peak in the incidence of the two conditions occurs late in the sixth decade. In most series, both sexes are equally affected. Thirteen percent with ulcerative colitis and 5% with Crohn's disease were less than 11 years of age. Approximately one third of the patients are between the ages of 11 and 15. The male-to-female ratio is almost 1:1. A tendency appears for Crohn's disease to develop later than ulcerative colitis.

Crohn's disease in black patients may be more common than is generally appreciated, the disease generally appears to be associated with more severe complications than is observed in whites.

## DIFFERENTIAL DIAGNOSIS: ULCERATIVE COLITIS VERSUS CROHN'S DISEASE

Ulcerative colitis and Crohn's disease can usually be distinguished on the basis of the clinical course, symptomatology, manifestations, and endoscopic findings. Ulcerative colitis is a disease characterized by exacerbations and remissions. In contrast, the individual with Crohn's disease has less clear-cut periods of flare-up and remission; the disease often tends to run a more smoldering course. Frequently, the patient is really not well and yet is not sufficiently ill to warrant hospitalization. Table 29.1 summarizes a number of the characteristic features that can help to differentiate between the two conditions.

Rectal bleeding is virtually a *sine qua non* for the diagnosis of ulcerative colitis, but is much less frequently seen in Crohn's colitis. In fact, 25% of patients with Crohn's disease never manifest bleeding. However, in rare instances, massive lower gastrointestinal bleeding may be associated with Crohn's disease.

Ulcerative colitis is confined to the colon and rectum; Crohn's disease can occur anywhere in the digestive tract—from the mouth to the anus. Anorectal disease, in particular (fissures, abscesses, and fistulas), is more commonly noted in patients with Crohn's disease than in those with ulcerative colitis (see Chapters 9, 10, and 11). The diagnosis is often suggested on examination of the perianal skin.

**TABLE 29.1.** *Features of nonspecific inflammatory bowel disease*

|  | Ulcerative colitis | Crohn's disease |
|---|---|---|
| Course | Exacerbations and remissions | Smoldering |
| Bleeding | Virtually always | Uncommon |
| Abdominal pain | Uncommon | Common |
| Perianal disease | Rare | Up to 40% |
| Fistulas | Never | Occasional |
| Abdominal mass | Never | Occasional |
| Carcinoma | Increased association | Increased, but less than in ulcerative colitis |
| Extraintestinal manifestations | Not unusual | Not unusual |
| **Radiologic and endoscopic** | | |
| **Distribution** | In continuity with rectum | Skip areas often observed |
| | Uniform distribution | Often eccentric |
| | Rectal involvement always | Often rectal sparing |
| Small bowel | Spared (backwash only) | Often involved |
| Stricture | Rare, virtually always malignant | Frequent, virtually always benign |
| Mucosa | Contact bleeding; superficial ulcers; pseudopolyps | Longitudinal ulcers; fissuring; cobblestone appearance |
| **Microscopic** | | |
| Extent | Mucosa and submucosa | Transmural |
| Granulomas | Never | Common |
| Dysplasia | Yes | Yes |
| Lymph nodes | Reactive | With granulomas |
| Crypt abscesses | Present | Present |
| Mucus production | Decreased | Increased |

Proctosigmoidoscopic examination can be of value in differentiating between the two conditions. The rectum is always diseased during attacks of ulcerative colitis. Characteristic changes include contact bleeding, granularity, and ulceration. In Crohn's colitis, 40% of the patients have sparing of the rectum, irrespective of anal or perianal involvement. However, when the rectum is involved by Crohn's disease, differentiation between the two can be difficult.

Extracolonic manifestations, presumably, have been found only with ulcerative colitis, but it is now recognized that these can be observed in both conditions. They are discussed in Chapter 30.

It may not be possible to differentiate between the two diseases, either by radiologic or clinical means. In approximately 10% to 15% of cases, distinction cannot be made even pathologically; these patients are thus placed into the so-called "indeterminate" category (see Chapter 30).

## Physical Examination

Physical examination is usually unrewarding in patients with ulcerative colitis who do not have fulminant disease. Abdominal tenderness and distension usually are absent. No masses are palpable. However, in the acutely ill person, abdominal distension may be associated with toxic megacolon. Diffuse tenderness may be apparent and, if perforation has ensued, all the usual signs and symptoms of an intraabdominal catastrophe may be noted.

## Endoscopic Examination

Proctosigmoidoscopy, flexible sigmoidoscopy, and colonoscopy are important tools for evaluating the bowel and for confirming the presence or absence of IBD. Proctosigmoidoscopic examination is particularly useful in differentiating Crohn's disease from ulcerative colitis; the rectum is always diseased during attacks of ulcerative colitis. The earliest manifestation of inflammation is the loss of a normal vessel pattern. This is a result of edema of the bowel wall. Contact bleeding, granularity, and ulceration are more obvious signs of inflammatory disease

In individuals with distal disease (i.e., ulcerative proctitis or proctosigmoiditis), complete endoscopic examination by means of the colonoscope is unnecessary at the time of presentation. The extent of disease can usually be determined with the rigid instrument or the flexible sigmoidoscope. The presence of diffuse, confluent, symmetric disease from the dentate line cephalad to the limit of the inflammatory reaction is consistent with ulcerative proctitis or proctosigmoiditis, depending on the extent of involvement. In individuals with *treated* ulcerative colitis, the finding of rectal sparing or patchiness should not necessarily indicate a change in the diagnosis to Crohn's disease. If the patient's symptoms are appropriate to the endoscopic findings, treatment can be initiated without further contrast study or colonoscopy. Conversely, if the patient's disease extends beyond the limit of the endoscopic procedure performed, at some point total colonic evaluation will be necessary.

Colonoscopy has virtually replaced barium enema examination for the evaluation of IBD. Generally, endoscopic examination will identify more proximal inflammatory changes than will the radiologic study. Furthermore, histologic examination of random biopsy specimens often reveals more proximal disease than was suspected by endoscopic examination. It is important to perform biopsies distal to obvious inflammatory changes if the rectum appears to be spared, because of the possible discovery that the rectum is not truly normal. This may cause the physician to reassess the accuracy of a diagnosis of Crohn's disease, based on what was initially thought to be a lack of rectal involvement.

## *Preparation*

Often, colonoscopy can be performed without prior bowel cleansing in patients with mild to active IBD, with essentially the same comprehensive evaluation achieved as when a full preparation is used. In the patient who has a history of IBD, the preparation for colonoscopy includes a modified diet; clear liquids are suggested for 24 hours. Vigorous cleansing enemas, such as those used in the evaluation of a noninflamed colon, are contraindicated. For someone with a relatively active colitis, no laxative is suggested. In more severe cases, a clear liquid diet as the sole modality for bowel preparation is probably the safest alternative. If the colitis is minimal or relatively inactive, a reduced dose of a laxative is suggested, although it is probably wiser to use a balanced electrolyte solution (e.g., Colyte, GoLYTELY).

## *Appearance*

Ulcerative colitis and Crohn's disease are usually recognized endoscopically by excluding IBD of specific causes, such as amebic colitis, ischemic colitis, pseudomembranous colitis, and so forth. Other sources of confusion include radiation changes, the solitary ulcer syndrome, and the differentiation between the two nonspecific IBD themselves Biopsy can be helpful because histologic changes suggestive of Crohn's disease in particular may be apparent; up to 20% of such patients may exhibit granulomas. In patients with ulcerative colitis, rectal biopsy is extremely important for recognizing dysplasia, especially in those with long-standing disease (see *Relationship to Carcinoma*).

A number of colonoscopic features have been described in the differential diagnosis of IBD. Patients with ulcerative colitis always have rectal involvement from the anal verge cephalad in continuity with whatever proximal involvement is present. Erythema of the colonic wall is one of the early manifestations. More obvious changes include granularity, friability, bleeding, edema with interhaustral septal thickening and blunting, ulceration, mucosal bridging, the presence of pseudopolyps, and the superimposition of carcinoma.

With granulomatous colitis, the major colonoscopic finding usually includes a normal rectum; asymmetry or eccentricity of involvement; cobblestone appearance, normal vasculature because friability is not usually encountered except in advanced disease; bowel wall edema, as seen in ulcerative colitis; normal mucosa intervening between areas of ulceration, serpiginous or rake ulcers, which may course for several centimeters; pseudopolyps (as in ulcerative colitis), and skip areas.

The most useful endoscopic features in the differential diagnosis are discontinuous involvement, anal lesions, and the cobblestone appearance of the mucosa for Crohn's disease, and erosions or microulcers and granularity for ulcerative colitis.

Additional biopsy specimens for the evaluation of a patient with IBD should be obtained from an area that appears macroscopically to be relatively uninvolved. The true extent of the inflammation, as well as the significance of the presence of granulomas (granulomas may be seen in patients with ulcerative colitis underlying an ulcer), can then be interpreted properly.

### Colonoscopy Versus Barium Enema

In general, colonoscopy permits identification of segmental involvement and microulceration better than does barium enema. However, radiographic studies yield more information about haustra, especially in the right colon. The procedure is contraindicated in patients with acute exacerbation of the colitis and, certainly, in those who have a toxic megacolon. Erosions, mucosal edema, and vascular injection may not be detected by barium enema.

### Radiographic Features

*Plane Films.* In any evaluation of a patient with IBD, the importance of a plane x-ray film of the abdomen should not be underestimated. The importance of a plane film of the abdomen is further increased in those who have toxic dilatation, a condition usually seen in the transverse colon (Fig. 29.1). When the radiographic appearance of toxic dilatation is noted, a barium enema examination is contraindicated, but serial abdominal films are clinically valuable. The effectiveness of medical therapy can be evaluated by determining the increase or decrease in the degree of dilatation.

*Barium Enema.* The radiologic findings during the acute phase of ulcerative colitis include edema, ulceration, and changes in colonic motility. Edema may be apparent even on the plane film of the abdomen. Initially, ulceration may be rather minimal and difficult to identify. As the disease becomes more fulminant, the ulceration becomes more obvious and may take on a "collar-button" appearance (Fig. 29.2). Edema and inflammation of the mucosa can result in the radiologic appearance that has been called "thumb-printing," a phenomenon characteristically observed in patients with ischemic colitis (Fig. 29.3).

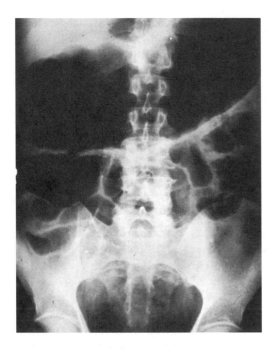

**FIG. 29.1.** Ulcerative colitis. This plane abdominal x-ray film reveals marked dilatation of the transverse colon (toxic megacolon). (From Corman ML, Veidenheimer MC, Nugent FW, et al. *Diseases of the anus, rectum and colon.* Part II: Nonspecific inflammatory bowel disease. New York: Medcom, 1976, with permission.)

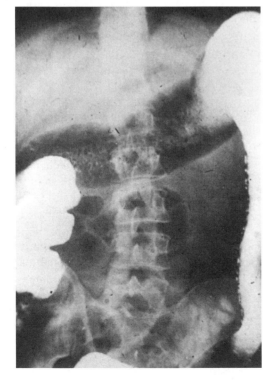

**FIG. 29.2.** Acute ulcerative colitis. Note the loss of haustral markings up to and including the mid-ascending colon and numerous discrete ulcerations deep in the submucosa along the descending colon. (From Corman ML, Veidenheimer MC, Nugent FW, et al. *Diseases of the anus, rectum and colon.* Part II: Nonspecific inflammatory bowel disease. New York: Medcom, 1976, with permission.)

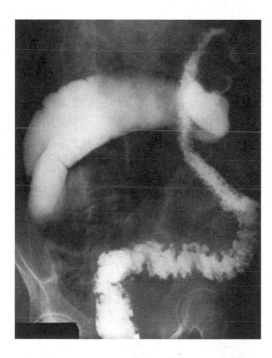

**FIG. 29.3.** Edema of the bowel wall in acute ulcerative colitis; flocculation of barium caused by mucus (*fuzzy appearance*) and thumb-printing in the region of the splenic flexure.

When the disease enters a more chronic phase, other features become characteristic on barium enema examination. These include fibrosis, which results in shortening of the bowel, depression of the flexures, pseudopolyposis, and stricture formation. The bowel wall is less distensible, and the motility pattern is disturbed. Diffuse, confluent, symmetric disease, beginning with the anorectal junction, is the hallmark of the radiologic manifestations of chronic ulcerative colitis (Fig. 29.4). The presence of polypoid lesions throughout the entire colon can be confusing to the uninitiated with the radiologic picture seen in familial polyposis. However, foreshortening of the bowel may be evident, particularly at the flexures, and if the outline of the colon is carefully examined, numerous discrete ulcerations can usually be appreciated.

Benign strictures are uncommon in ulcerative colitis. Radiologic examination usually reveals a smoothly outlined, concentric lumen with tapering margins. Areas of spasm are frequently seen in ulcerative colitis and can be difficult to differentiate from stricture. The administration of propantheline (10 mg of Pro-Banthine) intravenously or glucagon (2 mg) intramuscularly may eliminate the stricture caused by such spasm. If the lumen is eccentric and the margins are irregular, a carcinoma must be suspected.

Another radiologic finding sometimes observed in patients with ulcerative colitis is "backwash ileitis." This is a very poor term because it implies that the ulcerative colitis has somehow regurgitated through the ileocecal valve to cause the disease in the distal ileum. This phenomenon has been demonstrated in

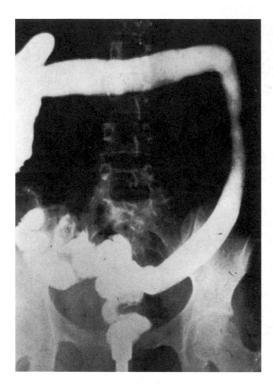

**FIG. 29.4.** Chronic ulcerative colitis: a classic example of diffuse, symmetric, confluent disease. Characteristically, the left side is more involved than the right. Note more foreshortening of the splenic flexure than of the hepatic flexure, and the suggestion of haustra on the right but not on the left. (From Corman ML, Veidenheimer MC, Nugent FW, et al. *Diseases of the anus, rectum and colon.* Part II: Nonspecific inflammatory bowel disease. New York: Medcom, 1976, with permission.)

approximately 10% of patients with ulcerative colitis. The changes can vary from lack of distensibility, as the head of pressure is increased when the barium is inserted, to ileal dilatation, narrowing, rigidity, and changes that can mimic those of regional enteritis.

Portal venous gas has been reported to be a benign, albeit unusual, consequence of air-contrast barium enema in patients with IBD. Although the implication of such an observation, when made in other patients, is that antibiotic treatment is required, it may not be necessary if the patient is without bacteremic symptoms.

### Computed Tomography

The advent of computed tomography (CT) has permitted direct visualization of the entire thickness of the bowel wall and mesentery, and determination of the presence or absence of fluid, fistula, or abscess. With the exception of its unique application to abscess drainage, the role of this study in the diagnosis and management of patients with IBD is controversial. Its advantages over contrast enema are primarily in delineating the presence and severity of pericolonic inflammation and in evaluating other organ diseases. Although the place of CT in IBD is still a matter of conjecture, it is unlikely to prove to be of benefit in patients with ulcerative colitis. Because Crohn's disease is a transmural process, greater application with this condition can be anticipated.

## *Ultrasonography*

Crohn's disease and ulcerative colitis can be detected by ultrasonography with a sensitivity of 86% and 89%, respectively. The primary benefit is in the demonstration of bowel wall thickening. However, because the study is less invasive than other alternatives and can be done without preparation, it can be used to reduce the frequency of repeated colonoscopic or barium enema studies in patients already known to harbor IBD.

## Pathology

### *Macroscopic Appearance*

Ulcerative colitis is a disease confined to the mucosa and submucosa of the bowel. The only exception to this occurs when transmural involvement produces so-called "toxic megacolon." The bowel wall is not thickened, no granulomas are present (except that a foreign body giant cell reaction is occasionally seen in an area of acute inflammation), and no skip areas are seen. The rectum is always involved, and the disease extends proximally for varying distances, but always with continuity of involvement to the proximal extent of the disease process. Characteristically, ulcerative colitis tends to involve the bowel more severely in a distal location than proximally. Despite extensive inflammatory reaction, the bowel wall retains its normal thickness. Longitudinal furrows of denuded mucosa that alternate with islands of heaped-up mucosa, the so-called "pseudopolyps" (Fig. 29.5) result from the confluence of numerous ulcers. Pseudopolyps are inflammatory polyps, not neoplastic

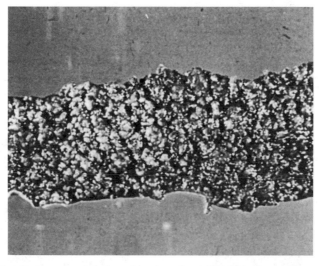

**FIG. 29.5.** Extensive pseudopolyps in active ulcerative colitis. Note the relative uniformity of the polyps in comparison with the varied sizes seen in familial polyposis (see Chapter 21). (From Corman ML, Veidenheimer MC, Nugent FW, et al. *Diseases of the anus, rectum and colon.* Part II: Nonspecific inflammatory bowel disease. New York: Medcom, 1976, with permission.)

lesions. These are seen during a quiescent phase of ulcerative colitis and are a later manifestation of this condition. They can be confused with familial polyposis (see Chapter 21), but the absence of normal mucosa between these polyps suggests the correct diagnosis.

The entire colon, including the cecum and appendix, may be involved. Characteristically, however, the disease does not affect the ileum. In fact, if the small bowel is involved for more than a few centimeters, the diagnosis is not ulcerative colitis. One exception to this is the so-called backwash ileitis seen occasionally when the entire colon is affected. This reversible condition, which may be demonstrated radiographically as edematous, thickened mucosal folds, is a nonspecific inflammatory reaction resulting from proximity of the ileum to the diseased colon.

The entire mucosa can be denuded in patients with long-standing, chronic ulcerative colitis. Under these circumstances, the physician may be lulled into a false sense of security, as the patient's symptoms are often minimal. It is unlikely that someone will experience discharge of mucus, diarrhea, or bleeding if no inflamed mucosa is present. It is this type of patient who is predisposed to the development of carcinoma (see *Relationship to Carcinoma*).

Toxic megacolon is a condition in which an acute inflammatory reaction extends throughout the entire thickness of the bowel wall to the serosa. Gangrene and perforation can result. This is the only manifestation of ulcerative colitis that is not limited to the mucosa and submucosa.

### *Histologic Appearance*

Ulcerative colitis is characterized histologically by an intense inflammation of the mucosa and submucosa, in addition to the presence of multiple crypt abscesses. Marked vascular engorgement accounts for the propensity to rectal bleeding (Fig. 29.6). An obvious decrease occurs in the production of mucus by the crypt epithelial cells (Fig. 29.7). Conversely, increased secretion of mucus is seen in patients with Crohn's disease.

If the bowel is cut longitudinally, it becomes apparent that the deeper parts of the colonic wall are spared. Confinement of the disease to the mucosa and submucosa is the most characteristic finding in ulcerative colitis. Abscesses can enlarge to undermine the mucosa, which can then be shed into the bowel lumen, leaving an ulcer behind. When multiple ulcers form, the remaining nonulcerated mucosa extends above the muscularis as polypoid projections, resulting in the well-known pseudopolyps of ulcerative colitis. If ulceration continues, the entire mucosa can become denuded, and broad areas of the submucosa can be exposed to the fecal stream.

In toxic megacolon, full-thickness involvement of the bowel, necrosis, and friability are seen.

Lymphoid hyperplasia involving the mucosa and submucosa occurs in up to 25% of patients with ulcerative colitis. This can be present beneath an area of relative inactivity.

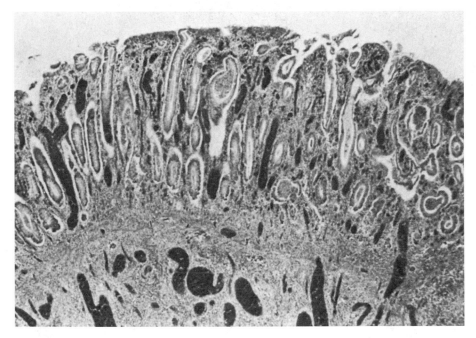

**FIG. 29.6.** Ulcerative colitis. Intense inflammation of the mucosa with multiple crypt abscesses. (Original magnification ×80; from Corman ML, Veidenheimer MC, Nugent FW, et al. *Diseases of the anus, rectum and colon*. Part II: Nonspecific inflammatory bowel disease. New York: Medcom, 1976, with permission.)

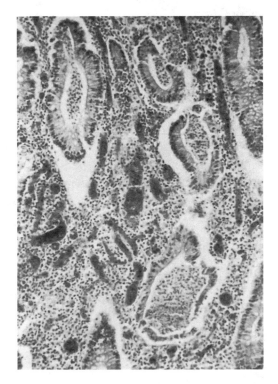

**FIG. 29.7.** Ulcerative colitis. Crypt abscesses with degeneration of crypt epithelium and communication between the crypt lumina and lamina propria. Note vascular engorgement and decrease in mucus production by crypt epithelial cells. (Original magnification ×280; from Corman ML, Veidenheimer MC, Nugent FW, et al. *Diseases of the anus, rectum and colon*. Part II: Nonspecific inflammatory bowel disease. New York: Medcom, 1976, with permission.)

Three features—an excess of histiocytes in combination with a villous or irregular aspect of the mucosal surface and granulomas—have a high predictive value in distinguishing ulcerative colitis from Crohn's disease.

### Antineutrophil Cytoplasmic Antibody Determination

A number of studies have shown that antineutrophil cytoplasmic antibodies (ANCA) with a perinuclear staining pattern (pANCA) are present in up to 86% of patients with ulcerative colitis. Theoretically, this autoimmunity may represent a possible pathogenetic mechanism for the development of ulcerative colitis. A set of marker antibodies is now available for the screening and differential diagnosis of ulcerative colitis and Crohn's disease (Prometheus, Inc., San Diego, CA, USA). Proven applications of this new technology include the following:

As an adjunct to clinical and tissue pathology in the differential diagnosis of inflammatory bowel disease

Confirmation of the correct diagnosis before surgery

Identification of those patients with left-sided ulcerative colitis that may be resistant to treatment

Identification of those patients susceptible to the development of pouchitis following ileal pouch-anal anastomosis

### Breath Pentane Analysis

Neutrophils, macrophages, and other cells are capable of producing free oxygen radicals that can stimulate lipid peroxidation, especially during periods of active inflammation. The production of pentane, the product of the peroxidation of polyunsaturated fatty acids, can be quantified by measuring the content of exhaled breath. Pentane analysis may be correlated with IBD activity.

### Leukocyte Scan

Abdominal scintigraphy by means of autologous-labeled leukocytes has been used to assess activity in IBD. Indium 111 ($^{111}$In) and technetium 99m ($^{99m}$Tc) have been helpful in this regard. With colonoscopy as the reference method, the maximal extent of colitis is correctly assessed by the scan in two thirds of patients, but rectal involvement is not perceived in 19%. The intensity of inflammatory activity correlates significantly with the colonoscopic assessment. The noninvasive nature of this particular approach makes it a reasonable alternative to other investigations of the extent and activity of IBD.

## SIGNS, SYMPTOMS, AND PRESENTATIONS

Patients with ulcerative colitis and Crohn's disease can present with minimal symptoms and moderate complaints, or they may have fulminant manifestations.

Considerable overlap is seen in the symptomatology of the two conditions, but with some differences in the presentation between the two. Rectal bleeding is always seen in patients with ulcerative colitis at some time during the course of the illness. Individuals with Crohn's disease also can bleed, but this is not as frequent a manifestation and may not be as severe. Abdominal pain can be mild or absent in patients with ulcerative colitis; it is rarely severe, except possibly when toxic megacolon supervenes. However, patients with Crohn's disease frequently have abdominal pain. An abdominal mass is occasionally found on physical examination in a patient with Crohn's disease, but it is never seen in a patient with ulcerative colitis.

The presence of diarrhea and the passage of mucus are frequently observed in both conditions and do not serve as distinguishing characteristics. Diarrhea can be manifested as two or three loose stools a day or as severe as 20 or more bowel movements within a 24-hour period. Often, patients with ulcerative colitis are more troubled by the frequency of the bowel movements than are those with Crohn's disease. Perhaps, this is because distal disease tends to be associated with more urgency and, in some cases, tenesmus. Patients with Crohn's disease may have rectal sparing and are less likely to experience urgency.

Anal disease is much more commonly seen in Crohn's colitis than in ulcerative colitis. The presence of anal pain, swelling, and discharge may be a presenting feature of the former condition and may be the only abnormality observed on examination and subsequent investigation (see Chapters 11 and 30).

Fever is usually not a concern in patients with ulcerative colitis unless the patient is severely ill (toxic megacolon). However, in patients with Crohn's disease, pyrexia is not uncommonly noted and is usually caused by an intraabdominal abscess or an undrained septic focus. Nausea and vomiting are not seen frequently in either condition, except with evidence of intestinal obstruction. Anorexia, weight loss, anemia, and general debility are associated with relatively long-standing or fulminant disease.

## Disease in the Elderly

The development of IBD in the elderly population has been a source of some confusion. Many older patients who have signs and symptoms suggestive of IBD are thought to have ischemic colitis. Conversely, patients thought to have IBD subsequently have been proved to have ischemia as the cause of their symptoms. In older persons, ulcerative colitis may have a sudden and fulminating onset that progresses to a fatal outcome.

## Disease in Children and Adolescents

Recent data suggest that the rising incidence of IBD in young people is entirely a consequence of Crohn's disease, a condition now more common than ulcerative colitis in this age group. When the condition occurs in children, there may be a more rapid onset and progression than when the disease occurs in young adults. Symptoms are the same as in adults, but toxic megacolon, bowel perforation, and massive hemorrhage are not uncommon sequelae. These youngsters often become chronically ill, have impaired growth and decreased mental acuity, and are less developed physically than their healthy peers. Growth failure, especially, is the result of prolonged inadequate caloric intake. Because of these concerns, implementation of an elemental diet and parenteral nutrition are often part of the management of patients in this age group (see *Medical Management*). However, to be maximally effective, therapy must be initiated before puberty. Furthermore, unless medical treatment can achieve a sustained remission, operative intervention may be the only appropriate method for addressing the problem of retarded development (see *Surgical Management*). Particular emphasis should be placed on the assessment of growth and development as well as psychological support for both patient and family.

### Disease in Pregnancy

Because IBD is common in patients of childbearing age, the possibility of becoming pregnant is often an issue in medical and surgical care. However, pregnancy is not that frequent an event in patients with IBD. The reason probably is related to the fact that these patients may suffer any number of hormonal imbalances as a result of acute and chronic illness, so that their ability to become pregnant is probably severely impaired.

However, ulcerative colitis and Crohn's disease do not adversely affect fertility, nor do they necessarily impede the progress of a pregnancy or the delivery of a normal, term infant. A greater incidence of low birthweight (<2,500 g) is seen in infants of mothers with ulcerative colitis than in a control population. Although no evidence is seen of an increased risk for pregnancy loss, the likelihood of preterm birth is greater.

What happens to the colitis in patients who are pregnant? Only 30% of patients who became pregnant during a quiescent phase of the colitis had an exacerbation of their disease, but a recrudescence developed in 60% when the pregnancy occurred during an active phase of the illness. In patients whose colitis developed initially during pregnancy or in the postpartum period, a particularly severe result was noted; more than 60% had worsening of their symptoms. In studies specifically in women with Crohn's disease, pregnancy entailed no increased risk for exacerbation of the bowel inflammation. However, an increased risk for premature delivery and spontaneous abortion was observed in those with active disease or in whom resection was required.

In the counseling of a patient with colitis who is contemplating pregnancy, no justification exists to suggest that attempts at conception be avoided, except when the possibility of teratogenic effects of a medication exists (e.g., metronidazole [Flagyl]). Certainly, immunosuppressive treatment should be avoided in a patient wishing to conceive.

Concerns are also expressed about the safety of drug therapy in men, which could damage sperm and theoretically be associated with teratogenicity. Infertility in men is commonly associated with sulfasalazine administration. Sperm analysis may be helpful in determining whether a problem in conception can be attributed to this cause.

As mentioned, women who have a quiescent form of the disease are unlikely to experience problems with the subsequent pregnancy and delivery. Conversely, if the patient is experiencing an exacerbation of the colitis, the illness itself may preclude the possibility of pregnancy. If the disease is more than moderately active, a temporary waiting period and introduction of appropriate medical therapy to secure a remission may be appropriate However, even in this situation, the chances of a normal pregnancy and delivery are 50%. Contraception need be considered only in those women whose disease is so severe that surgery is imminent. Even in the severely ill pregnant woman, no evidence suggests that the pregnancy cannot be brought to a successful conclusion with the birth of a healthy child.

If surgery becomes necessary during pregnancy, the method of treatment (medical or surgical) should be identical to that for a patient who is not pregnant. It has also been determined that azathioprine is safe and that termination of the pregnancy is not mandatory for those who conceive while taking the drug. If an operation becomes necessary, the procedure should be performed as if the patient were not pregnant, although major reconstructive surgery should probably be deferred. Closer to term, the enlarged uterus may preclude the possibility of performing even a conventional proctectomy; a staged operation, sparing the rectum, is therefore appropriate.

A high fetal and maternal mortality rate has been reported if surgical intervention becomes necessary for fulminant colitis. Successful childbirth has been reported following restorative proctocolectomy with pelvic ileal reservoir. Neither vaginal delivery nor cesarean section affected pouch functional outcome, but the frequency of nocturnal stools increased during the pregnancy and for 3 months thereafter. After a continent (Kock) ileostomy, problems encountered include an increased urge to empty the reservoir, especially in the last trimester, and some difficulties with intubation. In most patients, a vaginal delivery is successful, with cesarean section reserved for obstetric indications.

If pregnancy develops following proctocolectomy and ileostomy, the question arises whether the prospective mother should have a cesarean section or deliver vaginally. I believe that if the pregnant woman has an adequate pelvis for a normal vaginal delivery, this should be attempted. A cesarean section is not mandatory simply because the patient has an ileostomy, but if an episiotomy is performed, healing of the perineal wound may be delayed. However, my experience is that the obstetrician almost invariably will opt for a cesarean section.

## Extraintestinal Manifestations

See Chapter 30.

## COURSE AND PROGNOSIS

Nordenholtz et al. examined the causes of death in patients with Crohn's disease and ulcerative colitis through an analysis of death certificates in Rochester, New York. Of the total of 1,358 patients with IBD followed from 1973 through 1989, death certificates were recorded for 130 (59 with ulcerative colitis and 71 with Crohn's disease). Findings were 68% with Crohn's disease and 78% of those with ulcerative colitis died of causes unrelated to their IBD. Deaths caused by Crohn's disease decreased from 44% in the first 8-year period to 6% in the second. Colorectal cancer caused 14% of the deaths in patients with ulcerative colitis, three times more often than in persons with Crohn's disease. Excluding cancer, only two deaths were directly attributable to ulcerative colitis, both occurring within the first 2 years after diagnosis.

With respect to course and prognosis during a 25-year period, the distribution of disease activity is remarkably constant each year, with about 50% of individuals in clinical remission. After 10 years, the colectomy rate is 25%. With 25 years of follow-up, the cumulative probability of a relapsing course is 90%. The probability of maintaining working capacity up to 10 years is approximately 93%.

## RELATIONSHIP TO CARCINOMA

Crohn and Rosenberg initially described carcinoma of the colon arising in a patient with ulcerative colitis in 1925. Today, uniform agreement exists with respect to the association between chronic ulcerative colitis and the subsequent development of adenocarcinoma. Primary malignant lymphoma complicating ulcerative colitis, although extremely rare, is nevertheless also thought to be associated with ulcerative colitis.

A number of factors predispose a colitic patient to colon cancer. These include total colonic or pancolonic disease; prolonged duration of the illness (the earliest reported case is in a patient with the disease of 7 years' duration); continuous active disease, as opposed to intermittent symptoms; and possibly the severity of disease. An early age of onset probably poses no increased cancer risk, except that cancer risk often parallels duration. The cumulative risk for cancer increases with the duration of colitis, reaching 25% to 30% at 25 years, 35% at 30 years, 45% at 35 years, and 65% at 40 years. Colitis and cancers developed in patients with left-sided colitis about a decade later than in those with extensive disease, although the mean duration of the colitis before the development of cancer was virtually the same in both groups (~21 years), irrespective of the age at onset of the disease. The incidence of cancer in patients with ulcerative colitis has been variously reported to be between 2% and 5%. Patients with left-sided disease may fare better with respect to risk for the development of colorectal cancer. Generally, the incidence of carcinoma is the same in both sexes. Multicentricity of the cancers is a frequently reported phenomenon, with 25% or more of patients presenting with tumors in more than one location.

Another characteristic of colorectal cancer with ulcerative colitis is that the cancer often tends to be infiltrative and scirrhous. Visible tumor involving the mucosa may not be observed, even by careful endoscopic examination

A fourth pathologic feature of carcinoma arising in ulcerative colitis is the tendency of the lesion to be highly aggressive and poorly differentiated. More than one half of young patients with ulcerative colitis and colorectal cancers have colloid carcinomas with histologically apparent mucus-secreting tumors of the signet-ring cell type. The fact few or no symptom is present tends to lull both patient and physician into a false sense of security. As suggested, physical examination, barium enema, and even endoscopic evaluation can fail to identify the lesion. But when stricture occurs, the patient must be presumed to have a carcinoma until it can be proved otherwise (Figs. 29.8 and 29.9). The presence of a stricture in a patient with ulcerative colitis is an indication for operative intervention. In the Mayo Clinic series, 40% of patients with carcinoma in chronic ulcerative colitis had a Dukes' A or B growth, in comparison with a 63% incidence if carcinoma arose in the absence of the disease. Conversely, 60% with carcinoma and ulcerative colitis had Dukes' C and D lesions, in comparison with

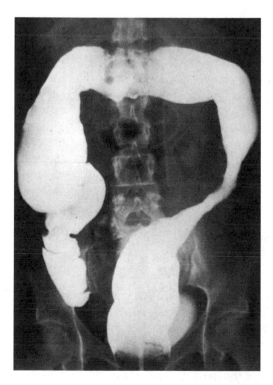

**FIG. 29.8.** Stricture in ulcerative colitis. Foreshortening of the lower descending and sigmoid colon with stricture. Laparotomy revealed extensive carcinoma, hepatic metastases, and two additional unsuspected primary cancers in the resected specimen. (From Corman ML, Veidenheimer MC, Nugent FW, et al. *Diseases of the anus, rectum and colon.* Part II: Nonspecific inflammatory bowel disease. New York: Medcom, 1976, with permission.)

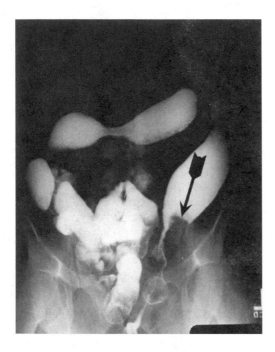

**FIG. 29.9.** Carcinoma in ulcerative colitis. Note the loss of haustrations, marked shortening, and sigmoid stricture. The tumor extends cephalad from the stricture to appear as a polypoid filling defect (*arrow*).

37% who had carcinoma alone. The mean age of these patients at the onset of the colitis was 26 years, with disease duration of 17 years before the development of malignancy; 23% exhibited multicentric tumors. Those whose carcinoma was identified incidentally during prophylactic colectomy had a 5-year survival of 72%, whereas those with clinical or radiographic evidence suggestive of cancer had a much poorer survival rate of 35%.

In comparing survival statistics with those of patients with noncolitic cancer, no statistically significant difference in survival rates is seen for the same stage of invasion. The poorer results are a consequence of the fact that a higher percentage of patients present with more advanced or incurable disease at the time of surgery. The prognosis for colitis-associated colorectal cancers, as for non-colitic cancers, is directly related to the degree of invasion

## Dysplasia

### Definition and Interpretation

Dysplasia can be mild, moderate, or severe; the correct interpretation of the biopsy results rests on the talent and experience of the pathologist.

The criteria for diagnosing dysplasia are problematic and vary from institution to institution. Dysplasia includes adenomatous and villous changes in the mucosa, irregular budding tubules beneath the muscularis mucosae, and cellular alterations consisting of a reduced number of goblet cells and the presence

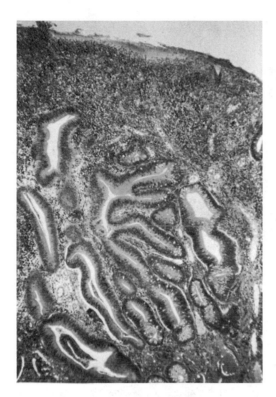

**FIG. 29.10.** Moderate dysplasia in a patient with ulcerative colitis. Note the loss of polarity and decreased mucus production. (Original magnification ×80; courtesy of Rudolf Garret, M.D.)

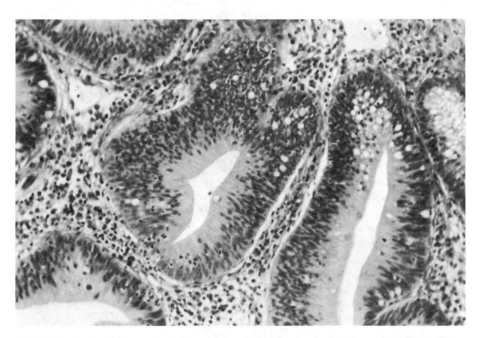

**FIG. 19.11.** Moderate dysplasia in ulcerative colitis. Loss of polarity and proliferation of epithelial cells. (Original magnification ×260; courtesy of Rudolf Garret, M.D.)

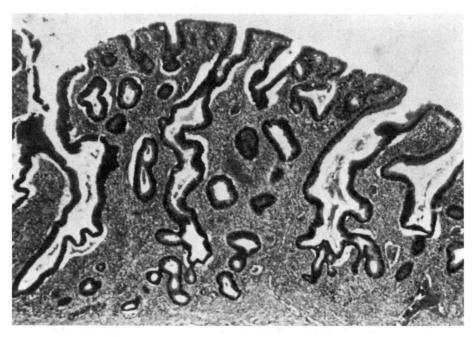

**FIG. 29.12.** Severe dysplasia. Atypical hyperplasia with irregularly shaped crypts lined by crowded cells with hyperchromatic nuclei. (Original magnification ×80; from Corman ML, Veidenheimer MC, Nugent FW, et al. *Diseases of the anus, rectum and colon.* Part II: Nonspecific inflammatory bowel disease. New York: Medcom, 1976, with permission.)

of hyperchromatic nuclei, stratified nucleoli, and coarse chromatin (Figs. 29. 10–29.12). The following criteria have been proposed:

Mild dysplasia
    Preservation of crypt architecture
    Nuclear stratification, but not reaching the luminal surface
    Nuclear crowding and hyperchromasia
    Mitoses in the upper portion of crypt
    Usually, moderate diminution of goblet cell mucin
Moderate dysplasia
    Distortion of crypt architecture, with branching and lateral buds
    Nuclear abnormalities, as in mild dysplasia, but stratification reaching the
        luminal surface
    Usually, depletion of goblet cell mucin
Marked dysplasia
    More marked distortion of crypt architecture, frequently with villous config-
        uration of surface epithelium
    Nuclear abnormalities, as in moderate dysplasia, but with loss of polarity fre-
        quently present
    Frequently, presence of "back-to-back" glands

The last category includes all abnormalities short of invasive carcinoma and encompasses what some might designate carcinoma *in situ*.

## Aneuploidy

Another method currently being explored to identify precancerous changes is flow cytometry. DNA aneuploidy correlates with the presence of dysplasia. Approximately 75% of dysplastic tissue demonstrates aneuploidy or polyploidy, whereas 95% of specimens of nondysplastic tissue exhibited diploidy. Flow cytometry may be usefully applied to complement histologic examination when dysplasia is suspected.

*Results.* As implied, one of the problems with the concept of dysplasia alone is interobserver and intraobserver variability. Sampling error, as well as total reliance on histologic information, has its own inherent limitations. Patients who demonstrate aneuploidy should probably have more extensive and frequent colonoscopic surveillance, whereas those who do not require less frequent investigations. The use of flow cytometry in surveillance programs might be of particular value for selecting individuals at an increased risk for the development of cancer.

## Results of Dysplasia Evaluation

Colonoscopic surveillance reduces colorectal carcinoma-related mortality by permitting the detection of carcinoma at an earlier Dukes' stage. The cumulative risk for the development of at least low-grade dysplasia is 14% after 25 years of disease.

## Dysplasia Surveillance Concerns

Although the increased risk for the development of colorectal cancer in individuals with longstanding ulcerative colitis is well known and accepted, in recent years, in particular, increased concern has been expressed about the utility of surveillance colonoscopy. First, the risk for progression to dysplasia has been found to be only 2.4% for individuals whose initial evaluation was negative. Therefore, surveillance might perhaps be less frequently applied for those patients. Of a greater concern, however, is that 32% of the patients with high-grade dysplasia were found to have invasive cancer. Conversely, when an unsuspected cancer is found at the time of surgery performed for dysplasia, it tends to be at a lower Dukes' stage than the cancer in patients in whom the diagnosis is made before surgery. For reasoned decisions to be made, it has been advised that patients be informed about the limitations of colonoscopic surveillance so that they can rationally take part in their management.

The cost-effectiveness of surveillance colonoscopy has become a hotly debated issue, and as of this writing, accord with respect to the appropriate frequency of such examinations is still an unattained ideal.

### Surveillance Method

With the description of the dysplastic phenomenon, surveillance is advised for those who have had a minimum of 7 years of total or subtotal colonic disease. These persons are then advised to have a total colonoscopy with biopsy of any demonstrable lesion. As suggested, the biopsy of a specific, elevated lesion will yield a much higher incidence of dysplasia. Multiple, random biopsy samples should be taken throughout the colon (10 are advised). This should be done every other year; more frequently, if dysplasia is identified. Histologic findings should be an indication for colectomy only if dysplasia is (a) severe, (b) consistent in more than one biopsy obtained at different sites, or (c) found in sequential biopsy specimens taken from an identifiable lesion. Preferably, biopsy specimens should be obtained in areas free from obvious inflammatory reaction.

*Comment*: It is certainly true that cost-to-benefit analysis has not been determined, incurable cancer may still supervene, patient compliance is problematic, and willingness of patients to commit themselves to a resection if the biopsy reveals dysplasia is doubtful. However, the alternative course is even less agreeable. Barium enema examination is useful only to demonstrate the macroscopic anatomy of the colon: loss of haustrations, shortening, and possible stricture. It is unlikely that this study will reveal a carcinoma earlier than will endoscopic examination with biopsy. Prophylactic colectomy after 8 to 10 years is one option; denial is another. However, until a better alternative is available, I shall continue to recommend the protocol as outlined, with the performance of flexible fiberoptic sigmoidoscopy in alternate years.

## Treatment of Carcinoma

If a carcinoma is identified in the rectum of a patient with ulcerative colitis, proctocolectomy is the treatment of choice. No attempt should be made to preserve the rectal mucosa. Alternative operations, however, include the continent ileostomy (Kock) and the ileoanal anastomosis with intervening pouch, provided that sphincter preservation does not compromise adequate tumor margins (see *Surgical Management*).

### Risk of Rectal Preservation Following Colectomy

With the rectum relatively spared, surgeons have occasionally attempted to preserve the rectum in the hope of some day reestablishing intestinal continuity. The rectum either would be oversewn or brought out as a mucous fistula. Another alternative operation is an ileorectal anastomosis, which maintains intestinal continuity but has the disadvantage of preserving potentially malignant rectal mucosa.

What is the risk for the development of cancer in the retained rectum? The number requiring rectal excision for all reasons ranges widely, with reports of 8% to 50% requiring subsequent proctectomy. The overall incidence ranges from 3.6% to 4.8 %, and the cumulative probability of a cancer developing in the rectum following subtotal colectomy is 13% to 17% at 25 years from the onset of disease, considerably less than when the colon is intact. Although the reports are reasonably favorable, careful endoscopic follow-up is a requisite. Others have also expressed their concern about the retained rectum after colectomy for ulcerative colitis.

Preexisting colonic cancer with severe dysplasia is a relative contraindication to rectal preservation. Frequent proctosigmoidoscopy and rectal biopsy is recommended to look for dysplasia.

If a biopsy demonstrates severe dysplasia, a repeated examination is suggested 3 months later. If sequential biopsy demonstrates severe dysplasia, excision of the rectum is recommended.

Evaluation of the rectum by means of proctosigmoidoscopy or flexible fiberoptic sigmoidoscopy can usually be done relatively easily in a patient whose rectum is in continuity with the intestinal tract. However, if someone has a mucous fistula or an oversewn rectal stump, it may be impossible to pass an instrument in the disused rectum after a time. These individuals are at great risk for the development of malignancy. If continuity has not been reestablished within 2 years following colectomy, serious consideration should be given to removing the rectum. However, even after a considerable period of time following ileostomy, a restorative proctectomy can be offered.

## MEDICAL MANAGEMENT

Treatment of nonspecific ulcerative proctitis and proctosigmoiditis can be rather difficult for a number of reasons: diagnostic uncertainty; empiric nature of the treatment; difficulty in correlating the response to therapy, especially when spontaneous resolution is common; variability of treatment duration; and differences of opinion with respect to the relative merits of the diverse approaches. Proximal extension occurs in approximately 10% of patients, almost always within 1 or 2 years of onset. However, in one group (between 15% and 30%), the course is characterized by multiple recurrences but without proximal extension. Surgical intervention is rarely indicated for persons with distal bowel disease. Therefore, reassurance should be the attitude of the physician and surgeon. No increased risk is seen for the development of malignancy in these people.

### Steroid Retention Enema

The rectal application of cortisone and hydrocortisone has been found to be beneficial in the management of patients with acute active colitis. Steroids are more potent than sulfasalazine in active colitis, inducing faster clinical, endoscopic, and pathologic improvement. Steroid retention enemas are often used initially and as the primary treatment for ulcerative proctitis. For a short time, a hydrocortisone enema is given once or twice daily. Enema kits containing 100 mg of hydrocortisone (Cortenema) or 40 mg of methylprednisolone acetate (Medrol Enpak) are convenient and effective for treating disease confined to the lower bowel. Frequently, retention enemas containing cortisone administered over 2 weeks will resolve the patient's complaints. The rapidity of the clinical response and a lack of complications usually encountered with systemic steroid therapy are the primary advantages of this method of treatment. The rectal instillation of steroids is advantageous, in that medication is applied directly to the involved mucosa, although it should be remembered that with persistent and frequent use, side effects associated with hyperadrenocorticism may ultimately develop. If this occurs, dosing should be reduced to alternate days so that within 2 or 3 weeks it can be discontinued. Some patients require longer treatment, and others have difficulty retaining the enema because of tenesmus or diarrhea. A number of studies have demonstrated both the efficacy of the retention enema (reaching quite proximal areas of the colon) and its favorable therapeutic benefit in comparison with low-dose oral steroids.

### Systemic Steroids

Oral steroids should be considered in patients who fail to respond to the aforementioned measures and who continue to bleed. A beginning dose of 20 mg of prednisone is suggested on a daily basis, which is then reduced by 5 mg after 1 week; ideally, the medication is completely withdrawn in a period of 4 to 6 weeks. Higher doses of steroids can be used transiently but are not recommended for prolonged use. Every attempt should be made to taper the level in a reasonable, nonprecipitous way.

One of the important aspects of education is to have the patient recognize that the condition can be relatively chronic and subject to exacerbations and remissions. In some individuals, bleeding persists for many months or even years. A common error is to augment the dose of prednisone or hydrocortisone in an attempt to eliminate every symptom. This inevitably eventuates in the consequences of hyperadrenocorticism.

The toxic effects of corticosteroids are related to the dose and the duration of treatment. Complications of steroid management include the masking of an acute abdominal problem (e.g., intestinal perforation), osteonecrosis, metabolic bone disease, and growth retardation in children. Corticosteroids can and have been used successfully during pregnancy without adverse side effects to the developing fetus. Because of attempts to modify the chemical structure of steroids and maximize their anti-inflammatory properties, and the desirability of limiting systemic use, most physicians, at least initially, prescribe rectal steroids whenever possible. Newer products, in which systemic absorption is limited through the attachment of prednisolone to a carrier or through an increase in hepatic metabolism after colonic absorption, have demonstrated improved efficacy, with reduced impact on the hypothalamic-pituitary-adrenal axis and consequent reduction of systemic metabolic problems.

Although the primary drugs for the treatment of both ulcerative colitis and Crohn's disease are identical, the approach to therapy for the two conditions is very different. For example, because ulcerative colitis is a disease subject to exacerbations and remissions, the physician endeavors to withdraw steroids as soon as the patient's condition permits. Crohn's disease, however, tends to pursue a more smoldering course, with less clearly defined exacerbations and remissions—hence, continuous low-dose steroid therapy is often required.

Because the therapy for both ulcerative colitis and Crohn's disease depends on the patient's symptoms, treatment must be individualized. Factors that contribute to medical management decisions with respect to ulcerative colitis include the extent of inflammatory disease, duration of illness, and status of disease (exacerbation or remission). Patients with ulcerative colitis tend to have the most severe manifestations early in the course of the illness, with the possibility of cancer developing being the primary concern at a later time. The prognosis of patients with Crohn's disease, however, worsens as active disease persists.

### Sulfasalazine, 5-Aminosalicylic Acid, Olsalazine, Mesalamine, and Paraaminosalicylic Acid

Sulfasalazine (Azulfidine, Salazopyrin) has for many years been the standard drug for preventing exacerbations of ulcerative colitis. Initially, it was thought that breakdown by bacteria in the bowel produced sulfapyridine, an antibiotic, and that this was the basis for the therapeutic effect. It is now known, however, that multiple pharmacologically active roles (e.g., inhibition of prostaglandin synthesis, inhibition of proteolytic enzymes, and immunosuppression) exist. The oral dosage is usually begun at 2 g/d, up to a maximum of 4 g/d. Increasing the dose further can lead to unpleasant side effects from the sulfapyridine moiety— skin rash, bone marrow depression, nausea, headache, and malaise—even at low doses. Folic acid deficiency can develop and go unrecognized; therefore, daily supplements are recommended. Other side effects of greater consequence include hemolysis in patients with glucose-6-phosphate dehydrogenase deficiency, exfoliative skin disorders, and temporary infertility in men. This is the only drug proved to have prophylactic benefits in the treatment of ulcerative colitis. More recent studies suggest that 5-aminosalicylic acid (5-ASA) is the most important active ingredient of sulfasalazine, at least with respect to its therapeutic effect, if not its preventive role. A total of 4 g of 5-ASA in a 100-mL retention enema can be given to patients who do not tolerate sulfasalazine. The generic name for 5-ASA is mesalamine in the United States and mesalazine in the United Kingdom and Europe. Mesalamine (Rowasa, Pentasa, Claversal, Salofalk) has been recommended and approved as a rectal suspension enema containing 4 g in 60 mL.

Oral 5-ASA (olsalazine sodium [Dipentum]; mesalamine [Pentasa, Asacol, Rowasa, Claversal, Salofalk]) requires the addition of an azo bond or an acrylic resin coating to prevent absorption in the small intestine. A number of studies have shown that the drug is well tolerated and effective for treating mild to moderately active ulcerative colitis and for maintaining remission. Delivery depends either on the azo reductase capability of the colonic microflora or the time-release properties of the encapsulation. The most troublesome consequences appear to be nausea and diarrhea. An isomer of 5-ASA, 4-ASA (paraaminosalicylic acid), has also been suggested as a retention enema for the treatment of distal colitis because of its stability in aqueous solution, its safety, and its low frequency of side effects. Another application of 5-ASA is in suppository form. The remission rate is essentially the same as that observed in individuals treated with sulfasalazine.

## Sucralfate Enema

Sucralfate, a basic aluminum salt of sucrose octasulphate, has been demonstrated to be an effective drug in the management of peptic ulcer disease. It achieves its therapeutic effectiveness by adhering to mucosal surfaces, increasing prostaglandin levels, increasing mucosal blood flow, and stimulating secretion of mucus. In experimental studies of chemically produced colitis in rats, encouraging results were observed. Further trials are awaited.

## Butyrate Enema

Short-chain fatty acid irrigation has been demonstrated to be of benefit in the management of individuals with so-called "diversion colitis" (see Chapter 33). Butyrate, as an endproduct of bacterial fermentation in the large bowel, profoundly affects the colonic epithelium in ulcerative colitis. Decreased frequency of bowel action is observed, in addition to a marked reduction in bleeding.

## Nicotine

As the search for the cause of IBD continues, the association between cigarette smoking and a more favorable clinical course in ulcerative colitis remains the sole epidemiologic feature that distinguishes it from Crohn's disease. An improvement with remission was demonstrated in a treated group in comparison with a placebo group. The most common complaints attributed to nicotine included nausea, lightheadedness, headache, and sleep disturbance. The addition of transdermal nicotine to conventional maintenance therapy may reduce symptoms in persons with active ulcerative colitis. The mechanism for the effect of nicotine is unknown.

## Immunosuppression

Immunomodulatory drugs are now generally accepted as appropriate for long-term management in certain patients with IBD. The rationale for their use is based on the observations concerning the implication of immune mechanisms in the pathogenesis of the disease.

### *Azathioprine and Mercaptopurine*

Two agents that have been demonstrated to be effective are 6-mercaptopurine (6-MP) and its analogue, azathioprine. Azathioprine is rapidly absorbed and converted to mercaptopurine in red cells. Subsequent hepatic conversion produces active metabolites that inhibit purine ribonucleotide and, therefore, DNA synthesis. The mechanism of action is believed to be inhibition of lymphocyte function, primarily that of T cells.

Probably the largest experience with the use of these agents comes from the Lenox Hill Hospital and the Mount Sinai School of Medicine in New York City. During 18 years of observation from this unit, a total of 81 patients with resistant ulcerative colitis were treated with 6-MP. All had failed therapy with sulfasalazine and steroids. The mean treatment period was 1.8 years, and the overall response rate was 61%. A low incidence of toxicity was encountered. One of the concerns with both of these agents is the development of pancreatitis, a complication that has been reported in up to 15% of patients. In addition, both cause bone marrow suppression, particularly neutropenia. Because this is dose-related and is essentially an ongoing concern, blood counts monitoring should be done at least four times a year. Although concern has been expressed about the carcinogenic and teratogenic potential of these agents, especially the development of lymphoma, controlled trials have failed to support this anxiety.

### *Cyclosporine*

The slow onset of action of azathioprine and mercaptopurine in patients with IBD has led to trials of more potent immunosuppressive drugs, such as cyclosporine. The primary indications for the use of this agent are acute, severe ulcerative colitis and refractory Crohn's disease. The primary side effect is renal dysfunction. Other complications include neurotoxicity, seizures, and opportunistic infections. Currently, cyclosporine is reserved for the treatment of severe, refractory disease when surgery is not appropriate or before other treatments have taken effect.

### **Antidiarrheal Agents**

The addition of "slowing" medications may be appropriate for the patient having frequent bowel movements out of proportion to the degree of inflammatory involvement of the rectum. Products such as diphenoxylate (Lomotil), loperamide (Imodium), codeine, and deodorized tincture of opium, individually or in combination, can be helpful. If an individual harbors an active colitis, slowing medications should be avoided, as they can precipitate a toxic megacolon. In patients who have ileal disease or who have undergone ileal resection, cholestyramine (Questran) also causes a reduction in diarrhea by adsorbing and combining with bile acids in the intestine to form an insoluble compound that is excreted in the feces.

## Dietary Measures

Additional medical measures include dietary restrictions. This usually involves the omission of all foods that tend to produce increased frequency of bowel movements (e.g., fruits, milk products [especially if the patient has a lactose intolerance], and fiber).

## Counseling

The possible value of psychiatric counseling has been discussed. Although the disease may not be of psychogenic origin, sufficient evidence suggests that stress and emotions may play a role in exacerbation or remission of the condition. In addition to the medication and dietary measures presented, it is often helpful to supplement these conventional medical approaches with psychotherapy and other supportive care.

## The Acutely Ill Patient

### *Signs and Symptoms in Acutely Ill Patients*

Patients with acute, fulminating, "toxic" megacolon may present with minimal symptoms or be critically ill. High fever, tachycardia, and abdominal pain are frequently noted. However, clinical signs and symptoms can be masked by the patient's medications, especially steroids. Keep in mind the possibility of perforation, even in the absence of colonic dilatation.

### *Medical Management of the Acutely Ill Patients*

Acute medical management of the acutely ill patient includes dietary restriction, intravenous fluids, protein replacement, blood transfusions, and the steroid therapy of choice. Some controversy exists over the relative merits of adrenocorticotropic hormone (ACTH) and hydrocortisone or methylprednisolone. Some physicians believe that ACTH is more effective in controlling the acute disease. The initial dose recommended is 40 U in 1,000 mL, over 8 hours. Therefore, a total dose of 120 U is given during a 24-hour period. If the physician prefers, the equivalent of 300 mg of hydrocortisone (~60 mg of prednisone) is recommended. Intravenous hydrocortisone, however, requires either continuous administration or intravenous bolus injections no less frequently than every 4 hours. After this period of time, the blood level falls to inadequate therapeutic levels. If cortisone acetate is given intramuscularly, however, the effective therapeutic level can be maintained for a longer period of time. This, of course, is inconvenient and uncomfortable for the patient. With a good response, the medication can be reduced at the rate of 5 mg (prednisone) every 4 or 5 days, or it may be tapered more rapidly.

### Parenteral Nutrition

Neither an elemental diet nor total parental nutrition decreases the inflammation associated with ulcerative colitis. However, increasing evidence suggests that patients frequently are hospitalized with varying states of malnutrition. As a consequence, hyperalimentation, either parenteral or oral, has been recommended in a supportive role for patients with IBD. Specifically, elemental diets and total parenteral nutrition with bowel rest improved the symptoms, inflammatory sequelae, and nutritional status in individuals with Crohn's disease more readily than in those with ulcerative colitis (see Chapter 30). With IBD, the rationale for implementing intravenous hyperalimentation is that the bowel is "put to rest." If this were attempted without supplementary intravenous caloric intake, the patient's nutritional status would rapidly deteriorate. Intravenous hyperalimentation, therefore, permits the patient with IBD to be managed with bowel rest and simultaneously provides adequate amino acids and calories for anabolism. If surgery is felt to be inevitable, however, total parenteral nutrition should be limited to those who are severely malnourished unless other specific indications are seen for this treatment.

*Comment*: I use total parenteral nutrition only in those patients for whom surgery should be avoided, or in whom the nutritional status is so poor that a very high rate of morbidity and mortality is anticipated. The concept of short-term intravenous hyperalimentation in preparation for bowel surgery may have certain theoretic advantages, but expeditiously performed surgery should allow an earlier commencement of oral intake, a much preferred method of supplying calories. Furthermore, intravenous hyperalimentation is costly and not without morbidity.

### Results of Medical Management of Acutely Ill Patients

Clinical remission can be achieved, on average, in 62% of acutely ill patients, whereas 38% will come to early colectomy. Remission can be maintained in from 38% to 71% of patients who achieved success during an acute management episode.

### Additional Treatments in Acute Illness

The usual supportive measures—intravenous fluid replacement, and blood, colloid, and steroid therapy—should be supplemented with broad-spectrum antibiotic coverage. The single most important guide in the management of a patient with acute toxic dilatation is the assessment obtained with plane abdominal x-ray studies. With serial abdominal films, the effectiveness of medical management can be evaluated. If the dilatation decreases, be reasonably assured that surgery can be deferred. Conversely, if colonic dilatation progresses or fails to improve during the period of maximum therapy, surgical intervention is advised.

Any medications that "slow" gastrointestinal activity (e.g., anticholinergics or opiates) are discontinued. A nasogastric tube is suggested. Placing the patient on the abdomen for a few minutes every 2 or 3 hours may help to distribute the gas, moving it into the rectum. Rectal tubes have also been advocated, but these are potentially dangerous in that they can cause a perforation of the sigmoid colon. Barium enema examination and colonoscopy are contraindicated; in fact, barium enema study has been reported to precipitate toxic megacolon. A high incidence of recurrent toxic dilatation and perforation and the requirement for emergency or urgent operation have been reported. This is in contrast to the group of patients with severe, acute colitis without dilatation, who can usually be effectively managed by nonsurgical means.

## SURGICAL MANAGEMENT

### Indications

Surgery for ulcerative colitis is indicated for toxic megacolon, perforation, hemorrhage, intolerable extracolonic manifestations, and the possibility of malignant degeneration. In addition, because proctocolectomy is curative, resection may be advised for intractable symptoms, even in the absence of a complication. Conversely, operative treatment for Crohn's disease is advised primarily for complications. Perforation usually occurs in the patient who exhibits toxic dilatation of the colon. Diagnosis can usually be made readily on the basis of physical examination and a decubitus film of the abdomen. A walled-off perforation may become evident at the time of laparotomy and can be converted to a free perforation as the bowel is mobilized. Although it is well recognized that ulcerative colitis can be associated with toxic megacolon and perforation, Crohn's disease can also. These complications tend to occur early in the course of the illness, before thickening of the bowel wall develops.

Hemorrhage is occasionally an indication for surgery in ulcerative colitis; it is unusual in Crohn's disease. Conversely, the presence of a fistula virtually excludes the diagnosis of ulcerative colitis. Usually, even massive hemorrhage can be controlled by medical means. It should be remembered, however, that a subtotal or total colectomy without proctectomy may not succeed in arresting the bleeding; it may be necessary to perform a proctectomy subsequently to control hemorrhage. Intractability is by far the most common indication for surgery in ulcerative colitis. These patients usually harbor total or nearly total colonic disease. Even patients with lesser involvement can come to elective surgery, especially those in the older age group (>60 years of age). These patients seem to tolerate their bowel problems less satisfactorily. It has been said that, ideally, one should be sick enough for long enough to "earn" an ileostomy—that is, a person should feel that the physical and psychological burden of caring for a stoma is indeed justified. Today, with the available alternative of a sphincter-saving approach, a tendency is seen to intervene surgically sooner. Irrespective of the choice of operation, no justification exists for deferring an operation until a patient is virtually moribund. Regrettably, referral to the surgeon after such procrastination results in the physician's self-fulfilling prophesy: high morbidity and mortality. The presence of cancer or the risk for malignant change as an indication for surgery has been previously discussed. Colonoscopic monitoring is still the preferred alternative, with operation reserved for those patients found to have persistent severe dysplasia on two consecutive examinations. Other indications for surgery include growth retardation and extraintestinal manifestations (e.g., pyoderma gangrenosum), erythema nodosum, liver function abnormalities, eye complications, and joint disturbances (see Chapter 30).

## Preparation of the Patient

Preparation of the patient for elective surgery is not significantly different, whether the procedure is resection for IBD or surgery for cancer. It is wise, however, to limit the amount of laxative administered. In fact, if a patient is troubled by diarrhea, a preoperative cathartic should be avoided. On the morning of surgery, an enema should be carefully administered until the returns are clear; this is the only mechanical preparation advised for patients with severe bowel frequency problems. Patients who are to have small-bowel resection do not require a mechanical preparation unless the possibility of colonic resection also exists. The antibiotic preparation should be the same as that described in Chapter 22.

Because most individuals who are to have surgery for IBD have been on steroids for varying periods of time, it is imperative that adequate perioperative "coverage" be maintained to prevent the complications of adrenal insufficiency. Unless the patient was on short-term prednisone therapy many months before the operation, steroid protection should be afforded, even if corticosteroids were withdrawn up to 2 years previously.

In an emergency situation, it is obviously impossible to prepare the bowel adequately, particularly for toxic megacolon. Preoperative preparation includes the correction of any fluid and electrolyte abnormalities, blood replacement as necessary, placement of a nasogastric tube, insertion of a Foley catheter, and possibly a central venous catheter.

Preoperative stoma marking should be accomplished for everyone who is to have surgery for IBD, and it is absolutely imperative if an ileostomy is contemplated. An improperly located stoma, one that does not permit convenient management, can cause a patient to become significantly disabled and reclusive. The techniques of stomal construction are discussed in Chapter 31, as are the complications of ileostomy and colostomy.

The optimal site is selected with the patient sitting, supine, and standing. It should be away from bony promontories, scars, and the umbilicus. The ileostomy should always be brought through the split thickness of the rectus muscle (Fig. 29.13).

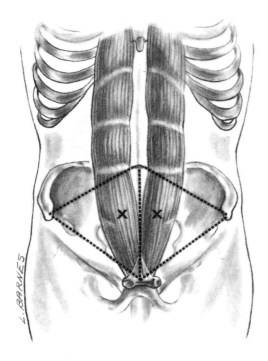

**FIG. 29.13.** When a site for ileostomy is chosen, scars, bony prominences, and the umbilicus must be avoided.

## Choice of Operation

Five basic operations for the surgical treatment of ulcerative colitis are (1) proctocolectomy and conventional ileostomy; (2) total or subtotal colectomy with rectal preservation (ileorectal anastomosis, mucous fistula, or closure of rectal stump); (3) total proctocolectomy with ileoanal anastomosis; (4) procto-colectomy with reservoir ileostomy (Kock); and (5) total abdominal procto-colectomy with ileoanal anastomosis and intervening pouch (Parks, Utsunomiya, Fonkalsrud, Peck). In patients with toxic megacolon, a sixth option is a diverting loop ileostomy with a decompressive skin-level ("blowhole") colostomy.

The incision for all colon resections, including operations for IBD, always should be midline. The reasons for this, which have been discussed, include rapid and facile entry into the peritoneal cavity, good exposure of all areas within the abdomen, and, most importantly, accessibility of both sides of the abdomen for possible stomal placement. If a paramedian incision is used, that side of the abdomen is excluded for possible location of an ileostomy.

The incision is made usually in the hypogastrium with supraumbilical exten-sion for varying distances. Incision to the level of the xyphoid may be required if splenic flexure mobilization is difficult. Abdominal exploration usually reveals the extent of pathology in patients with Crohn's disease, as this is a trans-mural inflammatory process and the serosa is virtually always involved. However, in patients with ulcerative colitis, one may be singularly unimpressed with the extent of disease as it appears from the serosal aspect. The surgeon may appreciate only tortuosity of the vessels, pallor on the serosal aspect, and, of course, in the case of longstanding, chronic ulcerative colitis, bowel shortening.

When operating for ulcerative colitis, a preconceived plan for the surgery should be in place. Conversely, in patients with Crohn's disease, it is not uncommon to discover that involvement is more extensive than might have been appreciated by preoperative evaluation. In both conditions, inspect the entire small bowel for the possibility of other lesions.

### Proctocolectomy with Ileostomy

Proctocolectomy with ileostomy is the conventional operative approach to the treatment of patients with ulcerative colitis and most patients with granulomatous colitis in which the rectum or anus is involved. However, it is interesting to note that few reports have been made on the management of IBD by this operation in the past 20 years. This was initially a consequence, of course, of the development of the continent, reservoir ileostomy (Kock). Currently, most literature on surgery for ulcerative colitis addresses the techniques and results of the various pouch-anal alternatives. However, proctocolectomy and conventional ileostomy should be considered the benchmark procedure with which all other operations are compared. It has been established as a safe, curative approach that permits the patient to live a virtually normal lifestyle.

The technique of proctocolectomy essentially combines the operations discussed in Chapters 22 and 23: total abdominal colectomy with proctectomy, using either the classic Miles approach or, ideally, the perineolithotomy position (synchronous combined). Some minor differences are important to consider, however. First, this is not a cancer operation; hence, it is not necessary to remove a large area of mesentery containing the lymphatic structures. Furthermore, it is not appropriate for the surgeon to excise the parietal peritoneum widely, as is often done for carcinoma of the rectum. The peritoneal cut can be made directly on the bowel wall, thereby expediting the dissection.

Another difference in surgical technique when removing the colon and rectum for IBD, is rectal mobilization. Erection is a parasympathetically mediated response that is transmitted through the nervi erigentes; these nerves arise from the second, third, and fourth sacral roots. Parasympathetic nerve injury can result in impotence, whereas injury to the presacral (sympathetic) nerves interferes with ejaculation. The presacral nerves originate from the thoracic and lumbar segments of the spinal cord and can be identified with a modicum of effort to do so. Because a ready plane of dissection exists between the mesentery of the rectum and the sacrum, I prefer to visualize the presacral nerves directly, displace them posteriorly, and proceed in this plane, as is done with proctectomy for carcinoma. To accomplish this safely, it is important to begin the dissection sharply with a scissors in the hollow of the sacrum rather than to initiate mobilization of the rectum from the promontory bluntly by means of the hand. After the dissection has proceeded well below the sacral promontory, it is then appropriate to complete the mobilization by blunt dissection.

An organized approach to the operation minimizes morbidity and mortality. Having ascertained the extent of the disease, proceed with mobilization of the sigmoid colon and rectum. At this time, the perineal surgeon commences that part of the operation. After completion of the proctectomy, the rectum is delivered to the abdominal operator and wrapped in a towel, and the rest of the colectomy is completed while the perineal surgeon closes the bottom end wound. Alternatively, the abdominal surgeon may elect to perform a total colectomy initially, calling the perineal surgeon in at the appropriate stage of the operation to complete the proctectomy.

If two teams are not available, the patient can be placed either in the perineolithotomy or in the supine position on the operating table, and the total abdominal colectomy is carried out. The rectum is divided and secured in a glove, the abdomen closed, the ileostomy created, and the perineal dissection performed with the patient either in the left lateral position or in the lithotomy position as described for the one-team approach for carcinoma of the rectum.

In contradistinction to what is done in proctectomy for carcinoma, the floor of the pelvis is not reconstituted. This results in a dead space that predisposes to the subsequent development of an abscess, perineal sinus, and delayed healing. Because it is not necessary to excise the levator muscle widely as is often done for cancer, it is always possible to reapproximate this and the external sphincter. The perineal dissection is done in a manner somewhat different from that for carcinoma. I prefer the intersphincteric dissection (Fig. 29.14), which permits a much smaller perineal wound. The procedure is carried out in the intersphincteric plane, between the internal and external anal sphincters. When the levator ani muscle is encountered, it is divided close to the rectum; the dissection is completed anteriorly in a manner identical to that for carcinoma of the rectum. A Silastic drain is placed into the pelvis, brought out through a stab wound in the buttock, and connected to continuous suction. Alternatively, a suprapubic suction drain can be employed. The levator ani muscle and external sphincter are then approximated and the skin closed.

Another method for performing an intersphincteric proctectomy is an endoanal mucosal stripping, such as is undertaken in conjunction with the ileopouch-anal procedure (see later). This leaves yet a smaller wound, but the operation can be associated with delayed healing. It is tedious to accomplish, and has the theoretic disadvantage of incomplete removal of the mucosa, thereby posing a potential risk for cancer and persistent perineal sinus.

Resection of the distal small bowel is sometimes necessary when proctocolectomy is performed for Crohn's disease, depending on whether the inflammatory process involves the intestine. Every effort should be made to preserve the full length of the small bowel. Even modest resection of the distal ileum can lead to malabsorption of nutrients as well as to loss of water and electrolytes.

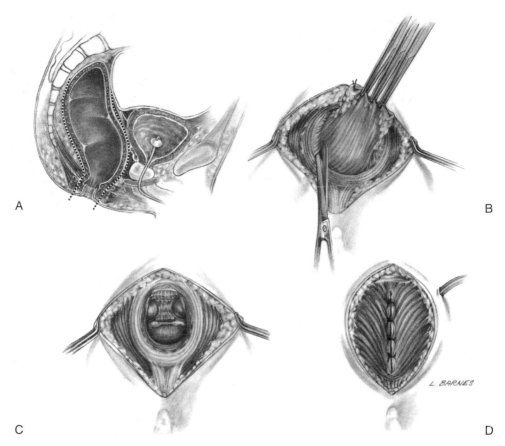

**FIG. 29.14.** Technique of intersphincteric proctectomy. **A.** Outline of the area removed. **B.** Dissection proceeds in the intersphincteric plane. **C.** Intact external sphincter and levatores following rectal removal. **D.** Closure of levatores with drainage.

In creating the ileostomy for patients with ulcerative colitis, I prefer an extraperitoneal approach. This technique permits total obliteration of the paraileostomy gutter, thereby avoiding the potential for herniation. It also facilitates subsequent entrance into the abdominal cavity without the risk for injuring the mesentery to the small bowel. Kocher clamps are placed on the cut edge of the parietal peritoneum. The peritoneum is then gently elevated and stripped off the abdominal wall to the point where the ileostomy site is located. An abdominal wall opening is then created, and the end of the ileum is delivered through the defect. The cut edge of the mesentery is then secured to the peritoneum that has been mobilized. Following closure of the abdomen, the ileostomy is matured.

An intraperitoneal ileostomy, a common alternative for most surgeons, is particularly recommended in patients who have proctocolectomy for granulomatous colitis, in those who have already had a portion of the terminal ileum removed, and in those for whom "stripping" of the parietal peritoneum is technically impossible. As suggested, the disadvantages are the technical difficulties associated with complete obliteration of the right lateral gutter; the inferior aspect of the distal ileum does not lend itself to closure in a satisfactory fashion, and entrance into the abdominal cavity from the right upper quadrant is impeded. Another option is to leave the lateral gutter open; as with sigmoid colostomy, it is better to have a very large opening than a small one. Some anchoring is nonetheless still required to avoid torsion of the distal ileum on itself (windlassing). A few sutures placed from the serosa of the ileum and its mesentery to the parietal peritoneum will usually prevent this complication.

## Complications

Most complications following proctocolectomy are not unique to the operation: wound infection, intraabdominal sepsis, wound dehiscence, ureteral and splenic injury, and urinary, pulmonary, and cardiovascular problems. These are discussed in Chapters 22 and 23. Complications attributed more specifically to this operation include stomal problems, intestinal obstruction, sexual dysfunction, and perineal wound difficulties.

*Stomal Problems.* Stomal complications and their management are discussed in Chapters 31 and 32. Complications with respect to recurrent Crohn's disease are discussed in Chapter 30.

*Intestinal Obstruction.* In patients in whom intestinal obstruction develops following ileostomy, consider a paraileostomy hernia as the cause of the problem. Initial conservative management includes nasogastric intubation and, possibly, an attempt to relieve the obstruction by irrigating the stoma. Occasionally, the obstruction is caused by inspissated fecal material or undigested food. As long as the patient is passing flatus, it is usually possible to delay surgical intervention. However, if a complete intestinal obstruction is present, early operation may be imperative. Often, the cause of the problem is a simple adhesion, but if a paraileostomy hernia with entrapment of the small intestine is the cause, the small bowel must be reduced and the defect closed.

The presence of a nonviable distal ileum usually is a consequence of torsion. Obviously, if the stoma itself is necrotic, the preoperative diagnosis is self-evident and resection of the stoma and nonviable bowel is necessary. Unless the area of nonviability is at least 25 cm from the ileostomy, no anastomotic attempt should be made. The stoma should be resected in continuity with the nonviable bowel and a new ileostomy created; this usually requires relocation to the left lower quadrant. Even though this means sacrificing additional intestine, the risk for an anastomotic leak is so great that preservation of this small segment is not justified.

*Sexual Dysfunction.* Sexual dysfunction (retrograde ejaculation and impotence) has been mentioned as an unfortunate sequela of proctectomy. Impotence after abdominoperineal resection for carcinoma of the rectum is not an uncommon problem, but one questions whether preservation of the rectum in IBD is justified solely because of this risk. The rate of impotence is 2.7%. In all reported series, the vast majority who are impotent are in the older age groups.

*Comment*: Impotence appears to be less the result of the type of operative approach, than of the age of the patient. It seems difficult to believe that careful attention to dissection close to the bowel wall is the reason for a low incidence of impotence, whereas the "radical" operation for cancer produces a high incidence. Although one cannot gainsay meticulous surgical technique, preoperative libido is probably a more important factor. Retrograde ejaculation occurs because of injury to the sympathetic nerves, a complication that has been variously reported to develop in up to 10% of male patients. More recent statistics suggest that, as with the problem of impotence, the complication is much less frequent in younger people. As stated, visualization and avoidance of the presacral nerves should make this complication a very rare occurrence indeed.

Sexual function in women has been less well surveyed than that of men, probably because no concern about impotence exists. Patients with a continent pouch may have a higher incidence of dyspareunia than those with an ileoanal anastomosis, presumably because of scarring or deformity associated with complete proctectomy.

Other concerns about sexual dysfunction are related primarily to the concept of an ileostomy itself—the need for an external appliance and the possibility of leakage—and its impact on sexuality and body image. These aspects are discussed in Chapters 31 and 32.

*Persistent Perineal Sinus.* Persistent perineal sinus is one of the most troubling sequelae of proctectomy for IBD. In a review of our experience with 160 patients who had proctectomy for this condition, the wounds of as many as 11% of patients with ulcerative colitis had not healed, and more than one third with Crohn's colitis had not healed by the end of the follow-up study.

A number of other factors can be associated with the development of this complication. In our experience, youth was felt to be a relevant consideration. All patients with ulcerative colitis who were more than 50 years of age and all with Crohn's colitis who were more than 60 years of age had healed perineal wounds. With respect to sex, women with ulcerative colitis were more likely to have the perineal wound heal per primum (97.5%), whereas only 82% of men achieved such healing. However, no statistically significant difference in rates of healing was seen when sex distributions in patients with Crohn's disease were compared.

Evaluation of the presence or absence of a stoma before proctectomy revealed that in patients with ulcerative colitis, diversion implied an excellent chance for healing. Interestingly, the opposite was true for those with Crohn's colitis.

Perineal disease, specifically fistula-in-ano (present at the time of proctectomy), was not a statistically significant factor in nonhealing. The rates of nonhealing were almost the same in both patients with ulcerative colitis and those with Crohn's colitis when a fistula was present. However, in the absence of a perianal fistula, a patient with Crohn's colitis did not heal as well as one with ulcerative colitis.

No significant role in prolonging perineal wound healing was found after the analysis of (a) the number of prior operations; (b) extent of disease; (c) emergent, urgent, or elective nature of the surgical procedure; (d) wound contamination; (e) presence or absence and duration of steroid therapy; (f) level of serum albumin; or (g) nutritional state of the patient.

In patients who have proctectomy for Crohn's disease, healing can be delayed longer than 1 year in almost 20% of cases.

The failure of perineal wounds to heal readily has stimulated considerable discussion and has served as an impetus for the development of a number of operative approaches to deal with the problem. Once a perineal sinus has developed, vigorous curettage, creating a pyramidal defect, should be done at 6-month intervals until healing is achieved. Other methods that have been advocated include a gracilis or inferior gluteal myocutaneous flap, semimembranous muscle graft, rectus abdominis flap, use of an omental graft, skin grafting, and the application of a fibrin adhesive.

*Perineal Pain and Phantom Sensations.* Phantom sensations of the "need to have a bowel movement" are common after proctectomy. This difficulty is analogous to that which may occur following amputation of an extremity. The cerebral pathway still exists, so that an indeterminate stimulus to the perineum or pelvis can trigger this perception. Treatment is reassurance.

A more troublesome complaint is perineal pain. In contrast to pain that develops following proctectomy for rectal cancer, such pain is not caused by recurrent malignancy, and it is possible to reassure the patient accordingly. Usually, the discomfort can be attributed to a neuroma. If the usual supportive measures (heat, rest, foam rubber cushion, and analgesic medications) fail to relieve the symptoms, consider excising the perineal fat pad. Almost invariably, the pathologist (if asked) will cooperate and succeed in identifying a neuroma, but the clinical significance and long-term benefits are problematic. Relief can be immediate, but recurrence ensured, presumably because the nerve regenerates. Fortunately, if this occurs, the pain is usually not as severe as initially reported.

## Results

Proctocolectomy and ileostomy can be carried out today with minimal morbidity and mortality. The overall operative mortality for proctocolectomy and ileostomy is between 0.5% and 10%, with much lower rates achieved in elective cases, and rates as high as 30% under emergent conditions.

### Ileostomy-Colostomy for the Treatment of Toxic Megacolon

Because of the high mortality rate associated with the surgical treatment of toxic megacolon by colectomy, Turnbull et al. in 1971 advocated what they considered a lesser-risk procedure. This consisted of a diversionary loop ileostomy and two decompressive colostomies, one in the transverse colon and the other in the sigmoid. The colostomies, created at the skin level, were designed to vent the dilated colon as a "blowhole." The major impetus for suggesting this operative approach was to avoid inadvertent fecal soiling of the peritoneal cavity when a walled-off perforation had been liberated by mobilization of the bowel. The technique consists of making a small midline incision and identifying a loop of distal ileum. This is brought out through a previously marked site in the right lower quadrant (Fig 29.15). Ideally, the proximal limb is placed inferiorly and the distal limb superiorly, so that subsequent colon resection will not necessitate a change in the fixation of the distal ileum. Exploration of the right upper quadrant of the abdomen identifies the point of maximal dilatation of the transverse colon, and a small incision is made in the skin, fascia, and rectus muscle. If the sigmoid colon is dilated, it can also be decompressed by making a small incision in the left iliac fossa, permitting the bowel to bulge into the incision. In later reports from the Cleveland Clinic, however, this second blowhole has rarely been felt to be necessary. The abdomen is then closed, and the loop ileostomy is matured, emphasizing the proximal limb.

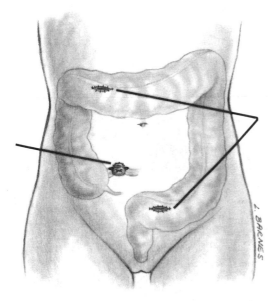

**FIG. 29.15.** Diverting ileostomy and decompression colostomies for toxic megacolon. (From Turnbull RB Jr, Hawk WA, Weakley FL. Surgical treatment of toxic megacolon: Ileostomy and colostomy to prepare patients for colectomy. *Am J Surg* 1971;122:325.)

Attention is then turned to the dilated transverse colon. Seromuscular sutures are placed into the colon and the peritoneum and rectus fascia with interrupted fine catgut. A second row of seromuscular sutures is placed between the bowel and the subcutaneous fat. The colon is then opened and the contents evacuated. With successful decompression, sutures can now be placed between the cut edge of the bowel and the skin. The same procedure can be used for the sigmoid colon, if an opening is necessary in this area.

This approach has several potential disadvantages. These include the necessity for further major abdominal surgery and possible continued bleeding if hemorrhage had been a presenting problem (approximately one fourth of these patients will continue to bleed postoperatively); also, if a septic focus persists, earlier surgical intervention than was first anticipated may be required. The procedure should not be performed in cases of free perforation but only when obvious acute colonic dilatation exists without peritonitis.

*Comment*: I am able to restrain my enthusiasm for the decompression and diversion technique in the treatment of toxic megacolon, primarily for the reasons alluded to above. It is a troublesome concept to commit the patient to at least one other operation when the procedure can be accomplished in one stage, removing the source of sepsis and liberating the patient from contending with at least two abdominal orifices. Drainage from upper and lower abdominal wounds may be a justifiable, albeit unaesthetic, experience if convinced that it is the only life-saving measure available. However, I believe that expeditious, well-conceived resection can accomplish the optimal goal. To deal with a sealed perforation, the transverse colon can be decompressed by simple needle aspiration before the splenic flexure is "attacked." Another alternative is to mobilize the sigmoid, descending, and transverse colon, to divide the bowel at the point of planned resection, and to exteriorize the segment so that minimal contamination will result if a sealed perforation is encountered. Finally, a certain impracticality exists when a "blowhole" colostomy is advised for decompression. In my experience, attempting to suture a profoundly dilated, possibly necrotic transverse colon is more than a frustrating experience—it is impossible.

### Total Colectomy with Rectal Preservation

Total abdominal colectomy with ileorectal or ileosigmoid anastomosis for ulcerative colitis has been advocated by a number of authors. Preservation of the rectum has been addressed earlier with respect to the risk of the subsequent development of malignancy in this segment. The technical aspect of total colectomy is identical to the surgical approach described in Chapter 22. Patients can be offered the option of reestablishment of intestinal continuity if the rectum is relatively free of disease. Under these circumstances, however, always recognize that the diagnosis can be somewhat in question. However, if the patient subsequently is proved to have Crohn's disease, this procedure might have been preferred. The relative merit of the ileorectal anastomosis for ulcerative colitis has diminished considerably, having been virtually replaced by the ileo-pouch-anal procedures (see later).

*Results*

A reduction in frequency of bowel movements to six or fewer within 24 hours was noted in 80% to 85% of cases. Subsequent proctectomy may become necessary for 25% to 55%; ileorectal anastomosis may be appropriate for selected patients with IBD, but the importance of cancer surveillance must be emphasized.

If the patient truly understands this risk and is willing to submit to frequent follow-up examinations, an ileorectal anastomosis should be considered for those in whom the rectum is not severely involved by inflammatory disease. However, if concern for possible development of carcinoma is sufficiently great, conventional proctocolectomy or a pouch-anal procedure should be considered.

## Other Restorative Operations

Other operations for ulcerative colitis that attempt to restore intestinal continuity are poor alternatives. Segmental resection of the sigmoid colon, right colon, and so forth will result uniformly in a 100% recurrence rate that will necessitate further resection. The only exception to the admonition against performing limited resection is for the patient who has severe proctitis or proctosigmoiditis. In an individual incapacitated as a consequence of urgency, tenesmus, incontinence, or bleeding, an abdominoperineal resection might be considered. It is understood, however, that palliation of symptoms does not necessarily preclude the possibility of subsequent recurrence.

## Ileoanal Anastomosis with or without Mucosal Proctectomy

Total colectomy and proctectomy, but with preservation of the anal canal and sphincter muscles, was described by Ravitch and Sabiston in 1947. The procedure fell into disrepute primarily because of the difficulties associated with frequent bowel movements and fecal incontinence. In 1977, Martin et al. described a procedure in children, whereby the entire colon was removed in the usual manner, but the mucosa was stripped from its rectal muscular sleeve and an anastomosis effected between the ileum and the anal canal. By this means, intestinal continuity was reestablished and all the potential disease-bearing area was extirpated. The procedure is theoretically suitable for patients with ulcerative colitis and for those with familial polyposis. However, this operation is not for patients with Crohn's disease.

### Operative Technique

Total abdominal colectomy is performed in the usual manner, and the bowel is resected as low as possible in the rectum. In current practice, the aim is to amputate the rectum as low as is possible, removing the residual mucosa (if any) by way of the perineal dissection. The procedure can be facilitated by infiltrating the submucosa with a dilute epinephrine solution. Because separation of the rectal mucosa can be difficult to accomplish in some patients, either because of friability or scarring, some advocate ultrasonic fragmentation and aspiration. Others prefer to evert the anorectal remnant, exposing the mucosa and excising the stump from the dentate line to the cut edge (Fig. 29.16). Another alternative is to use one of the modifications of the double-stapling technique (see later).

The ileal anastomosis is effected at the level of the dentate line using paired Gelpi retractors or an anal retractor (e.g., Parks, Lone Star) for exposure. Interrupted no. 3-0 long-term absorbable sutures are suggested to anchor the end of the ileum to the anal canal and underlying internal sphincter. A protecting loop ileostomy is virtually always advised.

### Results

Few current data are available for ileoanal anastomosis, because the modification that incorporates an intervening pouch has made this operation practically obsolete, except in children (see later).

The straight ileoanal anastomosis permits reestablishment of intestinal continuity, but with the distinct disadvantage of frequent bowel movements. It requires great motivation indeed on the part of the patient to avoid an ileostomy and be willing to accept seven or more bowel movements per day. Most surgeons have abandoned this procedure in favor of the ileoanal anastomosis with intervening pouch.

### Continent Ileostomy or Kock Procedure

It is self-evident that many patients have been dissatisfied with the encumbrance and emotional burden of wearing an ileostomy appliance. In 1969, Kock described a method of creating a reservoir from the terminal ileum; he subsequently modified it to create an intestinal obstruction by means of an intussuscepted portion of distal ileum, the so-called "nipple valve." Because no appliance is required, the stoma can be placed low on the abdominal wall and essentially flush with the skin. The procedure was enthusiastically received, but recently has been relegated virtually to historic interest, having been replaced by the pouch-anal operations (see later). Patients having this operation today are those for whom pouch-anal operations have failed or are inappropriate, or those who have previously had proctocolectomy and conventional ileostomy and wish to have the stoma revised.

### Technique

Two basic techniques can be used to construct the reservoir. One is analogous to the *S*-shaped reservoir, such as is described for the Parks procedure. This

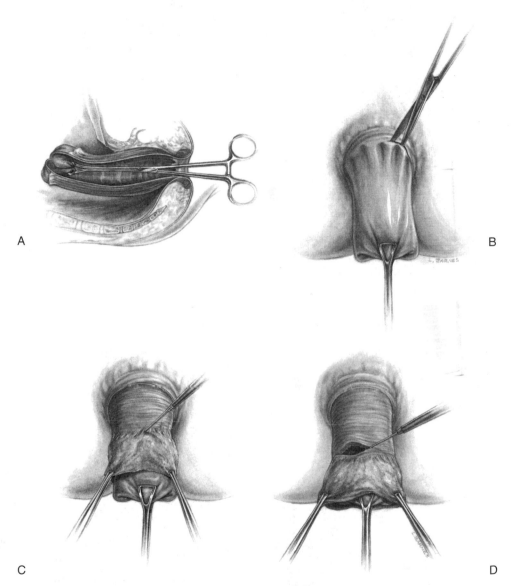

A

B

C

D

**FIG. 29.16.** Technique of eversion mucosectomy. **A.** The rectal stump is everted by placing a clamp on the proximal end. **B.** Mucosal stripping is begun from the dentate line. **C.** Mucosa is stripped using diathermy cautery or by scissors dissection. **D.** The mucosa and redundant muscular sleeve are excised.

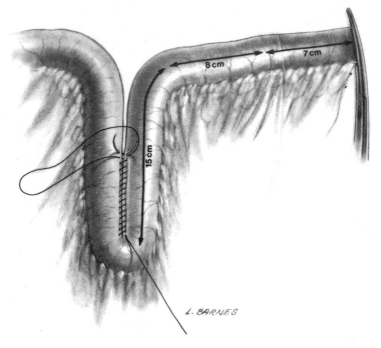

**FIG. 29.17.** Continent ileostomy. Apposition of the bowel.

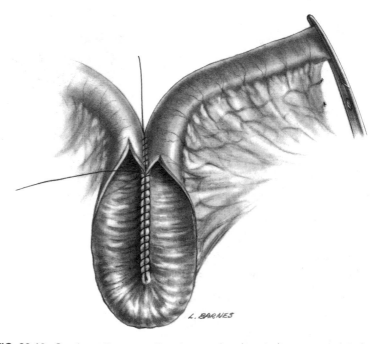

**FIG. 29.18.** Continent ileostomy. Bowel opened and posterior row completed.

method uses approximately 10 cm of ileum for each segment (three in all to create the pouch). An additional 18 to 20 cm is required to create the nipple valve and the conduit.

The Kock technique involves preparation of approximately a 50-cm segment of terminal ileum. A 30-cm segment is used to create the pouch and the remainder to make the valve and the external conduit. Figures 29.17–29.23 illustrate the procedure for preparing the continent (reservoir) ileostomy. An alternative to the conventional suturing method is to staple the pouch. Another modification is shown in Figure 29.30.

Before the ileostomy is "matured," test the competence of the nipple valve by occluding the afferent limb with a rubber-shod clamp. Then, insert a catheter through the nipple valve into the reservoir, and inflate the pouch with air. If the

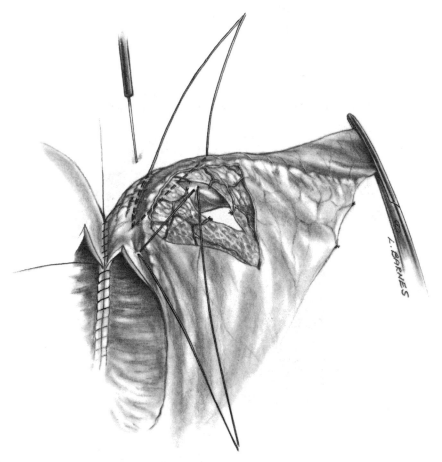

**FIG. 29.19.** Continent ileostomy. Cauterization or stripping of the ileal serosa and placement of sutures to rotate the mesentery 90°.

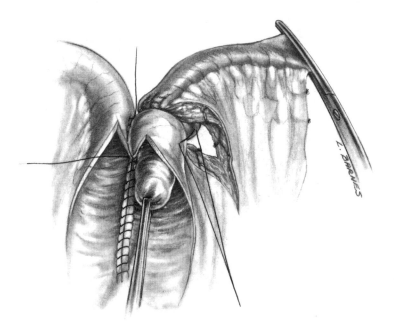

**FIG. 29.20.** Continent ileostomy. A nipple is created and sutures are secured.

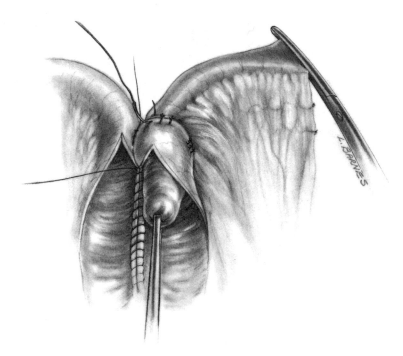

**FIG. 29.21.** Continent ileostomy. Silk sutures are placed from conduit to reservoir.

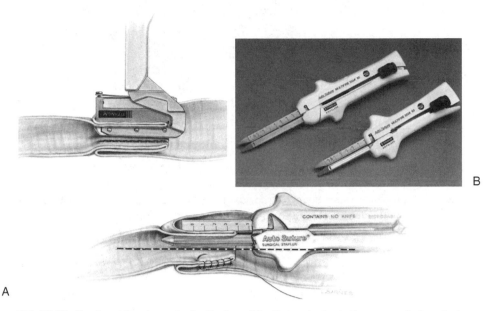

B

A

**FIG. 29.22.** Continent ileostomy. **A.** Application of the linear stapler to three areas in the nipple valve to prevent desusception. **B.** Alternatively, a SGIA-60 stapler (without the blade) or simple sutures can be used. The instruments without the knife are available in two sizes (*inset*). (Courtesy of United States Surgical Corp., Norwalk, CT, USA.)

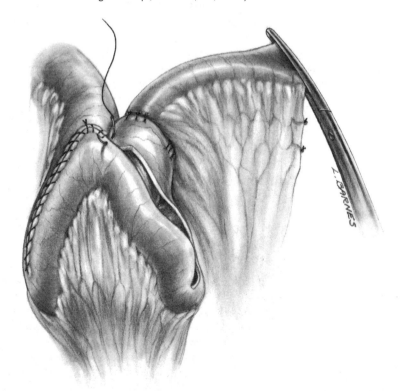

**FIG. 29.23.** Continent ileostomy. The reservoir is closed by folding over.

air fails to escape following catheter removal, assume that the valve is competent. The catheter is then replaced into the reservoir, and the air should dissipate.

The major problem with the Kock procedure is maintaining the position of the nipple; slippage is attributed to traction forces on the mesentery of the nipple during reservoir filling. A number of modifications have been proposed to address this complication, including implantation of Mersilene mesh to reinforce the nipple, magnetic closure using the Maclet device, stripping of the serosa, and even creation of a protecting loop ileostomy above the reservoir. The use of a fascial sling threaded through the mesentery has been suggested. Encircling the ileal outlet with a 1-cm strip of Marlex mesh or Teflon (passed through the mesentery of the reservoir and outlet) has been used, although this can cause other problems (e.g., fistula). A combination of triangular stripping of the mesenteric fat, serosal scarification, and rotation of the nipple valve segments has been demonstrated to be safe and effective in preventing nipple dessusception. The use of the CUSA (Cavitron Ultrasonic Surgical Aspirator, Cavitron Surgical Systems, Inc., Stamford, Connecticut) to strip the mesentery and remove the fat has also been suggested.

Another technique involves anchoring the nipple valve to the anterior pouch wall by stapling. A 2-cm transverse enterotomy is made in the anterior pouch wall just below the point where the intussuscepted nipple lies. The valve is then aligned with the anterior pouch wall away from the primary anterior suture line, and a single application of the linear stapler is used to anchor the nipple valve to the anterior pouch wall. The anvil of the stapler is brought through the transverse enterotomy from outside the pouch to pass along the inside of the nipple valve, thereby effecting a stapled anchorage. The anterior pouch wall and the enterotomy are then closed.

Barnett modified the procedure to prevent dessusception, using an adjacent segment of intestine to encircle the base of the valve as a "collar," a maneuver analogous to that of a Nissen gastric fundoplication. The lumen of the intestinal "collar" communicates with the pouch itself, allowing gas and fecal contents to enter. This acts to buttress the nipple valve and conduit, providing a greater degree of security against leakage. The technique is briefly described and illustrated in Figure 29.24.

### Postoperative Care

Before leaving the operating room, the surgeon places a heavy silk suture around a Silastic catheter that has been inserted into the pouch. This is secured to the skin, and a dressing is applied in such a manner that the catheter exits upward and gently curves into a drainage tube, and thence into a drainable bag. The straight exit of the catheter minimizes the risk for necrosis of the conduit should the catheter be under tension on one side. The dressing is left in place for 72 hours before the stoma is examined. An alternative is to use a Marlen continent ileostomy drainage system. The catheter can also be held in place by pass-

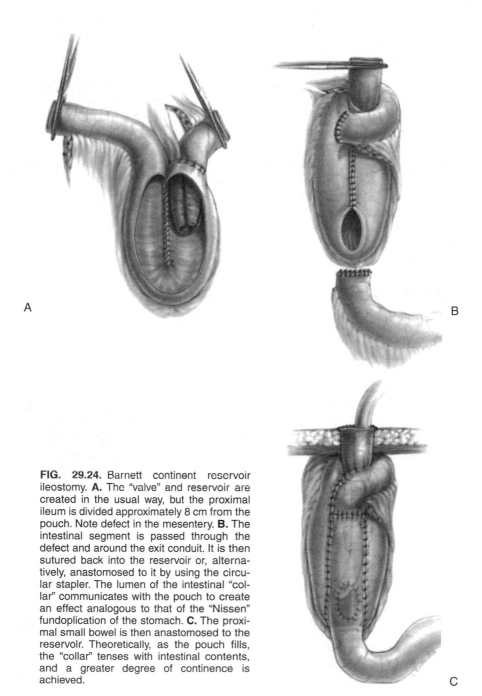

**FIG. 29.24.** Barnett continent reservoir ileostomy. **A.** The "valve" and reservoir are created in the usual way, but the proximal ileum is divided approximately 8 cm from the pouch. Note defect in the mesentery. **B.** The intestinal segment is passed through the defect and around the exit conduit. It is then sutured back into the reservoir or, alternatively, anastomosed to it by using the circular stapler. The lumen of the intestinal "collar" communicates with the pouch to create an effect analogous to that of the "Nissen" fundoplication of the stomach. **C.** The proximal small bowel is then anastomosed to the reservoir. Theoretically, as the pouch fills, the "collar" tenses with intestinal contents, and a greater degree of continence is achieved.

ing it through one of the perforations in a latex band, the type that is often used as a leg strap for a urine or bile bag.

Usually, only serosanguineous drainage occurs for the first several days; eventually this becomes bile-stained and then feculent. The patient is then begun on a progressive schedule of oral intake, but a low-residue diet is suggested to avoid plugging of the catheter. The drainage tube remains in place for 3 weeks, after which the patient is advised to clamp it for 10 to 15 minutes every 3 or 4 hours. During the night, it is left to drain continuously. After 1 month, intermittent catheterization is advised, initially every 3 or 4 hours and usually once during the night. After approximately 1 week of this regimen, nightly intubations are omitted and the interval for catheterization during the day is extended. Ultimately, the patient develops a time frequency based on convenience and the feeling of fullness that compels drainage of the reservoir. However, because radiologic studies reveal that reflux into the afferent limb increases with sensations of fullness and abdominal pressure, the patient should probably empty the reservoir at regular intervals.

Occasionally, formed fecal material and high-residue items (e.g., popcorn, mushrooms) require irrigation by means of a syringe, but this is usually unnecessary. A simple dressing is placed over the flush stoma, or one of the commercially available security pouches can be used.

### Complications

The greatest concern in the postoperative period is the possibility of leakage from one of the reservoir suture lines. Obviously, this can be of catastrophic consequence, requiring emergency surgical intervention. Initially, this complication was reported much more commonly than it is today. The reduced frequency can be attributed to the improved techniques of reservoir construction and the careful selection of patients for this procedure.

If surgical intervention becomes necessary in the immediate postoperative period for presumed suture-line leakage, every attempt should be made to preserve the ileal reservoir. This can usually be accomplished by a diverting proximal loop ileostomy and appropriate surgical drainage, with or without closure of the leak. Subsequent radiologic investigation may reveal that the fistula spontaneously closed even without repair.

However, if it appears that the reservoir is beyond salvation, it must be resected and a neoileostomy created. If the patient has had a procedure for what subsequently proves to be Crohn's disease, a suture-line leak has an ominous prognosis indeed. Under such circumstances, it is probably the wiser course to remove the pouch and create a new ileostomy.

Late complications of the continent ileostomy procedure are myriad: fecal incontinence resulting from reduction of the nipple valve, ileitis ("pouchitis"), recurrent Crohn's disease, catheter perforation, pouch fistula, detachment of the pouch from the abdominal wall, volvulus of the reservoir, urolithiasis, obstruction from inspissated material, stomal stenosis, and intestinal obstruction from a lost catheter.

*Nipple Valve Slippage.* As stated, the complication associated with reduction of the nipple valve and resultant incontinence is the most troublesome and most frequently observed late management problem (Fig. 29.25). Difficulty with intubation of the reservoir is suggestive of dessusception. The kinking of the intraabdominal portion of the distal ileum may in itself create a partial small-bowel obstruction. Under these circumstances, however, the patient usually is incontinent but not obstructed.

Physiologic studies of the nipple valve and pouch reveal that electric and motor patterns of the undistended ileum are similar with both types of ileostomy, but the anatomic and motor properties of the pouch allow it to accept far larger intraluminal volumes, both during fasting and after feeding. Pressure studies on the pouch, nipple valve, and outlet demonstrate the presence of a high-pressure zone in the nipple valve relative to the pouch. Distension of the pouch with air causes a tonic contraction that travels from the pouch along the intestinal layers of the intussuscepted nipple valve and the outlet. It is postulated that this is the mechanism for dessusception of the nipple valve, a complication that may be

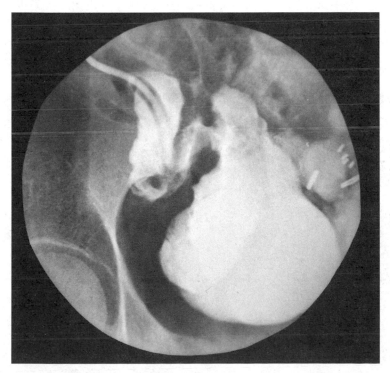

**FIG. 29. 25.** Dessuscepted nipple can be readily appreciated on this "pouchogram." Acute angulation precludes catheterization even with no leakage.

avoided by frequent intubation of the pouch. Other studies have demonstrated the functions of the mucosa and smooth muscle of the continent ileal pouch to be similar to those of normal ileum.

The diagnosis of nipple valve slippage can usually be made clinically. However, it is valuable to confirm the position of the nipple radiographically. This can be done by a barium enema study through the stoma or by upper gastrointestinal roentgenography (Fig. 29.26). The radiographic feature of a normal continent ileostomy on a plane abdominal film is the presence of a lobulated, gas-filled structure in the middle or right lower abdomen. With contrast material, the terminal, invaginated ileal segment resembles an inverted nipple protruding into the pouch. Barium enema examination can reveal the size of the reservoir; the effluent can be measured and the adequacy of the emptying confirmed. Other complications of continent ileostomy (e.g., small-bowel obstruction, anastomotic leakage, intraabdominal abscess, fistula formation, failure of the reservoir to dilate, and the presence of recurrent Crohn's disease) can also be confirmed radiographically.

Reduction of the nipple valve and kinking of the conduit are usually the causes of obstruction at the level of the reservoir. Revision is required to relieve the problem. Although the purpose of the operation, of course, is to create an intestinal obstruction, one of the distinct disadvantages is the need to have a catheter readily available. If a patient loses it and is unable to obtain one, a serious problem ensues. Relief of the obstruction cannot be obtained unless proper

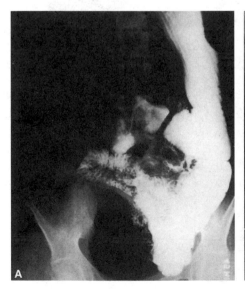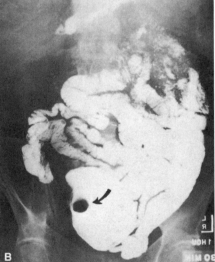

**FIG. 29.26.** Continent ileostomy. Small-bowel series. **A.** Normal pouch filling the pelvis on the right side. **B.** Normal reservoir and nipple valve (*arrow*).

equipment is available. Patients who enjoy outings away from civilization are well advised to secure the catheter on their person with great care.

*Pouchitis.* Pouch ileitis or "pouchitis" occurs at some time in 7% to 43% of patients with a continent ileostomy. Manifestations include a flulike syndrome, fever, diarrhea, bleeding, abdominal pain, generalized toxicity, and severe ileitis. Increased ileostomy output requiring more frequent intubation is a common presentation. The condition is believed caused by a change in the flora of the pouch, particularly an overgrowth of anaerobic organisms. Interestingly, this complication is rare in patients who have the procedure for familial polyposis. Barium enema study is usually not helpful, although thickening of the mucosal folds may be apparent. Endoscopic examination will usually reveal contact bleeding, friability, and an erythematous, ulcerated mucosa. Oral metronidazole (Flagyl) is the recommended treatment. Continuous drainage of the reservoir can have an ameliorative effect but, in the rare situation, it may be necessary to remove the pouch. Recurrence is not uncommon, and under these circumstances consider the possibility of Crohn's disease. Many of these patients respond rapidly to steroids. The condition is also seen in patients who have had an ileal reservoir-anal anastomosis created (see later).

*Other Complications.* Other unusual complications of the reservoir and nipple valve have been reported. These include the development of an enormous ileal pouch (the result of chronic outlet obstruction), and volvulus with obstruction leading to perforation. A case of invasive adenocarcinoma in a reservoir that had been in place for 17 years has also been reported.

Hemorrhage from the nipple valve or reservoir has also been reported. This can be caused by trauma during insertion of the catheter (perforation of the pouch can actually occur), but it is usually associated with a nonspecific inflammation of the mucosa, so-called "pouchitis."

Detachment of the pouch from the anterior abdominal wall has been reported to produce angulation of the efferent limb and difficulty intubating the pouch. Operative correction is required.

Urolithiasis is a well-known associated complication in patients who have had conventional ileostomy. Patients with pouch have similar urine volumes, pH levels, and uric acid concentrations, and would appear to be at the same level of risk for stone formation. Study of patients who have documented malabsorption or symptoms of a malfunctioning pouch reveals that the number of jejunal and ileal anaerobic bacteria decrease during treatment with metronidazole, implicating overgrowth of anaerobic bacterial flora in the pathogenesis of the syndrome.

Bile acid excretion rates are significantly increased in those with a continent ileostomy and an ileal resection. Also, continent ileostomy is associated with a significantly increased percentage of water content and a reduction in the pH of the ileal effluent.

*Nipple Valve Revision.* The nipple can be reconstructed by performing an enterotomy in the reservoir, reintussuscepting the distal ileum, and resecuring it. However, it may not be possible to accomplish this maneuver because of necrosis of the ileum, inadequate length of the conduit, or bowel injury during the process of mobilization. Under these circumstances, a new nipple can be created without sacrificing the reservoir. This is achieved by using the afferent limb, oversewing the old efferent conduit opening, and performing an anastomosis of the proximal ileum to another part of the reservoir. This is the method usually required to convert a reservoir-ileoanal anastomosis (Parks) to a continent ileostomy (Kock). In the former operation, usually an insufficient length of terminal ileum remains (that had been anastomosed to the anal canal) to create a nipple valve and conduit. By oversewing the efferent end and using the proximal bowel to create a new nipple and conduit, the reservoir can be preserved. Conversely, if the sphincter muscles have been preserved, it may be possible to convert a Kock pouch to a reservoir-anal anastomosis. If a short mesentery precludes the possibility of constructing a pelvic pouch, a temporary continent ileostomy can be performed with the expectation that the expanded reservoir may subsequently permit conversion.

Noninvasive means for maintaining continence after the valve has dessuscepted include insertion of various balloon tubes (e.g., an endotracheal tube) or, my own preference, a Prager balloon plug.

## Results

Many studies from numerous centers have been published, with many providing follow-up reports. These clearly demonstrate a high level of early complications (15% to 25%), and considerably fewer in later series (5% to 10%), reflecting a learning curve. Nipple slippage seems to be the most commonly reported complication, with up to 46% of complications being accounted for by this problem, although some authors have reported as few as 4%. Increased weight gain may have been a contributing factor, as the patients were generally well and had a much more fatty mesentery when operated on the second time. Subsequent revision of the nipple valve was required in as many as 50% of cases, and excision of the pouch in 7% to 10%. Revision was required less often in women, in younger patients, and in those with a primary proctocolectomy and continent ileostomy. If a malfunctioning valve develops, ideally it should be revised rather than a new one created; revision was felt to be technically simpler, and the long-term results were comparable.

Anastomotic leak has been shown in 6% to 12% of cases, and mortality rates are reported to be around 2%. Pouchitis is common, with 30% to 50% of patients experiencing this complication at some time.

However, continence is generally good—most reporting between 90% and 100%—and a high level of patient satisfaction persists even though the complication rate is high. McLeod and Fazio have noted that 97% of their patients would choose revisional surgery rather than have the continent ileostomy removed.

Morphologic and histochemical studies performed on the continent ileostomy reservoir for up to 10 years after its construction reveal no alarming changes in terms of dysplasia, fibrosis, or progressive atrophy. Histochemical investigation of the mucosa reveals largely unchanged, strong enzymatic activity involved in both oxidative metabolism and secretory functions.

*Comment*: Most observers experienced with the continent ileostomy believe that the operation offers a reasonably satisfactory alternative to the conventional procedure. The encumbrance of an appliance, the occasional "accidents" with appliance management, the unaesthetic proboscis on the abdominal wall, sexual inhibition, and psychological embarrassment have stimulated many patients to seek an alternative procedure. However, despite the many improvements in surgical technique, the procedure is still fraught with numerous complications. The Kock pouch is not for everyone. It is contraindicated in patients with Crohn's disease (although some authors have suggested that the Kock continent ileostomy be considered for patients with Crohn's disease, provided no evidence is seen of recurrence for 5 years), and the results in older people and those who are somewhat obese are poor. However, the quality of life for individuals who have elected the continent ileostomy is unquestionably improved in most cases. But, the matter seems rather academic; with the exception of conversion from conventional ileostomy, the operation has been virtually replaced by the pouch-anal procedures.

### *Total Proctocolectomy and Ileoanal Anastomosis with Intervening Pouch, or Parks Procedure; Pouch-Anal Procedure; Ileo-Pouch-Anal Procedure; Restorative Proctocolectomy*

As discussed, total abdominal proctocolectomy with ileoanal anastomosis is associated with frequent bowel movements, urgency, and fecal incontinence in a high percentage of cases. To address this problem, Valiente and Bacon, in 1955, described the application of an intervening pouch with an ileoanal anastomosis in experimental animals. With the success of the ileal reservoir as developed by Kock, Parks and Nicholls in 1978 reported an operation combining the application of an ileal pouch that eliminated propulsive activity and acted as a storage organ with preservation of the entire sphincter mechanism. In the past 20 years, the preponderance of publications on the surgical management of ulcerative colitis have addressed variations on this procedure, the morbidity, the physiologic effects, and the functional results.

### *Technique (S Type)*

The patient is placed in the perineolithotomy position as if for an abdominoperineal resection. Following completion of the colectomy and excision of the rectum as far distally as is possible (see previous section), an ileal reservoir is created. The distal ileum is transected with the GIA stapler as close to the cecum as is possible. Tension on the ileal mesentery is a potential problem because the bowel must be brought virtually to the perianal skin. If the tip of the conduit (or pouch) reaches 6 cm below the pubic symphysis, the dentate line will be satisfactorily reached.

Complete mobilization of the mesentery up to the level of the duodenum is imperative. The ileal artery can be divided to achieve additional length, and the parietal peritoneum of the distal ileum may be incised.

Parks and Nicholls suggested that an S-type reservoir be created (Fig. 29.27). In this modification, the terminal 50 cm of ileum is measured and folded twice to give three segments of bowel, the proximal two of which are 15 cm long and the distal segment 20 cm long (Fig. 29.27A). A 5-cm length of ileum projects beyond the pouch, which is the area to be used for the anastomosis. The ileum is

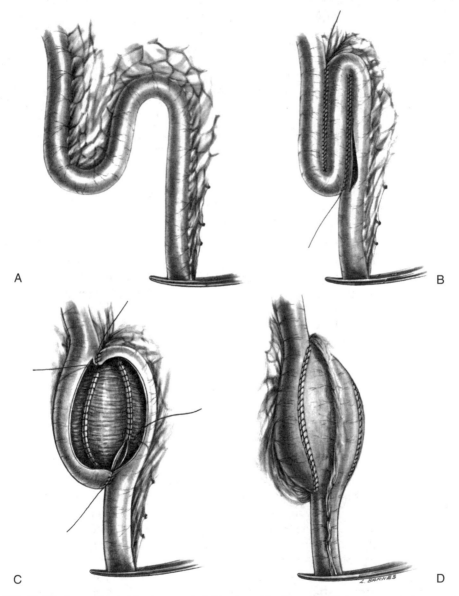

A

B

C

D

**FIG. 29.27.** S-type (Parks) ileal reservoir. **A.** The bowel is aligned. **B.** The antimesenteric aspect is opened after serosal apposition. **C.** Suturing of the adjacent walls. **D.** The reservoir is completed with an ileoanal anastomosis.

opened on its antimesenteric border (Fig. 29.27B), and the adjacent loops are sutured (Fig. 29.27C). An interrupted technique can be used, but a continuous suture of no. 3-0 long-term absorbable material is more expeditious. The two outer edges are then folded across to complete the pouch, with the closure effected using the same suture material (Fig. 29.27D).

Another alternative for pouch construction is to use a stapling technique (see later). This is a much more rapid approach, but it has the theoretic disadvantage of more tissue inversion and, therefore, decreased reservoir capacity.

The anastomosis is performed via the transanal approach by using an anal retractor, paired Gelpi retractors placed at right angles, or a self-retaining Lone Star retractor. In contrast to earlier suggestions, most surgeons today make no attempt to preserve a muscular sleeve. The full thickness of the ileum is sutured to the anal canal at the level of the dentate line, incorporating the underlying internal anal sphincter muscle. Alternatively, an anastomosis can be performed in the anal canal by using the circular stapling device, with or without a double-stapling approach, but care must be taken to avoid placing the staple line too low (see later).

### Concomitant Ileostomy

Irrespective of the type of pouch constructed, a loop ileostomy is usually advised to protect the anastomosis but some surgeons have selectively performed the procedure without a diversionary stoma. The construction and closure of an ileostomy is not without morbidity (see Chapter 31) and may actually increase the risk for postoperative bowel obstruction. Suggested criteria for considering this option are absolute lack of tension on the anastomosis, good blood supply to the terminal ileum, good general health, and no recent steroid use.

### Technique (J Type)

Another option, the so-called J pouch, was initially suggested by Utsunomiya et al. This type of pouch is prepared by selecting the point at which the ileal loop reaches the lowest level in the pelvis, usually about 20 to 30 cm from the end of the ileum. The length of the pouch is variable but generally is approximately 20 cm.

As mentioned, one of the critical concerns in the performance of the reservoir-anal techniques is the creation of an anastomosis that is free of tension. Optimally, the approach to mesenteric lengthening is best achieved by (a) division of the terminal ileum as close to the cecum as is possible; (b) mobilization of the mesentery of the small bowel to the third portion of the duodenum; and (c) selection of the apex of the J reservoir. The objective is to extend the mesentery 6 cm beyond the pubic symphysis. Mesenteric lengthening can be achieved through a number of possible maneuvers. In the first instance, care should be taken to divide the mesentery as close to the colon as possible to preserve the branches of the ileocolic artery. If incisions along the mesenteric peritoneum produce inadequate length and a window must be created, blood supply to the pouch can still be preserved.

Apposition of the loop can be performed by using a continuous double-layer suture technique, thereby creating a long, side-to-side anastomosis (Fig. 29.28). Alternatively, the GIA stapling device can be used to create the reservoir. Newer stapling instruments have been introduced that permit easier pouch construction, a long (8-cm) GIA. The stapler can be inserted in the middle of each limb or optimally through the apex. Care must be taken to pull the mesentery away from the bowel to avoid its incorporation in the line of staples. This opening can then be used for insertion of the proximal anvil. With this technique, it is necessary to pass the instrument cephalad once or twice more, using an intussuscepting maneuver. The endoscopic stapler has been suggested to create the J reservoir, as the length of this instrument allows the device to be applied multiple times without the problem of intussuscepting the intestine. Others have even suggested performing the operation laparoscopically; however, this is no mean achievement. When done in this manner, it appears to be associated with a higher morbidity than when the conventional, open technique is used.

### Effecting the Anastomosis

With the apical purse-string suture in place, another purse-string suture is placed at the top of the anal canal, incorporating the internal sphincter. The sutures are then secured, and the circular stapler is fired. Of course, a suture technique, such as has been described, can be used to complete the pouch-anal anastomosis.

Another method for completing the anastomosis is the double-stapling technique. This is analogous to the method used for effecting a low anastomosis for cancer of the rectum (see Chapter 23). The pouch construction is the same as described above, but linear closure of the rectal stump is performed instead of a purse string being used. Some have criticized the double-stapling technique as inadequate for removing the rectal mucosa. Some fear the possibility of malignancy arising in the remaining glandular epithelium and are also concerned about symptoms from residual inflammation. Furthermore, preservation of the anal transitional zone may actually preserve the disease. However, it is clear that the more maneuvers are used and the anal canal stretched, the more likely there will be an adverse impact on bowel control. Where and how to place the anastomosis remains a matter of some controversy.

Another method for creating an anastomosis is performed transanally by means of a purse-string suture. This is often a tedious maneuver and risks excessive dilatation and stretching of the sphincter mechanism. Additionally, eversion of the rectum might be performed to reestablish intestinal continuity and to facilitate a mucosectomy, if this is to be considered. The problem, as alluded to above, is that eversion is not associated with as good a functional outcome when compared with a stapled anastomosis prepared without eversion.

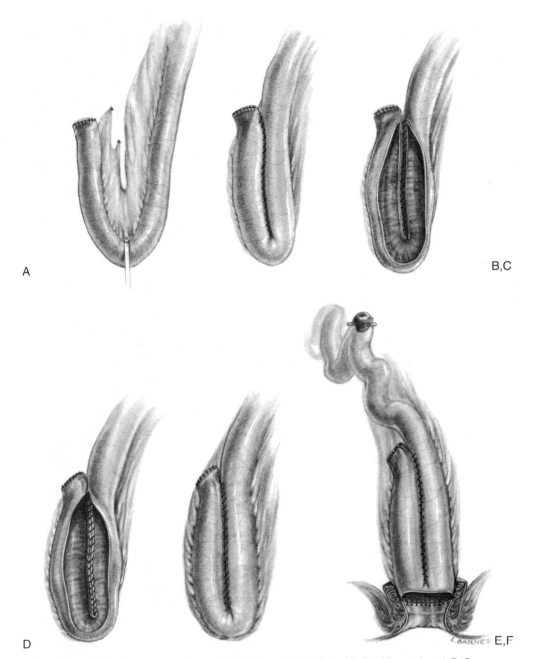

**FIG. 29.28.** Pouch-anal procedure (J type). **A.** Limbs identified with distal ileum closed. **B.** Seromuscular apposition. **C.** Long enterotomy. **D.** Closure of posterior wall. **E.** Closure of anterior wall. **F.** Completed anastomosis of pouch to anus with protecting loop ileostomy.

The stapling technique has permitted relatively effortless pouch construction and anastomosis, and because of this, an overwhelming majority of surgeons performing this operation prefer it.

### Technique (Lateral Ileal)

Fonkalsrud offered another option for creating an ileoanal-pouch anastomosis—the lateral ileal reservoir. This method is accomplished by dividing and oversewing the proximal end of the ileum approximately 25 to 30 cm above the peritoneal reflection. I believe an ileal reservoir of 14 to 16 cm in length appears to provide optimal function. A temporary end-ileostomy is then used for diversion (Fig. 29.29A). A lateral reservoir is constructed over the entire length of the original segment at a subsequent operation (Fig. 29.29B). Fonkalsrud's approach seems to be used essentially only by himself and has never achieved the popularity of the other alternatives. In fact, Fonkalsrud himself has moved virtually exclusively to the J pouch during the past 5 years.

### Other Approaches

One of the concerns about the S reservoir is the fact that many patients require catheterization of the pouch to effect evacuation. Conversely, the J pouch, although eliminating the requirement for catheterization, has been thought to be associated with increased stool frequency because of a smaller reservoir capacity (see later). To address these problems, another modification has been proposed, the so-called quadruple-loop or W reservoir. The terminal 50 cm of small bowel is folded into four loops, each 12 cm long, forming a *W*-shaped configuration (Fig. 29.30). The S pouch can also be constructed with the stapling instruments. As with the J pouch, the reservoir itself can be anastomosed to the anal canal.

### Ileal Kock Pouch

Kock et al. reported the application of the standard, double-folded ileal reservoir (Kock pouch) as a pouch-anal alternative. Six patients had interposition of the pouch between the ileum and the anus following colectomy and mucosal proctectomy. After the ileostomy was closed, the range of bowel evacuations was three to five per 24-hour period. The large reservoir capacity and the low pressure were believed to explain the excellent functional results. Further experience with this approach seems warranted.

### Postoperative Management

Following closure of the ileostomy, patients almost inevitably are troubled by frequent bowel movements and, perhaps, problems with continence. It is impor-

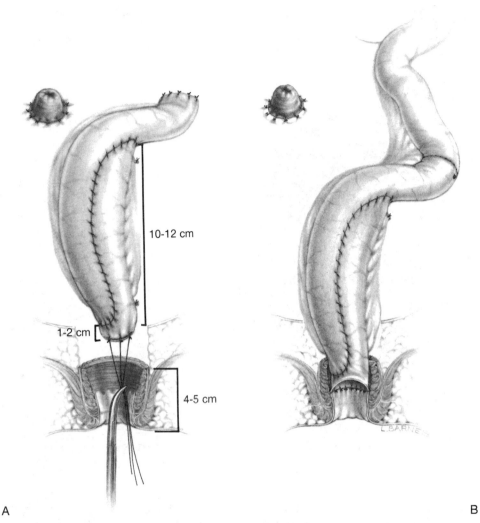

10-12 cm

1-2 cm

4-5 cm

A

B

**FIG. 29.29.** Lateral ileal reservoir (Fonkalsrud). **A.** Ileal reservoir is created using a side-to-side technique, either by hand-sewing or with the long GIA instrument. **B.** The ileal spout is drawn through the rectal muscle cuff to the anus and the ileoanal anastomosis is effected. Note that Fonkalsrud prefers to use an end-ileostomy. (From Fonkalsrud EW, Phillips JD. Reconstruction of malfunctioning ileoanal pouch procedures as an alternative to permanent ileostomy. *Am J Surg* 1990;160:245.)

tant, therefore, to prepare the patient emotionally for these consequences and to offer management alternatives. As with ostomates, an enterostomal therapist is an invaluable resource for counseling patients. They are given a list of foods that may increase or decrease stool output and frequency. Foods that have been demonstrated to exacerbate gastrointestinal disturbances are apple juice, raw fruits, raw vegetables, popcorn, seeds, nuts, beans, corn, beer, caffeine, choco-

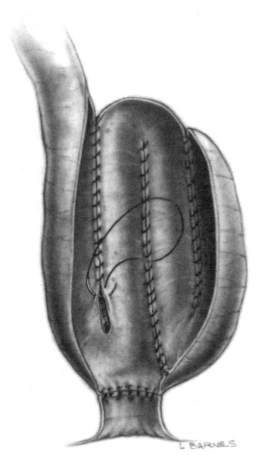

**FIG. 29.30.** Quadruple reservoir—hand-sewn.

late, milk and milk products, and spicy foods. The diet can be supplemented by one of the liquid nutrition products (e.g., Ensure). Ample fluid intake is strongly encouraged to avoid dehydration. Supplementary medication in the form of "slowing" agents is often helpful (e.g., loperamide [Imodium], diphenoxylate [Lomotil], deodorized tincture of opium, paregoric, codeine). A bulking agent (e.g., psyllium) can be added, and cholestyramine (Questran) may be ameliorative. Topical agents for perianal irritation may be required. An aggressive approach to the medical management of these patients is necessary to give them confidence until time permits bowel function to become relatively stabilized.

## Complications of Pouch Procedures

Despite the magnitude of the operation, operative mortality has been remarkably low—virtually anecdotal. In a review from the Mayo Clinic involving 1,603 patients who had proctocolectomy with pouch-anal reconstruction, 3 deaths occurred postoperatively (0.2%), and none of these were directly related to the intestinal disease. Late deaths occurred in 29 patients (1.8%). These were primarily related to carcinogenic and extracolonic manifestations of underlying or unrelated coexisting diseases and events. However, all published reports recognize that ileoanal-reservoir operations are associated with a high frequency of complications, often well in excess of 50%. These include pouchitis, anal stenosis, intestinal obstruction, "cuff abscess," stomal problems, ileus, fistulas, sepsis, hemorrhage, evacuation problems, ischemia, and a host of others. Generally, complications are more frequent in the early experience with the operation than in the later. Despite what may appear to be indomitable problems, every effort should be made to preserve the pouch. The success with various salvage operations has been reported by a number of investigators (see later).

*Perforation.* With the techniques currently used to create the reservoir, pouch perforation itself has become relatively unusual. The rate has been constant at approximately 1% to 4%, but the requirement for reservoir excision as a consequence of this complication has decreased as experience has been gained. Perforation of the terminal ileal appendage of the J pouch has also been noted. To avoid this complication, it is probably wise to secure the distal ileum to the reservoir or to amputate any terminal ileal appendage after pouch construction. Parenthetically, perforation of the pouch as a consequence of blunt trauma to the abdomen has also been noted.

*Anastomotic Leak.* Anastomotic leak is usually caused by one of several factors (tension on the suture line, ischemic necrosis, or sepsis) and is virtually always associated with the subsequent development of an anal stricture. It is because of the risk for this complication that a protecting ileostomy is usually advised. A 10% to 14% anal anastomotic leak rate has been described. However, because most centers have adopted a stapling technique, very little has been reported recently with respect to this particular complication. Whether this is because of the application of protecting ileostomy by most surgeons or the failure to pursue appropriate investigation of patients within the first few weeks after operation is not known. Still, leaks following a stapled anastomosis seem to have a better prognosis than those that occur following hand-sewn anastomosis. It is generally agreed that the major causes for pouch failure are poor functional results, pelvic sepsis, and unsuspected Crohn's disease

*Pelvic and "Cuff" Abscess.* Pelvic abscess was observed in 11% of patients in the earlier Mayo Clinic series and some surgeons favor preservation of the omentum to limit the risk for septic complications. Cuff abscess, specifically, which results from the creation of a long muscular sleeve, was a frequently recognized problem when this technique was popularized. Because all surgeons now endeavor to limit the length of the mucosectomy, this complication has become much less common.

*Intestinal Obstruction.* Intestinal obstruction, one of the most frequent problems after this operation, develops in 16% to 22% of patients. The obstruction can be caused by adhesions, internal hernia, reservoir angulation, or outlet problems, or it may be related to the loop ileostomy. As discussed in Chapter 22, the frequency of abdominal adhesions leading to intestinal obstruction precipitated a prospective, randomized trial with the use of a sodium hyaluronate-based bioresorbable membrane. By direct, standardized peritoneal visualization before closure of the ileostomy, this membrane was demonstrated to be safe, and it also significantly reduced the incidence, extent, and severity of postoperative abdominal adhesions.

The most common point of obstruction appears to be at closure of the ileostomy (50%). The ileostomy should not be rotated to facilitate emptying, as this seems to predispose to subsequent obstruction in a number of patients. Small-bowel obstruction is also often attributed to acute angulation of the afferent limb at the pouch inlet. Bypass of the obstructed segment from the distal ileum to the pouch is not only possible, but it also constitutes safe and effective management. Duodenal obstruction resulting from arteriomesenteric obstruction (superior mesenteric artery syndrome) has also been reported.

*Stomal Complications.* Ileostomy complications (e.g., stomal retraction, high ileostomy output, and parastomal hernia) are at least as frequent as the problems encountered relative to the pouch or the anastomosis. Dehydration requiring readmission to the hospital occurred in 20%. More than one half have problems with appliance management; retraction is seen in about 15%. Other complications include prolapse, fistula, and abscess; ileostomy dysfunction alone was noted in approximately 10%. As mentioned, some experienced surgeons have suggested that a temporary ileostomy can be avoided in selected patients. However, it has been demonstrated that patients with incomplete fecal diversion have a significantly higher incidence of pouch-anal anastomotic complications (44%) than those who have had complete diversion (14%).

*Ileal Pouch-Anal and Ileal Pouch-Vaginal Fistulas.* Fistula between the pouch and the vagina is an uncommon complication following the pouch-anal operations. Although no clear documentation is found for the cause, it is likely to be trauma during the anterior dissection, either at the time of mobilization of the rectum through the abdomen, or when the transanal dissection is done. In the latter situation, it is suspected that a woman with an ectopic anus (anterior displacement) is most vulnerable (see Chapter 13). Another possibility that must be considered is Crohn's disease, in which an incidence of 6% to 7% of this complication has been noted. Fistulas from the ileoanal reservoir to the perianal skin develop in approximately 5%, and fistulas from the reservoir or anastomotic line to other sites can be found in an additional 4%. Treatment options are essentially those that have been described for the management of this condition when it is not associated with a pouch procedure (see Chapters 12 and 13). These include transanal, transabdominal, and transvaginal closure; endoanal advancement flap; seton division; fecal diversion; and gracilis muscle interposition. Most surgeons prefer endovaginal or endoileal flap advancement. It may be necessary, however, to consider temporary ileostomy and reconstruction or even removal of the pouch. Late presentation of vaginal fistula is more frequently associated with Crohn's disease and is unlikely to result in pouch salvage. Impairment of bowel control following conventional fistula surgery in women is the rule rather than the exception. The likelihood of keeping the patient's ileoanal reservoir with this complication is therefore problematic.

*Anal Stricture.* Anal (anastomotic) stricture occurred in approximately 8% to 14%. The presence of an anal stricture may be the most significant factor contributing to a less-than-satisfactory functional result. Treatment consists usually of dilatation, but persistent symptoms may require an anoplasty (see Chapter 8) or a pouch advancement and neoileoanal anastomosis.

*Pouchitis.* Pouchitis, a term coined by Kock to describe the reservoir ileitis seen with the continent ileostomy, is a well-recognized complication of all pouch procedures, about as frequently noted as small-bowel obstruction. The condition is usually manifested by increased output of liquid stool, sometimes with blood, a low-grade fever, weakness, and malaise. The problem is believed caused by stasis of feces in the pouch with overgrowth of anaerobic organisms. The general impression is that pouchitis occurs rarely when the various reservoir procedures have been performed for familial polyposis, which develops in 30% to 50% of those with ulcerative colitis and 5% to 6% with familial polyposis. It has been suggested, therefore, that the likely cause is related somehow to that of ulcerative colitis. The cause of the condition has been investigated at a number of centers. Some support a role for mucosal ischemia and production of oxygen free radicals and have employed allopurinol, a xanthine oxidase inhibitor, and found that this agent either terminated an episode of acute pouchitis or prevented pouchitis from recurring in approximately 50% of patients. Smokers appear to have significantly fewer episodes of pouchitis when compared with nonsmokers and former smokers. Finally, the finding that pANCA occur more frequently in patients with chronic pouchitis suggests the possibility that this antibody may mark a genetically distinct subset of ulcerative colitis patients who are predisposed to the subsequent development of pouchitis.

Two apparently distinct patterns of presentation are seen based on the clinical course: those with two or fewer episodes and those with more than two. The Lahey Clinic has reported that those in the former group responded generally to antianaerobic organism therapy, whereas only 25% in the latter group did so. The authors also identified a subset of patients with so-called "short-segment pouchitis." They attribute this to retained rectal mucosa and have treated the problem successfully with topical steroid preparations.

Treatment usually consists of oral metronidazole or enemas containing steroids or salicylate derivatives, but recurrence is not uncommon (see earlier). Solitary pouch ulceration has also been described. Recurrent or intractable disease should alert the physician to the possibility of Crohn's disease involvement.

*Skin Irritation.* Severe perianal skin irritation is reported to occur in up to 10% of patients, likely caused by frequent bowel action and incontinence. Bowel management programs, including bulking agents and diphenoxylate hydrochloride (Lomotil) or loperamide (Imodium), have usually been advised. Topical application of 5% cholestyramine ointment in polyethylene glycol base has been reported to be helpful. Some are concerned that patients with presumed ulcerative colitis and significant perianal disease, in fact, may have Crohn's disease. However, a pelvic pouch procedure still may be an acceptable surgical alternative in those patients known to have ulcerative colitis but with perianal disease, because the overall pouch failure rate has not been demonstrated to be significantly increased.

*Malignancy.* One of the concerns expressed is the risk for the development of carcinoma if the rectal mucosa regenerates (see earlier discussion). Examination of pathologic specimens of the ileoanal anastomoses has demonstrated that reepithelialization of the rectal sleeve does not occur, although a few isolated rectal mucosal cells can be seen. The rectal muscle cuff is bound to ileal serosa by dense fibrous tissue and active rectal mucosal disease, dysplasia, or reepithelialization is not observed. With less attention to mucosectomy and with no attempt to preserve a muscular sleeve, the concern for the subsequent development of malignancy should be minimal. Whether concern for malignant transformation of the mucosa is justified will need to be clarified during the next several years.

With respect to whether restorative proctocolectomy is appropriate for patients found to harbor a carcinoma with ulcerative colitis or polyposis, it is probably prudent to delay the pouch construction until a later date because of the potential difficulty of intraoperative staging and the possible requirement for adjuvant therapy.

*Other Malignant Tumors.* As mentioned, adenocarcinoma has been described in the reservoir of a Kock pouch. Currently, no such tumor has been identified in the reservoir of a pouch-anal reconstruction. However, Nyam et al. have described a patient in whom a large-cell lymphoma developed in the pouch following this operation.

*Recurrent Disease.* The development of Crohn's disease following restorative proctocolectomy or Kock pouch implies an initial error in diagnosis (see earlier). The concern about the performance of reservoir procedures for Crohn's disease has been previously discussed and is further addressed in Chapter 30.

*Evacuation Problems.* The problems of bowel obstruction and evacuation difficulties have been discussed. Failure to evacuate adequately is usually associated with a long efferent limb, a particular concern with the S-type pouch procedure (Fig. 29.31; see *Results*). It is because of this complication that every effort should be made to place the reservoir as close to the anal canal as is reasonably possible. Treatment of this complication requires take-down of the anastomosis and shortening of the efferent limb.

*Impotence and Infertility.* As with conventional proctocolectomy and ileostomy, impotence does not seem to be an important issue, primarily because

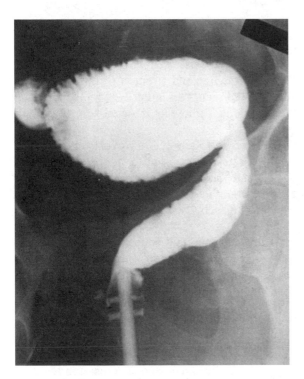

**FIG. 29.31.** Long efferent limb of pouch-ileoanal procedure predisposes to difficulties in evacuation. Pouchogram demonstrates part of the reservoir to be inferior to the pouch outlet.

of the young age of most patients. However, approximately 10% of men are found to have retrograde ejaculation. No impairment of bladder function was identified in patients of either sex.

*Other Complications.* The usual complications experienced with any major abdominal procedure have been reported following the various pouch-anal procedures. These include adrenal insufficiency, hepatitis, pneumothorax, gastrointestinal bleeding, pancreatitis, cholecystitis, deep vein thrombosis, and brachial palsy, as well as, of course, wound infection. Whether the incidence is higher in comparison with other gastrointestinal operations is problematic.

### Pregnancy and Childbirth

Stool frequency, incontinence, and pad usage are significantly increased during pregnancy, but postpartum function is the same as before pregnancy. The incidence of pouch-related complications compares favorably with that of conventional ileostomy and Kock pouch. The incidence of cesarean section, however, is higher. The type of delivery should be influenced by obstetric concerns only, not by issues relative to the ileal pouch-anal anastomosis procedure.

## Physiologic Studies and Laboratory Evaluation

*Anal Manometry: Determination of Reservoir Capacity and Compliance.* With normal sphincter function, continence correlates with reservoir capacity and compliance as well as with the frequency and strength of intrinsic bowel contractions. Others have demonstrated that the integrity of the sphincter mechanism can be satisfactorily maintained following ileoanal-reservoir operations.

Incontinent patients usually have lower resting pressures; extended anal canal relaxation; higher-amplitude, high-pressure waves; and a nonresponsive anal canal, all indicating a reversal of the anal canal pressure gradient. Incontinence is most likely a consequence of several factors, including a weak and less responsive anal canal, strong pouch motor activity, and dysfunctional coordination between pouch and anal canal.

Median resting anal canal pressure and maximal squeeze pressure are significantly lower in patients with pouch when compared with a control population. However, better results can be achieved with respect to voluntary control if the surgeon limits the potential for injury to the internal sphincter by avoiding anal dilatation and mucosectomy. This must be balanced with the concern for residual mucosa predisposing to the development of dysplasia and carcinoma.

The frequency of defecation appears inversely correlated to both the capacity and the compliance of the pouch. Patients who can postpone defecation for more than 30 minutes have higher anal squeeze pressures and empty their pouches more completely than those who experienced leakage. The best clinical results are associated with a high anal pressure and with a large volume, high compliance, and complete emptying of the pouch.

*Electromyography.* Recovery of internal sphincter electromyography activity and resting anal pressure is progressive and associated with a gradual decrease in stool frequency.

*Motility.* Most of the electric and motor properties of the terminal ileum are retained after surgery, but pouch motility is reduced. Patients who have poor functional results—incontinence and stool frequency—often have rapid pouch filling and an inability to evacuate completely.

*Pouchography and Scintigraphy.* Normal pouchograms can be obtained in 85% of patients, whereas pouchograms of the remaining 15% will reveal pouch leaks and other abnormal findings. Abnormal pouchograms are associated with an overall long-term failure rate of 23%, in comparison with a 6% long-term failure rate for patients with normal findings; pouchograms may have a long-term clinical predictive value.

*Anal Sensation.* Excision of the anal transition zone does not eliminate the ability to discriminate but other authors have found that anal sensation and discriminatory function were significantly better without mucosal proctectomy. Still others have demonstrated improved sensation to be associated with preservation of the anal transition zone, but correlation with the actual functional results was not obtained.

*Bacteriology.* Jejunal bacterial overgrowth is associated with an increased stool output, azotorrhea, and a poor clinical result.

*Absorption.* One of the concerns expressed with respect to the various pouch-anal alternatives is the problem of absorptive capacity and consequent nutritional disturbance. It has been observed that almost all patients after colectomy have supersaturated bile with cholesterol crystals, findings that are usually seen in persons with cholesterol gallstones. Otherwise, nutritional parameters and absorption appear to be essentially normal.

### Bowel Frequency and Continence

Interpretation of the results of the varied approaches to the assessment of ileoanal pouch function is obviously based subjectively. The four characteristics generally evaluated include spontaneity of defecation, ability to defer defecation, continence, and stool frequency.

A plethora of articles have been published on the functional results of the pouch-anal procedures. The general consensus is that this operation, with its various modifications, offers the best quality of life when compared with the alternatives. Tables 29.2 and 29.3 summarize the experiences from a number of institutions that address the issues of bowel frequency and control after restorative proctocolectomy.

### Comparisons of Reservoir Design

Much effort has been directed to comparing the functional outcome of patients who have had restorative proctocolectomy with creation of a variety of

**TABLE 29.2.** *Bowel frequency following pouch-anal procedures*

| Institution | Year | Patients (n) | Primary pouch | Daily evacuations: Total (mean) | Night (mean) | Day (mean) |
|---|---|---|---|---|---|---|
| Mayo Clinic | 1994 | 1,400 | J | 6 | 0–1 | 5–6 |
| St. Mark's Hospital | 1994 | 110 | J, S | 6 | 0–1 | 5 |
| Cleveland Clinic | 1995 | 521 | J | 6 | NS | NS |
| Cleveland Clinic (FL) | 1995 | 107 | J | 6.6 | 1.2 | 5.4 |
| University of Wisconsin | 1992 | 109 | W | 4.9 | NS | NS |
| Lahey Clinic | 1993 | 382 | J | 7 | 1 | 6 |
| University of Chicago | 1993 | 50 | J | 6 | NS | NS |
| Radcliffe Hospital | 1997 | 177 | J | 5 | 0–1 | 4.5 |

NS, not stated.
J, S, W indicate pouch type (see text for description of each).

**TABLE 29.3.** *Bowel control following pouch-anal procedures*

| Institution | Year | Patients (n) | Primary pouch | Excellent/ Good (%) | Impaired (%) |
|---|---|---|---|---|---|
| Mayo Clinic | 1994 | 1,400 | J | 48 | 52 |
| St. Mark's Hospital | 1994 | 110 | J, S | 45 | 55 |
| Cleveland Clinic | 1995 | 521 | J | 71 | 29 |
| Cleaveland Clinic (FL) | 1995 | 107 | J | 87 | 13 |
| University of Wisconsin | 1992 | 109 | W | 61 | 39 |
| Lahey Clinic | 1993 | 382 | J | 90 | 10 |
| University of Chicago | 1993 | 50 | J | 54 | 46 |

pelvic ileal reservoirs. Although the choice of reservoir is largely a function of the surgeon's personal preference, a number of options are available, including the duplicated J, triplicated S, quadruplicated W, and lateral, as well as modified versions of them. Four factors correlate significantly with an ideal functional result. These are maximal resting anal pressure, sensory threshold in the upper and middle anal canal, compliance of the ileal reservoir, and the presence of a pouch-anal inhibitory reflex. The quality of anal continence depends on a compliant ileal reservoir and a strong, sensitive anal sphincter. A number of studies have been conducted to investigate the advantages and drawbacks of each design.

Although some authors have concluded that W ileal reservoirs exhibit optimal function and compliance properties when compared with lower-capacity designs, many other studies demonstrate little difference. Their findings support the use of a small, duplicated ileal reservoir, which is simple to construct using linear stapling techniques.

Although the S-pouch generally enjoys good compliance, it is complicated by an increased difficulty in spontaneous evacuation, and many patients need routine catheterization to effect evacuation.

*Comment*: The ileal reservoir with endoanal anastomosis has become relatively standardized, at least with respect to the value of the procedure in the surgical management of individuals with ulcerative colitis and the polyposis syndromes. No question, most patients are satisfied with the functional results and to some extent serve as their own controls (as most have a protecting ileostomy for a time). However, these so-called control patients have a less-than-satisfactory loop ileostomy; it is more proximally located than a conventional end-stoma, and the effluent, therefore, is more liquid. Furthermore, despite meticulous attention to creating a loop ileostomy, surgeons often find that a consistently salutary stoma is an unachieved ideal. Thus said, however, a report from the Mayo Clinic compared the quality of life after conventional (Brooke) ileostomy with that after the pouch-anal procedure. After adjusting for age, diagnosis, and reoperation rate, logistic regression analysis of performance scores in seven different categories were used to discriminate between operations. The authors concluded that patients experience significant advantages with respect to their daily activities and quality of life with the pouch-anal procedure in comparison with the standard end-ileostomy.

Consider also the obvious fact that, despite many surgeons' increased experience with the technique, the procedure continues to have a high morbidity, albeit much lower than the initial experiences indicated. Mortality, however, is low, primarily because an ileostomy is usually accomplished until the pouch-anal or pouch-ileoanal anastomosis has healed.

Analysis of the numerous reports in the literature reveals a considerable variability in operative technique between surgeons and institutions. Furthermore, with rare exception, the failure to randomize patients also inhibits accurate assessment of the relative merits and risks of the plethora of approaches. Still, a number of appropriate conclusions can be drawn. Before agreeing to perform this procedure as an alternative to conventional ileostomy or reservoir ileostomy, determine that the patient is highly motivated to accept the consequences: frequent bowel movements (a minimum of four to six stools per day and the possible requirement for intubation if an S pouch is elected), as well as the risk for soilage and incontinence. It can take up to 1 year for a patient to achieve reasonable stability with respect to bowel function and frequency.

A number of factors may make restorative proctocolectomy with an intervening pouch technically difficult or impossible to accomplish. For example, obesity tends to be associated with a shortened mesentery; this may preclude the possibility of bringing the ileum down to effect an appropriate anastomosis. It may not be possible to position the reservoir in the pelvis if there is considerable fatty tissue or if there is narrowing of the inlet. Generally, the terminal ileum reaches the dentate line more readily in the S pouch than when the J reservoir is used. The patient, therefore, must understand that technical factors or unanticipated pathology may necessitate an alternative surgical approach.

Because of the risk for recurrence, the operation should not be performed in patients with Crohn's disease (see Chapter 30). Toxic megacolon is also a contraindication for embarking on this procedure at the time of emergency intervention. The wiser course in the latter situation is to perform a total colectomy and conventional ileostomy with rectal preservation, returning later to perform the restorative procedure. Older age is in itself not an absolute contraindication for the operation, but most agree that because the aging process has a pejorative effect on sphincter muscle function, the procedure should probably be limited to patients younger than 60 years of age, although this is by no means a requirement.

With respect to the type of pouch to be constructed, a trade-off seems to have evolved: the increased incidence of a need to intubate the S pouch versus the theoretically lowered capacity (and therefore increased frequency of defecation) of the J reservoir. Conversely, many reports suggest that the size of the reservoir is of limited importance.

Preoperative physiologic studies that evaluate anal squeeze pressure or at least subjectively assess the effectiveness of the sphincter mechanism should be considered before an ileal reservoir anastomosis is performed. The real question is whether preoperative physiologic studies help to predict the functional results following restorative proctocolectomy. Older patients, and those with a poor resting tone or suboptimal maximal squeeze pressure, might be forewarned that continence could be less than satisfactory.

We have certainly reached the point with the endoanal pouch procedures where they deserve complete legitimacy in our surgical armamentarium. Until relatively recently, I had been concerned that the complexity of the operation mandated that it be performed only by surgeons with a sufficiently large number of patients to gain adequate experience with the technique. However, with the stapled J pouch and the application of the double-stapling technique for effecting the anastomosis, the technical aspects of the surgery are relatively well standardized and can be performed by most general surgeons. However, the admonition concerning who should perform these restorative procedures still has validity. The major problem now is not so much surgical technique as the requirement for an obsessive, competently applied, follow-up program, as well as the obvious commitment of the surgeon to such a regimen. It appears today, that conventional ileostomy will be used primarily for patients with Crohn's disease, for older patients, for those with failed pouch procedures, and for those who are not motivated to assume the burdens of the pouch alternative.

# 30

# Crohn's Disease and Indeterminate Colitis

## CROHN'S DISEASE

Crohn's disease of the bowel was initially described by Crohn, Ginzburg, and Oppenheimer in 1932, at which time they noted a transmural inflammatory condition of the terminal ileum.

### Incidence, Epidemiology, Etiology, and Pathogenesis

The incidence, epidemiology, and theories concerning the cause and pathogenesis of Crohn's disease are discussed in Chapter 29. It is interesting to note that *Mycobacterium paratuberculosis* DNA has been found in Crohn's diseased tissue. The concept of a bacterial cause for inflammatory bowel disease (IBD) was discussed in Chapter 29, a concept that has generally been refuted. In one study, however, *M. paratuberculosis* was identified in 65% of specimens in individuals with Crohn's disease, but in only 4.3% of those with ulcerative colitis. The control tissues were found to have this DNA element in 12.5%. It was concluded that these observations are consistent with a causative role for *M. paratuberculosis* in Crohn's disease.

Another recent observation involves the identification of genes associated with IBD. Certainly, Crohn's disease appears to be influenced by a wide range of genetic and environmental factors.

### Physical Examination

In contrast to individuals with ulcerative colitis, even in the absence of toxic megacolon, a patient with Crohn's disease may demonstrate obvious findings on physical examination. Although it is true that anorectal disease can occur with ulcerative colitis, it is much more common in those with Crohn's disease. The diagnosis is often suspected on examination of the perianal skin. Simple inspection will often uncover the edematous tags, fissures, abscess, or fistulas charac-

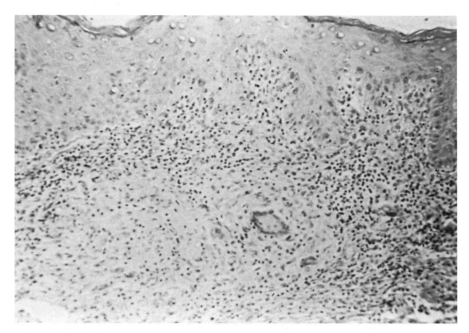

**FIG. 30.1.** This section from a macroscopically normal anus reveals a submucosal granuloma. The patient subsequently proved to have Crohn's disease. (Original magnification ×80; from Corman ML, Veidenheimer MC, Nugent FW, et al. *Diseases of the anus, rectum and colon. Part II: Non-specific inflammatory bowel disease.* New York: Medcom, 1976, with permission.)

teristically seen in this condition. The anal canal may be stenotic, fibrotic, and thickened on digital examination. If an anal fissure is apparent, severe pain is noted. Pelvic examination in a woman may reveal a rectovaginal fistula, and bimanual examination may show the presence of a pelvic mass. A biopsy of a sinus tract or an abscess cavity may show the granulomas characteristic of Crohn's colitis (Fig. 30.1).

Abdominal findings are more common in patients with Crohn's disease than in those with ulcerative colitis. A mass may be felt in the right iliac fossa, a common observation when regional enteritis involves the terminal ileum. A large, mesenteric abscess can often be palpated. Crohn's colitis, however, usually is not associated with clinically demonstrable abdominal abnormalities.

## Endoscopic Examination

Proctosigmoidoscopic examination is often helpful in differentiating between ulcerative colitis and Crohn's disease. The rectum is always diseased during attacks of ulcerative colitis, whereas with Crohn's colitis, 40% of patients have sparing of the rectum, irrespective of anal or perianal involvement. But when the rectum is involved by Crohn's disease, differentiation between the two may be very difficult.

A corollary to this observation is to perform biopsies distal to obvious inflammatory changes if the rectum appears to be spared, because the rectum may be discovered not to be truly normal. This may prompt a reassessment of the accuracy of a diagnosis of Crohn's disease for what was initially thought to be lack of rectal involvement. Biopsy can be helpful because histologic changes suggestive of Crohn's disease, in particular, may be apparent; up to 20% of such patients may exhibit granulomata.

Colonoscopy is recommended for five indications: differential diagnosis, resolution of radiographic abnormalities (e.g., filling defects and strictures), preoperative and postoperative evaluation in Crohn's disease, examination of stomas, and screening for premalignant and malignant changes. With granulomatous colitis, the following major colonoscopic findings may be observed: (a) a normal rectum, although this is not always the case; (b) asymmetry or eccentricity of involvement; (c) cobblestone appearance; (d) normal vasculature; (e) edema of the bowel wall, as seen in ulcerative colitis; (f) normal mucosa intervening between areas of ulceration; (g) serpiginous ulcers, which can course for several centimeters; (h) pseudopolyps, as in ulcerative colitis; and (i) skip areas (lack of continuity of involvement) (Fig. 30.2).

Unfortunately, interpretation is frequently difficult if biopsies are obtained by means of proctosigmoidoscopy or colonoscopy. In comparison with barium enema examination, the segmental nature of the involvement is more apparent by means of colonoscopy; microulceration is also more evident than by radiologic means. Radiographs yield more information about the haustra, especially in the right colon. Colonoscopy permitted a histologic diagnosis in 24% of patients, but granulomas were found in only 5% to 10%. The most useful lesion

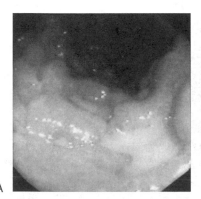 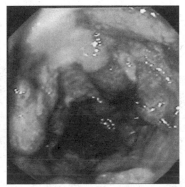

A                                                                                                      B

**FIG. 30.2.** Colonoscopic changes in Crohn's disease. **A.** Deep ulceration with pus can be seen; the colon is relatively spared more distally. **B.** Florid inflammatory changes with longitudinal furrows (i.e., rake ulcers) constitute the characteristic appearance of granulomatous colitis.

found on colonoscopic mucosal biopsy of patients with Crohn's disease is a granuloma. The limiting factor in establishing the correct diagnosis by means of biopsy, however, is the small size of the specimen. Hence, the physician or surgeon, having the benefit of clinical evaluation and the history, is often in the better position to make the correct diagnosis.

## Radiographic Features

As mentioned, Crohn's disease can occur anywhere in the alimentary tract. The disease tends to be segmental and asymmetric. Radiologic findings include skip lesions, contour defects, longitudinal ulcers, transverse fissures, eccentric involvement, pseudodiverticula, narrowing or stricture formation, pseudopolypoid changes that may be cobblestonelike, sinus tracts, and fistulas.

A plain film of the abdomen can be useful in the early stages of Crohn's colitis. Although toxic megacolon is much less common in Crohn's disease than it

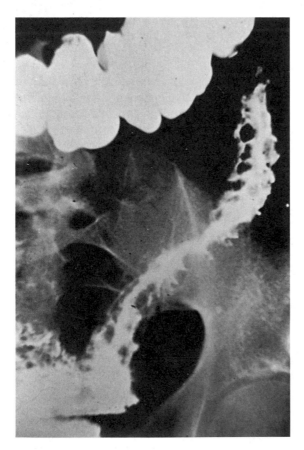

**FIG. 30.3.** Crohn's colitis. Coarse cobblestoning of the left colon with intramural fistula traversing longitudinally along the bowel wall. (From Corman ML, Veidenheimer MC, Nugent FW, et al. *Diseases of the anus, rectum and colon. Part II: Nonspecific inflammatory bowel disease.* New York: Medcom, 1976, with permission.)

is in ulcerative colitis, acute toxic dilatation can occur before any firm cicatrix has formed in the bowel wall.

The postevacuation film is most useful in identifying numerous discrete ulcers. Small ulcerations can combine to produce large, longitudinal ulcers, and when the longitudinal ulcers combine with transverse fissures, they produce the cobblestone appearance seen radiologically (Fig. 30.3). Intramural fistulas can result from the coalescing of the numerous longitudinal ulcers, which in turn can produce a double-lumen appearance. Ulcerations can penetrate beyond the contour of the bowel and present as numerous long spicules or as sinus tracts (Fig. 30.4). These deep fissures can be confused with diverticula; with experience, however, the physician should readily differentiate them.

Although the standard barium enema examination has been routinely used in the past to evaluate IBD, more recent evidence suggests that the air-contrast technique is preferred. Radiologists have prided themselves on their ability to identify the sometimes unusual radiographic features of IBD; these include mucosal bridging and aphthoid ulcers.

Strictures are of variable lengths and can be extensive indeed. When a stricture occurs in Crohn's disease, it does not imply a malignant association such as

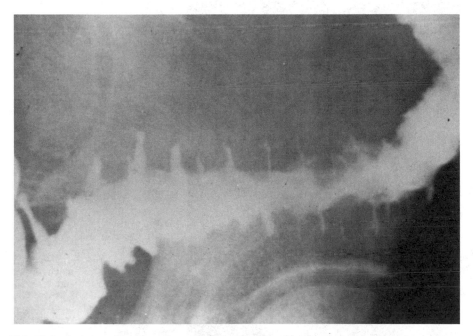

**FIG. 30.4.** Crohn's colitis. Deep fissuring of the bowel wall in the sigmoid colon, giving a thorn-like appearance. (From Corman ML, Veidenheimer MC, Nugent FW, et al. *Diseases of the anus, rectum and colon. Part II: Non-specific inflammatory bowel disease.* New York: Medcom, 1976, with permission.)

when it is seen in a patient with ulcerative colitis. However, individuals with Crohn's disease have been shown to have an increased risk for the development of malignancy (see *Relationship to Carcinoma*). Differential diagnosis between a Crohn's stricture and that of a carcinoma is usually not difficult. Close inspection often reveals that the bowel in adjacent areas is ulcerated (Fig. 30.5). Although a scirrhous carcinoma must always be considered in the differential diagnosis, the lack of associated ulceration or inflammatory changes elsewhere in the colon usually clarifies the dilemma.

A most difficult problem is to differentiate radiographically Crohn's disease from tuberculosis (see Chapter 33). When the condition is confined to the ileocecal region, it is virtually impossible to distinguish between the two diseases.

Upper gastrointestinal and small bowel x-ray films are extremely useful for evaluating IBD in this area of the alimentary tract, especially because no truly adequate nonoperative endoscopic examination of the small intestine is available, except for the very distal ileum. Evaluation of the terminal ileum is best obtained by reflux on barium enema examination, but unfortunately as many as 20% of patients will not demonstrate this phenomenon. Alternatively, a small-bowel follow-through study or an enteroclysis with good spot films can be used.

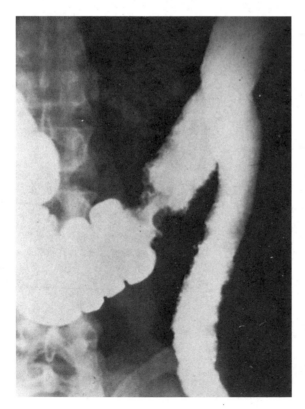

**FIG. 30.5.** Crohn's colitis with transverse colon stricture, an "apple core" lesion suggestive of carcinoma. Note, however, that the distal bowel is ulcerated. (From Corman ML, Veidenheimer MC, Nugent FW, et al. *Diseases of the anus, rectum and colon. Part II: Non-specific inflammatory bowel disease.* New York: Medcom, 1976, with permission.)

Crohn's disease of the terminal ileum has a characteristic appearance. Thickening of the bowel wall narrows the lumen, resulting in a degree of obstruction in some patients. This is the most frequent cause of abdominal pain in individuals with Crohn's disease. The radiologic appearance of the terminal ileum has been described as a "string sign" (Fig. 30.6). Involvement of the terminal ileum may be seen as an isolated finding or can be associated with multiple diseased areas throughout the small intestine (Fig. 30.7). In contrast to radiologic evaluation of the colon for Crohn's disease, it is virtually impossible to differentiate a benign from a malignant stricture in the small intestine. As with carcinoma of the small bowel in an individual without Crohn's disease, the prognosis is extremely poor.

Fistulous complications are frequently seen in patients with Crohn's disease. Communication between the ileum and colon is the most common, but other types of fistulas have been observed, including coloduodenal, and those to pelvic organs.

Barium enema has been used to evaluate the anal canal in patients with Crohn's disease. Whereas direct visual examination is more accurate, character-

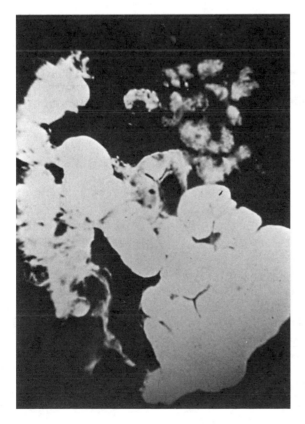

**FIG. 30.6.** Distal ileal Crohn's disease. Edema and thickening of the bowel wall produce the characteristic "string sign." (From Corman ML, Veidenheimer MC, Nugent FW, et al. *Diseases of the anus, rectum and colon. Part II: Non-specific inflammatory bowel disease.* New York: Medcom, 1976, with permission.)

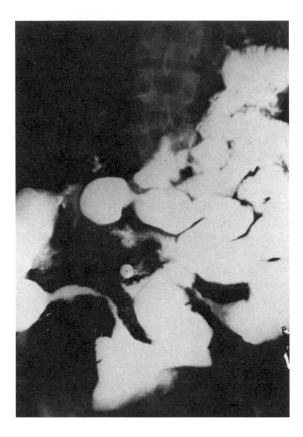

**FIG. 30.7.** Small bowel Crohn's disease. Terminal ileal disease in addition to multiple skip areas. (From Corman ML, Veidenheimer MC, Nugent FW, et al. *Diseases of the anus, rectum and colon. Part II: Nonspecific inflammatory bowel disease.* New York: Medcom, 1976, with permission.)

istic changes can be identified by careful radiologic examination of the area. The hallmark of a radiologically normal anal canal is the presence of straight, smooth lines of barium between the folds, whereas in an abnormal anal canal can be seen distortion of the folds, ulcers, fissures, sinus tracts, and fistulas.

Ultrasound examination is of limited value in patients with IBD, because of the presence of considerable artifact associated with the loops of bowel. The presence of air or fluid in the intestine and adhesed loops can simulate a septic focus. Diagnosis by ultrasound reflects primarily the thickening of the gastrointestinal wall itself, perceived as a characteristic "target" appearance. Transrectal ultrasound sharply delineates the rectal wall and may detect unsuspected abscesses and fistulas in the pararectal and paraanal tissues (see Chapters 4 and 6).

Computed tomography (CT) can demonstrate thickening of the colon, nodularity, adenopathy, and intraabdominal abscess. Presence of a fistula, especially an enterocutaneous communication, has also been demonstrable by means of CT scan. In most cases, however, adequate evaluation of the intraabdominal pathology can be obtained by means of endoscopic examination and by standard contrast techniques.

The most common findings are inflammation of fat planes (73%), bowel wall thickening (30%), fistulas or sinus tracts (22%), and abscesses (14%). More than one third had abnormal CT manifestations below the symphysis pubis, so it is necessary to emphasize the importance of scanning sequences to the perineum in individuals with Crohn's disease.

## Specialized Laboratory Studies

A number of specialized laboratory studies have been advised, primarily for evaluation of Crohn's disease. Some have suggested the use of an indium-labeled leukocyte scan to distinguish patients for whom medical therapy may be preferable from those who may be optimally treated by surgery. In active Crohn's disease, labeled leukocytes are excreted into the bowel lumen from the inflamed mucosa. Patients with positive scans, therefore, have higher values of indices of disease activity. As an anatomic indicator of acute granulocytic infiltration of the intestinal mucosa and submucosa, this scan has a 97% rate of sensitivity and a 100% rate of specificity. The study may be applied best to individuals with fulminant disease, especially those who cannot safely be put through the rigors of endoscopy or barium contrast radiologic evaluation.

A significant correlation has been described with recurrence and alteration of acid 1-glycoprotein, 2-globulin, and erythrocyte sedimentation rate in comparison with the patients who remained in remission. Also, it has been demonstrated that patients with Crohn's disease requiring operative treatment often have a severe peripheral lymphopenia.

### *Pathology*

#### *Macroscopic Appearance*

Crohn's disease can have protean clinical and pathologic manifestations. The condition can be confined to the colon alone or can involve only the anal canal. Fistulas, segmental involvement, rectal sparing, perianal disease, and abscess formation are all characteristic of granulomatous colitis.

Some of the earliest changes in the serosal aspect of the small intestine involved by Crohn's disease may be immediately recognizable if the patient is submitted to surgery. Subserosal extension of fat around the surface of the bowel ("fat-wrapping") and a prominent vascular pattern in the serosa are characteristic of the disease (Fig. 30.8). The serosal surface may be granular and bleed easily on any intraoperative abrasion. It has been demonstrated that fat-wrapping correlates best with transmural inflammation and represents part of the connective tissue changes that accompany intestinal Crohn's disease.

The disease frequently affects the bowel in a segmental fashion. This can produce extensive skip areas, limited involvement to an area of the bowel, or even a focal, isolated stricture.

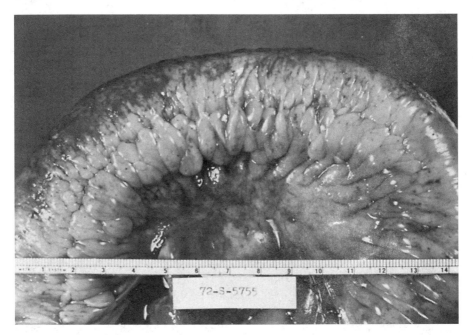

**FIG. 30.8.** Ileal Crohn's disease. Subserosal inflammation and "fat-wrapping" are evident. (From Corman ML, Veidenheimer MC, Nugent FW, et al. *Diseases of the anus, rectum and colon. Part II: Non-specific inflammatory bowel disease.* New York: Medcom, 1976, with permission.)

Classically, Crohn's colitis involves the intestine in an asymmetric fashion. Areas of the bowel may demonstrate disease on the mucosal aspect with sparing of adjacent sites, leaving islands of somewhat edematous but otherwise nonulcerated mucosa. Ulceration in an irregular fashion with large areas of uninvolved mucosa interspersed between broad, twisting lesions is characteristic. The relative sparing between ulcers is not seen in ulcerative colitis. Another characteristic feature of the macroscopic appearance of Crohn's disease is the thickening of the bowel wall. Involvement through all the layers, along with the cobblestone appearance of the mucosa, has been described as "stones in a running brook."

Crohn's colitis frequently involves the colon and ileum in continuity. Conversely, cecal ulceration can be seen primarily with ileal disease. Occasionally, the ileal disease terminates abruptly at the ileocecal valve, sparing the large bowel. Thickening of the bowel wall can produce sufficient narrowing to precipitate intestinal obstruction or to impede the passage of swallowed seeds or nuts. Gallstone ileus has even been reported to produce obstruction at a point of stenosis caused by Crohn's disease.

A common manifestation of Crohn's disease is fistula formation. Fistulas can occur into any adjacent organ, such as the small or large bowel, bladder, vagina, uterus, ureter, or skin. Burrowing of the fissures deep into the bowel wall predisposes to fistula formation. Fistulas occur more commonly in the mesocolic aspect of the bowel than on the antimesocolic border.

Occasionally, diffuse mucosal disease produces a pseudopolypoid pattern similar to that of chronic ulcerative colitis. Giant pseudopolyps can actually mimic neoplasms clinically and radiographically. The condition is most likely the result of fusion of numerous fingerlike pseudopolyps.

### Histologic Appearance

The three primary histopathologic findings in patients with Crohn's colitis are transmural inflammation and fibrosis, granulomas, and narrow, deeply penetrating ulcers or "fissures." The mucosal inflammation of Crohn's disease differs from that of ulcerative colitis in that, typically, fewer crypt abscesses and less congestion are seen, and the goblet cell population is better preserved.

Granulomas can occur in any part of the bowel wall and are usually identified in approximately two thirds of all patients with Crohn's colitis. If a biopsy is performed in an attempt to differentiate between the two inflammatory conditions, the material should be obtained from a noninflamed area, if possible (Fig. 30.9); a granuloma may be apparent with ulcerative colitis in an area of acute inflammation. Multiple biopsy specimens are suggested because submucosal lesions

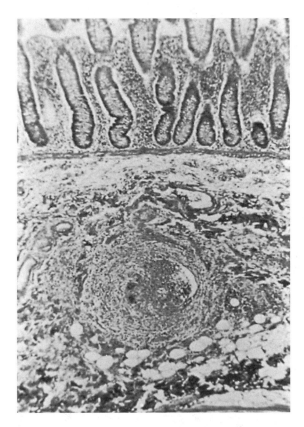

**FIG. 30.9.** Crohn's disease. Submucosal granuloma. Note that the overlying mucosa has inflammatory cells in the lamina propria but no crypt abscess or ulceration. (Original magnification ×80.) (From Corman ML, Veidenheimer MC, Nugent FW, et al. *Diseases of the anus, rectum and colon. Part II: Nonspecific inflammatory bowel disease.* New York: Medcom, 1976, with permission.)

tend to be very small (microgranulomas). The microscopic appearance of the granuloma is not diagnostic, and the possibility of an infectious agent should always be considered. Granulomas can also occur in the liver and in the omentum as well as in other sites.

Narrow, deeply penetrating ulcers or "fissures" are the third characteristic feature of Crohn's disease. The fissures, which can penetrate through the inner circular layer of the muscularis, are visible on the radiographs after a barium enema as spicules. A sinus tract present in the fat adjacent to the bowel wall indicates that one of the fissures has penetrated through the wall. When this occurs, a sinus can burrow into another organ to produce a fistula.

Information about the pathology of IBD has been further gleaned by electron microscopy. Early epithelial changes can be identified using this modality in areas that appear to be uninvolved. These include necrosis of individual columnar epithelial cells; budding of the tips of microvilli; thickening, shortening, irregularity, and fusion of intestinal villi; numerous Paneth's cells; hyperplasia of goblet cells; and augmented mucous secretion. Findings from other studies such as tissue-enzyme analysis, jejunal-surface pH, and differences in sodium flux and mucosal potential imply that the disease often is far more extensive than is recognized by other, more conventional means, and certainly much more extensive than is usually apparent at the time of surgery.

Another observation is the increased secretion of mucus by the bowel in Crohn's disease as compared with decreased colonic mucus in ulcerative colitis. The decrease may be explained by destruction of the epithelial cells. A number of biochemical changes have also been observed.

## Signs, Symptoms, and Presentations

Patients with Crohn's disease can present with minimal symptoms and moderate complaints, or they can have fulminant manifestations. The considerable overlap in the presentations of ulcerative colitis and Crohn's disease is addressed in Chapter 29. For example, individuals with Crohn's disease may bleed, but this is not as frequent a presentation and may not be as severe. However, life-threatening hemorrhage has been reported. Abdominal pain may be mild or absent in patients with ulcerative colitis, but those with Crohn's disease frequently complain of pain. This can be colicky in nature and be associated with intestinal obstruction, or it can be continual and related to the presence of a septic process within the abdomen. An abdominal mass is not uncommonly found on physical examination in a patient with Crohn's disease, but it is never seen in a patient with ulcerative colitis.

Diarrhea is usually a more troublesome concern in patients with ulcerative colitis. This is, perhaps, because distal disease tends to be associated with more urgency and, in some cases, tenesmus. Patients with Crohn's disease may have rectal sparing and are less likely to experience this urgency. Conversely, with rectal involvement, patients with Crohn's disease experience symptoms similar to those with ulcerative colitis.

As mentioned, anal disease is much more commonly seen in patients with Crohn's colitis than with ulcerative colitis. The presence of anal pain, swelling, and discharge may be a presenting feature of the former condition and may be the only abnormality observed on examination and on subsequent investigation. Between 20% and 35% or so of patients may be so afflicted. Anal fissure may account for 30% of anal manifestations; fistula in 30%, an abscess in 20%, and multiple presentations in about 20%. Crohn's colitis is much more frequently associated with an anal lesion than was Crohn's disease of the small bowel (50% vs. 15%). A high level of suspicion should exist if noting characteristic edematous tags, blue discoloration of the skin, an eccentrically located fissure, a broad-based ulcer, a rigid or strictured canal, or an anal fistula, especially if the patient reports gastrointestinal symptoms.

Fever is usually not a concern in patients with ulcerative colitis unless the patient is severely ill (toxic megacolon). However, in those with Crohn's disease, pyrexia is not uncommonly noted, and is usually caused by an intraabdominal abscess or undrained septic focus. Nausea and vomiting are not noted frequently in either condition unless evidence of intestinal obstruction is seen. Anorexia, weight loss, anemia, and general debility are associated with relatively long-standing or fulminant disease.

### Disease in Children and Adolescents

Crohn's disease occurring in children may have a more rapid onset and progression than when the disease occurs in young adults. These youngsters often become chronically ill, have growth impairment, decreased mental acuity, and are less developed physically than their healthy peers. It is because of these concerns that implementation of either an elemental dict or parenteral nutrition is an especially important part of the management of patients in this age group (see *Medical Management*). However, to be maximally effective, therapy must be initiated before puberty. Furthermore, unless medical treatment can achieve a sustained remission, operative intervention may be the only effective means for addressing the problem of retarded development (see later).

Children and adolescents with colonic disease are much more likely than adults to require resection, often after a relatively short period of illness. Growth retardation as an indication for surgery may be one of the reasons for this difference.

As with adults, the efficacy of surgery for Crohn's disease in children seems to depend mainly on disease location and, perhaps, the choice of surgical procedure, itself. Assessment of growth and development, psychological support for both the patient and the family, and close cooperation between the physician and the surgeon are important concepts in the management of these young people.

### Disease in Pregnancy

See Chapter 29.

## Extraintestinal Manifestations

Increasing evidence supports the statement that inflammatory disease of the intestine is a systemic problem rather than one localized to the small or large bowel. In a population-based study from Sweden of 1,274 patients with ulcerative colitis, the overall prevalence of extracolonic diagnoses was 21%. As discussed in Chapter 29, many etiologic concepts have been considered, but regardless of the sequence of pathologic changes in the colon, little question remains about the presence of related events, at times profound, in distant areas of the body. The joints, skin, liver, kidneys, eyes, mouth, blood, nervous system, and, of course, other areas of the alimentary tract can be sites of lesions that, at least in the extraintestinal manifestations, often seem dependent on the presence of diseased bowel. So broad indeed is the spectrum of Crohn's disease that specialists in dentistry, ear nose and throat (ENT), ophthalmology, and dermatology must be prepared to recognize its manifestations. Because so many of the complications in other areas of the body are exclusively seen in Crohn's disease, the discussion is placed within this chapter. However, as will be seen, many of the extraintestinal manifestations can be seen in ulcerative colitis also.

### *Oral Manifestations*

Inflammatory changes in the mouth can be the initial site of involvement of Crohn's disease. These included recurrent aphthous ulcers, pyoderma gangrenosum, pyostomatitis vegetans, hemorrhagic ulceration, glossitis, macroglossia, and moniliasis. Up to 20% of patients have been described as having oral lesions. The most frequently affected areas and their respective appearances are the buccal mucosa (a cobblestone pattern); the vestibule (linear, hyperplastic folds); and the lips (diffusely swollen and indurated).

Aphthous ulcers usually parallel the course or activity of the IBD: The more active the disease, the more likely this complication develops. Biopsy usually shows a chronic inflammatory reaction.

Pyostomatitis vegetans is an unusual manifestation of IBD. Papillary projections of mucous membrane can be seen separated by small areas of ulceration (Fig. 30.10). Biopsy may reveal suprabasal separation of the oral epithelium and infiltration with eosinophils.

The recognition of the specific oral granuloma is important because it may be the first manifestation of Crohn's disease.

### *Treatment*

Because the lesions are resistant to local therapy, general measures are advised to soothe the oral discomfort. The symptoms and clinical findings of oral problems are often ameliorated with appropriate treatment of the intestinal disease.

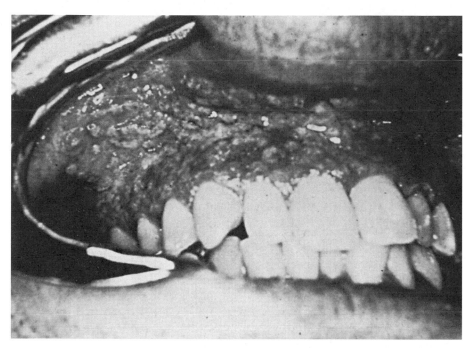

**FIG. 30.10.** Pyostomatitis vegetans. Involvement of the gingival mucosa by papillary projections. (From Corman ML, Veidenheimer MC, Nugent FW, et al. *Diseases of the anus, rectum and colon. Part II: Nonspecific inflammatory bowel disease.* New York: Medcom, 1976, with permission.)

## Esophageal Involvement

Patients with Crohn's disease of the esophagus will present with symptoms not unlike those associated with other lesions of that organ (e.g., carcinoma). Substernal discomfort, dysphagia, epigastric pain, weight loss, nausea, and vomiting are all part of the clinical spectrum. Other gastrointestinal symptoms are usually caused by disease elsewhere in the alimentary tract. Remember, dysphagia and the demonstration of an esophageal ulcer or esophagitis in a patient with known Crohn's disease can be caused by reflux esophagitis, certain drugs or corrosive agents, pressure from a nasogastric tube, an infectious agent, sarcoidosis, or Behçet's disease. In point of fact, many published reports of esophageal Crohn's disease cannot be supported by critical review.

Physical examination is usually unrewarding with respect to esophageal involvement. Diagnosis is usually made by a high index of suspicion and radiologic investigation, which obviously would include a barium swallow. This study may reveal thickened mucosal folds, multiple ulcerations, or, most commonly, a stricture. This last finding makes differentiation from carcinoma difficult, except that the presence of disease elsewhere or the relatively young age of the patient should lead to suspicion of an inflammatory process.

Endoscopic examination usually reveals hyperemia, with possibly either an ulcerated mucosa or the presence of an inflammatory stricture. Biopsies usually show an inflammatory reaction, but the absence of granulomata does not exclude the diagnosis of Crohn's disease.

### *Treatment*

Treatment usually consists of the standard medical management appropriate for Crohn's disease of the small or large bowel (e.g., steroids; see Chapter 29 and below). Resection is rarely indicated.

### Gastroduodenal Crohn's Disease

Crohn's disease involving the stomach and duodenum may not be as rare as originally suspected. Random endoscopic biopsies of the stomach and duodenal mucosa in patients with Crohn's disease frequently demonstrate the presence of microscopic alterations consistent with this inflammatory process in the upper gastrointestinal tract. Clinically, evident IBD of the gastroduodenal area is believed to occur in approximately 2% or 3% of all patients with Crohn's disease. The condition can occur without involvement elsewhere in the gastrointestinal tract, but this is extremely uncommon.

Patients usually present with epigastric abdominal symptoms exacerbated by eating—nausea, vomiting, and weight loss. Symptoms may resemble those of ulcer disease. Obstruction, perforation, fistula, and hemorrhage can occur. A fistula into the stomach characteristically produces symptoms of feculent vomiting, eructation, and odor. Duodenocolic fistula is a recognized complication of duodenal disease; in evaluating patients with this finding, however, it is important to ascertain whether the fistula arose from inflammatory disease of the intestinal tract outside of the duodenum or from the duodenum, itself. Most observers agree that gastroenteric and duodenoenteric fistulas are almost always result from intestinal disease.

Radiologic investigation may reveal antral inflammation, contiguous disease in the duodenum, cobblestone mucosal appearance with thickened folds, reduced distensibility or stricture, and ulceration. Barium enema examination is the preferred study to identify a fistula between the upper gastrointestinal tract and the colon.

Endoscopic examination may reveal ulceration, cobblestoning, or stricture. As with esophageal disease, the absence of granulomata does not necessarily mean that the patient does not have Crohn's disease.

### *Treatment*

Treatment usually consists of antacids and $H_2$ receptor blockers (an ulcer regimen), steroids, sulfasalazine (Azulfidine), hyperalimentation, and possibly surgical intervention. The primary indications for operation are the presence of a fistula and obstruction. If hemorrhage cannot be controlled by medical means, either resectional surgery or oversewing the bleeding point is the treatment of choice. Usually, however, surgery for primary gastroduodenal Crohn's disease is unnecessary.

### Management of Duodenal Stricture

A number of cases and reviews have been published on the evaluation and management of duodenal stricture as it affects this area. Gastrojejunostomy was used as the preferred treatment for those with this duodenal complication, initially, without vagotomy. Since it has been demonstrated that one third who had bypass required reoperation, usually for marginal ulceration or for gastroduodenal obstruction. Most surgeons now recommend that a vagotomy be performed. Many surgeons feel that whenever technically possible, strictureplasty (see later) is the optimal treatment for duodenal stenosis rather than bypass.

### Management of Gastric and Duodenal Fistulas

When a fistula develops as a consequence of intestinal disease, simple closure of the stomach or duodenum is all that is usually required, along with resection of the involved bowel segment. Gastric fistulas are always caused by disease in the intestine. Treatment of the gastric opening is wedge excision. Occasionally, the opening in the duodenum occurs in an area that is difficult to close (e.g., adjacent to the pancreas). In this situation and when a large defect is created, an omental or jejunal patch, or a duodenojejunostomy may be necessary.

### Results

As these conditions are uncommon, few large series exist. Most investigators conclude that irrespective of medical or surgical treatment, duodenal Crohn's disease follows a more benign course than when it affects the small bowel or colon.

### Pancreatic Manifestations

Pancreatitis or pancreatic insufficiency has occasionally been reported with IBD, but this had been felt to be coincidental. Be aware, however, of the risk of pancreatitis that may be associated with the administration of mercaptopurine (Purinethol). The following factors may indicate possibly important clinical distinctions:

Abdominal pain was absent or moderate and probably caused by bowel involvement.
Pancreatic calcifications were absent.

Those patients with pancreatic insufficiency had essentially normal pancreatograms.

More information is necessary to be able to establish with certainty whether pancreatic disease is truly an extraintestinal manifestation of IBD.

## Hepatobiliary Disease

Liver function studies and liver biopsy often show abnormal results in both ulcerative colitis and Crohn's disease patients. The most common is an elevation of the serum alkaline phosphatase, occurring in 30%. The reasons for the association between hepatobiliary disease and IBD are not known, but a number of studies have postulated that recurrent cholangitis results from a portal bacteremia from the interrupted intestinal mucosa, in addition to a probable genetic predisposition. Hepatoportal venous gas has been seen in patients with known Crohn's disease.

Cholelithiasis has been reported in up to one third of patients with IBD, especially in those with Crohn's ileitis. The explanation for this association is believed to involve the enterohepatic circulation. Disease or resection of the terminal ileum leads to loss or malabsorption of bile acids. Because the solubility of cholesterol depends on bile acids, excessive loss can precipitate this substance, which, in turn, can cause stone formation. Another explanation may be the colonization of the terminal ileum by anaerobic bacteria that deconjugate the bile acids to less well-absorbed substances. It is not clear, however, that a higher incidence of gallstones is seen in patients with Crohn's disease than in individuals with ulcerative colitis. Because of the high prevalence of cholelithiasis in the population, gallbladder imaging has been recommended preoperatively and in the follow-up of patients with IBD.

Fatty degeneration is probably the most frequently encountered microscopic abnormality. The incidence has been reported to be as high as 80%, which may be caused by the relatively poor nutritional state of many colitic patients. Occasionally, a granuloma may be seen. Treatment is directed toward correction of the malnutrition.

Another common histologic manifestation of liver disease is pericholangitis. A more accurate term is "portal triaditis," because of involvement of bile ductules, portal venules, lymphatics, and hepatic parenchyma. The condition can present with jaundice, abdominal pain, fever, and pruritus. Many patients, however, are asymptomatic. Bacterial infection and an autoimmune process have been implicated as possible causative factors. No specific treatment is currently available for this condition.

Although cirrhosis is an uncommon complication of IBD, it had been felt to cause 10% of deaths. Patients may develop the characteristic stigmata of portal hypertension, including bleeding esophageal varices and ileostomy hemorrhage (see Chapter 31).

Chronic, active hepatitis occurs in only 1% of patients with IBD; conversely, the incidence of IBD in patients with chronic active hepatitis varies from 4% to 30%. Patients have been reported improvement following removal of diseased bowel.

One of the most serious, albeit rare, consequences of IBD that occurs as a complication of both ulcerative colitis and Crohn's disease is primary sclerosing cholangitis. This condition has been diagnosed in 3.7% of individuals with ulcerative colitis. As many as 70% of patients with primary sclerosing cholangitis have IBD. The importance of identifying such individuals cannot be overestimated. It has been suggested that even the preclinical manifestations of IBD may subject that individual to an increased risk for the development of malignancy.

Primary sclerosing cholangitis has been much more common in patients with ulcerative colitis than in those with Crohn's disease. The cause is unknown, but toxins, infectious agents, altered immunity, and a genetic predisposition have been suggested. To establish this diagnosis, the patient should have no history of biliary surgery or gallstones, no diffuse involvement of the extrahepatic biliary ducts, and the absence of subsequent development of cholangiocarcinoma. Symptoms include right upper quadrant abdominal pain, vomiting, jaundice, and pruritus. Laboratory studies demonstrate the usual changes suggestive of an obstructive jaundice. Cholangiogram reveals a strictured bile duct (Fig. 30.11). When the sclerosing cholangitis has been established, removal of the diseased colon does not reverse the condition.

The disease is progressive and ultimately fatal, except if a liver transplantation is performed. It has been demonstrated that liver replacement and immunosuppression in those with sclerosing cholangitis and ulcerative colitis do not alter the course of the colonic disease. Some patients who have undergone liver transplant also appear to rapidly develop colorectal malignancy. These individuals require frequent, long-term surveillance following transplant. This suggests that the immunosuppressive agents used to manage individuals who have had orthotopic liver transplantation may have a pejorative effect on the colon through increased predisposition for the development of malignancy.

Interestingly, despite massive immunosuppression associated with transplanting small intestine, histologically confirmed recurrent Crohn's disease has been demonstrated in the transplanted bowel.

Because of the profoundly serious consequences of progressive cholangitis, a case may be made for "prophylactic" removal of the inflammatory bowel process if early changes in the biliary tract are observed. This has been suggested even when the gastrointestinal manifestations are minimal, but no good evidence supports implementation of this concept.

Carcinoma of the bile duct arising in a patient with ulcerative colitis is a rare complication. The condition is more common in men and is usually seen in patients who have had a prolonged history of colitis. Patients report a history of typical biliary obstruction with painless jaundice, weight loss, and pruritic symptoms. Diagnosis is usually confirmed by intravenous cholangiogram, ultra-

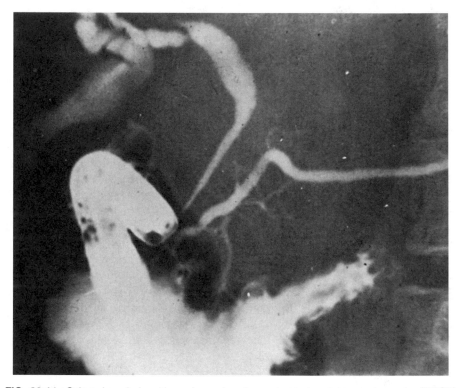

**FIG. 30.11.** Sclerosing cholangitis endoscopic retrograde cholangiopancreatography (ERCP) demonstrates narrowing of the distal common bile duct with complete obstruction at the level of the common hepatic duct. (From Corman ML, Veidenheimer MC, Nugent FW, et al. *Diseases of the anus, rectum and colon. Part II: Nonspecific inflammatory bowel disease.* New York: Medcom, 1976, with permission.)

sound demonstration of dilated intrahepatic ducts, and endoscopic retrograde cholangiography. Prognosis is poor, with biliary diversion the usual surgical approach. A number of cases of carcinoma of the gallbladder have been described in individuals with sclerosing cholangitis and ulcerative colitis.

## Cutaneous Manifestations

### *Pyoderma Gangrenosum*

Pyoderma gangrenosum is a condition found exclusively in individuals with IBD but, fortunately, is uncommon, occurring in no more than 2% of patients. Most patients have active intestinal disease at the time the pyoderma develops, although, in rare cases, the skin lesions may antedate apparent bowel involvement. Clinically, the lesion appears as a spreading, undermining ulceration that has a characteristic violaceous border (Figs. 30.12 and 30.13). It is usually found on the extremities, the most common location being the anterior tibial area. However, the ulcers can occur on the trunk, buttocks, and other places. Usually, only one or two lesions are present, but these can be of considerable size.

Biopsy shows no definite characteristics that would identify the ulcer as being specific for a complication associated with IBD. A vasculitis has been suggested as a possible cause.

Treatment consists of administration of systemic steroids; occasionally intralesional steroids; and, of course, the management of the colitis. Successful response to topical disodium cromoglycate (DSG) has been reported. Because DSG is known to prevent the release of histamine from mast cells, an allergic component may be involved in the mechanism for its efficacy. Topical measures also should include appropriate antibiotics if culture suggests the value of such treatment or if lymphangitis or cellulitis is present. As with so many other extra-colonic manifestations, the course of the pyoderma parallels the clinical progress of the intestinal disease. Rarely, does the skin condition assume such significance that colectomy must be performed.

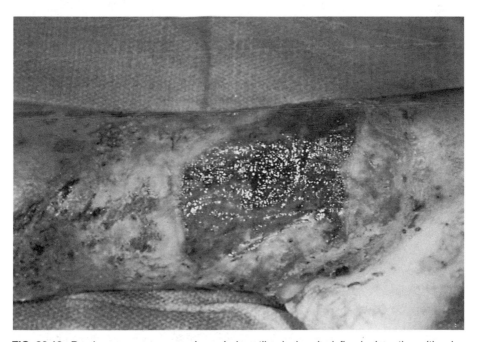

**FIG. 30.12.** Pyoderma gangrenosum. Irregularly outlined, sharply defined, ulceration with edematous edges and pyodermatous base in a patient with ulcerative colitis. (Courtesy of Rudolf Garret, M.D.)

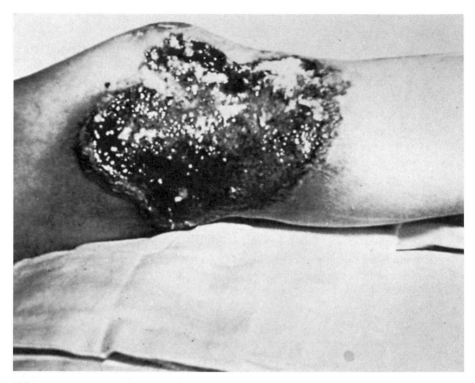

**FIG. 30.13.** Pyoderma gangrenosum. An undermined ulcer with a violaceous border. (From Corman ML, Veidenheimer MC, Nugent FW, et al. *Diseases of the anus, rectum and colon. Part II: Non-specific inflammatory bowel disease.* New York: Medcom, 1976, with permission.)

### Polyarteritis Nodosa

Polyarteritis nodosa is a rare cutaneous manifestation of Crohn's disease. The presence of erythematous and tender nodules in the extremities should lead one to suspect the diagnosis. Biopsy or excision may reveal an arteritis with luminal narrowing by fibrinous thrombus. The relationship of the cutaneous manifestation to systemic polyarteritis nodosa is controversial.

### Erythema Nodosum

Erythema nodosum is another cutaneous manifestation that is relatively uncommonly seen with IBD; up to 5% of patients are afflicted. Of these patients, 90% will have active bowel disease at the time skin lesions developed. In some, erythema nodosum typically occurs as a single episode and lasts for several days, and is associated with active bowel disease and joint symptoms. Tender, subcutaneous nodules are usually seen on the pretibial aspects of the legs. As with other extracolonic manifestations, the clinical course usually parallels that of the intestinal disease.

## Psoriasis

An increased risk exists for the development of psoriasis in patients with IBD. In a report by Yates et al., the prevalence of psoriasis in Crohn's disease (11.2%) and in ulcerative colitis (5.7%) was significantly greater than that of the control group (1.5%). The increased association of the two conditions, as well as the higher rate of psoriasis in first-degree relatives of Crohn's patients, implies the possibility of a genetic link.

## Cutaneous Crohn's Disease

Crohn's disease of the skin can develop with the characteristic histologic feature of the bowel condition—specifically granulomatous inflammation of the dermis. When this occurs other than by direct extension from the gastrointestinal tract, it has been given what I consider to be a poor but now accepted term, "metastatic cutaneous Crohn's disease." Only a few cases have been reported. Biopsy is required to establish the diagnosis, with differentiation from sarcoidosis a potential problem. The two diseases have similar cutaneous findings. Treatment by means of intralesional steroid therapy has been attempted with usually transient improvement. Therapeutic benefit has also been achieved with oral metronidazole (Flagyl).

## Arthritis and Rheumatologic Conditions

Depending on the interpretation of what truly constitutes arthritic or rheumatologic conditions associated with IBD, as many as four clinical patterns are seen: a peripheral joint synovitis closely related to the activity of the bowel disease (15% to 20% of patients); second, ankylosing spondylitis (3% to 6%), in which the relationship with the bowel disorder is less clearly defined; third, a bilateral symmetric sacroiliitis (5% to 15%); and fourth, a category that includes rheumatic complications, such as granulomas of bones and joints, clubbing, periostitis, osteomalacia, osteoporosis, septic arthritis, and complications of corticosteroid therapy.

## Colitic Arthritis

Colitic arthritis or "enteropathic" arthritis is the most common joint manifestation of IBD; it is seen more frequently with Crohn's disease than with ulcerative colitis. The large joints are primarily involved (knees, ankles, elbows, and wrists). They may be swollen, warm, and red. The appearance may not be dissimilar to that of rheumatoid arthritis, but it is nondeforming and seronegative; that is, rheumatoid factor is absent from the blood. Although any joint can be affected, small joints are affected less frequently (Fig. 30.14).

Symptoms of the arthritis usually develop after the IBD has been diagnosed and tend to parallel the course of the intestinal disease. The inflammation is usu-

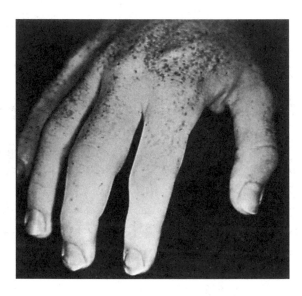

**FIG. 30.14.** Colitic arthritis. Proximal interphalangeal joint involvement in a 20-year-old man with acute ulcerative colitis. (From Corman ML, Veidenheimer MC, Nugent FW, et al. *Diseases of the anus, rectum and colon. Part II: Non-specific inflammatory bowel disease.* New York: Medcom, 1976, with permission.)

ally adequately controlled by antiinflammatory agents or by steroids. The arthritis completely resolves after colectomy.

### Rheumatoid Spondylitis

As stated, other joint disorders that can be encountered are severe arthralgias and rheumatoid spondylitis. The incidence of rheumatoid spondylitis is considerably higher in patients with IBD than in the general population; estimates range in excess of 20 times. The well-known gender incidence (4:1 ratio of men to women) is reversed when rheumatoid spondylitis complicates IBD. A genetic association between the two diseases has been demonstrated. In contradistinction to most other extracolonic manifestations, spondylitis does not parallel the activity of the bowel disease. The incidence is similar in Crohn's disease and ulcerative colitis.

The patient initially develops pain in the lumbosacral region, but the discomfort can rapidly progress to involve the thoracic and cervical spine. As ankylosis progresses, the patient exhibits the characteristic dorsal kyphosis. Interestingly, isolated asymptomatic sacroiliitis occurs more often than does spinal involvement (4% to 18%).

Treatment consists of physiotherapy, antiinflammatory agents, and steroids. Colectomy is not indicated for the treatment of the arthritic manifestations.

### Hypertrophic Osteoarthropathy or Finger Clubbing

Finger clubbing, which has also been reported in association with IBD, can regress after resection of the involved bowel segment, and usually correlates with disease activity.

## Polymyositis

Polymyositis has been reported on rare occasions to be a condition associated with IBD, especially ulcerative colitis. As with other unusual extraintestinal manifestations, always exercise concern about the possibility that the manifestation may be simply coincidental. Still, because of the possible autoimmune cause of the two conditions, a causal link is considered plausible.

## Bronchopulmonary Disease

Pulmonary manifestations have been said to be associated with IBD, including bronchiectasis, granulomatous lung disease, interstitial fibrosis, and sulfasalazine pneumonitis.

## Ocular Manifestations

Ocular disease, including orbital congestion, uveitis, conjunctivitis, iritis, and keratitis, is found in up to 10% of patients with IBD. The most common ocular lesion is episcleritis, an inflammation overlying the sclera, under the conjunctiva. A thickened, deep red appearance is usually noted in one segment of the eye. Burning, itching, and pain are the primary symptoms, but the patient often seeks medical attention because of the appearance. Steroids and antiinflammatory agents are the treatments of choice. Episcleritis is often associated with exacerbations of the underlying IBD, but is unrelated to extent or severity. Because of the complications that may lead to a chorioretinitis, ophthalmologic consultation is advised.

Uveitis usually produces ocular pain, blurred vision, and headache, and can occur whether the underlying disease is symptomatic or in remission. The diagnosis is established by slit-lamp examination. Treatment consists of pupillary dilatation to relieve spasm, an eye patch, and the application of topical corticosteroids.

## Amyloidosis

Secondary amyloidosis, when recognized, occurs almost exclusively with Crohn's disease. The diagnosis has been made usually at postmortem examination, although confirmation has been established on a few patients who presented with renal failure and had renal biopsy. In the absence of kidney dysfunction, a search for secondary amyloidosis is probably not justified. The application of rectal biopsy for establishing the diagnosis is discussed in Chapter 25. Regression of proteinuria and other manifestations of renal as well as hepatic dysfunction have been reported following bowel resection.

## Urologic Complications

Urologic complications are commonly seen in association with IBD. These include chronic interstitial nephritis, chronic pyelonephritis, acute tubular necrosis, urinary fistulas, ureteral obstruction, and nephrolithiasis.

Ureteral obstruction is much more frequently identified in association with Crohn's disease than with ulcerative colitis. The incidence has been reported to be as high as 50% in this group of patients. An inflammatory mass involving the terminal ileum and, occasionally, the sigmoid colon can produce extrinsic compression of the distal ureters; the right is more frequently involved than the left. The result is hydroureter, hydronephrosis, and, possibly, caliectasis. Symptoms related to the urinary tract may be minimal; if present, they may actually be caused by compression of the bladder by an inflammatory mass rather than from the obstruction of a ureter. Flank pain is suggestive of ureteral obstruction.

Treatment involves removal of the mass that is causing the compression. Complete resolution can be expected, assuming that the obstruction has not produced irreversible renal damage. Preoperative identification of ureteral dilatation should warn the surgeon that a meticulous dissection may be required to avoid ureteral injury. The preoperative placement of ureteral catheters should be considered.

Nephrolithiasis and bladder calculi are seen in at least 5% of individuals with IBD. Following proctocolectomy and ileostomy, patients are still at risk for the development of nephrolithiasis. Many factors contribute to the development of calculi in chronic IBD: decreased urine volume, increased crystalloid concentration, urinary electrolyte and pH changes, and recurrent urinary tract infections. A more acidic urine favors precipitation of urates and, as a result, uric acid calculi are more common in patients with IBD than in the "normal" population of stone formers. Intestinal absorption of oxylate is increased when ileal disease is present, and this is a further reason for formation of stones. Ileostomy patients were demonstrated to have a significantly lowered urinary pH and volume, and a higher concentration of calcium, oxylate, and uric acid. An adequate urinary volume should be maintained by encouraging the patient to consume sufficient water to increase urinary volume without increasing ileostomy output, by alkalinization in selected patients, by a diet low in oxylate and fat, and by "slowing" medications to reduce the ileostomy volume.

## Psoas Abscess

Psoas abscess has long been recognized as a complication of Crohn's disease, but it has also been found, albeit rarely, with ulcerative colitis. When seen as a consequence of Crohn's disease, it may be the result of a fistula or abscess from the terminal ileum on the right side or of disease of the jejunum or sigmoid on the left. The usual symptom is pain in the iliac fossa, abdomen, groin, or hip. Chills and fever, abdominal or flank mass, and an associated cutaneous fistula may be apparent. Drainage of the abscess with appropriate bowel resection is the preferred treatment, in addition to adequate, prolonged antibiotic coverage. Extension of the septic process, with establishment of a spinal extradural abscess requiring emergency laminectomy has been reported.

## Cardiac Complications

Cardiac complications in association with IBD are extremely unusual; pericarditis is certainly the most frequently described. Heart block may, in some individuals, be a complication of ulcerative colitis and not a coincidental association. Others believe that IBD can be considered an independent risk factor for the development of bacterial endocarditis. Therefore, endocarditis prophylaxis should be considered, according to some investigators, even in the absence of primary cardiac factors predisposing to the development of bacterial endocarditis.

## Other Manifestations

A number of other conditions have been suggested to be associated with nonspecific IBD. Evidence of Crohn's disease has been found in voluntary muscle, the larynx, and the ovary. Whether these and other manifestations, such as hyperthyroidism, hyperparathyroidism, and hematologic problems, are coincidental has not been clearly established.

## Relationship to Carcinoma

For many years, it was felt that the risk for the development of carcinoma was not increased in patients who had Crohn's disease. However, an accumulation of published reports beginning in the 1960s seems to indicate an exponential increase in the frequency of this observation. Some have suggested that the observations are merely coincidental. Most investigators, however, accept the thesis that such a relationship does indeed exist. This association is not equivalent to that which has been observed in longstanding, chronic ulcerative colitis, however.

It is difficult to assess the true incidence of Crohn's disease and carcinoma in the small intestine because small bowel carcinoma is such a rare condition. However, the association appears genuine and is based on several observations.

A different distribution of small bowel cancer is seen in Crohn's disease when compared with cancer of the small intestine that occurs in the absence of this inflammatory condition. In Crohn's disease, two thirds of the small bowel cancers occur in the ileum, whereas no more than 30% occur in this area when it is not involved by disease. In the large intestine, Crohn's disease with cancer is usually found in the right side of the colon, as compared with the usual more distal bowel involvement in the general population. Additional features of carcinoma in Crohn's disease include multifocal lesions and metachronous intestinal and extraintestinal cancers. Patients who develop carcinoma in Crohn's disease are usually relatively young; more than one half with colonic cancer are less than 40 years of age. A long duration of illness also appears to be an underlying factor, and perhaps a 10-fold greater risk exists of developing colon cancer in this circumstance than in the general population.

The likelihood of the development of carcinoma is greatly enhanced in patients who have had intestinal bypass. This is particularly true when chronic inflammatory disease persists for many years. The mortality rate of patients who develop cancer in excluded bowel is high (>80%), probably because it is recognized late in the progression of the disease. Even without an exclusion or bypass procedure having been performed, survival is poor with small bowel cancer. The mean survival rate is only 6 months compared with 65 months for those individuals with large bowel cancer. The observation of new signs and symptoms after a prolonged period of quiescence, particularly with longstanding disease, and especially if the patient previously had an exclusion or bypass procedure, should prompt vigorous evaluation for the possible presence of a malignancy.

Anal Crohn's disease also appears to be associated with an increased risk for the development of anal carcinoma. A relationship also appears to exist with intestinal-cutaneous fistulas, although the question always remains whether the fistula is secondary to an underlying malignancy in the intestine. Whether the anal or abdominal fistula causes malignant change to occur by "irritation" or by a stimulus to mucosal regeneration is a matter for conjecture.

Although carcinoma arising at the stomal site in patients with polyposis or ulcerative colitis has been described, only recently has the complication been reported in Crohn's disease. In both of the cases, dysplasia was identified in adjacent tissue.

### *Dysplasia*

As with carcinoma in ulcerative colitis, radiologic diagnosis of malignant change in patients with Crohn's disease is virtually impossible. Endoscopic examination likewise is of little benefit in establishing the diagnosis. However, dysplasia, if present, probably is as significant a finding as it is with ulcerative colitis. Unfortunately, with the exception of the very distal ileum, the small intestine does not lend itself well to investigation by means of biopsy, particularly if the segment is excluded. It is probably a reasonable precaution to recall all patients who have had a bypass or an exclusion procedure and evaluate them for possible resection.

Some authors have suggested that surveillance of the colon should commence after 10 years of disease. How frequently this should be done remains to be determined, but the issues and concerns expressed in Chapter 29 should be well heeded.

### *Other Malignancies*

The issue of extraintestinal malignancies with IBD is a matter of some controversy. Whether the association is valid or merely coincidental is still not a resolved issue. Concomitant malignant melanoma and lymphoma have been suggested to be more than mere coincidence, perhaps related to immunosuppression from the disease, itself, or from medical treatment.

## Medical Management

Clinical remission, on average, is achieved in 65% of individuals with Crohn's disease. Current medical therapy for severe Crohn's colitis seems to spare many patients early colectomy, but few clinical trials support the use of various therapeutic regimens. The Crohn's Disease Activity Index, which consists of the clinical variables correlated with physician's assessment of the patient's well-being, while being validated, has been criticized on other grounds because of its subjectivity and interobserver variability. Approaches to the management of patients include lifestyle, dietary, and pharmaceuticals, each of which can independently aid in the management of the asymptomatic individual with Crohn's disease.

### Aminosalicylates

The primary drugs traditionally used for the treatment of Crohn's disease are sulfasalazine and steroids (see Chapter 29). However, if the patient is ill enough to require hospitalization, intravenous administration of a steroid is recommended. A dramatic response is often observed with intravenous steroid administration; a mass may rapidly disappear, or a patient's acute abdominal symptoms may resolve.

A double-blind study of the effectiveness of sulfasalazine compared with 6-methylprednisolone in patients with Crohn's disease revealed that the addition of the former drug offered no advantage. Yet, most physicians continue to recommend that sulfasalazine be used. Even when the patient is recovering from resective surgery, with no evidence for continued abdominal disease, sulfasalazine is usually recommended. The maintenance of remission following resective therapy for Crohn's disease continues to be a topic of concern among internists, gastroenterologists, and surgeons. Symptomatic relapses occur at a rate of 40% to 70% in most series within 2 years following resective therapy. Oral mesalamine (Pentasa) for maintenance therapy appears to make a significant difference in the incidence of endoscopic lesions and severity in a treated group compared with a placebo. A similar favorable result was observed in individuals who were treated with oral 5-ASA (Asacol).

### Metronidazole (Flagyl)

Metronidazole, initially introduced for the treatment of *Trichomonas vaginalis* infections, was subsequently demonstrated to be an effective antibiotic against anaerobic organisms. It was also found to have activity against gram-positive and gram-negative bacteria. The drug is a substituted imidazole that is rapidly absorbed orally and rectally; it can also be given intravenously in the acutely ill patient.

Metronidazole has been demonstrated to be slightly more effective than sulfasalazine. A number of theories suggesting the mechanism of its action have been proposed: immunosuppression, an effect on wound healing, stimulation of leukocyte chemotaxis, and, of course, its antimicrobial effect. Although metronidazole may be beneficial for some patients with intestinal disease, it does not appear to have a therapeutic potential for preventing relapse of Crohn's disease. Patients having prolonged treatment need to be closely monitored for the development of peripheral neuropathy.

Metronidazole has been suggested to be particularly useful in the management of anal and perianal Crohn's disease. Drainage, erythema, and induration diminish dramatically in most patients so treated, with complete healing obtained in more than one half of those who are maintained on therapy. Dosage reduction may be associated with recurrent disease activity, but healing occurs promptly when the full dosage of metronidazole is reinstituted.

### Antituberculous Chemotherapy

Crohn's disease had been thought to resemble tuberculosis in many respects, and multiple attempts to isolate microbacteria have been made, albeit unsuccessfully. Double-blind, randomized trials involving rifampin, isoniazid, and ethambutol, or placebo, have demonstrated no tangible benefit from these agents.

### Immunosuppressive Agents

Because of the supposition that IBD is an autoimmune condition, treatment with immunosuppressive drugs has been recommended. The two agents that have been used extensively are 6-mercaptopurine and its analogue, azathioprine. Although immunosuppressive drugs have been shown to be effective in both ulcerative colitis and Crohn's disease, and with few exceptions the complications have been reversible, many physicians, perhaps inappropriately, fear to employ this modality in the management of their patients. However, the drugs are effective, with about two thirds of patients experiencing improvement. Furthermore, the combination with prednisolone is superior to that of treatment with prednisolone alone, in that more frequent remissions are observed and with lower doses of prednisolone. The drugs are not felt to be effective in the treatment of fulminant disease, but should be used in those individuals who can tolerate the relatively slow response to treatment (commonly, at least 6 months). They have been recommended for the treatment of perianal disease, small bowel obstruction (when surgery is contraindicated), and fistula complications, and for the management of Crohn's disease children. Prophylaxis after two surgical resections is another possible indication.

Complications include bone marrow suppression, liver abnormalities (including liver necrosis), pancreatitis, and hair loss. The initial concern about the possible induction of cancer does not seem to be justified on the basis of almost 20 years of experience. The steroid-sparing effects are felt to be of particular benefit in this group of patients. In all probability, the use of immunosuppressive agents is of comparable value in the management of ulcerative colitis.

In addition to the aforementioned drugs, methotrexate, a folic acid antagonist, has been used in the treatment of IBD. Preliminary results have been encouraging, with significant improvement observed with respect to symptomotology and the reduced requirement for prednisone.

Cyclosporine, a drug that has been widely used in organ transplantation, has been subjected to evaluation in the management of Crohn's disease. Currently, the use of cyclosporine in IBD must still be considered experimental, but preliminary results are encouraging, and the medication appears to be well tolerated.

### Enteric-Coated Fish Oil

The antiinflammatory effect of fish oil has been well documented to reduce production of a number of agents (e.g., leukotriene $B_4$ and thromboxane $A_2$), which have been observed in the inflamed intestinal mucosa of patients with Crohn's disease. Inhibition of the synthesis of cytokines and tumor necrosis factor has also been demonstrated with fish oil.

### Antibody Therapy

It has been thought that tumor necrosis factor-alpha (TNF-$\alpha$) has an important role in the pathogenesis of Crohn's disease. Early data suggest that antibody neutralization of TNF-$\alpha$ is a potentially effective strategy in the management of Crohn's disease. Further studies will be necessary to confirm this observation.

### Monoclonal Antibody Therapy

The concept of monoclonal antibody therapy is based on the development of antibodies to TNF-$\alpha$ to prevent or reduce inflammation in animals. Early studies have demonstrated statistically significant differences the clinical response when compared with the placebo group. Further trials are pending.

### Withdrawal of Smoking

Smoking has a pejorative effect on the clinical course of individuals with Crohn's disease. Irrespective of the way the course of Crohn's disease is analyzed, it is much less favorable for those individuals who smoke, especially if they are heavy smokers. As part of the therapeutic regimen, therefore, patients with Crohn's disease should be dissuaded from smoking.

### Intravenous Hyperalimentation

Hyperalimentation, either parenteral (TPN) or oral (enteral) has been recommended in a supportive role for patients with Crohn's disease. The rationale is to replenish nutritional deficits, to allow bowel rest for healing and "repair," and to provide perioperative support for healing in an attempt to reduce morbidity and mortality. There appears to be no lasting benefit for hyperalimentation as a primary method of therapy for patients with IBD, particularly for those with Crohn's disease. But if the purpose of the treatment is to defer surgical intervention so that it can be pursued on an elective basis, hyperalimentation should be considered.

An extensive review by Payne-James and Silk can be summarized by the statement, "Evidence at present indicates that TPN [total parental nutrition] in Crohn's disease should be restricted to a supportive role, rather than employed as primary therapy."

### Home Hyperalimentation

One additional application of hyperalimentation needs to be addressed— home parenteral nutrition—for the patient who has a short bowel syndrome, a potential consequence of multiple or extensive resections for Crohn's disease. In 1990 alone, TPN represented $937,000,000 or one third of the home intravenous market (according to Total Pharmaceutical Care, Inc., Santa Barbara, CA, USA).

Almost all patients who require rehospitalization do so because of problems with the catheter, and mortality usually results from the underlying disease process rather than therapy. Catheter-related sepsis occurs at a rate equivalent to one episode per 3 catheter-years. More than one half of patients have had at least one or more hyperalimentation-related complication—catheter sepsis, blocked or damaged catheters, and dehydration or electrolyte imbalance. The only valued nutritional parameters in monitoring patient well-being are body weight and serum albumin. Although this therapeutic modality is extremely tedious for the patient, it does permit an improvement in the quality of life.

### Oral or Enteral Nutrition

The place of an elemental diet in the management of Crohn's disease has been evaluated. Some suggest that the remission rate is comparable to that achieved with steroids. Failure to tolerate the diet is, of course, one potential problem. Obviously, if the patient fulfills the same criteria for treatment as those selected for ambulatory hyperalimentation, it would seem that the preferred alternative is oral management, if indeed it can be adequately achieved.

### Somatostatin

Somatostatin, a tetradecapeptide, growth-hormone release-inhibiting factor, has been found to have a powerful inhibitory action on gastrointestinal endocrine and exocrine secretions. As a consequence of its ability to profoundly decrease the volume and the enzyme content of the gastrointestinal tract, the drug has been used in the management of intestinal fistulas. It, therefore, has particular merit for the treatment of patients with Crohn's disease, especially those individuals who have fistula complications. Continuous intravenous infusion of somatostatin (250 µg/h) has been demonstrated to result in reduced output and, in some cases, spontaneous fistula closure. The synthetic analogue, SMS 901-225 (Sandostatin), has been developed to provide a longer half-life with less influence on insulin secretion. It has also been shown to prolong gastrointestinal transit time and to improve water and electrolyte absorption. The drug is supplied in 1-mL ampules containing 100 µg and is administered subcutaneously at a dose of 1 mL every 8 hours.

### Growth Hormone, Glutamine, and Diet

A new method of treatment for individuals with short bowel syndrome has been suggested through the administration of growth hormone, glutamine, and a specialized diet. With this regimen, parenteral nutrition requirements have been reduced in 80% of patients treated. Furthermore, approximately 40% are relieved of the TPN requirement completely. The theory concerning the efficacy of treatment is based on the fact that intestinal growth and adaptation are mediated, in part, by factors extrinsic to the gastrointestinal tract, such as growth hormone and thyroxine. Furthermore, the amino acid glutamine is a primary energy source for the gastrointestinal tract by exerting trophic effects on the bowel and through stimulation of nutrient absorption. Additional experience is anticipated with interest.

## Surgical Management of Short Bowel Syndrome

For the sake of completeness, it is worth mentioning surgical approaches are available for the treatment of patients with the short bowel syndrome. Some are considered experimental, such as intestinal transplantation and the growing of new intestinal mucosa by means of serosal patching. Other options include intestinal tapering and lengthening, creating intestinal valves and sphincters, constructing antiperistaltic intestinal segments, intestinal pacing, and the implementing recirculating intestinal loops. It is not within the purview of this text to detail all of the potential options.

### Operative Management

#### Indications

Operative treatment for Crohn's disease is advised primarily for complications (abscess, fistula, perforation, and obstruction, because surgical intervention may not cure the patient. Severe inanition, extraintestinal manifestations, and the presence or risk of malignancy are uncommon indications for surgery in this condition. It is well established that ulcerative colitis can produce toxic mega-colon and perforation, but it is important to recognize that early in the course of the illness, Crohn's disease can produce these conditions as well. Free perfora-tion of the small bowel in Crohn's disease has been reported to occur in approx-imately 1% of hospitalized patients.

Hemorrhage is rarely an indication for surgery with Crohn's disease, although the approach to surgical intervention tends to be somewhat more conservative when compared with ulcerative colitis. Because the latter condition can be cured with resection, less procrastination occurs if hemorrhage is profuse. A more cir-cumspect attitude generally pervades with Crohn's disease.

The presence of an abscess or fistula virtually excludes the diagnosis of ulcer-ative colitis. Internal and external fistulas associated with Crohn's disease are usually indications for surgical intervention. As stated, TPN may succeed in effecting temporary closure, and the place of somatostatin has likewise been addressed; however, patients almost invariably develop symptoms severe enough to justify surgical intervention.

Abscess formation is usually a consequence of fistula in Crohn's disease with up to 20% of patients having surgery for intraabdominal abscess. The most fre-quent site of origin is the terminal ileum, with the abscess located in the right lower quadrant.

Stricture is a common feature of Crohn's disease and a frequent indication for surgery. A number of reports suggest that abnormalities of collagen metabolism may be important in the pathogenesis of both fistulas and strictures and, in fact, may predate gross pathologic changes.

*Appendicitis.* Crohn's disease confined to the appendix is an unusual entity, with less than 100 cases reported in the literature. The disease is found most commonly in the second and third decades. The signs and symptoms mimic that of acute appendicitis, with 27% having a palpable mass. A protracted preopera-tive history of symptoms should alert the surgeon to this possibility. No incident of subsequent fecal fistula has been reported. Crohn's disease confined to the appendix appears to have a favorable prognosis.

*Acute Ileitis.* Occasionally, a patient has a laparotomy for presumed appen-dicitis and found to have distal ileal Crohn's disease (acute ileitis). Some con-troversy exists about the appropriate management under these circumstances. If the patient has abdominal pain for less than 1 week, appendectomy is followed by minimal complications. For those who have symptoms longer than this period, incidental appendectomy is followed by an 83% incidence of fistula or sinus tract arising, not from the appendiceal stump but from the terminal ileum. Most surgeons agree that the fistula arises from the ileum unless the cecum is involved with the disease. After initial ileocolic resection, one half of patients require no further resection, with a mean follow-up of more than 12 years. Con-versely, 92% of those who do not have resection require ileocolic resection for intractability or complications of Crohn's disease. I prefer to perform an appendectomy if I am convinced that the cecum is normal; it simplifies the differential diagnosis in the subsequent evaluation of abdominal pain. In reality, however, acute appendicitis not related to the underlying Crohn's disease is extremely rare. When it does occur, it is likely to be associated with a long delay before surgical treatment is initiated. Certainly, exercise caution if terminal ileitis is identified at the time of operation for what was presumed to be acute appendicitis. It may be easier to advise than to perform, but the surgeon should not attempt to "break up" adhesions to the abdominal wall under these circumstances, because of the risk of precipitating an abscess or a fecal fistula.

Always be aware of the differential diagnosis of terminal ileitis. A self-limited process caused by *Yersinia enterocolitica* should be considered, as should the diagnosis of *Campylobacter*.

## Anal Manifestations

Anorectal abscess and anal fistula are frequent complications of Crohn's disease, especially when the condition involves the colon or rectum. If the disease is confined to the small intestine, however, anal manifestations are less common. In the absence of other areas of involvement, anorectal disease, itself, is rarely an indication for surgical intervention outside of the anus and perineum. However, in those patients with fecal incontinence, or in whom a rectovaginal or anovaginal fistula develops, radical surgery may be indicated for these complications alone. Under these circumstances, a permanent ileostomy or colostomy is usually required, but a temporary diversionary procedure may permit the surgeon to perform a reconstruction on selected patients.

Definitive surgery has been recommended and has been successfully performed in patients with anal fistulas in Crohn's disease. The success that these authors have had is certainly, I believe, because of careful patient selection. It is important to make the distinction between anal Crohn's disease and a fistula-in-ano arising in the patient who has IBD without anal involvement. In this latter group, definitive anal surgery can be done with reasonable expectation of healing. This is particularly true if the involved bowel segment either has been resected or is quiescent. Conversely, healing of wounds in a patient with anal Crohn's disease or with active disease elsewhere in the gastrointestinal tract will often lead to chronic, draining, indolent, and painful ulcers, which create more problems in management than did the original complaint. To assess adequately the extent of disease, examination under anesthesia may be required. Endoscopic or radiologic evaluation of the entire gastrointestinal tract is a requisite before definitive surgery is considered in a patient with known or suspected anal Crohn's disease.

The optimal form of therapy for anal Crohn's is medical management and simple drainage of an abscess, when it occurs. Long-term catheter or seton drainage may offer the best palliation for recurrent suppuration. Treatment by local depot methylprednisolone injection (Depo Medrol, 40 to 80 mg) has been attempted with some success in alleviating severe anal pain.

### Patient Preparation

See Chapter 29.

### Operative Approaches

Regardless of the choice of operation and irrespective of how radical the extirpation, surgery for Crohn's disease is primarily palliative, not curative. Therefore, operative intervention is recommended essentially for the complications that have been previously discussed. For individuals with Crohn's disease involving the colon and rectum, proctocolectomy with ileostomy is considered the appropriate operation, although preservation of the rectum may be contemplated if this area is relatively spared. When Crohn's disease affects other segments of the gastrointestinal tract, the choice of operation depends on the location and the extent of disease. Most surgeons believe that the ileo-pouch–anal procedures and the Kock operation are contraindicated in individuals with granulomatous colitis.

### General Principles

Exploration of the abdomen usually reveals the extent of pathology in those with Crohn's disease, because this is a transmural inflammatory process, and the serosa is virtually always involved. In fact, it is not uncommon to discover that the disease is more extensive than can be appreciated by preoperative evaluation. Conversely, with ulcerative colitis, the severity of inflammation is usually unimpressive as perceived from the serosal aspect.

The small intestine should be carefully examined, and the areas of disease identified and marked with sutures, if necessary. This is a particularly important principle if more than one segment is to be resected. Measurement of the length of residual normal and diseased bowel (if left behind) is helpful if further surgery is to be considered later.

Some surgeons, at one time, had thought it prudent to remove enlarged lymph nodes, believing that the nodes harbor a factor that predisposes the individual to recurrent disease. No evidence suggests that this is the case, and the surgeon is not advised to pursue a more radical excision in an effort to eliminate this tissue.

In patients with Crohn's disease, retroperitoneal inflammation can pose some risk for ureteral injury during mobilization of the right colon or the rectosigmoid. Care should be taken during this maneuver to identify the ureter and to keep it out of harm's way. Likewise, duodenal injury is possible, particularly if transmural involvement by Crohn's disease causes fixation of the bowel to the second and third portions of the duodenum. Careful dissection between these structures must be performed: drop the duodenum posteriorly until it is well out of the area of dissection. Shortening and thickening of the mesentery of the right colon and proximal transverse colon also predisposes the duodenum to possible injury. By clamping the blood vessels on one side only, dividing the mesentery on the bowel side, the side wall of the duodenum is less likely to be incorporated. Back-bleeding can then be addressed with the bowel delivered away from the area of potential injury. A finger-fracture technique can be used in the dissection of the small and large bowel mesentery, similar to that described for hepatic resection, identifying the vessels after the mesentery has been separated.

### Proctocolectomy with Ileostomy

Proctocolectomy with ileostomy is the conventional operative approach for the treatment of ulcerative colitis and for most patients with granulomatous colitis in which the rectum or anus is involved. Resection of the distal small bowel is sometimes necessary when proctocolectomy is done for Crohn's disease, depending on whether the inflammatory process involves the small bowel. Even modest resection of the distal ileum can lead to rapid small-bowel transit and malabsorption of nutrients as well as water and electrolyte loss. Do not remove any normal small bowel and limit the resection of ileum to the minimal length necessary for extirpation of macroscopic disease.

An intraperitoneal ileostomy is the recommended technique for stomal creation in a patient with granulomatous colitis, in those who have already had a portion of the terminal ileum removed, and in those for whom "stripping" of the parietal peritoneum is technically impossible. The relative disadvantages of this procedure when compared with the extraperitoneal approach are mitigated by the occasional requirement for revision as a consequence of recurrent disease. This is easier to accomplish with an intraperitoneal ileostomy.

### *Complications*

Most complications of proctocolectomy are not specific for this operation and are discussed in Chapters 22, 23, and 29. Sexual dysfunction, intestinal obstruction, and perineal difficulties are addressed in Chapter 29.

### *Stomal Problems*

Stomal problems and their management are discussed in Chapters 31 and 32. A special concern is recurrence in the ileum or in the ileostomy following proctocolectomy for Crohn's disease. Although proctocolectomy is usually curative when granulomatous colitis is confined to the colon, rectum, and anus, between 10% and 20% of patients will develop a proximal recurrence, usually at or just above the ileostomy. The development of a paraileostomy abscess in a patient who has had resection for Crohn's disease implies recurrence until proved otherwise. Evaluation can include endoscopic examination of the ileostomy, radiologic investigation by a barium enema through the stoma, or both.

Treatment almost always requires resection of the involved ileum and ileostomy with relocation of the stoma to another site. In the acute situation, it may be possible to drain the abscess by inserting a clamp at the mucocutaneous junction and liberating the pus. This, then, can be incorporated in the ileostomy appliance with a drain left in the cavity. Alternatively, if the abscess "points" at some distance from the ileostomy, drainage should be effected outside of the appliance faceplate. Every attempt should be made to avoid draining the abscess directly under the faceplate; such a maneuver will inevitably make management of the ileostomy effluent difficult.

### Recurrent Crohn's Disease

Recurrent Crohn's disease can develop at any time following resection for the condition, even as early as a few days postoperatively.

## Results

Recurrence following proctocolectomy for Crohn's disease, when the disease is confined to the colon, has been reported to be between 10% and 20%. The prognosis appears to be better if total proctocolectomy is performed as compared with restoration of intestinal continuity. Cumulative reoperation rates at 5 and 10 years of 19% and 24%, respectively, have been described. The recurrence rates following restorative surgery in the small and large bowel are discussed later.

Today, proctocolectomy and ileostomy can be carried out with minimal morbidity and mortality. Elective resection should carry with it an operative mortality no greater than 1% or 2%.

## Ileostomy

The indications and technique for ileostomy, with and without so-called "blowhole" colostomy are discussed in Chapter 29. Although its application for the management of toxic megacolon in patients with ulcerative colitis is generally appreciated, it can also be usefully applied to those individuals whose disease fails to respond to medical therapy or who have specific problems (e.g., perianal sepsis). As many as 90% to 95% of patients may be improved by simple diversion. Definitive resection can then be done at a later stage. Patients who had fecal diversion for colonic Crohn's disease may have a sustained period of remission. Furthermore, diversion is associated with a significant reduction of steroid requirements and a significant improvement in the blood count as well as the serum albumin.

### Ileorectal Anastomosis

For patients with colonic Crohn's disease and rectal sparing, colectomy and ileorectal anastomosis is the optimal procedure. The operation may still be applicable, however, for patients with mild or moderate rectal inflammation and, obviously, for those individuals anxious to avoid an ileostomy. The technique is described in Chapter 22.

## *Results*

Interpretation of the results of colonic resection is often difficult, because some authors make recommendations based on comparing limited, segmental resection of the colon with that of total colectomy. The requirement for subsequent proctectomy is similar for both patients with ulcerative colitis and those with Crohn's disease (24% vs. 29%, respectively). However, quality of life is felt to be satisfactory in only one third of those with Crohn's disease, as opposed to more than 50% of those with ulcerative colitis.

The need for reoperation because of recurrence has been calculated actuarially to be 50% after 16 to 20 years. Recurrence rates are slightly higher, ranging from 65% to 80%, but not all required further operative intervention, and intestinal continuity could still be maintained in most.

*Comment*: I believe ileorectal anastomosis for Crohn's colitis is the procedure of choice when the rectum is relatively spared and when the patient does not have significant anal disease. With the passage of time, approximately one third will develop symptoms severe enough to require either proctectomy or diversion. Even those individuals who must have a second procedure can still be relatively well served by temporarily avoiding an ileostomy. The problem, of course, is to select the appropriate patients—an exceedingly difficult task. One is often surprised at the degree of inflammatory reaction a patient may harbor in the rectum or indeed in the anal region and still, for a time, have a relatively salutary result following a restorative operation. However, patients who demonstrate pelvic sepsis, an intraabdominal abscess, or a fistula to the rectum should probably have a diverting loop ileostomy to protect the anastomosis. This is obviously a surgical decision, and each patient must be treated on an individual basis. Preoperative decision-making can be facilitated by determining rectal capacity and compliance. These physiologic studies are discussed in Chapters 4 and 6.

Those who are troubled by frequent bowel movements can often be helped by the addition of a bulk agent containing psyllium, as well as "slowing" medications (e.g., codeine, deodorized tincture of opium, and diphenoxylate with atropine sulfate [Lomotil] or loperamide [Imodium]). If resection of the distal ileum were performed, cholestyramine (Questran) may help control diarrhea.

## Segmental Colon Resection

With Crohn's disease, restoration of intestinal continuity is certainly a viable option under many circumstances, depending on the location and the extent of involvement. Because the condition can occur anywhere in the gastrointestinal tract, it is difficult to discuss the operative choices as they pertain solely to the colon and rectum. A reasonable approach is probably to perform three basic sphincter-saving operations for colonic disease: right hemicolectomy for ileocolonic and right-sided involvement; total or subtotal colectomy for disease involving at least one half of the colon; and sigmoid colectomy or anterior resection, when the disease is limited to this area.

## Results

Results of segmental resection suggest that recurrence rates and requirement for reoperation are similar to those of total colectomy with restoration of continuity.

### Resection with Exclusion of Rectum, Hartmann Procedure, and Ileostomy

Resection of the colon without reestablishment of intestinal continuity is a reasonable option in the management of Crohn's colitis. The 10-year risk of subsequent proctectomy is 50% to 80%. The early necessity for resection in many cases (as many as 50%) has led some authors to suggest that early completion proctectomy or primary total proctocolectomy should be seriously considered in this group of patients.

### Management of Small Bowel Crohn's Disease

The indications for surgery for regional enteritis include inanition, intraabdominal sepsis, intestinal obstruction, fistulas, urologic complications, and extraintestinal manifestations. The most common indication for surgical treatment is chronic obstruction (35%), followed by internal fistulas (30%), intractability (22%), and abscess formation (11%). As discussed, occasionally a patient has laparotomy with a presumed diagnosis of acute appendicitis. The appendix may be safely removed with no evidence of cecal disease. Conversely, if the cecum appears to be involved by the inflammatory process, appendectomy can result in a fecal fistula. Laparotomy alone can lead to a fistula through handling of the diseased bowel, presumably from disrupting microperforations of the distal ileum. In any event, resection of the ileum is not advised under these circumstances, as fewer than 10% of patients develop subsequent identifiable ileitis.

When an operation is indicated for other than acute ileitis, the involved segment is resected. The choice of operative procedure depends on the intraabdominal findings. As mentioned, it is not usually difficult to identify the area of involvement, because of the macroscopic appearance of the serosal surface of the bowel fat wrapping, inflammatory changes, stricture, and so on. Still, it is discouraging to note that as many as 65% of patients operated on for Crohn's disease have lesions of the small intestine undetected by the surgeon but which can be identified by perioperative endoscopy of the whole small bowel. It appears then that recurrence may not truly represent recurrence in every case, but persistent disease.

Types of operations include limited small-bowel resection, multiple small-bowel resections (with enteroenterostomy, diversion, or both), bypass, strictureplasty, balloon dilatation, and resection of distal ileum in continuity with cecum, right colon, most or all of the colon, and, of course, with proctocolectomy.

## Resection

Small-bowel resection is usually a straightforward procedure, an operation that is familiar to all surgeons. A special concern is the often remarkable thickness of the mesentery. It is sometimes helpful simply to divide the mesentery without the use of clamps, maintaining pressure on the blood supply with the fingers, and then performing suture ligation of the cut ends of the vessels. This will certainly expedite what can be the tedious dissection often associated with hematoma formation. A finger fracture technique has been mentioned earlier. Transillumination of the mesentery is another method for identifying the blood supply to the bowel. It is a particularly useful method when creating an ileostomy or performing a pouch procedure. Although it has been said that the small bowel can be safely reapproximated with chewing gum and baling wire, an interrupted single-layer technique or stapling method is suggested.

Resection is usually done, leaving a minimal normal bowel margin of 5 or 6 cm. If multiple "skip" areas are present, attempt to remove or bypass only the most constricting portions that may be causing the symptoms. If two segments are involved in relative proximity (e.g., <30 cm), it is probably safer to perform an *en bloc* resection of both segments rather than to perform two anastomoses. Laparoscopic-assisted intestinal resection has been applied for the surgical management of Crohn's disease with success. Patients who have a documented mass or radiographic evidence of fistulas are poor candidates for this approach.

## Strictureplasty

Radical excision of the small bowel in an attempt to remove all obvious disease can result in profound disturbances in fluid and electrolytes as well as severe malnutrition. In recent years, *strictureplasty* has been suggested as an alternative in this situation. The procedure was originally advocated for the treatment of tubercular strictures, but has been successfully applied to the management of extensive Crohn's. The primary indications are the presence of multiple, relatively short strictures, and the need to conserve intestinal length because of extensive disease or prior resection. The procedures advocated for pyloroplasty (either Heineke–Mikulicz for short strictures or Finney for long ones) can be used (Figs. 30.15 and 30.16). An interrupted single-layer technique is less likely to cause luminal narrowing, and patching the suture line to the serosa of the adjacent

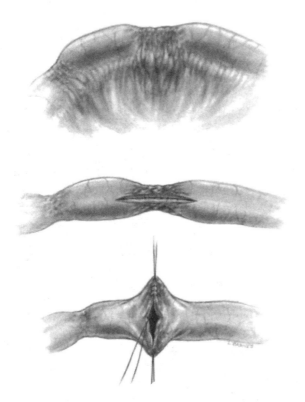

**FIG. 30.15.** Strictureplasty for Crohn's disease. Short stricture treated by the technique analogous to Heineke–Mikulicz pyloroplasty. Longitudinal enterotomy is closed transversely using interrupted no. 3-0 long-term absorbable sutures.

bowel helps prevent leakage (Fig. 30.17). As with all operations designed to coapt intestine, a stapler modification can also be used, but the presence of thickened bowel may preclude the application of this instrument (Figs. 30.18 and 30.19). A 2-cm bougie or Foley catheter may help identify all areas of significant narrowing. Strictureplasty can be combined with limited small-bowel resection and bypass, all within the same individual, depending on the operative findings.

Another alternative to the management of colonic strictures is balloon dilatation. This technique has been performed successfully via the colonoscope using Riglex TTS dilating balloons. One of the concerns that has been expressed is the possibility of performing strictureplasty in the presence of cancer arising in Crohn's disease. It, therefore, would seem prudent to perform a small biopsy of the full thickness of the bowel before completing the procedure, obtaining frozen sections to confirm the absence of malignant change.

*Results*

The Cleveland Clinic group has reported what is arguably the world's largest experience with strictureplasty. The latest publication involves 162 patients hav-

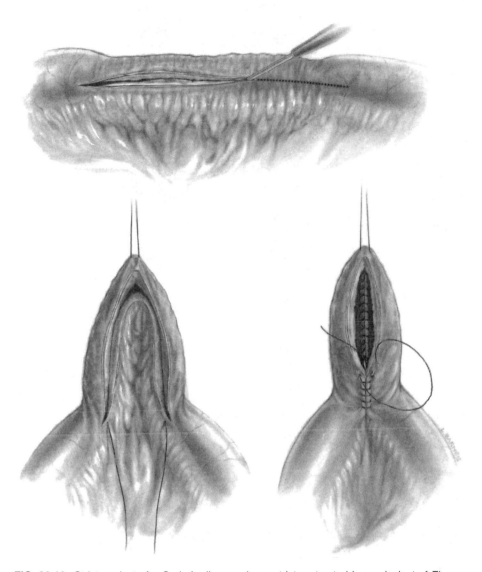

**FIG. 30.16.** Strictureplasty for Crohn's disease. Long stricture treated by equivalent of Finney "pyloroplasty" technique. A long antimesenteric incision is made over the stricture site and carried into the normal bowel.

ing a total of 698 strictureplasties. The mean number performed for each individual was three. No deaths were reported. The cumulative 5-year incidence of reoperation for recurrence was 28% with a mean follow-up of 42 months. Symptoms of obstruction were relieved in 98% of the patients. Reoperative rates were comparable to resection. For patients treated by strictureplasty alone, the cumu-

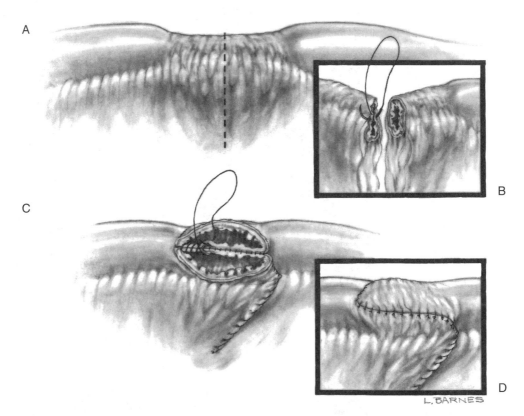

**FIG. 30.17.** Crohn's stricture. **(A)** Severe narrowing of a long segment of small bowel. **(B)** The bowel is transected. **(C)** Suturing of the two ends by means of a two-layer, hand-sewn running suture. Approximation of the two segments in a parallel fashion. **(D)** Completion of side-to-side ileal-ileal anastomosis. The original lumen has been doubled, thus sparing half the length of the intestine. (From Taschieri AM, Cristaldi M, Elli M, et al. Description of new bowel-sparing techniques for long strictures of Crohn's disease. *Am J Surg* 1997;173:509.)

lative reoperation rate at 5 years was 31%, whereas for those who had concomitant bowel resection it was 27.2%.

### *Management of Enteric Fistulas*

Approximately 30% of patients with Crohn's disease will develop a fistula; one third of these will be external. An external fistula may be the manifestation in which the patient presents initially, but it is obviously much more commonly recognized as a postoperative complication. The nonsurgical approach to this

**FIG. 30.19.** Stapled strictureplasty. **A.** The bowel is opened in a longitudinal fashion. **B, C.** Utilizing a linear stapler and overlapping staple lines, the strictureplasty is performed.

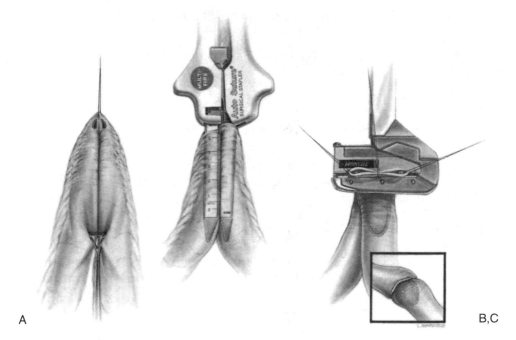

**FIG. 30.18.** Stapled strictureplasty for Crohn's disease. **A.** The midpoint of the stricture becomes the apex; the bowel is held in position by a suture or a Babcock clamp. Two small enterotomies are created. **B.** The two limbs of the stapler are inserted and fired. The stapler instrument size can be changed to accommodate the length of the stricture. **C.** The linear stapler is fired. A biopsy specimen can be obtained by trimming the residual tissue (*inset*).

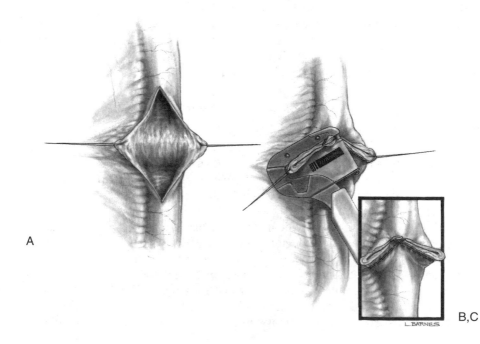

problem has been discussed. The principles of surgical and metabolic management include the following:

Drainage of the septic process
Correction of any metabolic deficits
Identification of anatomy and the pathologic process
Resection

When an enteroenteric fistula is identified, it is important to try to ascertain whether the bowel is primarily or secondarily involved by Crohn's disease. For example, in the latter situation, resection of the segment of intestine that is not actually diseased can often be avoided. Such a circumstance arises when the involved terminal ileum creates an ileosigmoid fistula. The ileum is resected done by dividing the fistulous communication to the sigmoid colon. Whether resection of the sigmoid is appropriate depends on the degree of inflammatory reaction; if the opening can simply be sutured, no resection is advised.

If a vesical fistula develops, management of the bladder is essentially the same as that described when the communication is a consequence of radiation injury. Because no disease affects the bladder itself, no specific measures aside from urinary drainage are indicated. Cystoscopy is the most accurate investigative procedure for identifying such a fistula.

### Bypass or Exclusion

A bypass or exclusion procedure has been advocated for distal ileal and cecal Crohn's disease. These operations are open to criticism because of the high incidence of persistent septic problems and the association with the subsequent development of carcinoma (see earlier). One exception to the caution of applying bypass is for patients with duodenal Crohn's disease. A gastroenterostomy is often advised in this circumstance, but a strictureplasty should definitely be considered.

### Continent or Kock Ileostomy

As I stated, the application of the continent ileostomy in the management of granulomatous colitis is contraindicated. Recurrence in the reservoir or distal ileum occurs in approximately 50%. Although generally the functional results are reasonably satisfactory, the incidence of postoperative and late complications is significantly higher than observed in those who have the procedure for ulcerative colitis.

Some "courageous" surgeons, however, believe that the procedure can be applied selectively to some individuals with this disease. The usual circumstance is the patient who had proctocolectomy and conventional ileostomy a number of years previously with no evidence of recurrence in the interval. With this scenario, willingness is seen to accept the risks and, with appropriate patient consent, proceed to a continent ileostomy. Most surgeons willing to pursue this course would demand a 5-year disease-free period. The risk of recurrence is probably at least 50%, and many may ultimately require excision of the pouch.

## Ileo-Pouch–Anal Procedure

The experience with the ileo-pouch–anal procedure to manage enteric fistulas is based primarily on those who had the operation for presumed ulcerative colitis only to discover after examination of the surgical specimen that the diagnosis was in error. Another group of patients subsequently develops Crohn's disease, even though retrospective analysis of the specimen failed to demonstrate the diagnosis. The results suggest two distinct categories of patients: those with preoperative stigmata of Crohn's disease, and those whose Crohn's disease was not suspected, but only discovered on the basis of the histologic evaluation. Patients in whom any preoperative suggestion of Crohn's disease exists, clinically or pathologically, have very poor results following this operation. In the short term, at least, if the clinical diagnosis of ulcerative colitis seems assured, early results following the ileo-pouch–anal procedure are significantly better with postoperative, histologically proved Crohn's disease than when Crohn's disease is suspected preoperatively. On the basis of the poor results observed in most of the patients found to have Crohn's disease postoperatively, the Toronto General Hospital group counsel that the pelvic pouch procedure should not knowingly be performed in these individuals. Virtually all reputable surgeons refuse to perform reservoir procedures in patients with Crohn's disease, even when the disease has been limited to the colon, and despite no evidence of small bowel recurrence with long-term follow-up.

*Results.* At some time, a number of factors have been suggested to contribute to an increased risk for recurrence after resection: site of involvement, age at onset of disease, age at first resection, gender, prior resection, extent of resection, presence or absence of gross or microscopic disease at the resection margin, immunologic factors (T-cell and total lymphocyte counts), blood transfusion, choice of operation, pathological variables, and probably others. Clearly, recurrence is unaffected by the width of the resection margin from macroscopically involved bowel. Furthermore, generally recurrence rates are not increased when microscopic Crohn's disease is present at the resection margins. However, some believe that the presence of granulomas is associated with a statistically significant increased risk for the development of recurrence. A close correlation also appears to exist between the duration of postoperative recurrence with the extent of presurgical disease. Others confirm that disease extent has prognostic value with respect to the risk of symptomatic recurrence, whereas the length of resection margins does not appear to influence this risk. All of these findings reaffirm the importance of a conservative approach to resection margin in individuals with Crohn's disease. Ileostomy, itself, seems to be associated with a significantly lower early recurrence risk than for colon anastomoses. Others suggest that the fecal stream and reflux of colonic contents are important factors in determining the pattern of recurrence.

The protocol for following patients who have had resection identify early recurrence has never been clearly established nor is it without considerable controversy. A variety of approaches include regular follow-up visits, periodic endoscopic evaluation, long-term drug therapy, and radiologic and laboratory investigations. The fecal excretion of 1-antitrypsin has been felt to be a reliable marker of intestinal protein loss; it, therefore, has been evaluated for its efficacy as an early indicator for recurrence in Crohn's disease.

The Cleveland Clinic has been associated with more papers, and with greater numbers of patients, than any other institution. Results of a study involving 615 consecutive patients seen at that institution revealed the following primary clinical patterns: ileocolic, 41%; small intestine, 28.6%; colon, 27%; and anorectal, 3.4%. At 10 years, more than 90% of patients with ileocolitis had surgery, and nearly 70% of patients with ileal or colonic disease required operation. Those with ileocolic disease had the highest rate of recurrence requiring another operation (53%), compared with 45% for colonic and 44% for small intestinal patterns. Fazio and Wu conclude with the following main characteristics of patients with Crohn's disease:

Most have surgery at some point.

Reoperation is always a possibility.

Prognosis with respect to recurrence differs, based on the initial pattern of presentation.

## Mortality

General opinion, which has been borne out by multiple reviews, is that Crohn's disease does not significantly increase long-term mortality, a factor that needs to be conveyed to actuaries, insurers, and those individuals who advise employers.

## INDETERMINATE COLITIS

The differential diagnosis between ulcerative colitis and granulomatous colitis can usually be made on the basis of clinical, radiologic, endoscopic, and pathologic criteria. However, perhaps up to 15% of patients develop nonspecific IBD of a type that cannot clearly be labeled as one or the other, often because of overlapping features. These individuals, therefore, have been classified as having an indeterminate colitis.

Indeterminate (not "indeterminant") colitis is essentially a pathologic diagnosis—often with equivocal or contradictory histologic observations. Many of these patients have surgery on an urgent basis. Insufficient opportunity—clinically, radiologically, or endoscopically—exists to clarify the nature of the disease. It follows, then, that the disease activity affects the evaluation of morphologic features and that, given the opportunity, repeat evaluation during a quiescent phase may clarify any confusion.

Diagnosis of Crohn's colitis is made by either the clinician (preoperatively or intraoperatively) or by the pathologist. It is the latter individual who is responsible for creating the diagnosis of indeterminate colitis. Typical features in patients otherwise thought to have ulcerative colitis include "intermittent" ulceration, relative rectal sparing, preservation of goblet-cell population, and deep fissuring. Absence of granulomas in certain patients with presumed Crohn's disease also may place the patient in an indeterminate category. The additional criteria of extensive mucosal and submucosal ulceration separated by normal colonic mucosa, nonaggregate, full-thickness inflammation; increased vascularity in the base of the ulceration; and the absence of both crypt abscesses and transmural lymphoid aggregates have been suggested as well.

A particularly compelling caution against restorative proctocolectomy is the presence of an anal fistula or perineal disease. If the clinical diagnosis is suspected it is wise to stage the procedure. The problem with this admonition is that either the definitive diagnosis may never be clarified or that Crohn's disease may not be evident until the rectum has been removed. Therefore, the importance of multiple biopsies cannot be overestimated. Because small, colonoscopic biopsies may be inadequate, deeper biopsy by means of the rigid proctosigmoidoscope is preferred.

Consider also total abdominal proctocolectomy, leaving a minimal rectal remnant. This important technical consideration, performing the resection of the rectum as low as is possible, facilitates the subsequent procedure—either proctectomy or a restorative operation.

Until further data become available, utilization of the pouch procedure in these individuals requires circumspection.

## CONCLUSION

The results of surgery for Crohn's disease are less than satisfactory. The concept that repeated resections will ultimately cure the patient is obviously erroneous. It is evident that as additional operations are required, the likelihood of recurrence is actually increased.

Therefore, surgical intervention must be limited to those patients who have complications severe enough to justify an operation. Longstanding disease is not yet a surgical indication, as it classically has been for ulcerative colitis. Because it is not clear what the actual prognostic validity of the concept of dysplasia is in patients with granulomatous colitis, and because the incidence of malignant change is low, long duration of disease is not, itself, an indication for surgical intervention. However, recent opinions suggest that when dysplastic changes are identified, resection should be advised. Bypass procedures and exclusion operations should not be performed, except in the critically ill patient. If carried out, definitive resection should be done at the earliest possible time. Strictureplasty should be applied rarely, and then only in those for whom a resection would result in significant disability, such as the requirement for intravenous alimentation.

Because important endoscopic lesions can be present without clinical symptoms, periodic colonoscopy should be part of the follow-up evaluation of all patients who have had an anastomosis in the colon for Crohn's disease.

The future is not altogether bleak, however. A number of new medical approaches are being suggested; some, such as in the area of immunosuppression, are being pursued in clinical trials. It is hoped that within the next few years successful medical management can be anticipated and that surgery for this condition will be relegated to that of a historical curiosity.

# 31

# Intestinal Stomas

## PREPARING THE PATIENT

Overcoming ignorance and fear is often the most important issue that must be addressed by the surgeon in preparing an individual for a stoma. The surgeon must confront the fear of the disease itself, the potential for complications, and, indeed, the possible mortality; these issues must be addressed as part of a comprehensive rehabilitative program. It is often helpful to provide literature concerning the nature of the surgery and the reasonableness of living with a colostomy or an ileostomy. In addition, it is often helpful to have an individual of similar age, gender, and socioeconomic position serve to acquaint a patient with the concept of living and functioning normally with a stoma. Whenever possible, the enterostomal therapist should be involved with the preoperative counseling, not necessarily to provide detailed stomal care at that time, but instead information about the wide variety of ostomy products available (see Chapter 32).

### Stomal Marking

The location of the stoma has a direct bearing on subsequent ostomy management. Establishing the stomal site before surgery is usually done by the surgeon, but in many instances can be delegated to a trained enterostomal therapist.

The stoma should always be placed at the summit of the infraumbilical bulge and within the rectus muscle, avoiding the groin, waistline, costal margins, umbilicus, skin folds, and scars, and leaving a 5-cm margin of smooth skin around the site. When the site is being marked, it is helpful to have the patient lie in the supine position and tense the abdominal muscles. This allows one to feel the lateral border of the rectus muscle. A triangle is formed by drawing an imaginary line from the umbilicus to the pubis, one from the umbilicus to the anterosuperior iliac spine, and another from the pubis to the anterosuperior iliac spine (the inguinal ligament). The stoma usually should be in the center. The faceplate should be taped over the site and the patient should stand, sit, and bend with the faceplate in place. Slight adjustments may be required because of interference from skin creases and from adiposity.

Another factor to consider is the patient's preference for clothing style, especially where the belt is worn, because stomas must be placed below the waist and preferably below the belt line. Should an individual require two stomas, the new opening must be placed either above or below the existing one. I prefer simply to scratch a mark onto the proposed location. The use of a pen is not advised, because such marks will be obliterated during the abdominal preparation.

The aforementioned considerations are applicable to all intestinal stomas—ileostomy, sigmoid colostomy, transverse colostomy, and urinary conduit.

## LAPAROSCOPIC INTESTINAL STOMAS

A number of papers have been published attesting that this approach is well tolerated and can be performed safely and effectively. Obvious advantages include the avoidance of a laparotomy and still maintaining the ability to precisely identify and orient the pertinent bowel segment. The technical approach to performing this technique is discussed in Chapter 27.

## SIGMOID COLOSTOMY

The possible indications for either a permanent or a temporary stoma in this area include carcinoma of the rectum, diverticulitis, Crohn's disease, congenital anomalies, anal incontinence, and colorectal trauma.

The technique for creating a satisfactory end sigmoid colostomy has been described previously as it pertains to the abdominoperineal resection for carcinoma of the rectum (see Chapter 23). It is important that the colon be brought through the split rectus muscle and sutured to the skin without tension. A "flush" colostomy can be performed with reasonable safety because the colostomy effluent is noncorrosive, but this technique is not advised. With the patient's possible weight gain, the stoma tends to retract. This makes appliance management more difficult. Hence, the stoma should be permitted to pout slightly, but not to the extent of a conventional ileostomy.

### Complications

The principles of proper stomal construction have already been outlined. If these are attended to, the risk of colostomy complications will be minimized.

#### *Ischemia and Stomal Necrosis*

Ischemia and stomal necrosis obviously result from inadequate blood supply. Recognition of stomal ischemia should not be difficult. If the mucosa looks blue, it probably is ischemic. If the stoma is nonviable, the bowel can retract into the peritoneal cavity. Peritonitis can ensue and necessitate emergency surgical intervention. Less critical, the sigmoid colostomy can retract and the stool presents in the lower portion of the abdominal incision, tracking subcutaneously from the original opening in the rectus fascia. In a less ominous consequence, the stoma separates from the skin at the area of nonviability, with a resultant stricture.

## Management

If the patient cannot cope with the retraction or stenosis, revision is required. Dilatation alone of a skin-level stenosis is not recommended. A formal laparotomy with colostomy resection and the creation of a new stoma are necessary if adequate length cannot be established by a limited approach. However, an attempt should be made to circumcise the colostomy, to free up the bowel, and to resuture it.

Rarely, the stenosis occurs at the fascial level. This is usually results from an inadequate opening in the fascia itself or to vascular compromise. Treatment requires mobilization of the bowel, enlargement of the opening in the fascia, and resuture of the colon.

## Results

Only a limited number of papers are available in contemporary writings. Local excision of the scar tissue at the mucocutaneous junction has been reported as one treatment option, with a 61% success rate for relief of the stenosis.

## Paracolostomy Abscess and Perforation

Paracolostomy abscess is an unusual postoperative complication. The problem can occur after ileostomy maturation when sutures are placed too deeply and penetrate the bowel lumen at the time of eversion. This can also develop as a consequence of recurrence of Crohn's disease

This complication can also be the result of stomal retraction with fecal contamination of the subcutaneous tissue. More commonly, improper irrigation technique can lead to perforation and abscess. Either the irrigating fluid or the device used for insertion into the stoma perforates the bowel.

Symptoms include an unrewarding irrigation, which is often associated with immediate abdominal pain. Obvious sepsis can supervene with evidence of cellulitis of the abdominal wall. If the process dissects into the peritoneal cavity or had started within the abdomen, it can lead to generalized peritonitis.

## Management

Abscess with perforation is a major septic problem that usually requires an urgent operation and extensive debridement, drainage, stomal relocation, and, in some situations, a proximal colostomy or ileostomy.

### *Hemorrhage*

Colostomy hemorrhage is extremely unusual in the immediate postoperative period. However, in the event of underlying portal hypertension from cirrhosis secondary to alcohol ingestion or sclerosing cholangitis, the mucosa of the exposed bowel is predisposed to the possibility of considerable bleeding. The bleeding originates from enterostomal varices located at the level of the mucocutaneous junction, a consequence of communication with the high-pressure venous network of the superior and inferior mesenteric veins. Erosion of the varix or trauma can exacerbate the hemorrhage.

### *Treatment*

Direct pressure is usually the initial approach. Other suggested alternatives include suture ligation of the bleeding areas, beta blockade, and injection sclerotherapy. If these attempts fail, portasystemic shunting may be required to control major hemorrhage. Others have performed mucocutaneous disconnections down to the level of the fascia. The varix is then divided and ligated. Good results have been reported.

### *Prolapse*

Prolapse occurs much more frequently in those who have had a loop colostomy than in those with an end stoma. It can occur early or late in the postoperative phase. The cause can be an oversized opening in the abdominal wall, a redundant sigmoid loop leading to the stoma, sudden increased abdominal pressure, a rigid appliance worn with a tight belt, the presence of a redundant colon, or simply the stoma initially created too long. The condition is frequently associated with a pericolostomy hernia.

### *Treatment*

In the absence of an associated hernia, treatment of a prolapse usually does not require a laparotomy. If the prolapse occurs relatively soon after it has been constructed, the colostomy is circumcised at the mucocutaneous junction and the bowel liberated, resected, and resutured. If the prolapse occurs several months after the initial operation, the incision should be made into the mucosa rather than into the skin. The blood supply from the adjacent skin will be sufficient to maintain viability of the stoma, and an anastomosis is actually effected between the distal colon and the residual mucosa. It is important to liberate as much intraabdominal colon as possible and to resect it to avoid recurrent prolapse. Some surgeons have applied a modification of the Delorme procedure as an alternative approach.

Acute stomal prolapse is not uncommon but does require immediate attention to reduce it. This is usually accomplished by gentle pressure as described in

Chapter 17. As with osmotic therapy through the use of sugar applied to the prolapse, the same treatment has been demonstrated to be effective for the acute, irreducible stomal prolapse.

## Results

Colostomy prolapse represents up to 13% of the stomal complications requiring operation. Local fixation procedures have failed to prevent recurrent prolapse in up to 65% of cases, but if successful, the operation avoids a larger and more morbid procedure.

## Peristomal Hernia

The usual reason for a peristomal hernia is the placement of the stoma in a pararectus location. It has been reported that the prevalence of this complication is 2.8% in those brought through the muscle and 21.6% in those placed laterally, a highly significant difference. Other possible causes of peristomal hernia include locating the stoma in the incision itself and the creation of too large an opening in the abdominal wall, weight gain, the effects of the aging process, other systemic diseases, and nutritional problems.

### Treatment

The choices of operative approaches to the repair of a peristomal hernia are usually dictated by its size. Relatively small defects can be repaired by direct suture, circumcising the colostomy, repairing the abdominal wall, and rematuring the stoma. This technique is suggested only if the colostomy has been created in the proper location (i.e., through the split rectus muscle). If a small hernia is present in conjunction with an improperly located stoma, the colostomy should probably be relocated, either by laparotomy or by an intraperitoneal tunneling method. The use of the umbilical site is not a unique concept. Some surgeons prefer to create the colostomy in the umbilicus initially because of their low incidence of complications. If an umbilical colostomy is created, the technique of construction is essentially the same, but it is important to remove all of the skin that tends to turn inward.

It is always better, when possible, to use the patient's own tissue for repair. Reconstruction of larger or massive hernias, however, usually requires insertion of a synthetic material (e.g., Marlex mesh, Dacron prosthesis, or Gore-Tex). In repairing the hernia, some surgeons prefer to maintain the stoma at the original location, using the mesh around the colostomy. Others bring the bowel through the middle of the material. I prefer to use mesh, if necessary, to effect the repair and to relocate the stoma elsewhere. Although the possibility of sepsis occurring if a prosthetic material is placed in a contaminated field always exists, this is rarely a concern.

### Results

One study identified 42 individuals who underwent repair of paracolostomy hernia, an incidence of 34% of all operative stomal complications. Local repair failed in 47%, but changing the stoma site to the umbilicus or right side of the abdomen was more successful (57%). Some surgeons feel that stomal relocation is superior to direct fascial repair. Furthermore, for those that recur, a prosthetic material is the most successful for effecting a cure. Most individuals, however, are relatively asymptomatic; hence, operative intervention is not necessarily a requisite.

### Recurrent Disease

The primary condition can recur at the stoma site. For example, if Crohn's disease recurs, then medical management of the underlying disease process may resolve the inflammation and ameliorate the patient's complaints. However, because of diarrhea and the inability to maintain an appliance satisfactorily, a more extensive bowel resection and, possibly ileostomy may be required (see *Ileostomy Complications*).

Recurrent malignancy can be caused by tumor implantation at the time of the resection or an inadequate resection margin or a second primary lesion. Radical resection of the involved area, including part of the abdominal wall with relocation of the stoma, is the recommended treatment.

## Alternative Techniques for Sigmoid Colostomy Creation and Management

### Maturation by Stapling

In addition to the conventional maturation technique for sigmoid colostomy, the circular stapling device has been advocated for performing an end colostomy. This permits a geometrically perfect opening but does not prevent the development of stoma complications related to ischemia, tension, and improper location.

### Technique

A small opening is created just large enough to pass the center rod without the anvil. A purse string is created of the distal colon in the usual manner and the anvil inserted into the bowel. The cartridge and anvil are approximated, and the instrument is fired. It is a colocutaneous anastomosis by means of the circular stapling device.

In another stapler application, ordinary skin staples are used to mature the stoma. They are then removed on the tenth postoperative day.

### Primary Insertion of Mesh Implant

The prosthetic mesh is appropriately tailored and a window created of adequate size to permit the colon to pass through. The mesh is secured to the peritoneum and posterior fascia. It is debatable whether this approach is necessary. I believe that a properly located and matured stoma is unlikely to pose a subsequent problem.

### Continent Colostomy

The search for continence in a colostomy has stimulated many attempts to control bowel movements by means of prosthetic devices. They can be considered in four categories: external devices, surgical technique alone, surgical technique with passive implanted devices, and surgical technique with active implanted devices. These include the Kock continent colostomy, which has been largely abandoned, except for a continent cecostomy. The balloon plug, the magnetic ring colostomy device, and the Prager implantable ring are no longer available because of the complications of erosion and necrosis of the bowel or stoma.

Others have used intestinal smooth muscle to form a wrap around the stoma. In a large series of more than 500 patients, 40 did not require an appliance, and only 5 required removal of the surgical implant.

### Colostomy Irrigation

Colostomy irrigation is a method of bowel control offered to selected patients with sigmoid or descending colon colostomies. Success depends on personal interest, bowel habits before surgery, manual dexterity, available toilet facilities, and lifestyle. The following selection criteria have been suggested for patients for whom colostomy irrigation is suited.

Permanent descending or sigmoid colostomy
Physically and mentally capable of performing self-care
Motivated to learn the procedure and adhere to a schedule
No prior history of inflammatory bowel disease (IBD), radiation therapy (to the
    abdomen or pelvis), or other major intestinal resection
A history of regular bowel pattern or constipation
Availability of bathroom facilities, including running water

Irrigation techniques are often taught on the fifth or sixth postoperative day, and for some individuals, a few months following the operation. It is advisable to learn the technique, but the decision whether to use irrigation should be personal. Stomal management problems such as hernia and stenosis, as well as an individual's poor eyesight, impaired dexterity, fear of the irrigation procedure, and resentment of the time necessary, militate against irrigating.

### Method

A nipple, cone, or catheter is inserted into the stoma. The cone tip is now being used more frequently for colostomy irrigation than the catheter, not only because of less risk of perforating the bowel, but also because it provides a dam to prevent backflow. The colon does not need to be washed out; the bowel is merely stimulated with the irrigant to produce evacuation. The height of the bag should be adjusted to permit a steady flow into the stoma. Tepid water (750 to 1,000 mL) is slowly instilled over a 5- to 10-minute period. Experiment with different irrigation volumes to determine the most efficacious program for each patient. After waiting approximately 1 minute, the patient removes the cone, and the water and stool are permitted to pass through the irrigation sleeve into the toilet bowl. Most of the returns are usually collected within 15 minutes. The collecting sleeve can then be closed while the patient tends to other activities. After about 45 minutes, the irrigant usually will have been expelled. With time, the patient may require irrigations only every 48 hours or even every 72 hours. Some, however, may never be able to irrigate satisfactorily and require a pouch all of the time. Under these circumstances, it is difficult to justify the time and effort expended to perform this task.

## TRANSVERSE COLOSTOMY

### Indications

Transverse colostomy is a procedure often used on a temporary basis for a number of reasons: obstructing or perforating lesions of the colon, trauma, anastomotic leak, congenital anomalies, fecal incontinence, and to protect the anastomosis. With improvement of suturing and stapling techniques, however, this last indication has become less applicable.

### Technique

#### *Loop Colostomy*

If a transverse colostomy is undertaken in an emergency situation, it should be accompanied by a full exploratory laparotomy, identifying the nature of the pathology. Ideally, the colostomy should be created as distally as possible and, if performed in the transverse colon, should be done on the left side to reduce the risk of efferent limb prolapse. By placing the opening in the left transverse colon, the splenic flexure tethers the bowel and limits the risk of this complication.

The transverse colostomy should be brought through the split rectus muscle, over a rod or bridge. The omentum is freed from the colon for a sufficient distance to permit exteriorization without tension. The colostomy is then "matured" by opening it longitudinally and suturing the bowel edge to the skin. The bridge or rod can be removed as soon as sufficient edema is present to maintain exteriorization of the colon.

### *Adequacy of Diversion*

A properly constructed loop transverse colostomy is a fully diverting stoma. Unless the proximal limb retracts, it is impossible for the stool to pass into the distal limb. Three factors have been identified as responsible for the failure of loop colostomies to be fully diverting:

1. Retraction
2. Reduction of a prolapsed loop colostomy (invariably associated with retraction)
3. Improper technique for diverting

### *Divided Colostomy*

Theoretic concern about inadequate diversion can be addressed by "stapling" the distal end, or by dividing the colon, creating an end transverse colostomy, and performing a side-to-side colon anastomosis of the distal segment. This last method, an alternative to the concept of a "double-barreled" stoma, is time-consuming to create and may require a laparotomy to close.

The so-called "end-loop colostomy" is another option; the proximal limb and the antimesenteric corner of the distal limb are drawn through the abdominal wall following staple division of the bowel. In an obese patient, it is sometimes impossible to deliver the transverse colon out as a loop. Accordingly, the bowel is divided and the distal end oversewn. The colostomy is then created using the end of the transverse colon, maturing it in a similar manner to that of a conventional sigmoid colostomy. Another alternative in such an individual is to perform a loop ileostomy (see later).

### Results of Loop Colostomy Construction

Embarking on a transverse colostomy cannot be considered a whimsical undertaking. The complication rate is reported to be 10% to 50% when this form of stoma is created.

The methods for preventing complications of transverse colostomy are similar to those of sigmoid colostomy. The size of the opening must be adequate to avoid edema, stricture, and obstruction. Ideally, the appropriate site should be selected before the operation, but this is not always possible if the colostomy construction was unanticipated. If the colostomy is created with the bowel under tension, it is likely to retract or to necrose. But a more common complication is colostomy prolapse, usually of the efferent limb. If a colostomy is brought through the abdominal incision, it will always prolapse.

### *Treatment of Loop Colostomy Prolapse.*

A number of methods have been devised to treat colostomy prolapse. One method described is the use of a smooth-backed button placed on the abdominal wall, with a nonabsorbable suture passed through the buttonhole, skin, fascia, and intestine. A finger in the lumen of the intestine helps to reduce the prolapse and to direct the entrance of the needle through the bowel. The result is to fix the reduced intestine firmly against the anterior abdominal wall, preventing further intussusception.

Others have described a purse-string suture to narrow the colostomy orifice. Another is a device that consists of attaching the base of a Gellhorn pessary to the faceplate of a colostomy appliance. Another option for treating prolapse is to circumcise the distal limb, divide the bowel, oversew it, and resuture the end colostomy stoma

*Comment*: One should endeavor to avoid, if at all possible, a permanent loop transverse colostomy. Occasionally, a so-called "temporary colostomy" may inevitably become permanent. This is usually because a distal anastomosis has failed to heal or the patient has developed other serious medical problems that preclude further surgical intervention. If a problem arises, the surgeon might consider one of the methods described to control prolapse of the efferent limb.

## Colostomy Closure

Much has been written about colostomy closure. To summarize: Early closure of the colostomy is associated with a high rate of morbidity and resection of the bowel, and in the experience of most surgeons, is more hazardous than simple closure. Wound infection is by far the most common complication; its avoidance, therefore, should be possible by delayed wound closure.

### *Technique*

The technique I prefer for colostomy closure is as follows. The patient is placed on a full bowel preparation, as if for colon resection. Both limbs of the colostomy and the rectum are irrigated the morning of surgery until the returns are clear. Broad-spectrum intravenous antibiotics are administered on call to the operating room, the same protocol that is employed for bowel resection.

The colostomy is circumcised by means of a diathermy cautery, leaving an attached cuff of skin. The bowel is dissected down to the level of the fascia. The peritoneal cavity is entered, clamps are placed on the fascia, and the bowel is liberated circumferentially from the fascia. The skin and any remaining fibrous tissue are then excised. Closure of the anterior wall of the bowel is then effected in a transverse fashion with interrupted, long-term absorbable sutures or by means of a stapling technique. If, however, edema and fibrosis prevent safe closure, the bowel is resected and an anastomosis performed, as with any colon resection. The fascia is then approximated with interrupted, heavy, long-term absorbable sutures. Because of the high risk of infection, the wound is left open for delayed primary closure. The wound is packed either with iodoform gauze or a Betadine-soaked sponge, and secondarily closed 3 or 4 days later. Postoperatively, the patient is maintained on intravenous fluids until oral intake can be tolerated. No nasogastric tube is advised.

## CECOSTOMY

A cecostomy is a decompressive procedure. It produces essentially a venting of the bowel and can be fashioned as an open procedure or by tube insertion, either percutaneously, or at laparotomy.

This form of stoma can be used to treat cecal volvulus, and colonic ileus (Ogilvie's syndrome). Other stomal options are preferred for other indications. If diversion of the fecal stream is desired, then an ileostomy should be considered. An ileostomy is also a better stoma when dealing with appliance management.

A cecostomy should optimally be accomplished by the exteriorization technique. If it is to be performed as a "blind" procedure for acute cecal dilatation, a small incision is made in the right lower quadrant in a manner similar to the approach used for appendectomy. However, instead of the muscle being split, the external and internal oblique and transversus abdominis are divided. The peritoneum is exposed and carefully incised. The cecum will tend to pout into the open wound, but if it is so distended that it cannot be delivered through the incision, it can be decompressed by needle or trocar aspiration. The seromuscular surface of the cecum is sutured to the abdominal wall with interrupted, long-term absorbable sutures. After the peritoneal cavity is walled off in this manner, the cecum is opened and the cut edge of the bowel is sutured to the full thickness of the skin in a manner similar to that used to mature a conventional colostomy.

Even when this technique is applied properly, appliance management can be extremely cumbersome. The effluent is corrosive and liquid. But because the cecostomy does not truly divert, drainage can actually be minimal. The paucity of recent literature on the subject is a testament to its lack of applicability and to its replacement by alternative diversionary procedures.

### Continent Cecostomy

Kock et al. performed a continent cecostomy on 30 patients by isolating the cecum from the remainder of the colon and providing the distal end with an intussuscepted valve constructed from an isolated segment of ileum. When comparing the functional results of the continent cecostomy with that of continent ileostomy, the latter is superior.

## ILEOSTOMY

An ileostomy is often used in the management of IBD (ulcerative colitis or Crohn's disease), familial polyposis, congenital anomalies, carcinomatosis, trauma, and as a diversion to protect a distal anastomosis. Siting of an ileostomy done by the same principle as that for a colostomy.

## Historic Perspective

The writings of Brooke, Crile, and Turnbull have influenced our current concepts of primary ileostomy maturation. This essentially involved covering the serosal surface of the ileostomy to prevent serositis and stricture formation.

## Technique

A disk of skin is excised from a previously marked site on the abdominal wall. Because a subcuticular technique is used instead of sutures through full-thickness skin, it is preferable to saucerize the skin obliquely when making the incision. This emphasizes the subcuticular aspect for easy suturing. The ileum is brought through the split rectus muscle protruding for a distance of about 4 or 5 cm. Following extraperitoneal or intraperitoneal fixation, the mesentery to the distal ileum is trimmed.

Three sutures are then placed, one on the antimesenteric aspect and one each on either side of the mesentery. A triangulation technique is recommended. This consists of a full-thickness suturing of the end of the bowel, the seromuscular aspect of the ileum (at the skin level), and the subcuticular skin. The seromuscular bite aids in the subsequent eversion of the bowel. Babcock clamps placed within the bowel lumen and at the end facilitate eversion. With proper length and appropriate eversion, the stoma is primarily matured. Interrupted, absorbable sutures are used to complete the construction.

## Complications: Prevention and Treatment

Complications following an ileostomy can result from a technical error on the part of the surgeon, such as improper location or a faulty maturation technique. Second, disease can cause subsequent stomal problems. Third, the patient, either through inadequate education, neglect, or misuse, can precipitate stomal problems that may necessitate surgical intervention.

### *Complications Due To Improper Maturation Techniques*

#### *Stenosis and Retraction*

Stenosis and retraction are the most common indications for revising an ileostomy. Between 18% and 30% of revisions are performed for these reasons. The primary causes are inadequate initial stomal length, vascular compromise, and improper skin excision. In addition to one of these factors, weight gain may also be responsible.

*Treatment.* Ideally, revision of a stenosis or retraction is accomplished without a formal abdominal operation. Unfortunately, retraction is a complication that sometimes requires a laparotomy to obtain the desired length of ileum necessary to create a satisfactory stoma. It is prudent, therefore, to warn the patient that this may be an eventuality.

Correction of the retraction or stenosis requires (a) excision of sufficient skin to create a proper-sized opening; and (b) mobilization of the bowel as much as is necessary to prepare a stoma of adequate length. Intraperitoneal freeing of the ileum is carried out as far as possible, and the stoma is matured in the usual manner. Some have suggested the implantation of three strips of polyglactin 910 (Vicryl) mesh, longitudinally fixed to the serosa before eversion, to prevent subsequent retraction. Others have used a GIA stapling device without the blade to prevent recurrence of retraction. This can be accomplished without an anesthetic, but only if the retraction is not of the fixed type. That is, the ileostomy protrudes for an appropriate length, but intermittently falls back to produce a flush or retracted stoma. With this technique, three rows of the stapler are fired the length of the ileostomy.

## Prolapse

Prolapse can be of two types, fixed (irreducible) and sliding. The sliding type implies inadequate abdominal fixation and indicates that mobilizing an ileostomy when performing a revision predisposes to subsequent problems with the sliding type of prolapse. Retraction is associated with leakage and with ensuing skin problems.

*Treatment.* If the stomal protrusion is not a true prolapse, but simply an ileostomy that was created too long initially, the ileal mucosa is incised, preserving the ileocutaneous junction, and the stoma is inverted. Redundant ileum is resected, and the stoma is matured in the usual manner. Do not attempt to perform an intraabdominal dissection so that the intraperitoneal fixation is not disrupted. Occasionally, however, with a sliding type of prolapse, so much small bowel is delivered that some form of intraperitoneal fixation is required. This can be accomplished by laparotomy, or consider the linear stapling method of fixation mentioned in the previous section.

## Fistula

Fistula is not an uncommon reason for ileostomy revision; 15% of revisions are performed for this indication. Causes of this complication are recurrent Crohn's disease erosion of the stoma by the faceplate of an appliance, or from deep placement of a suture. If caused by recurrent Crohn's disease, then resection and reconstruction of the stoma is required. For other causes, local therapy can be attempted.

## Seeding

Seeding of viable ileal mucosa can develop along the suture line if subcuticular sutures for maturation are not used. Such seeding can lead to persistent secretion and, consequently, to problems in fitting the appliance.

*Management.* The only effective management is excision, and even with this procedure the viable ileal mucosal cells may grow again to the surface from a deeply implanted location. Often, relocation of the stoma is required.

This is a totally preventable complication if a subcuticular suturing technique is used.

### Complications Due to Improper Placement

The aforementioned complications were caused by errors in the ileostomy maturation technique. Another cause of difficulty after stomal construction is the initial improper location of the stoma. The stoma must be placed through the rectus muscle, in an area where the patient can care for it properly, and wear the appliance with confidence, without the fear of leakage.

*Treatment.* If the stoma is improperly located and appliance management is unsatisfactory, relocation is necessary. This can be achieved by laparotomy, or by a tunneling method, without a complete abdominal exploration, as described for resiting a colostomy.

*Paraileostomy Hernia.* A paraileostomy hernia is reported to occur in up to 28% of patients who have an end ileostomy.

*Treatment.* Paraileostomy hernia, is a complication usually caused by an error in the location of the stoma. Repair is effected in a similar manner to that described for colostomy hernia, with or without mesh. Unfortunately, most such complications usually require relocation of the ileostomy.

Even in the absence of a parastomal hernia, additional pouch support can be achieved by the use of a belt, especially during lifting or exercise. For nonsurgical management of a hernia, the device is available up to 9 inches wide.

### Other Complications

#### Recurrent Crohn's Disease and Other Manifestations of IBD at the Ileostomy

Medical management of recurrent Crohn's disease in the stoma or more proximal bowel is discussed in Chapter 30. Conservative management includes debridement, curettage, unroofing, and pouching of the stoma with Telfa strips placed in the ulcer base with a conventional appliance or a Perry Model no. 51 device. Successful healing is anticipated. When medical therapy fails, surgical revision with possible relocation is necessary. Rotation or advancement skin grafts have also been used with some success.

#### Infectious Enteritides

*Campylobacter jejuni* has been reported to cause profound ulceration of the stoma in association with an acute ileitis. This case report emphasizes the importance of obtaining a stool culture in the evaluation of a patient with suspected recurrent IBD.

### Carcinoma at the Ileostomy

*Inflammatory Bowel Disease.* Carcinoma arising in an ileostomy can occur following seeding of viable tumor cells at the time of the original procedure, or as a consequence of some late-developing dysplastic phenomenon. The most common presenting signs and symptoms include bleeding, ulceration, and a friable mass at the ileostomy site.

Treatment requires *en bloc* resection of the stoma, adjacent mesentery, and abdominal wall, and the creation of a new ileostomy. Some suggest screening of asymptomatic patients with ileostomies of long standing by means of biopsy, looking for dysplastic or neoplastic changes.

### Familial Adenomatous Polyposis

Familial adenomatous polyposis (FAP) can be associated with tumors and tumorlike conditions throughout the gastrointestinal tract. Although most lesions in the small bowel are areas of lymphoid hyperplasia, adenomas have been reported to be present the ileum in 20% of cases studied. Such tumors may be evident on the stoma. Adenocarcinoma has also been reported. In light of the fact that the potential for malignant change has not been clearly defined, careful follow-up with ileoscopy and biopsy is recommended.

### Hemorrhage

Patients with cirrhosis and portal hypertension, have the potential for shunts developing within adhesions between the ileal (portal) veins and the anterior abdominal wall (systemic) veins. This can lead to ileostomy hemorrhage from parastomal varices. Sclerotherapy can be expected to afford only temporary. Successful shunting directed at relieving the portal hypertension should prevent subsequent hemorrhage, but the procedure may accelerate liver failure.

### Trauma

Trauma to the ileostomy can be accidental or deliberate. The risk of this complication is increased when the stoma is larger than necessary.

## Ileostomy in the Elderly

Advanced age does not appear to be a contraindication to ileostomy. However, older patients experience a greater frequency of appliance management difficulties.

### Patient Evaluation of Results: Lifestyle and Sexual Function

Many studies have addressed the psychologic and sexual aspects of patients who have undergone an operation resulting in an ileostomy or colostomy. Although some have shown no effect of the stoma, most report some degree of psychological (body image) and sexual problems (sterility and impotence). This suggests that the surgeon or enterostomal therapist should discuss these concerns with patients before performing permanent ostomy surgery. Certainly, an understanding surgeon as well as a knowledgeable enterostomal therapist and site visitor can create a climate in which the patient can feel at ease in asking for guidance on sexual matters.

## LOOP ILEOSTOMY

Loop ileostomy is a technique that is effective for the management of colonic obstruction, to protect a distal anastomosis, and to divert the fecal stream in the treatment of toxic megacolon. In addition, a loop ileostomy can be fashioned when an end ileal stoma is technically difficult to create. Such a problem arises with obese patients, in whom the mesentery may be shortened and thickened, and it can also be encountered when the distal ileum has been previously resected.

### Construction Technique

A disk of skin is excised in the same manner and at the same location as if for a conventional ileostomy. An appropriate portion of ileum is selected. A Penrose drain or red rubber catheter is placed around the intestine. The loop of small bowel is brought through the split rectus muscle. A catheter or rod supports the loop, and the bowel is opened at the level of the skin on the distal, nonfunctioning side. The stoma is created by eversion with interrupted mucosubcuticular sutures and may be facilitated by means of Babcock clamps. The rod is usually removed in 3 to 5 days, with the general appearance and the functional results identical to that obtained by conventional end ileostomy.

Others have proposed a divided ileostomy, analogous to that of the previously mentioned end-loop. Although this can often be accomplished with safety, a potential risk of compromise to the blood supply is present. The procedure has also been described laparoscopically (see Chapter 27).

### *Results*

A loop ileostomy is generally a temporary stoma. Complications include small bowel obstruction, retraction requiring revision, peristomal abscess, and appliance management problems.

## Technique for Closure

Closure can almost always be done without a complete laparotomy, circumcising the ileostomy as if for a revision. The proximal and distal bowel are mobilized and the intestine resected on the abdominal wall. The anastomosis can be sutured, or a side-to-side (functional end-to-end) anastomosis can be created using a stapler. The stapled anastomosis has the theoretic advantage of creating a much larger luminal diameter.

## *Results*

Complications of closure include anastomotic leak, hernia, and wound infection.

# 32

# Enterostomal Therapy

## PREOPERATIVE CARE

This has been discussed in Chapter 31.

## STOMAL FUNCTION AND CARE

Fecal and urinary diversion can be performed in patients for a variety of clinical indications and situations. A brief overview of these various stomas follows.

### Gastrointestinal Stomas

Stomas can be constructed from small bowel (e.g., jejunostomy, ileostomy, and continent ileostomy), or colon (e.g., cecostomy, and transverse, descending or sigmoid colostomy).

With the exception continent ileostomy, indications for the various stomas have been discussed in Chapter 31. Because of the development of the pelvic pouch procedure, the continent ileostomy is primarily performed for conversion of a permanent, conventional (Brooke) ileostomy and for those with a failed reservoir-anal procedure. It can be also offered to patients with anal incontinence.

#### Continent (Kock) Ileostomy

In the early postoperative period, one of the important concerns is to stabilize the defunctioning drainage catheter that is placed in the pouch to ensure that the pouch drains adequately.

To minimize tube blockage, gentle irrigation with 20 to 30 mL of normal saline is recommended, commencing in the recovery unit and continuing every 2 to 3 hours for the next few days. Intervals between irrigations can be increased, based on how well the tube is draining. It is extremely important to avoid overdistension of the pouch for the first few weeks following surgery to limit the likelihood of dessusception of the continent nipple valve. A bedside drainage bag or leg bag must be used to maintain constant drainage.

## Urinary Stomas

Urinary stomas include vesicostomy, ureterostomy, nephrostomy, and continent or noncontinent conduits. They are fashioned from ileum, jejunum, or colon. Continent urinary diversion requires pre- and postoperative management techniques similar to those of continent ileostomy. It is essential to avoid overdistension of the pouch before adequate fixation of the continent nipple has occurred. Consequently, the newly created urinary reservoir is decompressed by a cecostomy tube and bilateral urinary stents, and a catheter is placed into the plicated exit conduit. Depending on the surgeon's preference, the cecostomy tube is gently irrigated with 20 to 30 mL of normal saline every 2 to 3 hours. Stabilization of the tubes and drains can be achieved by a variety of tube anchoring devices. Use of constant drainage through a bedside drainage bag or leg bag is recommended for the first few weeks after surgery.

## OSTOMY MANAGEMENT

### Immediate Postoperative Period

Proper application of a pouching system should begin in the operating room. The appliance is fixed to clean, dry skin to protect the incision and the peristomal skin, and to contain stomal discharge. Pouch application, coupled with connection to gravity drainage, is indicated for urinary stomas.

A variety of one-piece or two-piece, disposable, odor-proof, pouching systems can be used (Table 32.1). By using a disposable measuring guide, and by sizing the aperture of the pouch within one-eighth inch (3 mm) of the base of the stomal mucosa, the peristomal skin can be protected and mucosal trauma prevented. A transparent, drainable pouch will permit the clinician to assess stoma viability as well as output. A closure clamp or tubing device is then securely applied. Viability and function should be assessed daily by the surgeon and enterostromal therapist (ET) nurse and by each shift of the nursing staff.

### Principles of Fitting

To provide some appreciation for the alternative methods of managing ostomies, it is important to have an understanding of ostomy collection devices. They consist of three primary parts—skin barrier, faceplate, and pouch, which are necessary for an effective collecting system. The newer generation of appliances incorporates these parts into a single, disposable or reusable system.

### Skin Protective Agent

A skin protective agent, such as Skin Prep (Smith & Nephew United) or Skin Gel (Hollister), provides a clear dressing that coats the skin. These agents pro-

**TABLE 32.1.** *Products to control odor*

| Internal | Form | Side effects |
|---|---|---|
| Activated charcoal | Capsules | Large dose can interfere with absorption of vitamins |
| | | Darkens stool |
| Chlorophyllin copper complex | Tablets | Absorbs some gas |
| | | Turns stool dark green |
| Bismuth subgallate | Tablets | Can cause toxicity if taken in large doses |
| Bismuth subcarbonate | Tablets | Constipation |

| External | Form | Description |
|---|---|---|
| Pouch deodorizing agents | Pouch Liquids Powder Tablets | May contain a combination of water, zinc ricinoleate, propylene glycol. Some contain silver nitrate, organic acids, urea and fragrance. |
| Air deodorizing agents | Aerosol Pump spray Liquids Solids | May contain water, ethanol, fragrance, and artificial colors. |
| Pouch cleaning/ deodorizing agents | | Used to clean and deodorize reusable stoma plates and pouches. May contain water, detergent, surfactants, liquid petroleum. Must rinse well. |
| Gas filters | Stick to 1- to 2-piece drainable pouches | Charcoal filter incorporated to deodorize gas Some plastic pouches may not permit a secure seal of the adhesive Not suitable for use with watery effluent. |

tect the skin from the irritation that can be caused by the ostomy device. They also augment adherence of an appliance and facilitate adhesive removal from reusable faceplates. These protective agents are available as gels, sprays, wipes, paint-on solutions, or pastes.

## Skin Barrier

A skin barrier is an adherent porous material that offers protection from the contents of the colon or ileum. The most commonly used skin barriers are discussed in the following sections.

### Karaya Products

Karaya is a resin that forms a protective base when combined with glycerin, thus inhibiting the corrosive effects of ileal contents. It is relatively insoluble and hydroscopic. It is refined and marketed in different forms, including powders, washers, wafers, and blankets, and mixed with natural clays. It is also manufactured in paste form, which provides an excellent means for filling in crevices created by abdominal folds near the stoma.

Karaya is nonallergenic, although the ingredients in some products can cause some sensitivity. If this is a problem, a change to a karaya product manufactured by another company may be all that is required.

One disadvantage of karaya products is the tendency to break down in the presence of urine. Therefore, they should never be used with urinary diversions. Karaya melts easily in heat or even when the patient has an elevated temperature. Thus, for ostomates who live in warm climates, a different skin barrier should be used (e.g., Stomahesive or Hollihesive). Generally, the use of karaya is advised less often than one of the products subsequently discussed. It is used less often today, having been replaced by more flexible products.

### Gelatin–Pectin Skin Barriers

Generally, the gelatin–pectin skin barriers have an advantage over the karaya products because they are more water-resistant and, therefore, permit a longer interval between appliance changes.

#### Stomahesive

Stomahesive is composed of gelatin, pectin, carboxymethylcellulose sodium, and polyisobutylene. It is nonallergenic and looks like a piece of American cheese. Its shiny surface is affixed to the appliance, and the sticky side is secured to the skin. It should be cut to fit around the stoma, leaving a 2- or 3-mm clearance; it can be used as a washer or as a whole wafer. The product is also available in a powder or a paste. Stomahesive can be applied directly onto excoriated skin and provides an excellent means for filling in crevices created by abdominal folds near the stoma.

A skin barrier such as Stomahesive is appropriate for intestinal as well as urinary tract diversions and should be placed on the skin immediately after the operation.

#### Durahesive

Durahesive is similar to Stomahesive, but it has specific hydrophyllic properties that absorb fluid from the effluent; this causes the product to swell or "turtleneck" around the stoma. It is a particularly advantageous barrier for urinary ostomies.

#### Hollihesive

Hollihesive is similar to Stomahesive, except that it is a bit more flexible and stickier to the touch. It, too, is available as a paste.

### Reliaseal

Reliaseal is similar in composition to Stomahesive. It has two adhesive sides, one covered with white paper and the other with blue. The white paper is peeled off and that side is placed directly on the skin; then, the blue paper covering is removed, and that side is placed directly on the faceplate of the pouch. Reliaseal is also an effective washer for an ileal conduit.

### Crixiline

Crixiline is an extremely sticky siliconelike barrier that comes in rings and sheets. This material also is available attached to a disposable, soft-backed, open- or closed-ended pouch called "Stomaplast-plus" with a micropore tape backing. This product is useful around drains. To achieve good adhesion, the skin must be dry.

### Other Barriers

United's Soft-Guard XL is pliable and resistant to breakdown. Coloplast manufactures Comfeel, and Nu-Hope has skin barrier wafers, precut round and oval washers, and paste strips for flexibility.

### Faceplate

The faceplate or mounting area is that part of the appliance that supports the pouch and attaches it to the body. It may be made of rubber, metal, paper, adhesive, or plastic. It can be flexible or hard—convex, flat, or concave.

### Adhesives

Adhesives are of two types: liquids (cements) and disks. Adhesive cements are generally made of acrylic or rubber, but are usually unnecessary. If used, they should be applied lightly and evenly as a single coat to the skin or to the barrier. Cement is occasionally recommended for a patient with a difficult abdominal contour or in whom a satisfactory seal cannot be established by another means.

### Pouch

Numerous disposable and reusable pouch systems are available. Selection depends on a variety of physical and psychosocial factors affecting the patient. The pouch can be made of synthetic material or of rubber. Some disposal pouches come with an adhesive or microporous tape backing and, in some instances, with a soft plastic faceplate and belt tabs.

Two-piece disposable appliances have become popular. They consist of a skin barrier with a plastic ring. A pouch with a ring snaps onto the barrier-ring, much like a Tupperware product.

The disadvantages of the disposable system include the possibility of a shorter wearing time, increased cost, and limitation to certain body configurations. A faceplate with a firm base provides better peristomal support, particularly in a patient with a "flabby" abdomen. A disposal pouch always requires a skin barrier to enhance the wearing time and to provide adequate skin protection.

Reusable or "permanent" appliances are available in one or two pieces, depending on whether the faceplate is detachable. A faceplate for any appliance must always have a means of securing it to the body, regardless of the type of skin barrier used. Attachment is usually accomplished through the use of precut, double-faced adhesive seals or disks.

A one-piece appliance may be preferred by patients with arthritis affecting the hands, those who have poor eyesight or who are blind, active youngsters who need a secure pouch construction with ease of application, patients with a neurologic deficit, and those with flush stomas. Disposable one-piece equipment often is available precut, so that the patient merely peels off the protective paper and affixes the appliance. However, the selection of a one-piece appliance may also be simply personal preference.

The main advantages of the two-piece system are cost-effectiveness and durability. An elastic ring around the neck of the pouch holds the appliance to the faceplate. The attachment of a double-faced adhesive disk to the back of the faceplate is the same as that with the one-piece appliance. Generally, the firmer the abdomen, the softer and flatter the faceplate should be. Most patients, with the exception of those who are very slender or who have firm abdomens, will need a slightly convex faceplate. In addition to the reusable system, many individuals maintain a supply of disposable pouches for an "emergency," for rapid change, or for camping and traveling.

### Belt and Tape

Many patients feel secure when wearing a belt, but this device is not meant to hold the appliance in place. It is intended merely to support the weight of the pouch. With few exceptions (e.g., active children or problem stomas where revision is not advisable), the use of belts should be discouraged.

An alternative to a belt, such as framing the faceplate or adhesive area with paper tape, is the preferred approach. For swimming or bathing, many types of waterproof tapes are available.

### Appliance Management

Establishing the optimal frequency for a pouch change requires individual adjustment and experimentation. In the immediate postoperative period, the pouch is changed more frequently than is required at a later time to permit stomal assessment and to provide instruction in self-care procedures. After discharge, the patient is encouraged to gradually extend the interval between pouch changes until optimal frequency can be determined. No one frequency is correct for pouch changing. The goal is to establish a routine to avoid leakage or skin irritation. This usually requires a frequency of every 5 to 7 days in a well-sited and well-constructed stoma.

The following factors are essential to a properly fitting appliance:

It must not leak contents nor cause odor.
It must not cause skin or stomal irritation.
It must be comfortable for all levels of activity.
It must not require a wardrobe change.
It must be unobtrusive.

With knowledge of a few basic principles, a satisfactory management protocol can be developed. What may seem complex in the beginning will be routine in a brief time as the patient gains confidence that the system will not leak and that it will enable the individual to return to productive activity.

### Patient and Family Education

Ideally, the timing of instruction should be based on learner readiness. Shorter lengths of hospitalization often accelerate the teaching process, but unfortunately, learning may not be enhanced. Support from family, friends, and home care nurses will ease the transition to home self-care. It is important that these support services build on the patient's previous knowledge to avoid fostering dependence.

Patients and families need to be supplied with a discharge folder that includes step-by-step written instructions specific for their type of ostomy and pouching system, along with stock numbers and ordering information, a list of dealers and manufacturers, referral phone numbers, and discharge instructions. Tables 32.2 and 32.3 are examples of patient instruction sheets distributed at the Cleveland Clinic Foundation.

If the patient is ever in an accident or unconscious, the nature of the ostomy should be communicated to emergency medical personnel. This is especially important for patients with continent diversions or pelvic pouches.

Before discharge those with continent diversions are instructed in catheter irrigation, stoma and skin care, and management of leg and bedside drainage bags. Preventing overdistension of the pouch must be emphasized.

### Prevention and Treatment of Skin Irritation

The corrosive effluent from an ileostomy demands careful appliance management. Additionally, mechanical irritation, allergic and nonallergic dermatitis,

**TABLE 32.2.** *How to change your disposable, one-piece,*
*cut-to-fit pouch with attached skin barrier*

---

Gather the following supplies:
 Washcloths or paper towels
 Nonoily soap (Ivory and Dial are recommended brands)
 Scissors
 Plastic bag or newspaper
 New pouch
 Accessory products
Prepare the new pouch
 Trace the pattern (sized to fit within ___" of stoma) onto the cover paper of the skin barrier.
 Cut out the skin barrier. Be careful not to cut through the front of the pouch.
 Remove the covers from the skin barrier and the adhesive surface of the pouch.
 Set the pouch aside, sticky side up.
Remove the worn pouch
 Holding the pouch upright, remove the clip from the end of the pouch.
 Empty the waste from the pouch into the toilet.
 Remove the worn pouch by:
  Applying light pressure on the skin with one hand.
  Gently pulling the pouch from the skin with the other hand.
 Wrap the worn pouch in newspaper, or place in a plastic bag and discard.
Cleanse the skin around the stoma
 Wash the area around the stoma with nonoily soap and warm water.
 Rinse the area thoroughly with warm water.
 Pat the skin dry with a washcloth or paper towel.
Apply the new pouch
 Center the pouch opening over the stoma and press into place.
 Smooth the sticky surface of the pouch onto the skin.
 Hold the pouch firmly in place for a few moments.
Close the pouch end securely
 Fasten the pouch end securely with the clip.

---

and various infections can predispose the ostomate to the risk of injury despite fastidious care and a properly fitting appliance. To prevent complications from developing, it is important for the patient to return annually for a stomal inspection. This provides the physician (or ET nurse) with an opportunity to remeasure the stoma and to evaluate the integrity of the peristomal skin. In addition, the patient can be informed about any new developments in equipment.

## Mild Irritation

Even mild skin irritation must be treated promptly to prevent serious consequences. Mild or moderate dermatitis can be treated by gently washing the peristomal skin with warm water. The area should be permitted to dry thoroughly. A hair dryer held about 1 foot away from the skin can be used. Karaya or Stomahesive powder should be dusted on the area, and the excess brushed off. After a skin protective agent is applied and permitted to dry, a skin barrier is used with a clean appliance.

**TABLE 32.3.** *How to change your disposable, two-piece pouch with cut-to-fit skin barrier flange*

Gather the following supplies:
  Washcloths or paper towels
  Nonoily soap (Ivory and Dial are recommended brands)
  Scissors
  Plastic bag or newspaper
  New pouch
  Skin barrier flange
  Accessory products
Prepare the new pouch
  Trace the pattern (sized to fit within ___" of stoma) on the cover paper of the
    skin barrier flange.
  Cut out the skin barrier flange.
  Remove the cover papers from the skin barrier and the adhesive surface of the flange.
  Set the skin barrier flange aside, sticky side up.
  Set the pouch next to the flange.
Remove the worn pouch
  Holding the pouch upright, remove the clip from the end of the pouch.
  Empty the waste from the pouch into the toilet.
  To remove the worn pouch and skin barrier:
    Apply light pressure on the skin with one hand.
    Gently pull the pouch from the skin with the other hand.
  Wrap the worn pouch in newspaper, or place in a plastic bag and discard.
Cleanse the skin around the stoma
  Wash the area around the stoma with nonoily soap and warm water.
  Rinse the area thorough with warm water.
  Pat skin dry with a washcloth or paper towel.
Apply the prepared pouch
  Center the skin barrier flange opening over the stoma and press into place.
  Smooth the sticky surface of the skin barrier flange onto the skin.
  Snap the pouch securely onto the skin barrier flange.
  Hold the pouch firmly in place for a few moments.
Close the pouch end securely
  Fasten the pouch end securely with the clip.

### Severe Irritation

Severe irritation can result from improper faceplate fitting, leakage, allergy to the adhesive product, or yeast infection. Cleansing the area with an antacid usually relieves the irritation. This is done by decanting the antacid (e.g., Amphogel, Maalox, Milk of Magnesia) and spreading it thinly over the skin. After drying, a skin protective agent is applied, followed by a skin barrier and a clean pouch. Occasionally, a small piece of Telfa can be placed over a draining area to prevent undermining of the skin barrier and to allow drainage to take place. This appliance must be changed daily until the problem resolves.

### Yeast and Fungal Infections

Problems with yeast or fungal infections often occur during warm weather or whenever moisture accumulates under the appliance. The area should be cleansed and dried gently, and a small amount of an antifungal powder applied to the affected area. The powder can be combined with an antacid to form a thick cream, which can be more effectively applied.

## Diet

Dietary modifications in patients with fecal and urinary diversions may be advisable. Generally, a low residue diet is suggested for the first 6 to 8 weeks following surgery. Patients with ileostomies may find it difficult to tolerate poorly digested foods, such as corn, nuts, and raw fruits and vegetables. These products can result in a food bolus obstruction at the ileostomy. Certain foods (e.g., applesauce, rice, and bananas) can decrease bowel frequency. Conversely, caffeine, fiber, spicy foods, and raw fruits and vegetables can increase function. Individuals with continent ileostomies need to keep the stool fairly liquid to allow passage of the effluent through the catheter. After the initial postoperative period, a patient with a urostomy has no dietary restrictions.

## Odor Control

Diet and personal hygiene probably are the most effective means of decreasing odor. A number of products are available that help to reduce odor. These can be used externally or taken orally.

## Sexual Concerns

Initially, most individuals are often more concerned with the practical aspects of managing their ostomies than with psychosexual concerns. In collaboration with the surgeon, the enterostomal therapist should address this topic as part of the patient's preoperative and postoperative counseling. Concerns about reproduction, sexual function, and interpersonal relationships are common. Teenagers may be especially reluctant to talk about dating, sex, and reproduction in front of their families. Women with pelvic pouches or perineal incisions often experience vaginal dryness. Use of a water-soluble lubricant during sexual intercourse may, therefore, be indicated. Support for gay or lesbian patients with ostomies can be obtained from Gay/Lesbian support group (GLO) of the United Ostomy Association.

## Discharge Planning

Discharge planning should begin at the time of admission to the hospital. Active communication among surgeon, nurse providing ostomy care, staff nurses, social worker, case manager, discharge planner, and the patient and family will ease the transition home. For an especially complex pouching system, it can be helpful for the hospital nurse and the home care or extended care facility nurse to make a joint visit before the patient's discharge from the hospital. Long-term follow-up will be based on the patient's underlying condition. It is recommended that the ET nurse or surgeon evaluate the stoma, pouching, skin, and overall rehabilitation at least once a year.

## Activity

Once recuperation from surgery is complete, patients should be encouraged to enjoy a full and active life. Heavy lifting and contact sports are best avoided because of the risk for hernia or stomal trauma. Otherwise, no physical restrictions are associated with fecal or urinary diversions.

# 33

## Miscellaneous Colitides

This chapter discusses a number of inflammatory conditions of the bowel that, generally speaking, are either infectious or noninfectious. The common denominator for all of these illnesses is an association with the symptom of diarrhea.

Although diarrheal disease is still one of the leading causes of morbidity and mortality, especially among children in the developing world, it is not an insignificant source of morbidity in Western countries. In the United States, adults experience an average of one and a half to two episodes per year. Although most diarrheal conditions are self-limiting, an acute onset of diarrheal disease may be the initial presentation of an underlying disorder that mandates thorough gastrointestinal investigation.

### NONINFECTIOUS COLITIDES

#### Eosinophilic Gastroenteritis or Eosinophilic Colitis

Eosinophilic gastroenteritis is a chronic inflammatory intestinal disease of unknown cause that is characterized by eosinophilia in the involved tissue and in the peripheral blood. Initial publications suggested an allergic association, but this has not been proved. The three major clinical patterns are as follows:

- Primary mucosal disease with enteric protein loss and malabsorption
- Predominant muscle layer disease with obstructive symptoms
- Primary subserosal disease with eosinophilic ascites

The gastric antrum and the proximal small intestine are most frequently involved; the colon is a rare location for the condition. Perianal disease has also been reported.

The most common presenting symptoms are abdominal pain and change in bowel habits. Nausea, vomiting, weight loss, and rectal bleeding are also frequently noted. If mucosal disease predominates, gastrointestinal bleeding, protein-losing enteropathy, diarrhea, and malabsorption are the common complaints. Serosal involvement can manifest as eosinophilic ascites. Large-bowel obstruction secondary to a colocolonic intussusception may also develop.

Tissue eosinophilia is a common feature of eosinophilic gastroenteritis. Although eosinophiles are a recognized manifestation in numerous gastrointestinal conditions, especially Crohn's disease and ulcerative colitis, no comparison can be made with the massive infiltration present in eosinophilic gastroenteritis and colitis.

When the condition occurs in the colon, radiologically, it may mimic tuberculosis, amebiasis, or Crohn's disease. Based on the few cases reported thus far, the proximal colon seems to have a greater predilection for involvement. Colonoscopic evaluation may reveal changes from erythema and friability, to granularity and narrowing. In addition to inflammatory bowel disease, the differential diagnosis should include infectious colitides, such as helminthiasis and amebiasis, systemic hypereosinophilia syndrome, milk protein colitis, vasculitis, and allergic gastroenteropathy. Evaluation of IgE levels can help in determining the possibility of allergen involvement.

Prognosis is generally good, with clinical, hematologic, roentgenographic, and histologic improvement occurring spontaneously or on steroid therapy. However, resection of the involved bowel may be required for unremitting symptoms or to exclude another diagnosis.

## Microscopic Colitis

Microscopic colitis is a condition in which patients with severe, watery diarrhea are found to have no detectable abnormality of the bowel, except by microscopic examination of biopsy specimens. No evidence is seen of an infective agent, ischemia, dietary predisposition, or endocrine abnormality. Anemia, increased erythrocyte sedimentation rate, hypokalemia, and hypoalbuminemia are common findings. Patients are usually middle-aged or elderly women, and all have watery diarrhea of lengthy duration as the predominant symptom associated with frequent problems of anal incontinence.

Diagnosis is based on histologic evaluation of rectal and colonic biopsy specimens. The changes consist of a pancolonic, diffuse, chronic inflammation of the lamina propria (Fig. 33.1). The inflammation is found to be remarkably uniform, indicating a total colitis.

Severe reduction of colonic fluid absorption probably contributes to the development of the chronic diarrhea. The condition may respond to antiinflammatory medication, but a pathophysiologic role for bile salt malabsorption may exist, because cholestyramine has also been demonstrably effective.

Some debate whether microscopic and collagenous colitis represent variants of the same condition.

## Collagenous Colitis

Collagenous colitis is a disease characterized clinically by profuse watery diarrhea and histologically by marked thickening of the colonic subepithelial

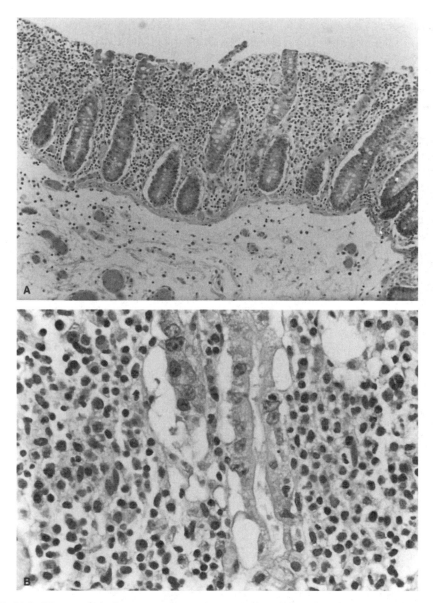

**FIG. 33.1.** Microscopic colitis. **A.** Heavy lymphocytic infiltration confined to the mucosa and filling the lamina propria. A decrease is seen in glandular mucus content as well as cryptoglandular distortion, but no suggestion of crypt abscess. (Original magnification ×330.) **B.** Higher magnification (×400) reveals infiltration of glands by lymphocytes.

basement membrane. It can also involve the terminal ileum. As with microscopic colitis, the patients are predominantly middle-aged to elderly women who are essentially well except for the diarrhea and abdominal pain. Findings are that 85% follow a chronic, intermittent course; nocturnal diarrhea is present in 25%, abdominal pain in 40%, and weight loss in 40%; and 40% have one or more associated diseases.

Endoscopic examination and radiologic studies have demonstrated a normal appearing mucosa in most individuals. However, edema, friability, pinpoint mucosal hemorrhages, and hyperemia are seen occasionally. As the disease progresses, the collagen can gradually increase and possibly act as a diffusion barrier, which can further exacerbate diarrheal symptoms (Fig. 33.2).

The pathogenesis of the condition and the subepithelial fibrosis characterizing the disease remain uncertain. Thickening of the subepithelial collagen layer may be a response to chronic inflammation or a local abnormality of collagen synthesis. It has been postulated that the disease may be attributable to reduced cell turnover, allowing fibrocytes to remain longer in the mature phase, hence producing more collagen and a thicker collagen plate. The possibility of this being another of the autoimmune conditions has also been suggested.

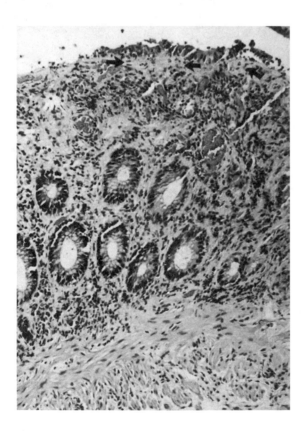

FIG. 33.2. Collagenous colitis. Note the deposit of collagen in the upper lamina propria (*arrows*) underneath the slightly denuded superficial epithelium. (Original magnification ×100; courtesy of Lauren M. Monda, M.D.)

Recommended treatments have included sulfasalazine, and for refractory cases, corticosteroids. Prednisolone is the most effective, with a response rate of more than 80%, but the required dose may be high and the effect may not be maintained following withdrawal. The response rate for antibiotics, cholestyramine, and loperamide are between 60% and 70%. Spontaneous resolution can occur. Very unusual refractory cases may benefit from surgical management, but the place of surgical intervention in this condition is extremely limited.

### Neutropenic Enterocolitis, Ileocecal Syndrome, and Typhlitis

Neutropenic enterocolitis, ileocecal syndrome, and typhlitis are labels for a syndrome associated with bowel wall necrosis, which can occur during treatment of hematologic malignancies, especially leukemia, lymphoma, and aplastic anemia. Profound neutropenia secondary to chemotherapy has been considered the hallmark of the disease and the major causative factor in its development. It has also been described as a complication of a rare benign hematologic disorder, cyclic neutropenia. This is a condition characterized by regular oscillations in blood neutrophil counts in which these cells periodically disappear from the circulation. Involvement of the process is most commonly seen in the terminal ileum, cecum, and right colon, possibly because of the higher concentration of lymphatic tissue in these areas.

Patients exhibit symptoms of diarrhea, abdominal pain, sepsis, and findings typical of acute appendicitis. Even when the pain is localized to the right lower quadrant, the rapidity of the appearance of toxicity, with tachycardia, fever, and delirium, can be extremely dramatic. Although the precise pathogenic mechanism is not understood, current evidence suggests that neutropenic ulceration of the bowel wall facilitates invasion and propagation of *Clostridium septicum*, and bowel necrosis and septicemia result.

With obvious peritoneal signs, treatment is surgical, and a resection is demanded. A high operative mortality rate must be anticipated because of the patient's underlying disease. However, most individuals with neutropenic enterocolitis have minimal, if any, abdominal symptoms and do not progress to develop necrosis, perforation, or peritonitis.

### Diversion Colitis, Disuse Colitis, and Starvation Colitis

Diverting the fecal stream and defunctionalizing the bowel can produce a noninfectious colitis. Generally, patients are asymptomatic, although mucous discharge and bleeding may be noted. An association of microcarcinoids with diversion colitis has also been reported. This occurrence has been attributed to neurogenic hyperplasia, which represents proliferation of a separate, neuron-associated, extraglandular population of endocrine cells.

Proctosigmoidoscopic findings are essentially that of a mild inflammatory bowel disease suggestive of ulcerative colitis. Microscopic alterations, however, tend to be focal, and include crypt abscesses, epithelial cell degeneration, acute and chronic inflammation in the lamina propria, and regenerative changes in the crypts. The histologic picture with the condition is variable, however. Crypt cell production rate has been determined to be less than one half that of controls; additionally, crypt length is lower as is crypt width. Pathologic evaluation of more severely diseased resected specimens may demonstrate diffuse nodularity caused by lymphoid hyperplasia and an inflammatory process confined to the mucosa and submucosa.

The mucosa of the intestinal tract is unique in that it draws nutrients from both the vasculature and the bowel lumen. Nutrition of the colonic epithelial cells is mainly from short-chain fatty acids produced by bacterial fermentation in the colonic lumen. Deficiency in these substances leads initially to mucosal hypoplasia and then to a more typical picture of nonspecific inflammatory bowel disease. Installation of a solution containing short-chain fatty acids twice daily results in the disappearance of symptoms and in the inflammatory changes observed at endoscopy within a period of 6 weeks. The condition can also be successfully treated through the use of 5-aminosalicylic acid enemas.

The affected bowel rapidly returns to a normal appearance following reestablishment of intestinal continuity.

### Disinfectant Colitis (Pseudolypomatosis)

Ryan and Potter have emphasized the poorly recognized entity of disinfectant colitis in causing injury to the colonic mucosa and creating a unique form of colitis. It has also been termed "pseudolypomatosis." Commercially available endoscope disinfecting solutions (e.g., glutaraldehyde and hydrogen peroxide), if allowed to contact the mucosa, can injure the crypt epithelium or mucosal stroma with resultant tissue necrosis. Patients may experience signs and symptoms of abdominal pain, fever, and bloody diarrhea. This usually commences 12 to 48 hours following endoscopy. The entity can become visible as opaque plaques or pseudomembranes, even when the colonoscopy is in progress. Based on experimental studies, it is felt that hydrogen peroxide alone is responsible for the unique form of colitis that has been termed *pseudolypomatosis* by pathologists (Fig. 33.3).

Although it is certainly important to be concerned about the serious implications of communicable diseases and strict attention must be paid to the appropriate disinfecting of endoscopes, adequate rinsing and thorough air-drying should prevent this complication. Recognition of this entity, especially when the endoscopist notes the sudden appearance of psedomembranelike plaques during a procedure, minutes before normal bowel was observed, should help to avoid confusion as to the diagnosis.

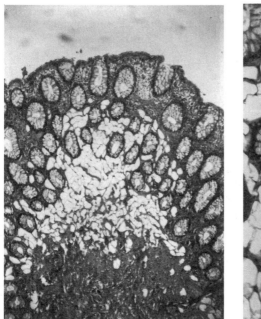 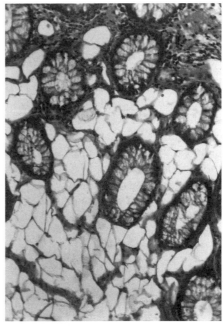

A B

**FIG. 33.3.** Disinfectant colitis (pseudolypomatosis). **A.** Colonic mucosa demonstrating spaces devoid of epithelial lining in the lamina propria. Note the similarity to pneumatosis coli. (Original magnification ×280.) **B.** Note the absence of nuclei. These are empty spaces, not lipocytes. (Original magnification ×560.)

## Corrosive Colitis

The oral administration of a host of corrosives is a well-recognized entity for which surgical intervention is often required. Less well recognized, however, is the installation of various toxic or corrosive materials by means of an enema. The most common is hydrogen peroxide, but detergent enemas, herbal medicines, acetic acid, ethyl alcohol, sodium hydroxide, and hydrofluoric acid have all been implicated. Drugs, such as ergotamine, can also be associated with inflammatory reaction and toxicity. Toxic exposure can result from conventional medical therapy, unconventional medical therapy, radiographic examination, colonoscopic examination (see previous discussion), deliberate self-mutilation, or accidental self-administration.

Rectal bleeding, diarrhea, and abdominal pain are frequent symptoms. Endoscopic examination usually reveals nonspecific changes consistent with inflammatory bowel disease, including erythema, ulceration, granularity, friability, and purulent exudate. A history of an exposure with the installation of medication or a toxic agent is obviously helpful.

Treatment is generally supportive, although emergency laparotomy and bowel resection may be required for fulminant acute colitis, stricture, or perforation.

## NSAID-Induced Colitis

Adverse effects of nonsteroidal antiinflammatory drugs (NSAIDs) on the upper gastrointestinal tract and small intestine are well recognized. Additionally, the ingestion of these agents can be associated with large bowel toxicity, which can lead to profuse diarrhea, chronic blood loss, anemia, and even fatality. The pathogenesis is thought related to inhibition of prostaglandin synthesis. In addition to the oral route, NSAID-induced suppository toxicity is well-recognized.

Ingestion of NSAIDs should certainly be considered in the differential diagnosis of colitis. Discontinuation of the medication will allow the findings to normalize. Additionally, the use of sulfasalazine has proved to be of some benefit.

## Toxic Epidermal Necrolysis

Toxic epidermal necrolysis is a rare and severe reaction to certain drugs that results in full-thickness epidermal necrosis of the skin. Other mucosal surfaces have been implicated, including the large bowel. The most common drugs that are associated with this condition include sulfonamides, penicillin, NSAIDs (see previous discussion), phenytoin anticonvulsants, and barbiturates.

Symptoms include abdominal pain and bloody diarrhea, usually at the same time as the development of the skin lesions. Several cases of colonic necrosis complicating this condition have been reported.

## INFECTIOUS COLITIDES

Viruses, bacteria, fungi, and a host of other parasites can cause infections of the gastrointestinal tract. The upper intestine tends to be attacked by organisms that produce toxins (e.g., *Vibrio cholerae*), whereas, in general, colon infection is associated with organisms that produce dysentery (e.g., *Shigella*). In the former situation, infection tends to leave the mucosa uninvolved, whereas in the latter, the intestinal mucosa is often ulcerated or destroyed. Upper intestinal organisms tend to produce diarrhea with severe dehydration; however, usually not septicemia. Those that affect the large bowel often produce severe abdominal pain, tenesmus, and signs and symptoms of generalized infection (e.g., malaise, pyrexia). A rapid onset is often caused by the presence of a toxin produced by a bacterium, rather than by the bacterium itself; this type of syndrome is occasionally associated with certain restaurant foods.

Most episodic diarrheas are caused by an infection acquired by ingesting fecally contaminated food or beverages. *Escherichia coli* is the most common pathogen, although many other bacteria, viruses, and protozoa have been implicated.

Recommended antimicrobial therapy for severe cases of diarrhea includes trimethoprim/sulfamethoxazole, trimethoprim alone, quinolones (e.g., ciprofloxacin [Cipro], norfloxacin [Noroxin]), or doxycycline, but most infectious diarrheas represent little more than a self-limited nuisance. A National Institute of Health panel of experts in 1990 recommended that antibiotics not be used as routine prophylaxis for traveler's diarrhea because of adverse drug reactions and increasing worldwide bacterial resistance. Instead, the conference endorsed the use of two tablets of bismuth subsalicylate three to four times a day for this purpose.

Comprehensive microbiologic testing and thorough gastrointestinal studies are impractical and expensive for every individual with the complaint of diarrhea. No investigations, except perhaps a rigid or flexible sigmoidoscopy and biopsy, are required for younger patients if the weight is stable and the stool is free of occult blood. A few individuals do require a more extensive evaluation, but that decision is based on the physician's clinical judgment.

In this section, the various diarrheas of potential interest to the surgeon are discussed: presentation, diagnosis, and therapy.

## Bacterial Infections

### *Antibiotic-Associated Colitis, Pseudomembranous Colitis,* and Clostridium Difficile *Colitis*

In recent years, a marked increase has been seen in the number of surgical patients who develop antibiotic-associated colitis and associated complications. Generally, this has been attributed to a heightened awareness of the condition, better diagnostic methods, the more widespread use of broad-spectrum antibiotics, and the increasing number of patients who are elderly or immunocompromised

Any patient who develops diarrhea, either during or after receiving antibiotic therapy, must be considered at risk for this complication until proved otherwise, although it is certainly possible that a form of colitis may be unassociated with antibiotic therapy. Under these circumstances the process can be localized (e.g., cecum) and may mimic carcinoma. Diarrhea with or without blood and abdominal pain can commence within 48 hours after the administration of the drug. The condition can even occur up to 6 weeks following discontinuance of the medication. The incidence with inpatients is 0.1% to 1.0%. Virtually all antibiotics have been suggested to cause this syndrome (e.g., tetracycline, chloramphenicol, clindamycin, lincomycin, ampicillin). The condition has also been reported as a complication of sulfasalazine therapy in a patient with inflammatory bowel disease. The occurrence of this particular complication poses a considerable challenge in the differential diagnosis because the symptoms of the two diseases are so similar.

Those who appear to be at increased risk are individuals who are somewhat immunocompromised. Other factors associated with an increased risk of infection include advanced age, malignancy, chronic pulmonary disease, prolonged hospitalization (>4 weeks), transfer from another hospital, antibiotic course (>7 days), treatment with more than one antibiotic, immunosuppressive medication, chemotherapy, antiperistaltic medications, antacid therapy, an intensive care unit location, non–single-room accommodation, and those conditions in which the intestinal motility is altered.

### Evaluation

Current evidence suggests that the colitis is caused by a change in the flora of the colon and an overgrowth of toxin-producing strains of *Clostridium difficile*. The organism is a spore-forming, gram-positive anaerobic bacillus that is the component of the normal intestinal flora in approximately 3% of individuals. Because it is so difficult to isolate, a *C. difficile* cytotoxin assay is preferred, from which results are usually available within 24 hours. High toxin levels are an indication for specific therapy, but quantitative culture results have little diagnostic or therapeutic value. The presence of polymorphonuclear leukocytes in the stool is a helpful and rapid technique that makes suggests the diagnosis. A latex agglutination method is available for detecting the toxin in stool samples, but it may not be specific for this bacterium alone.

Proctosigmoidoscopic examination may reveal diffuse edema, multiple ulcerations, and the presence of the adherent, so-called "pseudomembranes" (Fig. 33.4). Colonoscopy may be necessary to make the diagnosis, particularly because no uncommonly right-sided involvement with a relatively normal distal bowel is seen. Biopsy of the lesion is not mandatory for confirming the diagnosis. However, with any question of the cause of the inflammatory change, tissue should be obtained (Fig. 33.5).

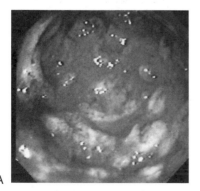 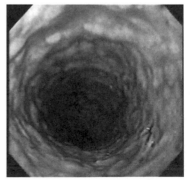

A                                                                                          B

**FIG. 33.4. A, B.** Colonoscopy clearly demonstrates the patterns of yellow and yellow white adherent plaques in pseudomembranous colitis.

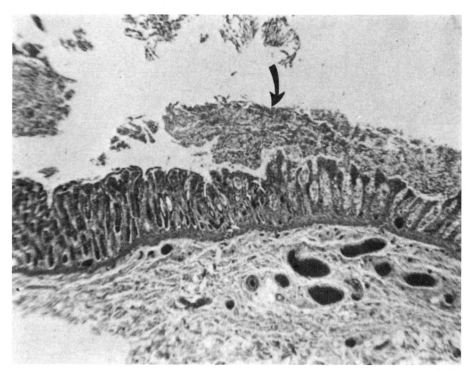

**FIG. 33.5.** Pseudomembranous colitis. Superficial necrosis (*arrow*) with acute inflammatory mucosal exudate. (Original magnification ×80.)

Barium enema examination may demonstrate "thumbprinting," which is caused by bowel wall edema. In more advanced stages, severe ulceration may be present (Fig. 33.6). The procedure, however, is relatively contraindicated in the acutely ill patient because of the risk of precipitating toxic megacolon or a perforation. Plain abdominal radiographs may reveal classic megacolon with or without small bowel dilatation. Differential diagnosis of such a radiologic picture must include Ogilvie's syndrome (colonic ileus), ischemia, and volvulus.

### Treatment

Treatment requires discontinuing the antibiotic, and fluid and electrolyte replacement. Because *C. difficile* is a transferable enteric pathogen, stool precautions for the duration of the illness are advised. However, depending on the severity of the manifestations, it may not be necessary to use specific antibiotic therapy. Medications that slow peristalsis should be avoided, because elimination of the toxin is inhibited. Those patients with pyrexia, abdominal signs and symptoms, leukocytosis, or who are elderly or debilitated, should be treated with van-

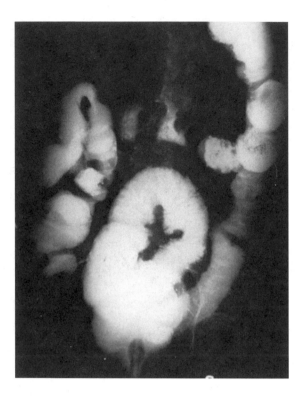

**FIG. 33.6.** Pseudomembranous colitis. Barium enema demonstrates extensive ulceration. Note the collar-button appearance of the ulcers extending into the bowel wall.

comycin. The drug can be given orally in a dosage of 125 to 250 mg every 6 hours for at least 5 days, but treatment for more than 10 days is rarely necessary. Improvement in symptoms usually occurs within 48 hours, but the diarrhea may not disappear for 1 week or more.

One of the concerns is how to administer the agent in an individual who is not able to take oral medication, because intravenous administration fails to achieve adequate therapeutic levels in the bowel. Some have recommended giving the drug via enema, using a solution of 500 mg in 1 L of saline every 8 hours. If this fails and the patient is not responding, performing a cecostomy or colostomy can provide a route for administration.

A number of physicians suggest that, especially in milder cases, bacitracin or metronidazole can be substituted. Cholestyramine, used alone, has also been shown to be effective.

One of the concerns with this disease is the possibility of relapse following therapy, a frequency that has been reported to be from 10% to 14%. Successful treatments with rectal installation of homologous feces as well as a mixture of ten different facultatively aerobic and anaerobic bacteria have been reported—so-called "biotherapy." It has been proposed that the absence of a *Bacteroides* species predisposes to the recrudescence of this illness.

The most frequent indication for operative intervention is perforation, although pseudomembranous colitis can be a terminal complication in someone with a malignancy. Acute abdominal signs and symptoms, in fact, can be the initial presenting manifestations in some individuals. Total colectomy with ileostomy is the preferred treatment for a perforation or for fulminant disease. At laparotomy, the external appearance of the colon can be deceptively normal. This finding should not influence the surgical procedure. With sepsis or a dilated bowel, in the absence of necrosis or perforation, a diversionary ileostomy, alone, may be adequate surgical management. The mortality rate for this disease can be as high as 100%, especially if a less than subtotal colectomy is performed. Even in cases of aggressive surgical management, mortality rates of 15% are seen.

### Campylobacter Enteritis

*Campylobacter jejuni*, one of the major causes of infectious diarrhea in the United States today, is also an important cause of diarrhea throughout the world. The organism is a curved or "gull-wing" microaerophilic, gram-positive rod. Transmission occurs by way of the fecal-oral route through contaminated fruit and water or by direct contact with infected animals or persons. The organism is not uncommonly isolated from hospitalized patients who have diarrhea.

Symptoms and findings may be difficult to differentiate from those of other diseases affecting the intestinal tract. Abdominal pain, fever, nausea, and vomiting may be associated.

Proctosigmoidoscopic examination usually reveals an edematous, inflamed mucosa. Histologic examination of biopsy specimens is nonspecific. A double-contrast barium enema may demonstrate aphthoid ulcers and a stippled appearance. Examination of the fecal specimen within 2 hours of passage by dark-field or phase-contrast microscopy may identify the organism. The presence of polymorphonuclear leukocytes in the fecal stream is not uncommon, but is not pathognomonic for the condition.

Usually, the infection is self-limited, but relapses are frequent. In severe cases, hospitalization and fluid and electrolyte replacement may be necessary. Ciprofloxacin (250 to 500 mg), orally four times a day for 7 days, is the recommended treatment, although erythromycin, tetracycline, doxycycline, gentamicin, and clindamycin can also be used. Appropriate stool precautions (particularly for hospitalized patients) are indicated, with proper disposal of contaminated linens and washing of hands. Toxic megacolon caused by a *Campylobacter* colitis necessitating total colectomy has been reported.

### Yersinia Enterocolitis

*Yersinia enterocolitica* is a relatively recently recognized cause of enteric infection. *Yersinia* enterocolitis is of particular interest to the surgeon because of its prevalence and because of its occasional confusion with regional enteritis. A former name for the causative organism was *Pasteurella pseudotuberculosis*, again implying confusion with another bacterial infection that tends to involve the ileocecal region. Epidemics caused by contamination of food, water, and milk have been reported.

The disease is caused by a facultatively anaerobic gram-negative coccoid bacillus resembling nonlactose-fermenting *Escherichia coli*. It grows optimally in a cold temperature. The diagnosis is established by isolation of the bacteria from the stool. Biotyping and serotyping according to O antigens have been the most helpful of the epidemiologic techniques.

The organism usually produces signs and symptoms of an acute gastroenteritis as a consequence of invasion of epithelial cells and the penetration of the intestinal mucosa; diarrhea is frequently observed in addition to abdominal pain. Drainage of the bacteria into regional lymph nodes accounts for the systemic complications. A syndrome simulating appendicitis is seen in 40% of the patients: fever, leukocytosis, right lower quadrant abdominal tenderness, and pain. The condition can produce generalized septicemia and metastatic abscesses in other organs. It can also present as a colonic abscess or toxic megacolon. The disease can pursue a chronic course for many weeks, particularly if not treated with appropriate antibiotics. Postinfection manifestations include erythema nodosum and reactive arthritis. Predisposing factors to the development of the infection include:

- Cirrhosis
- Hemochromatosis
- Acute iron poisoning
- Transfusion-dependent blood dyscrasias
- Immunosuppression
- Diabetes mellitus
- Malnutrition

Radiologic examination shows a coarse, irregular, nodular mucosal pattern in the terminal ileum. Ulcerations can be also noted. In contrast to Crohn's disease, the infection of the terminal ileum is usually confined to the mucosa and submucosa; the characteristic "string-sign" is absent. Endoscopic examination demonstrates signs of inflammatory disease in approximately one half the patients.

Recommended treatment includes antipseudomonal aminoglycosides, trimethoprim/sulfamethoxazole, ceftizoxime, or ceftriaxone, but antimicrobial therapy has not been proved to be essential or necessarily efficacious in the uncomplicated situation. However, when systemic illness supervenes or when the patient is immunocompromised, doxycycline or trimethoprim/sulfamethoxazole is advisable.

### Salmonellosis and Typhoid Fever

Typhoid fever is caused by the bacillus *Salmonella typhi*. This bacterium produces extensive epithelial invasion along the small bowel and colon, without destroying the intestinal mucosa. The bacteria breach the mucosa and submucosa in areas of an inflammatory reaction, and an endotoxin is produced on autolysis of the bacterial cell. Because the condition is endemic in many underdeveloped countries, the diagnosis is usually suggested when symptoms occur in such areas. However, in Western countries it is rarely considered. Humans are the only known reservoir, with transmission effected by the fecal-oral route, usually through contamination of water supplies. Stool culture may reveal the organism or, in the case of typhoid sepsis, blood culture may identify salmonella. Salmonella bacteremia, involving many serotypes, including typhi, has been recognized as an emerging concern in the acquired immunodeficiency syndrome (AIDS).

If the organism enters the bloodstream, severe septicemia can result. Characteristics of the febrile illness include fever, headache, delirium, spleen enlargement, abdominal pain, maculopapular rash, and leukopenia. Generalized hyperplasia of the entire reticuloendothelial system occurs, particularly in the Peyer's patches of the ileum and solitary lymph follicles of the cecum.

Acute cholecystitis can occur; this can progress to gangrene and perforation. Toxic megacolon and intestinal perforation can also complicate the disease and, on rare occasion, massive lower gastrointestinal hemorrhage can develop. The process is usually limited to the terminal 70 cm of ileum and proximal colon.

Abdominal examination may reveal mild tenderness or signs suggestive of a generalized peritonitis, if a perforation has ensued. Mortality rates of 8% to 32% have been reported, but are probably less in Western nations with combination antibiotic therapy and surgery. Medical management includes the use of parenteral or enteral nutrition and antibiotics (amoxicillin [1 g orally, three times a day for 3 to 14 days], ciprofloxacin, chloramphenicol, or trimethoprim-sulfa).

### Tuberculosis

Tuberculosis involving the intestinal tract can be caused either by *Mycobacterium tuberculosis* or *M. bovis*. In the former situation, the disease is primary to the lungs, and carried to the intestinal tract by swallowing of sputum. The latter organism produces the infection in association with swallowing unpasteurized milk. This condition is extremely unusual in most Western countries, because pasteurization of milk is standardized. However, more recently it has increased in countries such as the United Kingdom and the United States, a fact attributable to the large number of Asian immigrants. The proportion of extrapulmonary tuberculosis is much higher in patients with AIDS as well. The incidence, especially in urban areas, has been increasing steadily for the past 15 years. Peritoneal tuberculosis is presently the sixth most common site of extrapulmonary tuberculosis in the United States, followed by lymphatic genitourinary, bone and joint, miliary, and meningeal involvement.

When the disease does affect the intestinal tract, it is usually caused by the pulmonary strain and most commonly is localized to the ileocecal region.

Although the condition is most commonly seen in the proximal colon and ileum, segmental bowel involvement has occasionally been observed.

### Symptoms and Findings

The most common presenting complaints are abdominal pain, weight loss, and fever. This is usually confined to the hypogastrium and is most frequently localized to the right lower quadrant. Other symptoms include anorexia, fever, and weight loss. Tuberculous peritonitis, however, usually presents as an acute abdomen that mimics appendicitis, and is seen mainly in young children or adolescents. Ascites with abdominal pain and distension may be the first indication of this complication.

Physical examination may reveal the presence of a mass, usually in the right lower quadrant. In the rare situation when tuberculosis involves the rectum or anus, a stricture may be apparent. Depending on whether the lesion produces ulceration or stricture, it can simulate carcinoma.

### Evaluation

The diagnosis requires a high index of suspicion. Acid-fast bacilli will rarely be identified in the stool. Although a positive tuberculin test result can be useful, it does not establish the diagnosis with certainty.

Radiologic investigation is helpful but not necessarily diagnostic of tuberculosis. Barium enema study may reveal retrograde obstruction, stricture, or a "conical cecum." The terminal ileum can be normal, dilated, ulcerated, or strictured.

A nonspecific ultrasonic finding, the "pseudokidney sign," has also been identified in association with ileal tuberculosis. This is a pattern consisting of a strong echogenic center surrounded by a sonolucent rim, the common factor being bowel wall thickening. Computed tomographic (CT) evaluation may provide more insight into the disease process by identifying subclinical ascites, adenopathy, abscess, and thickening of the bowel wall. The distinction between tuberculosis and Crohn's disease may not be possible radiologically or endoscopically, although colonoscopy with biopsy has been suggested to be a useful tool.

Laparoscopy has been found to be a useful procedure for the diagnosis of tuberculous peritonitis. The laparoscopic appearance can be classified according to three types: (a) thickened peritoneum with miliary, yellowish white tubercles with or without adhesions; (b) thickened peritoneum only with or without adhesions; and (c) a fibroadhesive pattern. Visual diagnosis is accurate in 95% of patients.

### Histopathology

Generally, the macroscopic appearance of the cecum is indistinguishable from that of Crohn's disease, but the diagnosis may be established by histologic examination. The yield of biopsy-proved granulomas in tuberculous lesions is 100%, although acid-fast bacilli may not be recovered from any.

Examination of the resected specimen may reveal thickening of the bowel wall, mucosal ulceration, localized segmental disease, or skip lesions. The mucosal appearance may demonstrate characteristic transverse ulcers. The classic histologic criteria include the presence of submucosal or serosal Langhans' giant cells and caseous necrosis (Fig. 33.7). The organism may be demonstrated in the specimen or may be grown by guinea pig culture.

## Treatment

Conventional antituberculous agents are recommended in the uncomplicated case. Approximately one half of the patients with colonic or ileocolonic tuberculosis may be adequately treated with medical therapy alone. Possible regimens include a combination of isoniazid with ethambutol or rifampin. Others prefer pyrazinamide to ethambutol because of the lower incidence of side effects. Patients with ulcerating lesions are more likely to respond to medical management than are those with the hypertrophic form of the disease. As has been implied, abdominal tuberculosis can be cured medically if recognized early, but the nonspecific presentation that is often observed tends to delay the diagnosis

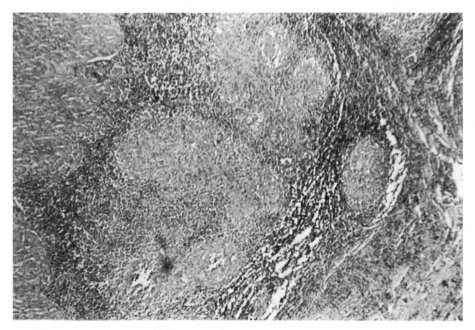

**FIG. 33.7.** Tuberculous granulomas (note caseous necrosis) in a mesenteric lymph node. (Original magnification ×180; courtesy of Rudolf Garret, M.D.)

in many instances. Surgical treatment should be limited to those patients with symptomatic, localized disease. Obviously, if the distinction cannot be made between tuberculosis and carcinoma by endoscopic means, a resection is indicated.

### *Gonococcal Proctitis*

Gonorrhea is a common, sexually transmitted, acute infectious disease of the mucous membranes affecting the urethra, vagina, and cervix, but rectal gonorrhea has been recognized only relatively recently. The disease is caused by the bacterium, *Neisseria gonorrhoeae* (the gonococcus), a gram-negative coccus occurring in pairs or clumps. Characteristically, the organism appears on smears as intracellular gram-negative diplococci (Fig. 33.8). To confirm the presence of the organism by culture, rectal swabs are inoculated on a selective chocolate agar (Thayer Martin) and sent to the laboratory without delay, where they are placed in a carbon dioxide jar and incubated.

In men, the disease is most commonly associated with the homosexual population and is transmitted by anal intercourse. However, in women, the disease is usually transferred to the rectum by discharge from the vagina. Usually, only the lower rectum is involved.

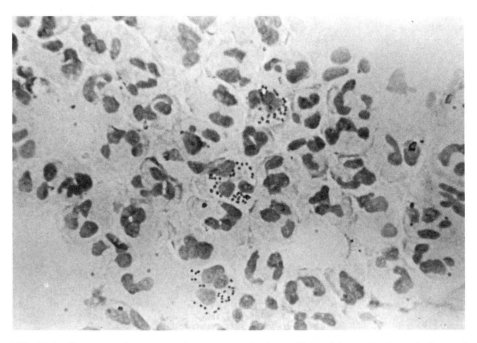

**FIG. 33.8.** Gonorrhea. Smear reveals gram-negative intracellular diplococci in the cytoplasm of polymorphonuclear cells. (Original magnification ×1,000.)

Eradication of the disease is particularly difficult because the patient may report no complaint. If symptoms are evident, they can include pruritus, mucous discharge, rectal bleeding, diarrhea, and concerns referable to either gonorrhea or syphilis in other sites. Disseminated disease can occur (septicemia), as well as pericarditis, endocarditis, meningitis, perihepatitis, and gonococcal arthritis. Characteristically, the arthritis produces an acute purulent effusion of a single joint.

Proctosigmoidoscopic examination will usually reveal edematous, friable mucosa with occasional areas of ulceration. Biopsy may show degeneration of the epithelium, capillary engorgement, and infiltration with inflammatory cells. However, in many persons, no identifiable lesion will be seen.

### Treatment

Treatment of rectal gonorrhea has been a particular problem, because of the greater difficulty in eradicating the organism from this area than from the genitourinary tract. Alternative regimens include procaine penicillin (4.8 million units), in two equally divided, simultaneous intramuscular injections, with probenecid (1 g) given orally prior to or at the time of penicillin injection. Alternatively, tetracycline (1.5 g) in an initial oral dose, followed by 500 mg four times a day for 4 days; or spectinomycin (2 g) by intramuscular injection. Other antibiotics suggested include kanamycin (2 g) intramuscularly, or cotrimoxazole orally, three tablets, twice daily for 3 days. Recently, ceftriaxone followed by a 10-day course of doxycycline has been recommended. The importance of close follow-up examination with culture to assess the adequacy of the therapy cannot be overestimated.

### Syphilis of the Rectum or Syphilitic Proctitis

Syphilis of the anal canal and perianal skin is a well-recognized clinical entity (see Chapter 19), but the manifestation of syphilitic proctitis is less familiar to most physicians. The condition occurs almost exclusively in the male homosexual population.

Symptoms include mucous discharge, bleeding, tenesmus, and change in bowel habits. Endoscopic examination may reveal a mass or an ulcerating lesion that is suggestive of carcinoma. Biopsies fail to reveal tumor, however. Anorectal lesions have been divided into four categories:

1. Anal ulceration
2. Rectal ulceration
3. Granulomatous (hyperplastic)
4. Miscellaneous (fixed, tumorlike)

Although the diagnosis can be confirmed by dark-field examination of the exudate, disclosing the presence of the treponemal organisms, this does require a high index of suspicion. Treatment is that which has been described in Chapter 19.

## Shigellosis

Shigellosis, also known as bacillary dysentery, is caused by the *Shigella* organism, a gram-negative, non–spore-forming rod (Fig. 33.9). The condition can present acutely, with fever, diarrhea, and severe dehydration. Whereas the condition is usually confined to the mucosa of the colon, more profound disease has been reported, including that of intestinal obstruction and toxic megacolon. This is another disease that is virtually epidemic in the male homosexual population and in those with AIDS.

The hallmark of the inflammatory reaction is invasion and destruction of the intestinal mucosa. Watery diarrhea is followed by severe abdominal pain, tenesmus, and rectal bleeding. The small bowel phase of the symptoms can be determined by an enterotoxin, whereas the invasive phase is typical of the large bowel.

Sigmoidoscopic examination may reveal the typical changes of a proctitis, with edema, friability, and ulceration. The appearance may be indistinguishable from that of nonspecific inflammatory bowel disease. The most satisfactory means for establishing the diagnosis is culture obtained by swabbing any ulcerating lesion during endoscopy; alternatively, mucus or fecal material can be used

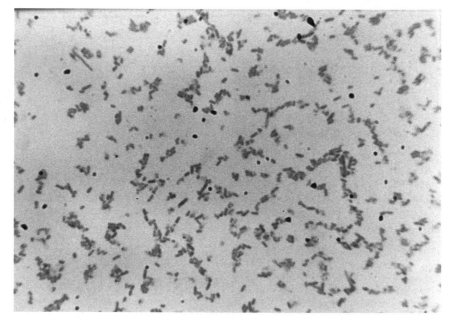

**FIG. 33.9.** Shigella. Gram-negative bacilli, which, on biochemical and serological testing, reveal *Shigella* organisms. (Original magnification ×1,060.)

for culture. Because the organism is somewhat labile, the plates should be inoculated as soon as possible.

Because of the usually self-limited nature of the condition, supportive measures may be the only treatment required, although some believe that all patients should undergo antibiotic therapy irrespective of the severity of symptoms. Trimethoprim-sulfamethoxazole (Bactrim, Septra) is the drug of choice (one double-strength tablet orally twice daily for 5 to 15 days); or ampicillin (500 mg orally, four times a day for 5 days may be substituted. Another option is ciprofloxacin (500 mg orally twice daily for 7 days). As with other infectious colitides, it is important to reevaluate the stool to ascertain that the bacterium has been eliminated.

### Brucellosis

Brucellosis is caused by the bacterium, *Brucella melitensis*, usually because of the consumption of unpasteurized goat's milk or cheese. Although relatively common in developing countries, it is rarely seen in the Western nations. On rare occasions, it can cause a severe colitis. The symptoms and endoscopic findings are essentially the same as those for other inflammatory bowel conditions. Culture of the purulent exudate will lead to the diagnosis. Treatment consists of tetracycline or doxycycline (Vibramycin).

### Actinomycosis

Actinomycosis is a suppurative, granulomatous disease that tends to form draining sinus tracts, discharging granules. The organism *Actinomyces israelii*, an anaerobic, gram-positive bacterium, is a normal inhabitant of the mouth, lungs, and intestinal tract. When the disease involves the colon or rectum, it usually presents with an abdominal mass, a fistula, or a sinus. Although ileocecal involvement is the most common intestinal manifestation, rectal stricture has also been reported. Differential diagnosis from a neoplasm can be very difficult.

Unless material is available for histologic study, the disease is usually not diagnosed until resection has been performed. Radiologic studies have not generally been useful in the preoperative assessment. However, CT can be helpful, demonstrating a solid mass with focal areas of attenuation, or a cystic mass with a thickened wall that enhances with infusion.

For actinomycosis confined to the colon, resection is the treatment of choice, in addition to antibiotic therapy (penicillin). Large doses are recommended over a prolonged period of time.

## VIRAL INFECTIONS

Viral infections that specifically attack the rectum or colon are extremely rare. However, three areas merit attention—AIDS, herpes simplex proctitis, and cytomegalovirus infection. The virus that causes the acquired immune deficiency syndrome (HIV) is important to address, because so many of the complications and manifestations of the disease affect the anus, rectum, and colon. The reason for this is the fact that the gastrointestinal tract is the largest lymphoid organ in the body, and as such is an enormous potential reservoir for HIV. The adverse consequences on the cellular and humoral defense mechanisms lead to a plethora of viral, bacterial, fungal, and protozoal infestations.

Chapter 20 contains a discussion of both AIDS and cytomegalovirus infection. The one remaining area, that of herpes simplex proctitis was addressed, to some extent, in Chapter 19. The following discussion, however, is limited to that of the inflammatory change in the rectum.

## Herpes Simplex Proctitis

Herpes simplex virus (HSV) proctitis is the most common cause of nongonococcal proctitis in sexually active male homosexuals. Herpes infections in patients with AIDS can also present as an ulcerative proctitis that remains confined to the rectum. The likelihood of having proctitis caused by the herpes virus is greater if the patient has tenesmus, anorectal pain, constipation, and perianal ulceration. Difficulty in urinating, sacral paresthesias, and diffuse ulceration of the distal rectal mucosa also suggest the nature of the condition. Intestinal perforation associated with intestinal herpes simplex infection has been reported.

Sigmoidoscopic examination reveals an acute proctitis, with a high index of suspicion as to the cause based on the fact that the individual is a homosexually active man. The diagnosis is established by immunoassay of the antibody to the virus. In addition, HSV can be isolated by culture from rectal swabs or biopsy specimens.

Acyclovir has been demonstrated to eradicate perirectal HSV infection. Acyclovir is also believed to be of benefit by affecting the natural history of recurrence of the proctitis after the initial episode.

## FUNGAL INFECTIONS

### Candidiasis or Moniliasis

Fungal infections of the gastrointestinal tract are extremely rare in the healthy person. Candidiasis usually occurs in immunosuppressed patients, those with severe debilitating disease, and those taking steroids; it can also develop following prolonged administration of broad-spectrum antibiotics, particularly the third generation cephalosporins. Diffuse fungal infections are common causes of death in patients with terminal cancer.

When the fungus affects the gastrointestinal tract, it usually produces diarrhea and, occasionally, abdominal pain. In addition, internal fistulas may develop. The diagnosis is established by identifying the yeast, spores, or pseudomycelia by microscopic examination. Biopsy may demonstrate the characteristic pseudohyphae (Fig. 33.10). Nystatin (500,000 to 1,000,000 U), orally, four times daily,

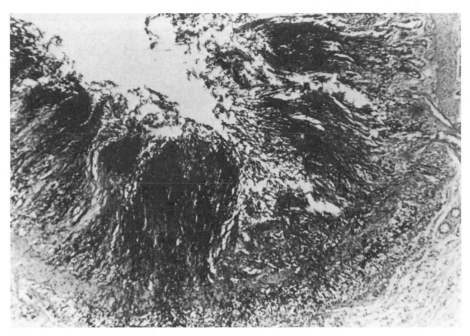

**FIG. 33.10.** Intestinal candidiasis (moniliasis). Postmortem biopsy demonstrates characteristic pseudohyphae replacing mucosa. (Original magnification ×180; courtesy of Rudolf Garret, M.D.)

is the usual treatment for intestinal candidiasis. Alternatively, ketoconazole (200 to 400 mg), once a day, or intravenous amphotericin B may be used (0.3 to 0.6 mg/kg body weight daily).

## Histoplasmosis

Histoplasmosis is caused by the dimorphic fungus, *Histoplasma capsulatum*, principally an intracellular mycosis of the reticuloendothelial system. It is endemic to areas of the Midwest, especially in the fertile river valleys. It is usually a subclinical infection in otherwise healthy individuals, but in immunocompromised persons disseminated disease can ensue. Although the lung is by far the most common organ involved, the condition can affect the entire gastrointestinal tract, especially the terminal ileum and proximal colon. When it involves this area, ulceration with bleeding, stricture, and even perforation may be seen. The condition is sometimes confused with colon carcinoma.

Endoscopic examination may reveal skip areas of inflammation, with plaques, ulcers, and pseudopolyps. Whereas biopsy may demonstrate the characteristic intracellular oval budding yeasts within the mucosa, serologic complement-fixation titers of 1:8 or greater are suggestive of the disease. Fungal culture of biopsy specimens will also confirm the diagnosis. If pathologic changes are correlated with the roentgenographic features, six patterns of gastrointestinal involvement have been described:

1. Malabsorptive (edema, diffuse inflammatory infiltrates)
2. Ulcerative
3. Polypoid (nodular hyperplasia of the lymphoid follicles)
4. Granulomatous (diffuse infiltrates)
5. Tumefactive (large granulomas)
6. Compressive (enlarged lymph nodes)

Common physical findings are peripheral lymphadenopathy and hepatosplenomegaly.

Ketoconazole is the recommended drug for those with pulmonary involvement who are not immunocompromised, but amphotericin B is suggested for individuals with such impairment or who have central nervous system disease. Diversion or resection of strictures may be indicated, in addition to aggressive long-term amphotericin-B therapy for those with AIDS.


## PARASITIC INFECTIONS

### Amebiasis

Whereas amebiasis is a worldwide disease that is most commonly found in the tropics, it is the most frequent parasitic condition encountered by surgeons in the United States. A patient will often believe that he or she has "amebiasis" based on a travel experience or contact with persons who are known to harbor the organism. The largest reservoir for *Entamoeba histolytica* infection is in the male homosexual population.


#### *Pathogenesis*

*Entamoeba histolytica* is caused by a protozoan that exists in the colon as either a trophozoite (Fig. 33.11) or as a cyst. The cytoplasm of the organism usually is very granular owing to ingestion of many bacteria, red blood cells, and other cellular debris (Fig. 33.12). Transmission occurs either through water or food contaminated by carriers of the cysts. The swallowed cysts pass into the small intestine where the trophozoites are released. These burrow into the mucosa and result in the characteristic flask-shaped ulcer. Ulcers are usually identified in the cecum and ascending colon, but the process can be diffuse throughout the bowel; it is rare for the small intestine to be involved.

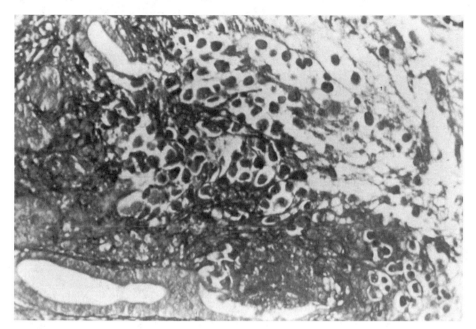

**FIG. 33.11.** *Entamoeba histolytica.* Trophozoites in an ulcer in the colon. (Original magnification ×280; courtesy of Rudolf Garret, M.D.)

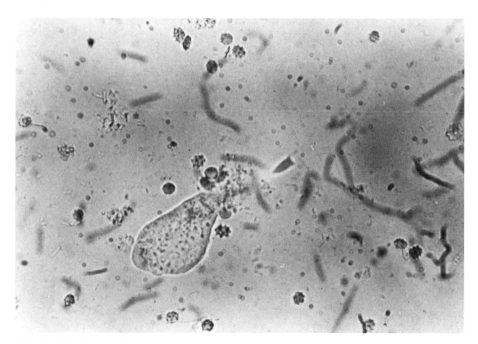

**FIG. 33.12.** *Entamoeba histolytica* ingesting red blood cells. (Wet preparation; original magnification ×360; courtesy of Rudolf Garret, M.D.)

### Symptoms and Findings

Symptoms of amebiasis may be minimal, or the disease can be acute and fulminant, and include crampy abdominal pain, tenesmus, and bloody stools. The most common complaint is diarrhea, which can be bloody and contain mucus. Bowel movements can be frequent, in excess of ten per day.

Physical examination may reveal abdominal tenderness, most marked in the hypogastrium. The liver can be enlarged, but hepatomegaly does not necessarily indicate the presence of a liver abscess. Toxic dilatation of the colon can develop in the fulminant condition, a clinical and radiologic manifestation not dissimilar to that occurring in ulcerative colitis. Perforation can supervene with generalized peritonitis. Extraintestinal amebiasis can lead to hepatitis, amebic abscess of the liver, pulmonary disease, and involvement of the pericardium, brain, and skin.

### Diagnosis

The diagnosis is established by microscopic examination of fresh stool specimens for the trophozoites. Of patients with symptomatic disease, 90% will demonstrate this finding. It is important that stool examination is done before any barium investigation; the use of mineral oil and broad-spectrum antibiotics also impedes the ability to identify the protozoan. In addition to stool culture and at least three stool examinations for eggs and parasites, amebic titer by indirect hemagglutination technique may establish the diagnosis.

Sigmoidoscopic examination is a valuable method for diagnosis; ulcerations are usually visible in the rectum in up to 85% of the cases. However, because the disease occurs more frequently in a proximal location than it does distally, a negative proctosigmoidoscopy does not rule out the diagnosis. Colonoscopy can be a useful technique for this reason. Although the histologic appearance is usually indistinguishable from nonspecific inflammatory bowel disease, the overhanging mucosa, undermining margins, or flask shape, along with the appropriate history, suggest amebic colitis. Occasionally, a granulomatous reaction leads to the formation of a mass, the so-called "ameboma." When this clinical picture is present, it can be difficult to differentiate an ameboma from that of granulomatous colitis or carcinoma.

Barium enema examination may reveal the so-called "collar-button ulcer," a cobblestone appearance, thumbprinting, and the signs of nonspecific inflammatory bowel disease. Amebiasis is almost always multifocal, so that a careful search throughout the length of the colon for other areas of infection is an important aspect of differential diagnosis. The presence of a stricture or tumorlike ameboma may confuse the interpretation; an ameboma can also involve the rectum.

### Management

The drugs of choice for the treatment of asymptomatic patients with intestinal amebiasis are iodoquinol (Yodoxin), furamide, and metronidazole. Other options that have been demonstrated to be efficacious include emetine hydrochloride, dehydroemetine, and paromomycin (Humatin). For severe intestinal disease, metronidazole (750 mg), three times daily for 10 days, followed by iodoquinol (650 mg), three times daily for 20 days, has been recommended.

If the patient requires surgical intervention for hemorrhage or for perforation, the involved bowel must be resected. Indications include the following:

- Free extraperitoneal perforation, impending perforation, or perforation during antiamebic chemotherapy
- Failure of perforation with a localized abscess to respond to antiamebic drugs
- Persistence or the development of abdominal distension, and abdominal tenderness in patients being treated
- Persistence of severe diarrhea after 5 days of chemotherapy
- Symptoms of postamebic colitis with unremitting anemia and hypoproteinemia

No general agreement exists to the best surgical approach, but the mortality rate in most series is at least 75%. Total abdominal colectomy may be required if multiple areas of perforation are identified. Because of the high risk of anastomotic leak, some suggest exteriorization or, at least, a concomitant diversionary procedure. Even in patients for whom an operation is considered, aggressive medical treatment is recommended because it may obviate the need for surgery, or improve the likelihood of survival following resection in this high-risk situation.

## Balantidiasis

Balantidiasis is caused by a protozoan, *Balantidium coli*, a ciliate that is the only member of the subphylum *Ciliophora* known to affect humans. The condition is found where sanitation is a problem. The trophozoite is large and occasionally is seen with the naked eye (Fig. 33.13). Locomotion is by means of longitudinal rows of cilia that cover the body and propel it forward with a spiral motion. A cyst develops when the organism is passed in the feces and is the source for dissemination of the disease.

After the cyst is ingested, it passes into the small intestine where it excysts, and the trophozoite then passes into the colon where it penetrates the intestinal epithelium. Ulcerations are produced, not dissimilar to those seen with amebic colitis. In fact, it is not uncommon for the two conditions to coexist.

The usual symptoms are abdominal discomfort, distension, flatulence, and a loose, offensive, pale stool. Mucus and blood may accompany the bowel movements. The disease may be self-limited with constipation alternating with diarrhea.

Proctosigmoidoscopic examination can reveal the same changes seen in amebiasis. The diagnosis is made by examination of a fresh stool specimen, but

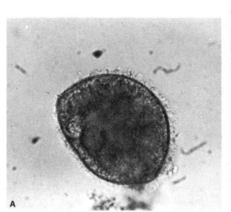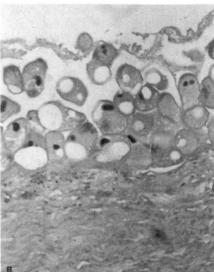

**FIG. 33.13.** *Balantidium coli.* **A.** Trophozoite. Note the cilia. **B.** Surface of the colonic mucosa replaced by trophozoites of *B. coli.* (Original magnification ×280; courtesy of Rudolf Garret, MD.)

patients with frequent bowel movements may pass only the trophozoites. An additional method for confirmation is to obtain the trophozoites by duodenal aspiration or by a recoverable nylon yarn swallowed in a weighted capsule.

A number of drugs are effective in the treatment of balantidiasis, including tetracycline either alone or in combination with mepacrine. Other alternatives include metronidazole, iodoquinol, and furazolidone (Furoxone). Treatment should be directed toward the asymptomatic carrier as well as to the patient with acute or chronic illness in order to eliminate the organism and to prevent its spread.

### Cryptosporidiosis

Cryptosporidia are protozoal parasites that primarily infect animals, but the disease has been recognized as an important infection in immunocompromised patients. It is the most frequent pathogen in patients who are HIV positive and have symptoms of diarrhea; in fact, the diagnosis of AIDS can be made if the infection lasts longer than 3 weeks. A high rate of infection is also seen among children in day-care facilities and among persons arriving from developing countries.

The organism can be transmitted by a variety of routes, including fecal-oral, hand-to-mouth, contaminated food, pets (especially cats), and water-borne. Human-to-human transmission, especially in a hospital population, is an important mechanism of dissemination. The gastrointestinal tract is predominantly

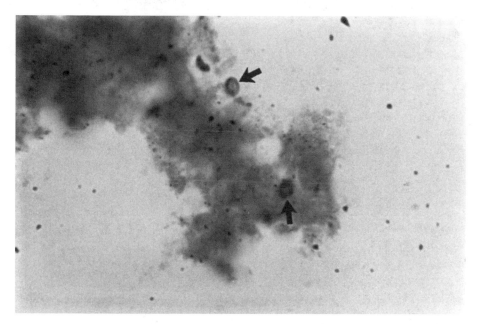

**FIG. 33.14.** Cryptosporidiosis. Small round to oval-shaped forms (*arrows*) usually seen by acid-fast stain or fluorescent staining techniques. (Original magnification ×1,000.)

affected, with the production of a severe, watery, debilitating, chronic diarrhea. Malabsorption, wasting, and weight loss may be evident. Abdominal pain, however, is unusual.

The diagnosis is based on demonstration of *Cryptosporidium* oocysts in the stool or in gastrointestinal mucosal biopsy specimens (Fig. 33.14). The most sensitive diagnostic method, however, uses a murine antibody to the oocyst wall. The protozoan appears to attach to the mucosa and may be surrounded by a host cell membrane, but no evidence is seen of invasion or tissue reaction.

Drug treatment with spiramycin, a macrolide antibiotic with a spectrum similar to that of erythromycin, has been recommended, and the recent use of zidovudine (AZT [Retrovir]) may hold some promise. However, because the clinical response has been disappointing, often only supportive measures (antidiarrheal agents and fluid replacement) are applicable in these patients at high risk.

### Giardiasis

Giardiasis is a disease caused by a flagellated protozoan, *Giardia lamblia*. It is a worldwide condition, with most patients being asymptomatic. So-called "traveler's diarrhea" is commonly attributed to this protozoan. Hikers and backpackers, drinking untreated water from mountain lakes and streams, where animals serve as a reservoir for the parasite, are at risk. It is probably the most common waterborne disease in the United States. An increased incidence is seen in the male homosexual population, in adults who care for children in diapers, and in those individuals who are institutionalized. Twenty percent to 50% of children under the age of 3 in daycare centers and 20% of homosexual men may be cyst passers.

As with balantidiasis, the protozoan exists both as a cyst and as a trophozoite. Infection results from ingestion of the cyst, which excysts in the small intestine. This can lead to a variety of histologic changes, ranging from minimal cellular infiltrates of the lamina propria, reduction in the height and the number of villi, loss of the brush border, and an increase in epithelial cell mitosis.

### Symptoms

If the patient is symptomatic, the most common complaint is diarrhea, but symptoms not unlike those of amebiasis may be reported. The mechanism of the diarrhea is poorly understood. Additionally, the patient may complain of nausea, abdominal cramps, flatulence, anorexia, and weight loss. Malabsorption may also be manifested. Although on rare occasions the disease can pursue a fulminating course, most infected individuals are asymptomatic carriers.

### Evaluation

Proctosigmoidoscopic examination may reveal changes impossible to differentiate from those of amebiasis. The diagnosis can be made by examination of scrapings of the base of the ulcer for the trophozoites. Loose stool contains only the trophozoites; in formed stool, however, cysts may be found as well (Fig. 33.15). Rectal biopsy can also be helpful in identifying the organism. A negative stool examination, however, does not exclude the diagnosis. A more accurate determination of the cause can be made by microscopic examination of the duodenal fluid or by a "string test." Most recently, a commercially available test, the ProSpecT/Giardia enzyme-linked immunosorbent assay (ELISA, Alexon, Inc., Mountain View, CA, USA) has been found to be 96% to 98% sensitive and 100% specific. This test is less expensive than the conventional egg and parasite series, it is 30% more sensitive, and the results are available more quickly.

### Treatment

The drugs of choice for the treatment of giardiasis are quinacrine hydrochloride (Atabrine [100 mg], three times daily for 5 days or metronidazole [250 mg], three times daily for 5 days), the latter being associated with a somewhat lower cure rate. Treatment of the asymptomatic carrier is somewhat controversial, but prudence would seem to dictate that both the asymptomatic person and the acute or chronically ill patient should have therapy to prevent spread of the disease. No chemoprophylactic agent exists.

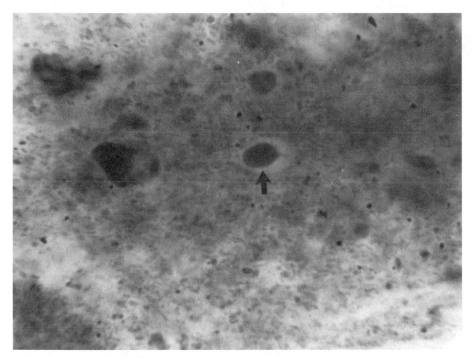

**FIG. 33.15.** Giardiasis. Oval-shaped parasite demonstrating retraction from cyst wall (*arrow*). Two nuclei can be appreciated. (Original magnification ×1,000.)

## Trypanosomiasis or Chagas' Disease

Chagas' disease is caused by *Trypanosoma cruzi*, which is transmitted by a reduviid bug. The trypanosomes are deposited from the feces of the bug when it is taking a blood meal. Phagocytosis of the invading organisms is performed by histiocytes in the skin, fat, and muscle; this is the so-called "leishmanial" form of the disease. Rupture of the cell causes escape of a large number of the trypanosomal forms into the circulation (Fig. 33.16). It had been thought that trypanosomiasis was a condition confined to Central and South America, but more recent evidence suggests that the disease is present in the United States, particularly in Texas.

Gastrointestinal manifestations occur from 2 to 20 years or more following initial infection. The colon and the esophagus are most frequently involved, although the stomach, small bowel, bladder, and ureters can be affected. Involvement of the myocardium and central nervous system can also develop. In the intestine, the release of the toxin destroys the submucosal and myenteric plexus, which can result in colonic dilatation. The patient can be severely constipated as the bowel becomes progressively dilated because of the neurologic abnormality and the presence of inspissated feces. Although obstipation may necessitate the frequent use of enemas,

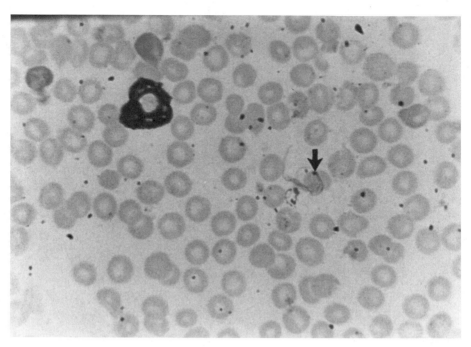

**FIG. 33.16.** Trypanosomiasis. *C*-shaped configuration found in human blood. Organism has prominent terminal kinetoplast (*arrow*). Intercellular location is typical of trypanosomes. (Original magnification ×1,000.)

often the patient compensates and is able to pursue a fairly normal existence. Volvulus, however, is a potential complication. In those individuals with chagasic megacolon, clinical signs and symptoms include severe pain and progressive abdominal distension, accompanied by fever, severe toxemia, and shock.

Radiologic examination may reveal an enormously dilated and elongated colon. In contradistinction to other forms of megacolon, the distribution can be segmental.

Resection of the aperistaltic esophagus or colon may be necessary if symptoms warrant. Because the colitis does not affect the rectum, colectomy with reestablishment of intestinal continuity can usually be performed, but because of the functional obstruction produced by the dyskinetic residual rectum, one of the pull-through procedures should be considered (see Chapters 18 and 23). Total colectomy with ileostomy is advised if toxic megacolon is the indication for the operation.

### Schistosomiasis or Bilharziosis

Schistosomiasis is a worldwide condition affecting perhaps 200 million people. The disease is caused by a trematode, a blood fluke seen in three forms:

*Schistosoma mansoni*, *S. japonicum*, and *S. haematobium*. A snail host is required to complete the life cycle. The disease is frequently seen in tropical and subtropical climates.

### Pathogenesis

The life cycle of the organism is of some interest. The infection is acquired by exposure to contaminated water containing the cercarial form (Fig. 33.17). The cercaria invades the skin, loses its tail, and enters the host's subcutaneous veins. From there it spreads to the heart and lungs and may produce a transient pneumonitis. Ultimately reaching the portal circulation, it grows, feeds, and differentiates into a male or a female form (Fig. 33.18). Following fertilization, the worms migrate together into the terminal mesenteric venules. There, the female deposits the fertilized eggs. The egg secretes a lytic substance that permits it to migrate through the surrounding tissue, into the intestinal lumen, and into the stool.

The three forms of the infestation are differentiated on the basis of the appearance of the *Schistosoma* eggs (Figs. 33.19 and 33.20). The *S. mansoni* egg has a

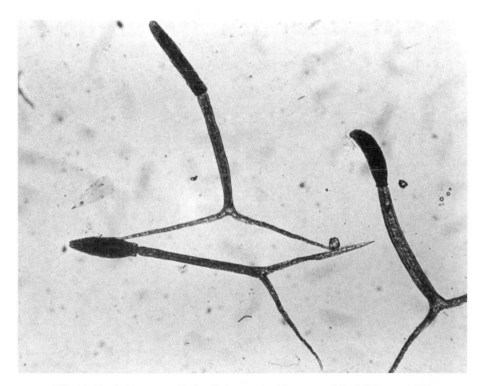

**FIG. 33.17.** *Schistosoma.* Fork-tailed cercaria. (Courtesy of Rudolf Garret, M.D.)

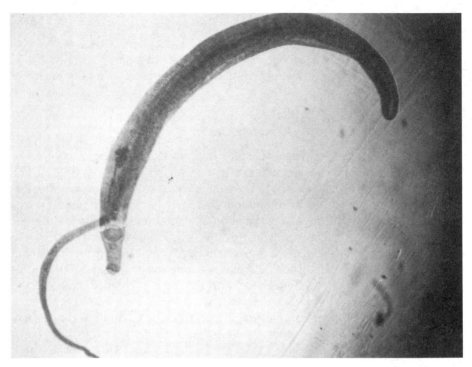

**FIG. 33.18.** *Schistosoma mansoni*, adult male and female. The female occupies the male's genital groove. (Courtesy of Rudolf Garret, M.D.)

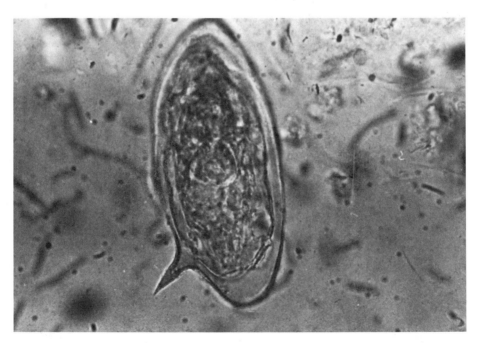

**FIG. 33.19.** *Schistosoma mansoni* egg. Note the lateral spine. (Courtesy of Rudolf Garret, M.D.)

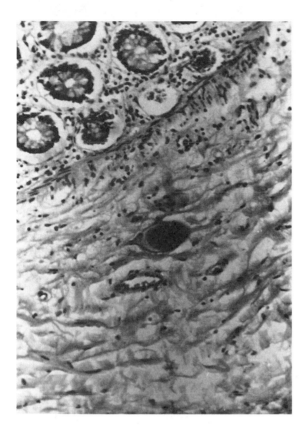

**FIG. 33.20.** *Schistosoma haematobium* egg in the rectal wall. Note the terminal spine. (Original magnification ×180; courtesy of Rudolf Garret, M.D.)

prominent lateral spine, the *S. haematobium* has a projecting terminal spine, and the *S. japonicum* has no definite spine. *S. japonicum* preferentially invades the superior mesenteric veins, thus involving the small intestine and ascending colon; *S. mansoni* usually invades the inferior mesenteric veins, perforating through the descending colon; and *S. haematobium* tends to invade the bladder vessels, thus producing symptoms in the bladder, pelvic organs, and rectum.

### Signs and Symptoms

Symptoms initially are referable to the skin. If migration through the bowel wall occurs, patients develop severe lower abdominal pain, diarrhea, rectal bleeding, and the passage of mucus. Other symptoms include fever, urticaria, and facial swelling.

Children are particularly susceptible to acute dysentery. Fibrosis and thickening can result, and polyp formation can also occur. Other complications include intussusception and rectal prolapse. Portal involvement can produce granulomas, hepatosplenomegaly, and portal hypertension. Central nervous system complications can also develop.

### Diagnosis

The diagnosis is usually made by identifying the eggs in fresh stool specimens. Rectal biopsy frequently reveals the presence of the eggs in the mucosa or submucosa. The diagnosis can also be made by a wet preparation; the biopsy specimen is compressed between two coverslips and examined for the eggs. A skin test and numerous serologic tests are also available for the diagnosis; the complement fixation test and indirect hemagglutination test may be valuable.

Colonoscopy with biopsy has been demonstrated to confirm the diagnosis, especially when eggs are present. Polyps are not uncommon, and because large or pedunculated ones tend not to regress but to cause persistent bleeding, polypectomy is recommended. However, additional polyps can be expected to regrow because the mucosa does not revert to normal. Rectocolic and urinary tract calcifications, as seen on radiologic studies, are felt to be associated with a clinically latent or mild form of schistosomiasis.

### Treatment

The medical management of schistosomiasis is risky. The drugs used differ, depending on which species is involved. A number of chemotherapeutic agents are variously effective; they include praziquantel, metriphonate, oxamniquine, sodium antimony dimercaptosuccinate (Astiban), antimony potassium tartrate (tartar emetic), stibophen (Fuadin), and niridazole.

Treating the complications of the colon involves a variety of resective and diversionary procedures. Anastomosis without a colostomy appears to be associated with a prohibitively high incidence of leakage.

### Relationship to Carcinoma

Patients with longstanding schistosomal colitis are at an increased risk for the development of carcinoma, but this applies primarily to *S. japonicum*. Slightly more than half of patients with schistosomal granulomatous disease of the large intestine, without obvious evidence of carcinoma, will have mild to severe dysplasia. These changes are felt to be presumptive evidence for the premalignant potential of schistosomal colitis, and analogous to those observed in patients with longstanding chronic ulcerative colitis.

### Relationship to Portal Hypertension

Cirrhosis with portal hypertension can produce massive hemorrhage from varices that requires portacaval shunting or variceal ligation. However, because of the high risk of these procedures, an approach has been recommended that involves cannulation of the portal vein, followed by trapping of the adult worms in a filter system. Administration of antimony potassium tartrate has been demonstrated to increase the yield of the worms removed by stimulating migration into the portal circulation.

## Ascariasis

Ascariasis is caused by a large roundworm, *Ascaris lumbricoides* (Fig. 33.21). The disease is an enormous problem; it is estimated that approximately 25% of the world's population is affected. The condition is endemic in tropical and subtropical areas, but epidemics have been reported in Europe and even in small, focal areas of the United States.

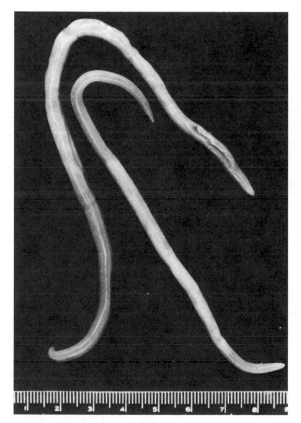

**FIG. 33.21.** *Ascaris lumbricoides*, adult worms. (Courtesy of Rudolf Garret, M.D.)

### Pathophysiology

Infection occurs from ingestion of the eggs in contaminated food and drink (Fig. 33.22). Following ingestion, the larvae emerge from the eggs and migrate through the wall of the small intestine into the portal venous system, passing through the liver and into the lungs. Ultimately, the larvae migrate through the capillaries, into the alveoli and the bronchioles, and are coughed up and swallowed. In the small intestine, they develop into the adult worm.

### Symptoms and Signs

Intestinal ascariasis usually produces crampy abdominal pain, but if the parasitic load is small, symptoms will be minimal. However, because of the large size of the adult worm, a number of complications referable to the gastrointestinal tract can ensue. Intestinal obstruction can result from blockage by a bolus of worms, particularly in the distal ileum, although it has been suggested that a major cause for obstruction can be spasm produced by irritation of the mucosal sensory receptors. Bowel perforation is unlikely to be caused by this condition, unless an associated ulceration of the intestine occurs, such as is seen with amebiasis or typhoid. Small-bowel volvulus can also occur. Additionally, allergic

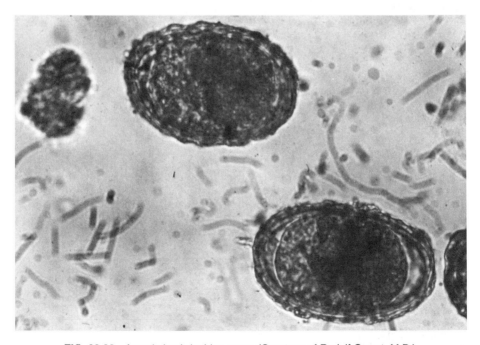

**FIG. 33.22.** *Ascaris lumbricoides*, eggs. (Courtesy of Rudolf Garret, M.D.)

reactions (asthma, urticaria, and conjunctivitis) can result from absorption of toxins from the worm.

Physical examination may reveal minimal signs; obviously in the presence of intestinal obstruction, however, abdominal distension and diffuse tenderness may be noted. Occasionally, perforation can ensue, and the patient will present with signs of peritonitis.

### *Diagnosis*

The diagnosis of ascariasis is made after finding the eggs, larvae, or adult worms. It usually takes approximately 2 months from the time of infection before the eggs appear in the stool. The worms can also be recovered from the sputum and occasionally from emesis. Laboratory studies are usually of no value, because the only significant abnormality is the presence of an eosinophilia.

X-ray films of the small bowel may reveal the presence of the worms in the distal ileum. Characteristically, the gastrointestinal tract of the worm can be identified because it is filled with the contrast material (Fig. 33.23). Ultra-

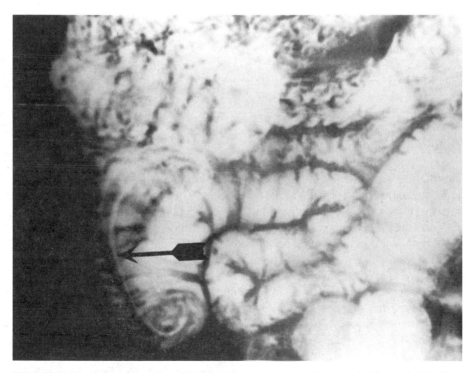

**FIG. 33.23.** Ascariasis. X-ray film of the small bowel demonstrates ascaris. The gastrointestinal tract of the worm can be identified (*arrow*).

sonography has been found to be useful in the diagnosis of intestinal obstruction secondary to ascariasis. Characteristic sonographic features of railway track sign and bulls-eye appearance are helpful in making the diagnosis.

### Treatment

Treatment with piperazine derivatives has been advocated, but it is associated with potentially serious side effects. Other recommended drugs include pyrantel pamoate, mebendazole, levamisole, thiabendazole, and fenbendazole.

In a patient with intestinal obstruction, in the absence of an acute surgical problem, nasogastric intubation is recommended, and consideration given to the placement of piperazine through the tube. If an operation is required and perforation has not occurred, it is best to attempt manipulation of the worms through the ileum into the cecum rather than to open the bowel. Resection is advised, if required, as opposed to enterotomy and extraction of the worms. The instillation of intraluminal vermifuge intraoperatively has been reported to minimize the risk of postoperative worm migration through suture lines and anastomoses. Early clinical diagnosis and prompt surgery for obstruction are important in reducing a high mortality rate in this potentially devastating condition.

### Strongyloidiasis

Strongyloidiasis is a parasitic disease often seen in tropical climates and caused by another roundworm, *Strongyloides stercoralis*. The condition usually occurs in the small bowel, but the colon is occasionally the site of involvement. Not too dissimilar to hookworm, the larvae penetrate the skin and are carried by way of the circulation to the lungs. They then rupture into the alveoli and develop into adolescent worms. The swallowed female invades the small intestinal mucosa where it remains, depositing eggs (Fig. 33.24).

Symptoms referable to the intestinal tract can be minimal, or the patient may complain of diarrhea, nausea, vomiting, and abdominal pain. Rectal pain and tenesmus have been reported in association with involvement in that area, and a proctitis may be present on sigmoidoscopy. The clinical syndrome of hyperinfection with this parasite (overwhelming proliferation of the worms) can be seen in immunocompromised patients and is characterized by profound abdominal symptoms and signs and by secondary infection. Those with lymphomas and leukemia are at greatest risk.

The diagnosis is established by examination of duodenal secretions; suction biopsy of the duodenum is a poor way of finding the parasite. Additionally, strongyloidiasis can be diagnosed by finding the larvae in the feces; this is the only intestinal nematode from which larvae rather than eggs are identified in the stool.

In the severe form of the disease, mortality is usually caused by dehydration and electrolyte imbalance, the result of vomiting and diarrhea. The drug of choice for the treatment of the condition is thiabendazole (Mintezol).

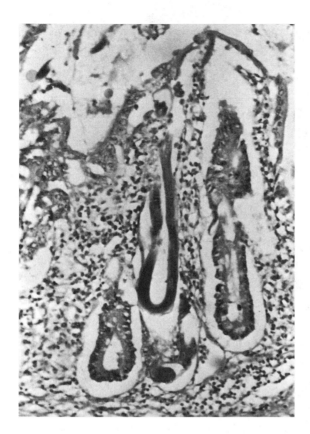

**FIG. 33.24.** *Strongyloides stercoralis.* Larvae and eggs in intestinal mucosa. (Original magnification ×280; courtesy of Rudolf Garret, M.D.)

## Trichuriasis

Trichuriasis is caused by the roundworm *Trichuris trichiura*, the so-called "whipworm." Its common name is misleading because the whip or tail is actually its head. In some areas of the world, up to 90% of the population is infected; it may be the most commonly recognized intestinal helminth in people returning from tropical areas.

The egg has a characteristic barrel shape with a nonstaining prominence at each end (Fig. 33.25). Ingestion of food or water containing the eggs is the method of contamination. In the intestinal tract, the eggs are digested, releasing larvae into the small intestine. The larvae reside in the mucosa for several days, and then relocate to the cecal area where they mature.

Patients can be virtually asymptomatic or have moderate or severe infective symptoms, depending on the extent of involvement. Lower abdominal pain, diarrhea, and rectal bleeding have been reported. Nausea, vomiting, flatulence, abdominal distension, headache, and weight loss are also noted.

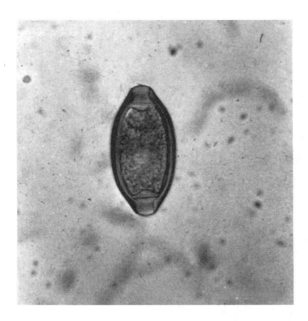

**FIG. 33.25.** *Trichuris trichiura* egg. Note the characteristic barrel shape with a "plug" at either end. (Courtesy of Rudolf Garret, M.D.)

Appendicitis and rectal prolapse can be consequences of whipworm infection. Rectal prolapse is thought to result from straining at defecation because of the massive number of worms in the rectum. The number of worms together, creating blockage of the appendiceal lumen, accounts for the signs and symptoms of appendicitis. *T. trichiura* eggs have also been identified in a patient with an anal abscess. Furthermore, the worm has been demonstrated to suck blood from the colon, and it is estimated that 0.005 mL may be lost per day per worm. Hence, severe infestation can cause anemia. However, significant blood loss in the adult has only rarely been recognized.

The diagnosis is made by the identification of the characteristic eggs in the stool. Egg counts are useful in determining the degree of infection and for evaluating the efficacy of treatment. Barium enema examination may reveal evidence of the worms on air-contrast study.

Treatment with mebendazole (Vermox) has been found to be highly effective against *Trichuris* as well as against other worms.

## Anisakiasis

Anisakiasis or herring worm disease is caused by the species of the marine roundworm, *Anisakis*. The adult nematodes are intestinal parasites of marine mammals, such as seals and dolphins. When inadequately prepared fish is eaten, the larvae penetrate the mucosa of the stomach, the small intestine, or even the colon. Patients present with acute abdominal pain together with an intestinal obstruction or appendicitis-like syndrome. Findings can mimic those of regional enteritis. Most symptoms of infection with this parasite will resolve spontaneously.

### Tapeworm (*Taenia Saginata*)

The beef tapeworm is by far the most common taeniid of humans; it is found throughout the world, except where meat is prohibited for religious reasons. The adult, a hermaphroditic cestode, can achieve several meters in length (Fig. 33.26). The eggs are spherical in shape and cannot be distinguished from those of the pork tapeworm (Fig. 33.27).

Abdominal discomfort, nausea, vomiting, cutaneous sensitivity, headache, and malaise are reported symptoms, but most infections are asymptomatic. Because of the large size of the worm, obstructive symptoms can occasionally develop.

Recommended treatment is with niclosamide or praziquantel.

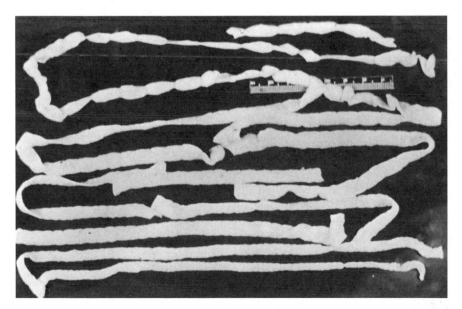

**FIG. 33.26.** *Taenia saginata*. Beef tapeworm adult. (Courtesy of Rudolf Garret, M.D.)

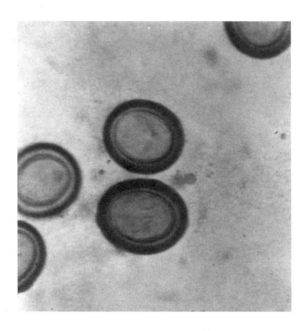

**FIG.    33.27.** *Taenia    saginata* eggs. (Courtesy of Rudolf Garret, M.D.)

# Subject Index